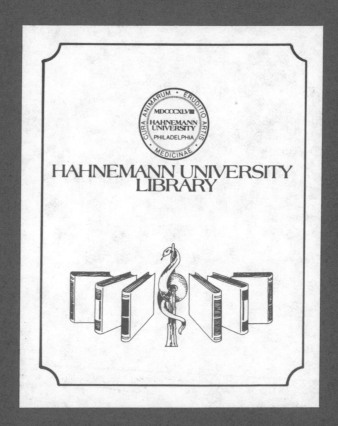

The Founders of Operative Surgery

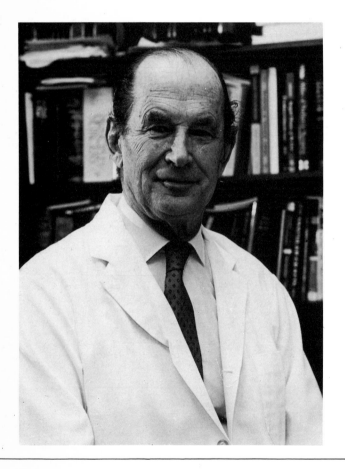

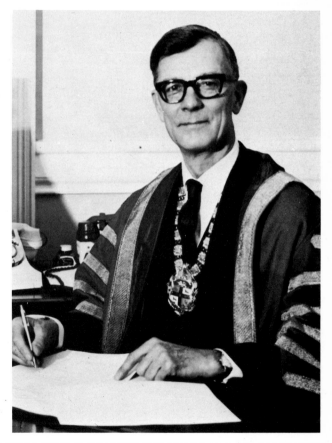

Charles Granville Rob MC, MChir, FRCS, FACS
Professor of Surgery, East Carolina University
Quondam: Professor of Surgery, St Mary's Hospital Medical
School, London 1950–1960;
Professor and Chairman, Department of Surgery, University of
Rochester, New York, 1960–1978

Lord Smith of Marlow KBE, MS, FRCS, Hon DSc
(Exeter and Leeds), Hon MD (Zurich), Hon FRACS,
Hon FRCS(Ed.), Hon FACS, Hon FRCS(Can.), Hon FRCSI,
Hon FRCS(SA), Hon FDS
Honorary Consulting Surgeon, St George's Hospital, London
Quondam: Surgeon, St George's Hospital, London,
1946–1978;
President of the Royal College of Surgeons of England,
1973–1977

Rob & Smith's
Operative Surgery

Urology
Fourth Edition

Rob & Smith's

Operative Surgery

General Editors

Hugh Dudley ChM, FRCS(Ed.), FRACS, FRCS
Professor of Surgery, St Mary's Hospital, London, UK

David C. Carter MD, FRCS(Ed.), FRCS(Glas.)
St Mungo Professor of Surgery, University of Glasgow;
Honorary Consultant Surgeon, Royal Infirmary, Glasgow, UK

Rob & Smith's

Operative Surgery

Urology

Fourth Edition

Edited by

W. Scott McDougal MD
Professor and Chairman, Department of Urology,
Vanderbilt University Medical Center, Nashville, Tennessee, USA

The C V Mosby Company
St Louis   Toronto

Butterworths
London   Boston   Durban   Singapore   Sydney   Toronto   Wellington

© Butterworths 1986

First edition published in eight volumes 1956–1958
Second edition published in fourteen volumes 1968–1971
Third edition published in nineteen volumes 1976–1981
Fourth edition published 1983–

British Library Cataloguing in Publication Data

Rob, Charles
    Rob & Smith's operative surgery. — 4th ed.
    Urology.
    1. Surgery
    I. Title   II. Smith, Rodney Smith, *Baron*
    III. McDougal, W. Scott.   IV. Rob, Charles.
    Operative surgery
    617   RD31

    ISBN 0-407-00658-3

Library of Congress Cataloging in Publication Data
(Revised for pt. 2)
Main entry under title:

Rob & Smith's operative surgery

    Rev. ed. of: Operative surgery. 3rd ed. 1976–
    Includes bibliographies and index
    Contents: [1] Alimentary tract and abdominal wall.
1. General principles, oesophagus, stomach, duodenum, small intestine, abdominal wall, hernia / edited by Hugh Dudley – –[2] Urology / edited by W. Scott McDougal.
    1. Surgery, Operative.   I. Rob, Charles.   II. Smith of Marlow, Rodney Smith, Baron, 1914– .   III. Dudley, Hugh Arnold Freeman.   IV. Pories, Walter J.
V. Carter, David C. (David Craig)   VI. Operative surgery. [DNLM: 1. Surgery, Operative.
WO 500 061 1982]
RD32.06   1983   617'.91   83-14465
ISBN 0-407-00651-6 (v. 1)

Photoset by Butterworths Litho Preparation Department
Printed by Blantyre Printing Ltd, London & Glasgow
Bound by Robert Hartnoll Ltd, Bodmin, Cornwall

Volumes and Editors

Alimentary Tract and Abdominal Wall

1 **General Principles · Oesophagus · Stomach · Duodenum · Small Intestine · Abdominal Wall · Hernia**

Hugh Dudley ChM, FRCS(Ed.), FRACS, FRCS
Professor of Surgery, St Mary's Hospital, London, UK

2 **Liver · Portal Hypertension · Spleen · Biliary Tract · Pancreas**

Hugh Dudley ChM, FRCS(Ed.), FRACS, FRCS
Professor of Surgery, St Mary's Hospital, London, UK

3 **Colon, Rectum and Anus**

Ian P. Todd MS, MD(Tor), FRCS, DCH
Consulting Surgeon, St Bartholomew's Hospital, London;
Consultant Surgeon, St Mark's Hospital and
King Edward VII Hospital for Officers, London, UK

L. P. Fielding MB, FRCS
Chief of Surgery, St Mary's Hospital, Waterbury, Connecticut, USA;
Associate Professor of Surgery, Yale University, Connecticut, USA

Cardiac Surgery

Stuart W. Jamieson MB, BS, FRCS
Assistant Professor of Cardiovascular Surgery,
Stanford University School of Medicine, California, USA

Norman E. Schumway MD, PhD, FRCS
Professor and Chairman, Department of Cardiovascular Surgery,
Stanford University School of Medicine, California, USA

The Ear

John C. Ballantyne FRCS, HonFRCSI, DLO
Consultant Ear, Nose and Throat Surgeon,
Royal Free and King Edward VII Hospital for Officers, London, UK
Honorary Consultant in Otolaryngology to the Army

Andrew Morrison FRCS, DLO
Senior Consultant Otolaryngologist, The London Hospital, UK

General Principles, Breast and Extracranial Endocrines

Hugh Dudley ChM, FRCS(Ed.), FRACS, FRCS
Professor of Surgery, St Mary's Hospital, London, UK

Walter J. Pories MD, FACS
Professor and Chairman, Department of Surgery, School of Medicine,
East Carolina University, Greenville, North Carolina, USA

Gynaecology and Obstetrics

J. M. Monaghan MB, FRCS(Ed.), MRCOG
Consultant Surgeon, Regional Department of Gynaecological Oncology,
Queen Elizabeth Hospital, Gateshead, UK

Plastic Surgery

T. L. Barclay ChM, FRCS
Consultant Plastic Surgeon, St Luke's Hospital,
Bradford, West Yorkshire, UK

Desmond A. Kernahan, MD
Chief, Division of Plastic Surgery,
The Children's Memorial Hospital, Chicago, Illinois, USA

Thoracic Surgery

J. W. Jackson MCh, FRCS
Formerly Consultant Thoracic Surgeon, Harefield Hospital, Middlesex, UK

D. K. C. Cooper MD, PhD, FRCS
Department of Cardiac Surgery, University of Cape Town
Medical School, Cape Town, South Africa

Trauma

John V. Robbs FRCS
Associate Professor of Surgery,
Department of Surgery, University of Natal, South Africa

Howard R. Champion FRCS
Chief, Trauma Service;
Director, Surgery Critical Care Services,
The Washington Hospital Center, Washington, DC, USA

Donald Trunkey MD
San Francisco General Hospital, San Francisco, California, USA

Urology

W. Scott McDougal MD
Professor and Chairman, Department of Urology,
Vanderbilt University Medical Center, Hashville, Tennessee, USA

Vascular Surgery

James A. DeWeese MD
Professor and Chairman, Division of Cardiothoracic Surgery,
University of Rochester Medical Center, Rochester, New York, USA

Contributors

Richard K. Babayan MD
Assistant Professor, Department of Urology, Boston University School of Medicine, Boston, Massachusetts, USA

Mahmoud M. Badr MCh, FRCS, FACS, FICS
Professor of Urology, Cairo University, Egypt

T. M. Barratt MB, FRCP
Consultant Paediatric Nephrologist, Hospital for Sick Children, Great Ormond Street, London; Professor of Paediatric Nephrology, Institute of Child Health, London, UK

Jonathan C. Boyd MD
Fellow in Urology, Section of Urology, Bowman Gray School of Medicine of Wake Forest University, Winston-Salem, North Carolina, USA

Herbert Brendler MD
Professor and Chairman, Department of Urology, The Mount Sinai Medical Center, New York, USA

William A. Brock MD, FACS, FAAP
Associate Clinical Professor of Surgery/Urology, School of Medicine, University of California, San Diego; Chief of Urology, Children's Hospital and Health Center, San Diego, California, USA

Kevin A. Burbige MD
Associate Director, Pediatric Urology and Assistant Professor of Urology, College of Physicians and Surgeons, New York, USA

Geoffrey D. Chisholm ChM, FRCS, FRCS(Ed)
Professor of Surgery, University of Edinburgh; Consultant Urological Surgeon, Western General Hospital, Edinburgh; Honorary Senior Lecturer, Institute of Urology, London, UK

J. C. Christoffersen MD, MA
Professor of Surgery and Director of Urology, Bispebjerg Hospital, Copenhagen, Denmark

S. Joseph Cohen FRCS, MRCP
Consultant Paediatric Surgeon and Urologist, Booth Hall Children's Hospital, Manchester; Royal Manchester Children's Hospital, Saint Mary's Hospital, Manchester; Lecturer in Paediatric Surgery, University of Manchester, UK

B. S. Crawford FRCS
Consultant Plastic Surgeon, Fulwood Hospital and the Children's Hospital, Sheffield, UK

E. Darracott Vaughan, Jr MD
James J. Colt Professor of Urology in Surgery, Cornell University Medical Center, New York; Attending Surgeon-in-charge, Disivion of Urology, The New York Hospital, USA

Emile de Backer MD
Conference Chairman, Catholic University of Louvain; Chief of Urology Service, The Institute of Saint Elizabeth, Brussels, Belgium

Hermann Dettmar MD
Director of the Urological Clinic, University of Düsseldorf, West Germany

John P. Donohoe MD
Professor and Chairman, Department of Urology, Indiana University Medical School, Indianapolis, Indiana, USA

Joseph B. Dowd MD
Chairman, Department of Urology, Lahey Clinic Medical Center, Burlington, Massachusetts, USA

Joseph R. Drago MD
Associate Professor of Surgery (Urology), Pennsylvania State University College of Medicine and The Milton S. Hershey Medical Center, Hershey, Pennsylvania, USA

F. d'Udekem MD
Department of Urology, University of Brussels, Belgium

Herbert B. Eckstein MD, MChir, FRCS
Consultant Paediatric Surgeon, Hospital for Sick Children, Great Ormond Street, London, UK

Robert C. Flanigan MD
Associate Professor of Surgery (Urology), University of Kentucky Medical Center, Lexington, Kentucky, USA

L. E. C. Franksson MD, PhD
Professor and Chairman of the Department of Surgery, Huddinge Hospital, Caroline Institute Medical School, Stockholm, Sweden

N. O. K. Gibbon MB, ChM, FRCS(Ed), FRCS
Consultant Urologist, formerly Head of the Urological Unit of the Royal Liverpool Hospital and Director of Urological Studies, University of Liverpool, UK

José Mª. Gil-Vernet
Department of Urology, University of Barcelona, Spain

Howard R. Goldstein MD
Pediatric Urologist and Clinical Assistant Professor of Surgery, UMDNJ-Rutgers Medical School at Camden, Cooper Hospital-University Medical Center, New Jersey, USA

J. G. Gow MD, ChM, FRCS
Consultant Urologist, Emeritus, Liverpool AHA (Teaching), UK

W. Gregoir MD
Chief of the Department of Urology, University of Brussels, Belgium

Lloyd H. Harrison MD, FACS
Professor of Surgery (Urology), Section of Urology, Bowman Gray School of Medicine of Wake Forest University, Winston-Salem, North Carolina, USA

Terry W. Hensle MD
Director, Pediatric Urology, and Associate Professor of Urology, College of Physicians and Surgeons, New York, USA

Stuart S. Howards MD
Professor of Urology and Associate Professor of Physiology, University of Virginia School of Medicine, Charlottesville, Virginia, USA

J. H. Johnston MB, FRCS, FRCSI, FACS
Urological Surgeon, Alder Hey Children's Hospital, Liverpool; Lecturer in Paediatric Urology, University of Liverpool, UK

George W. Kaplan MD, FACS, FAAP
Clinical Professor of Surgery/Urology, School of Medicine, University of California, San Diego; Chief of Pediatric Urology, University of California, San Diego; Senior Staff, Children's Hospital and Health Center, San Diego, California, USA

Evan J. Kass MD
Associate Professor of Urology and Child Health and Development, George Washington University School of Medicine and Health Sciences; Attending Pediatric Urologist, Children's Hospital National Medical Center, Washington, DC, USA

Robert J. Krane MD
Chairman, Department of Urology, Boston University School of Medicine, Boston, Massachusetts, USA

John A. Libertino MD
Director of Transplantation, Department of Urology; Vice Chairman, Division of Surgery, Lahey Clinic Medical Center, Burlington, Massachusetts, USA

Peter H. Lord MChir, FRCS
Consultant Surgeon, Wycombe General Hospital, High Wycombe, Buckinghamshire, UK

W. Scott McDougal MD
Professor and Chairman, Department of Urology, Vanderbilt University Medical Center, Nashville, Tennessee, USA

Warwick Macky OBE, MS, FRCS, FRACS
Urologist, Auckland Hospital, New Zealand

José A. Martínez-Piñeiro MD
Associate Professor in Urology, La Paz Hospital, Faculty of Medicine, Universidad Autónoma, Madrid, Spain

J. P. Mitchell CBE, TD, MS, FRCS, FRCS(Ed)
Honorary Professor of Surgery (Urology), University of Bristol, UK

Mohammed Mohiuddin MD
Associate Professor, Department of Radiation Therapy, Thomas Jefferson University Medical School, Philadelphia, Pennsylvania, USA

Drogo K. Montague MD, FACS
Head, Section of Urodynamics and Prosthetic Surgery, Department of Urology, Cleveland Clinic Foundation, Cleveland, Ohio, USA

S. G. Mulholland MD
Professor and Chairman, Department of Urology, Thomas Jefferson University Medical School, Philadelphia, Pennsylvania, USA

G. F. Murnaghan MD, ChM, FRCS(Ed), FRCS, FRACS
Professor of Surgery, University of New South Wales; Urological Surgeon to The Prince Henry and The Prince of Wales Hospitals; Consultant Urologist, The Royal South Sydney Hospital, Sydney and The Royal Hospital for Women, Paddington, New South Wales, Australia

J. Dermot O'Flynn MCh, FRCS, FRCSI
Consultant Urological Surgeon, Meath Hospital, Dublin; Lecturer in Urology, Trinity College, Dublin, Ireland

Richard G. Notley MS, FRCS
Senior Consultant Urological Surgeon, Royal Surrey County Hospital, Guildford, Surrey, UK

Andrew C. Novick MD
Chief, Renal Transplant Service, Department of Urology, Cleveland Clinic Foundation, Cleveland, Ohio, USA

L. Persky MD, FACS
Professor of Urology, University Hospitals of Cleveland, Cleveland, Ohio, USA

John P. Pryor MS, FRCS
Consultant Urologist, King's College and St Peter's Hospitals, London; Dean, Institute of Urology, University of London, London, UK

Alan B. Retik MD
Chief, Division of Urology, Children's Hospital Medical Center, Boston, Massachusetts; Professor of Surgery (Urology), Harvard Medical School, Massachusetts, USA

John R. Richardson, Jr MD
Clinical Associate Professor of Urology, Dartmouth-Hitchcock Medical School, Hanover, New Hampshire, USA

Robert A. Riehle, Jr MD
Assistant Professor of Surgery (Urology), Cornell University Medical Center, New York; Assistant Attending Surgeon, The New York Hospital, USA

Charles Rob MC, MD, MChir, FRCS
Professor of Surgery, Uniformed Services, University of the Health Services, Bethesda, Maryland, USA

C. J. Robson MD, FRCS (Can.), FACS
Professor of Urological Surgery, University of Toronto; Head, Division of Urological Surgery, Toronto General Hosputal; Consultant Urologist, Sunnybrook Hospital, Hospital for Sick Children and Women's College Hospital, Toronto, Canada

Thomas J. Rohner, Jr MD
Professor of Surgery (Urology), Chief, Division of Urology, Pennsylvania State University College of Medicine and The Milton S. Hershey Medical Center, Hershey, Pennsylvania, USA

Robert A. Roth MD
Department of Urology, Lahey Clinic Medical Center, Burlington, Massachusetts, USA

David C. Saypol MD
Resident, Department of Urology, University of Virginia School of Medicine, Charlottesville, Virginia, USA

Linda M. Dairiki Shortliffe MD
Assistant Professor of Surgery (Urology), Division of Urology, Stanford University School of Medicine, Stanford, California; Chief, Urology Section, Veterans Administration Medical Center, Palo Alto, California, USA

J. C. Smith MS, FRCS
Consultant Urological Surgeon, The Churchill Hospital, Oxford, UK

Thomas A. Stamey MD
Professor of Surgery (Urology), Chairman, Division of Urology, Stanford University School of Medicine, Stanford, California, USA

Stuart L. Stanton FRCS, MRCOG
Senior Lecturer in Obstetrics and Gynaecology, St George's Hospital Medical School, London; Consultant Obstetrician and Gynaecologist, St Helier Hospital, Carshalton, Surrey, UK

Richard Turner-Warwick FRCS, FACS
Senior Surgeon, The Middlesex Hospital; Senior Consultant Urological Surgeon, St Peter's Hospital Group; Senior Lecturer, Institute of Urology, University of London, UK

R. Dixon Walker MD
Professor of Surgery and Pediatrics and Director of Pediatric Urology, University of Florida College of Medicine, Gainesville, Florida, USA

J. E. A. Wickham MS, FRCS
Director of the Academic Unit, Institute of Urology, University of London; Senior Consultant Urological Surgeon, St Bartholomew's Hospital, London; Consultant Surgeon, St Peter's Hospital Group, London, UK

R. E. Williams MD, ChM, FRCS(Ed.), FRCS
Consultant Urologist, The General Infirmary and St James's University Hospital, Leeds, UK

P. H. L. Worth MB, BChir, FRCS
Consultant Urologist, University College Hospital and St Peter's Hospital, London, UK

W. K. Yeates MD, MS, FRCS
Consultant Urologist, Freeman Hospital, Newcastle-upon-Tyne; Lecturer in Urology, University of Newcastle; Honorary Senior Lecturer, Institute of Urology, University of London, UK

Contributing Medical Artists

Janis Kay Atlee BFA, BS, AMI
Medical Illustrator, 509 Nursing Center, Kentucky 40508, USA

Michele Barker
Senior Medical Artist, Institute of Urology, London, UK

Sylvia Barker NDD, FRSA
Medical Illustration Department, John Radcliffe Hospital, Headington, Oxford, OX3 9DU, UK

Daniel S. Beisel MA
Medical Illustrator, Department of Educational Resources, The Milton S. Hershey Medical Center, Hershey, Pennsylvania 17033, USA

T. Bell
Department of Medical Illustration, East Carolina, University School of Medicine, Greenville, NC 27834, USA

D. H. Blundell
5 Greenfields Croft, Little Neston, South Wirral, L64 OT2, UK

Rudolf Brammer
Medical Artist, Stuttgarter Strasse 8, 7809 Denzlingen, West Germany

Mary Broihier
Medical Illustrations Department, Indiana University School of Medicine, Indianapolis, Indiana 46223, USA

Kenneth Louis Clark MS
Medical Illustrator, Department of Learning Resources, University of Florida College of Medicine, Gainesville, Florida, USA

Bayard H. Colyear III AMAMI
Medical Illustrator, Instructional Media, Stanford University Medical Center, Stanford, California 94305, USA

Arthur E. Cottrell
Medical Artist, Department of Medical Illustration, Southmead General Hospital, Bristol, Avon, UK

Michael J. Courtney
Medical Illustrator, 78 Alfred Road, Hastings, East Sussex, TN35 5HY, UK

Bill Crutchfield
Medical Illustrator, Children's Hospital National Medical Center, Washington DC, USA

Patrick M. Elliott
Medical Artist, 31 Moor Oaks Road, Broomhill, Sheffield, Yorkshire, S10 1BX, UK

Arthus Ellis
Medical Artist, School of Medicine, University of Auckland, New Zealand

Ronald J. Ervin BFA
Coordinator of Arts and Graphics Department, University of Virginia School of Medicine, Charlottesville, Virginia, USA

Urban Frank
Strandvägen 39, 196 30 Kungsängen, Sweden

Douglas P. Hammersley BA, FMAA
Audio Visual Centre, University of Newcastle Upon Tyne, Newcastle Upon Tyne, NE1 7RU, UK

Nancy Heim
Medical Illustrator, Department of Biomedical Communications, Cleveland Clinic Foundation, Cleveland, Ohio, USA

Barbara Hyams
82 Kingsland Road, Boxmoor, Hemel Hempstead, Herts, UK

Gary M. James
Department of Medical Illustration, Bristol Royal Infirmary, Bristol, BS2 8HW, UK

Susan I. Klug AB, MA
Medical and Biological Illustrator, 5562 Hobart Street, 401, Pittsburgh, PA 15217, USA

Robert N. Lane
Medical Artist, Studio 19a, Edith Grove, Chelsea, London, SW10, UK

Geoff Lyth
15 Gunthorpe Road, Lowdham, Notts, UK

Kevin Marks BA (Hons)
3 Hilltop Court, Grange Road, Upper Norwood, London SE19 3BQ, UK

Mary Margaret Peel
Medical Illustrator, Veterans Administration Medical Center, Nashville, Tennessee, USA

Jean Perry AIMBI
Department of Medical Illustration, North Manchester General Hospital, Crumpsall, Manchester, M8 6RB, UK

Harriet Phillips
Medical Art Service, Rd 2, Box 229, Warwick, New York 10990, USA

J. Pizer
Formerly Medical Artist, Western General Hospital, Edinburgh, EH4 2XU, Scotland

Barbara N. Rankin BA, AMI
2853 Coleridge Road, Cleveland Heights, Ohio 44118, USA

Franca Rubiu
Medical Artist, Department of Medical Illustration, The University of New South Wales, The Prince of Wales Hospital, Randwick, Sydney, NSW 2031, Australia

Cathy Slatter
Medical Illustrator, 16 Gravel Path, Berkhamstead, Herts, UK

Ambia Smith
Freelance Artist, Boston, Massachusetts, USA

Francis E. Steckel
1360 Trapelo Road, Waltham, Massachusetts 02154, USA

James Suchy
Art Department, Cleveland Clinic Foundation, Ohio, USA

T. R. Tarrant
Moorfields Eye Hospital, High Holborn, London, WC1V 7AN, UK

Ladislao Tinao
Chief, Department of Medical Illustrations of the Jimenez Diaz Foundation, Dr Fleming 4, Bajo A, Majadahonda, Madrid, Spain

Freda Wadsworth MBE, DRN, MFRS, FMAA
11 Burnham Court, Moscow Road, London, W2 4SW, UK

Philip Wilson
23 Normanhurst Road, St Paul's Cray, Orpington, Kent, BR5 3AL, UK

Contents

Preface

The purpose of this Fourth Edition is to provide the reader with lucid illustrations and descriptions of those operative procedures which the urologist in training and in practice commonly encounters. It is recognized that there are many different ways of performing the same procedure. Most procedures however are performed in a similar manner by urologists throughout the world, and although minor modifications may be preferred by some, there is general agreement as to the technique of the operative procedure. In these cases, only one procedure has been described. However, when one technique is not widely accepted, several methods are illustrated.

The volume has been considerably expanded since the previous edition. Many entirely new chapters are included on such topics as: retroperitoneal surgery, stone surgery, radical extirpative surgery for cancer, reconstructive surgery for congenital anomalies, surgery for infertility, and traumatic injuries of the genitourinary system. The remaining chapters have been expanded to include more detail or have been revised to make them current. This major expansion and revision was necessitated by the technological advances which have occurred in urology over the past 10 years. Moreover, since many urologists today practice the full breadth of the speciality, this volume has been made more comprehensive so that it may serve as a single source for these urologists. The 67 authors from countries throughout the world have given *Urology* an international perspective thus obviating provincial attitudes about specific procedures. I am indebted to all the contributors for their superb manuscripts.

I am deeply indebted to Mr J. D. Fergusson and Mr D. Innes Williams, who edited previous editions of this volume and who set a standard of excellence which this edition has attempted to equal. I also owe a great debt of gratitude to Butterworths, for their patience, counsel and editorial critique of both the illustrations and manuscripts. Finally, my deepest thanks to the general editors for their encouragement, patience and enthusiastic support, and to Professor Hugh Dudley for his editorial critique.

W. Scott McDougal

Illustrations by Mary Broihier

Retroperitoneal lymphadenectomy

John P. Donohue MD
Professor and Chairman, Department of Urology,
Indiana University Medical School, Indianapolis, Indiana, USA

Introduction

The most common indication for a systematic retroperitoneal lymphadenectomy is for staging and treatment of non-seminomatous testis cancer. There are two quite useful approaches, each with its own advantages. Leadbetter, Cooper and Chute[1] described the thoracoabdominal approach for staging testicular tumours. This has been promoted with some modifications by Fraley[2] and Skinner[3]. Advantages of this approach are: extraperitoneal exposure of the retroperitoneal structures with less postoperative ileus and easier high exposure on the ipsilateral side. It is particularly well suited to large bulky lesions in and around the renal hilum. Another advantage is that the most difficult portion of the dissection is placed in the middle of the operative field. The principles of the extraperitoneal approach have been described by Fraley[2].

It has been the practice of the author, to use the anterior approach because of a special interest in developing a bilateral dissection, including a dissection above each renal hilum, both right and left in every case. This is not as easily achieved through the thoracoabdominal route.

Several unusual clinical experiences, including a relapse in the suprarenal hilar zone in a young child following removal of lymph nodes that were normal in the infrahilar zone, indicated that a technique needed to be developed which would facilitate good simultaneous exposure in both renal hilar zones as well as in both infrahilar zones.

Post-mortem dissections of the retroperitoneum were done through a midline incision from the xiphoid to pubis to determine whether this approach could equal the high exposure afforded by the thoracoabdominal approach. It was found that by using special techniques of pancreatic mobilization and elevation, equivalent high exposure could be achieved, not only on the ipsilateral side, but also on the contralateral side. This was of particular interest because lymphangiogram studies suggested abundant cross-over of lymphatics right to left and left to right, involving the suprahilar zones[3-6].

The remainder of this chapter is devoted to the more commonly used anterior approach for retroperitoneal lymphadenectomy.

The anterior approach including bilateral suprarenal hilar dissection

Special preoperative preparation and medical notes

The patient is prepared with overnight intravenous hydration – the procedure used for donors for renal transplantation. No antibiotics are used either pre- or postoperatively.

The bladder is catheterized at the time of draping in surgery. The catheter is usually removed on the 2nd postoperative day. The patient is placed in the supine position either with the right arm suspended from an ether screen or with both arms extended. Mannitol 12.5–25 g is given intravenously during the first part of the operation to prevent the oliguria associated with extensive bilateral renovascular dissections. Topical 1 per cent xylocaine is used on the renal vessels during the dissection. Intraoperative administration of colloid to replace large third-space losses of lymph during the dissection is important to avoid misleadingly high haematocrit values. An increased need for crystalloid is also apparent, as the losses from the intravascular space into the large, raw third space created in the retroperitoneum can produce significant contractions of effective blood volume. Transfusions of whole blood are often unnecessary if enough colloid replacement is given in uncomplicated cases.

Preoperatively emphasis is placed on pulmonary physiotherapy to improve the patient's condition postoperatively. Again, no prophylactic antibiotics are used. If fever develops, appropriate cultures and investigations are made and then a drug is selected, but this is rarely necessary.

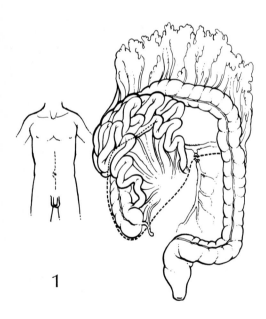

1

1

Exposure

The incision is midline, xiphoid to pubis. Drapes are sewn in place and a 27 cm (11 inch) circular plastic wound protector is used; two Balfour abdominal retractors are placed. The abdomen is explored carefully by palpation. The basic mesentric divisions are made in order to mobilize the entire small bowel and right colon so that they can be placed on the patient's chest in a plastic bowel bag. First, the hepatic flexure is taken down and then the mesocolon is incised from the foramen of Winslow to the caecum. It is important to extend this posterior peritoneal incision through the base of the foramen of Winslow, which covers the anterior surface of the vena cava, because later dissection must extend above this area.

After the right mesocolon has been divided, the incision is turned around and the root of the small bowel is incised cephalad to the ligament of Treitz. This incision is carried along the root of the bowel until the inferior mesenteric vein is encountered. This vein must be divided in order to carry the incision cephalad in an oblique manner further into the left upper quadrant, to run parallel to the inferior border of the pancreas. If the inferior mesenteric vein is not divided, it will restrict the exposure in this area. The pancreas can then be mobilized fully and retracted off the anterior surface of Gerota's fascia, which is separated bluntly and sharply from the undersurface of the bowel, the pancreatic head and body, duodenum and caecum. Mobilization is now complete and the bowel is placed on the chest in a bowel bag. We no longer recommend a routine appendectomy: the retroperitoneum is a rich culture medium postoperatively, and all potential sources of contamination should be avoided.

Suprarenal hilar dissection

Patients with retroperitoneal tissue entirely negative to inspection and palpation rarely have positive suprahilar nodes (*Tables 1* and *2*). Therefore, this element of the dissection is omitted entirely in the absence of gross nodal enlargement. On the other hand, there is a significant possibility of suprahilar nodal involvement in patients with lymph nodes that are grossly enlarged (greater than 2 cm in diameter). About 1 in every 4 cases will have most involvement in the deep posterior nodes – the para-aortic and often retrocrural. Therefore, this portion of the dissection is reserved until the end of the operation, when the renal vessels are well exposed and can be elevated simply by vein retractors to expose the deep posterior set of nodes at the foramina of L1–L2 bilaterally on the posterior body wall. These may extend in the retrocrural space up into the posterior mediastinum. If this can be detected preoperatively, a thoracoabdominal approach with a crural splitting incision is recommended for their removal. However, the crus can still be split and these nodes extracted while vascular and neural tributaries are clipped and cauterized from the anterior approach by elevating the renal vessels and the overlying pancreas with appropriate retractors.

Table 1 Incidence of positive nodes related to zone and stage B1, B2, B3: primary tumour right side

| Zone | Stage | | | |
	B1	B2	B3	Total
1 (R. paracaval)	3/26 (12%)	6/24 (25%)	8/8 (100%)	17/58 (29%)
2 (Precaval)	12/26 (46%)	23/24 (96%)	8/8 (100%)	46/58 (80%)
3 (Interaortocaval)	23/26 (88%)	23/24 (96%)	8/8 (100%)	54/58 (93%)
4 (Preaortic)	6/26 (23%)	21/24 (88%)	8/8 (100%)	35/58 (60%)
5 (L. para-aortic)	1/26 (4%)	3/24 (13%)	2/8 (25%)	6/58 (10%)
6 (R. suprahilar)	0/26 (0%)	8/24 (33%)	5/8 (63%)	13/58 (22%)
7 (L. suprahilar)	0/26 (0%)	3/24 (13%)	3/8 (38%)	6/58 (10%)
8 (R. iliac)	1/26 (4%)	4/24 (17%)	6/8 (75%)	11/58 (19%)
9 (L. iliac)	1/26 (4%)	2/24 (8%)	2/8 (25%)	5/58 (9%)
10 (Interiliac)	0/26 (0%)	2/24 (8%)	2/8 (25%)	5/58 (9%)
11 (Gonadal)	2/26 (0%)	3/24 (13%)	3/8 (38%)	8/58 (14%)

Table 2 Incidence of positive nodes related to zone and stage B1, B2, B3: primary tumour left side

| Zone | Stage | | | |
	B1	B2	B3	Total
1 (R. paracaval)	0/14 (0%)	1/19 (5%)	0/9 (5%)	1/42 (2%)
2 (Precaval)	0/14 (0%)	9/19 (47%)	5/9 (56%)	14/42 (33%)
3 (Interaortocaval)	4/14 (19%)	19/19 (100%)	8/9 (89%)	31/42 (74%)
4 (Preaortic)	10/14 (71%)	18/19 (95%)	9/9 (100%)	37/42 (88%)
5 (L. para-aortic)	11/14 (79%)	16/19 (84%)	9/9 (100%)	36/42 (86%)
6 (R. suprahilar)	1/14 (7%)	3/19 (16%)	6/9 (67%)	10/42 (24%)
7 (L. suprahilar)	2/14 (14%)	8/19 (42%)	9/9 (100%)	19/42 (45%)
8 (R. iliac)	0/14 (0%)	1/19 (5%)	1/9 (11%)	2/42 (48%)
9 (L. iliac)	2/14 (14%)	6/19 (32%)	6/9 (67%)	14/42 (33%)
10 (Interiliac)	0/14 (0%)	0/19 (0%)	1/9 (11%)	1/42 (2%)
11 (Gonadal)	2/14 (14%)	2/19 (11%)	3/9 (33%)	7/42 (17%)

2

The dissection can be started at the superior mesenteric artery. After being covered with a laparotomy pad, the head and body of the pancreas are elevated by two deep Harrington or Deaver retractors to expose further the superior mesenteric artery. The left colic mesentery has already been separated from Gerota's fascia and retracted laterally. This separation is continued inferiorly and facilitated by dividing the inferior mesenteric artery to enhance the exposure of the middle and inferior retroperitoneal space. The splanchnic nerves are divided between clips, as are the lymphatics from around the superior mesenteric artery. The dissection is carried down around the aorta and cephalad between the aorta and each crus of the diaphragm. Ganglia and lymphatics are clipped and divided on each crus. The dissection continues cephalad below the Harrington retractors and the tissue is drawn down and doubly clipped and divided as high as possible at the base of the diaphragm. Just above this, between the aorta and the vena cava, is the base of the cisterna chyli.

The right suprahilar dissection is continued across the crus of the diaphragm to the medial aspect of the inferior vena cava. This vessel is further dissected in the subadventitial plane to the medial border of the right adrenal gland which is separated from the specimen between vascular clips. The dissection is then carried down to the renal vessels. The adventitia of the renal artery and vein is divided. The dissection is carried out to the right renal hilum just beyond the bifurcation of the renal vessels. This block of nodal and ganglionic tissue is dissected sharply off the posterior body wall between vascular clips. Formerly this tissue was rotated below the renal vessels and kept *en bloc* with the infrahilar aortocaval package of nodes. Now, this tissue is submitted separately for analysis, in order to determine how many nodes there are in the right suprahilar zone. The normal range is 4–8. The major nodes are retrocrural and posterior para-aortic.

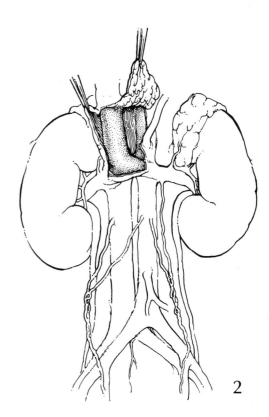

2

3

The left suphrahilar dissection is accomplished by dividing the left adrenal vein as it enters the renal vein and splitting the adventitia of the renal vein. This is carried out to the left renal hilum and up medial to the adrenal gland. It is clipped along the medial aspect of the adrenal gland and rotated and elevated out of the way to expose the renal hilum, the fat pad and the nodal tissue medial to the kidney. Then the tissue is mobilized off the posterior body wall by blunt and sharp dissection. The dissection on the aorta between the crura is carried cephalad obliquely about 4–6 cm above the left renal artery. Nodal tissue between the aorta and the body wall and the foramen of L1–L2 is an important and constant drainage point from the nodes just inferior to this at the left renal hilum. The several adrenal arterial branches from the aorta and the proximal left renal artery are divided between clips. Nodal and ganglionic tissue is peeled off the posterior body wall and, again, rotated either dorsal or ventral to the left renal artery from which it is mobilized in the subadventitial plane by sharp dissection. This tissue is submitted separately as the left suprarenal hilar package. The usual number of nodes here is 4–10. The major nodes are retrocrural and posterolateral to the aorta.

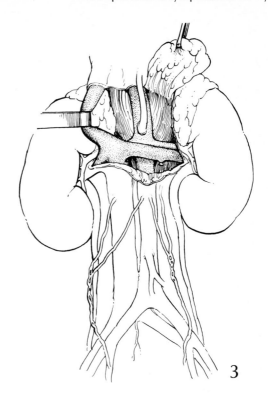

3

It is more convenient to save the suprahilar dissection until the infrahilar (main aortocaval) dissection is done. The major suprahilar nodes are posterior, at the foramina and medial to the crura of the diaphragm. Their exposure and removal is facilitated by prior complete aortic and caval mobilization, renal vascular dissection and removal of tissue from the posterior body wall. The extension of nodal tissue from infrahilar to suprahilar zones is readily appreciated by elevating the renal vessels with vein retractors. Also, the crural muscle fibres can be seen to cover these nodes. The crural muscle can be retracted or split to give access to large nodes, which occasionally occur. Usually, they can be grasped with broad Russian or Shingley forceps and extracted from this space, with care being taken to secure proximal lymphatic channels in vascular clips.

Infrarenal hilar dissection (aortocaval dissection)

4 & 5

This portion of the procedure has been well described in several sources[1,5,9,10]. The nodal package is split anteriorly down over the inferior vena cava and aorta. The specimen is then rotated off the vessels. The author believes that it is important to divide every lumbar vessel, both aortic and caval, to get complete mobilization and central vascular control. Another important manoeuvre is the squaring out of the upper corners of the nodal package at each renal hilum and taking the nodal package down off the posterior body wall at the foramen of L2–L3. The psoas fascia is stripped down parallel to the ureters which form the lateral borders of the dissection. The gonadal vein is divided on the left from the renal vein or on the right from the inferior vena cava. The involved gonadal vein is then followed to its origin in the groin, dissected out and submitted to the pathologist separately.

Care is taken to obtain the divided stump of the spermatic cord with its original ligatures, if at all possible. The vas deferens is clipped and divided so that the distal portion can be submitted with the spermatic vein and cord stump. On the left side the stump is then tunnelled under the left colic mesenteric artery. The aortic dissection is continued distally by dividing the inferior mesenteric artery. The left colic mesentery is then further mobilized off Gerota's fascia and the splanchnic nervous and venous connections are clipped where necessary to mobilize it thoroughly. This exposes the iliac areas from the medial approach without having to divide the left mesocolon. The left ureter is then easily seen over the pelvic brim. As noted earlier, the nodal packages are rotated off the anterior surfaces of both vessels, the dissection being advanced in the subadventitial planes. Each lumbar artery and vein is easily exposed and divided between 2/0 silk ligatures.

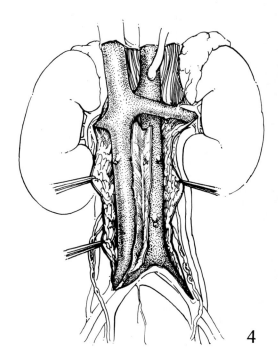

4

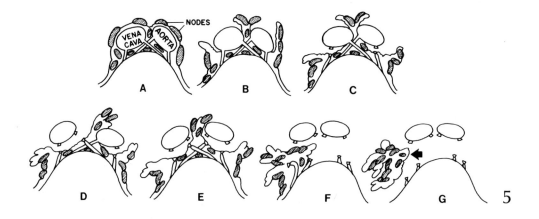

5

6 & 7

Now the great vessels are completely mobilized. The unfurled nodal package is held only by its posterior and lateral attachments. Each lumbar artery and venous penetration into the posterior body wall is divided between clips or ligatures. Bleeding venous tributaries are often controlled by electrocoagulation or additional suture ligature. Once the posterior attachments are divided at the foramina, the nodal package can be wiped off the anterior spinous ligaments with a gauze sponge and drawn under the vessels either medially or laterally. It is convenient to submit the aortocaval package of nodes for analysis separately and to submit the two iliac dissections later. The entire specimen used to be obtained *en bloc* and laid out on a predrawn template for the pathologist. There were some errors in nodal location once the tissue was placed in formalin, because occasionally the tissue would float off the paper template.

The iliac dissections extend several centimetres beyond the bifurcation of the hypogastric artery on either side. The same principle of nodal rotation beneath the vessels is employed. The anterior division of the arteries and veins is carried out and the tissue is rotated below these after the division of any lumbar attachments. It is important to mobilize the psoas muscle in retractors because the nodal chain in the paravertebral area here is often large but not clearly visible without mobilization of the psoas. Again, the right iliac and left iliac nodal packages are submitted separately.

The wound is thoroughly inspected and irrigated. When tumour invasion of the nodes is grossly evident, we irrigate with distilled water, which might lyse any tumour cells that might have been spilled in the wound during dissection. Then the mesenteric attachment is closed with running 0 chromic catgut beginning at the left posterior colonic mesentery in the left upper quadrant and proceeding below the pancreas to the ligament of Treitz. Closure is then carried down, closing the root of the small bowel from the caecum up to the foramen of Winslow. This helps prevent postoperative bowel complications and limits the escape of bloody lymphatic fluid into the peritoneal cavity. The omentum is drawn down over the bowel. The position of the Levin tube is checked. The midline incision is closed with interrupted 0 Prolene or Ethibond sutures. Buried knots are tied below the fascia to avoid uncomfortable nodules in the subcutaneous tissue in thin patients. Retention sutures are used in patients with grossly tumorous nodes who will have chemotherapy in several weeks, with some resultant delay in wound healing and increased abdominal pressure due to the vomiting caused by chemotherapy.

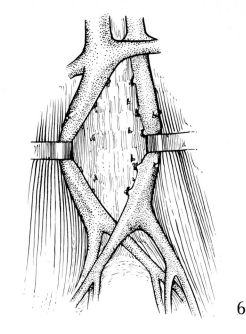

6

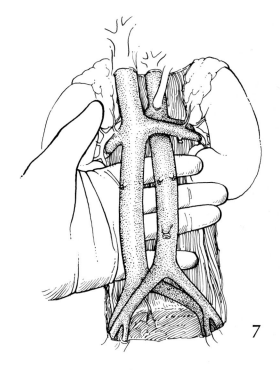

7

Cytoreductive surgery following chemotherapy

There are several special technical considerations when approaching the patient pretreated with combination chemotherapy for cytoreduction of masses and/or disseminated disease. Preoperative considerations include assessment of the bulk and location of the tumour by CT scan. This will direct the choice of incision. The very large persistent lesion in the hilar or suprahilar region is best approached by thoracoabdominal incision on the ipsilateral or involved side. If the disease is very extensive and equally bulky across the midline, the incision can be carried transabdominally. Also, preoperative pulmonary function studies and Po_2 values on room air are useful in assessing the patient's postoperative blood gases. Many patients tolerate relatively low Po_2s postoperatively because it represents their preoperative status quo. It is important to get them off the ventilator as soon as possible and to avoid excessive hydration with crystalloid[7,8].

At surgery, the bowel is reflected in the usual manner and set aside in a bowel bag for optimal exposure of the retroperitoneal mass lesion. The immense variety of histological subtypes in these tumour masses has already been demonstrated[9]. A simple biopsy will be insufficient in providing accurate tissue diagnosis. Therefore, a full retroperitoneal lymphadenectomy should be done for ideal clearance of potential tumour and complete histopathology sampling.

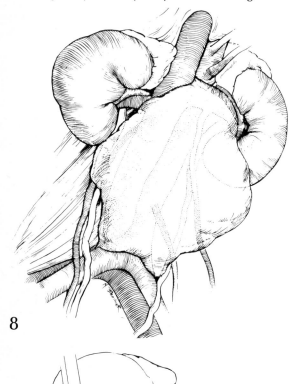

8

8

The illustration shows the common appearance of a large retroperitoneal tumour after chemotherapy has produced some cytoreduction. Note the relationships of the renal and gonadal vessels, and of the ureter and great vessels within the mass.

9

9

In order to do the complete operation in a retroperitoneum occupied by bulky disease, it is often necessary to dissect either below or on the adventitia of the great vessels and to reflect the tumour off in this manner. Usually sharp dissection with scissors and/or scalpel blade will effectively roll off a tumour, provided it is gently retracted with right-angle or other suitable clamps attached to the adventitia and tumour capsule. This is an extension of the split and roll technique used in ordinary lymphadenectomy (see *Illustrations 4* and *5*).

10

Again, the inferior mesenteric artery and the lumbar arteries are best divided after ligature and clipping respectively. This gives the vessels mobility and allows resection from the posterior body wall more safely.

The tumour mass can usually be separated from the ureter and the kidney. At times, however, these structures are inseparably bound within the tumour mass and are best removed *en bloc* with the tumour, provided the contralateral renal unit is established as functional and is not also involved with tumour. A plane of cleavage can often be established in the subadventitial plane, especially when dealing with the vena cava.

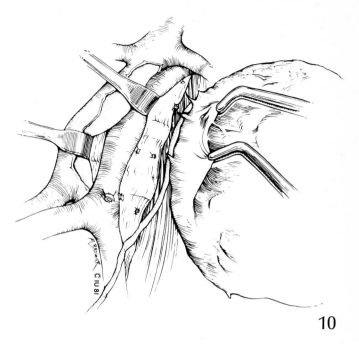

10

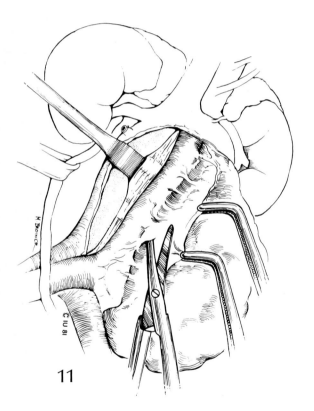

11

11

However, the aorta in certain cases is so diseased by tumour involvement of the wall and by post-chemotherapy changes that it is quite 'cheesy' and does not suture well. Therefore, it is best to leave an additional layer on the aortic side of the dissection so that fibrous tissue can support sutures placed in the aorta. Hence, pre- and para-aortic dissection should be in the extra-adventitial plane. Clamp dissection with electrocautery and splitting of tissue is also effective in the extra-adventitial plane (*see Illustration 9*).

Should the dissection prove technically impossible, or should the aorta give evidence of weakness or rupture, it should be replaced with a Dacron interposition tube graft or branched graft if the iliac vessels are also involved. The venous side is less of a problem. As long as the renal veins can be spared, the cava can be resected with impunity below this level, as is often done if it is quite involved with tumour. In such cases, the iliac lumbar contributions are spared whenever possible.

Results

At the time of writing some 300 patients have been staged with retroperitoneal lymphadenectomy as described above. Crude 2-year survival rates are available for 194 patients[10].

These patients can be divided roughly into two groups. The first group can be assigned to the 'pre-PVB' era (before platinum, vinblastine, bleomycin). There were 30 patients with Stage I disease, 3 of whom subsequently developed Stage III disease with pulmonary metastases. All 3 were saved by single agent chemotherapy (actinomycin D), pulmonary lobectomy, and, in one instance, chest local radiotherapy. These 30 patients continue well and disease-free. Another 28 patients were proved to be in Stage II, with nodal involvement in the retroperitoneum. Of these, 24 (86 per cent) survive clinically tumour-free. Their management formerly consisted of monthly chest radiographs and actinomycin D 1 mg intravenously daily for 4 consecutive days at monthly intervals for the first postoperative year. Therefore, 54 of the 58 patients with Stage I or II disease still survive clinically tumour-free for a cumulative survival rate of 93 per cent in this group of patients. This experience was reported in 1977[10] (see Table 4).

The second group represents the 'post-PVB' era (after the introduction of platinum-vinblastine-bleomycin for treatment of clinical relapse, i.e. Stage III disease). This group of 119 patients has also been reported[11, 12]. Again, these patients are divided into two major groups, histological Stage I and histological Stage II. The Stage II patients were treated in three different ways. One group was treated with surgery alone and followed carefully; another group was treated with single drug adjuvant actinomycin D, monthly for 1 year; and the third Stage II group was treated with adjuvant PVB as a pilot study. The dosages of platinum, vinblastine and bleomycin have been reported elsewhere[11].

All Stage I patients continue alive and well. None received adjuvant chemotherapy after retroperitoneal lymphadenectomy. Of the 57 Stage I patients, there were 4 relapses – at 3, 4, 10 and 22 months postoperatively. Each was saved with PVB chemotherapy at the time pulmonary metastases became evident. At present all 57 patients are in complete remission with no evidence of disease. Of the Stage II patients, 24 were treated with surgery alone. There were 7 relapses (30.4 per cent), all of which were treated with platinum, vinblastine and bleomycin at time of discovery. Of these, 23 show no evidence of disease. One died of unrelated causes and at post-mortem was tumour free. Another 31 patients were treated with adjuvant actinomycin D. There were 15 relapses (48.4 per cent), although the incidence of advanced disease seemed no higher in this group than in the surgery only group.

Table 3 Stage I and II non-seminominous germinal testicular tumours, 1973–1978 Indiana

Stage	Treatment	No. of patients	Relapse	Cure with PVB	Survival		
I	Surgery alone	57	4	4	57	57/57 (100%)	
II	Surgery alone	24	7	7	23*	53/55 (96%)	60/62 (96.7%)
II	Surgery + actinomycin D	31	15	13	30		
II	Surgery + PVB	7	0	–	7		

Table 4 Retroperitoneal lymphadenectomy results, Indiana

	Survival	
Era	Stage I	Stage II
Pre-PVB 1965–74	30/30 (100%)	24/28 (86%)
Post-PVB 1973–78	57/57 (100%)	60/62 (97%)

Thirty patients (96.8 per cent) show no evidence of disease, but one has died of progressive metastatic disease after initial partial remission. The third subset in Stage II was a small pilot group given adjuvant PVB. Seven such patients have been followed for a minimum of 24 months and all remain disease-free. We have reported these in more detail[14] (see Table 1). In summary, our 'post-PVB era' survival in Stage I remains 100 per cent and in Stage II is 96.7 per cent (Table 3). Table 4 summarizes survival rates for the pre- and post-PVB eras.

Summary

Several conclusions can be drawn. Chemotherapy is opening new avenues in the management of these patients. Patients with proven Stage I disease can be allowed to remain untreated provided there is close follow-up. Should Stage III disease develop, the patient can be saved with appropriate and aggressive combination chemotherapy. Patients with Stage I disease should have a 100 per cent survival rate if the retroperitoneum is dissected appropriately and the patient is closely followed postoperatively. Several options exist for the postoperative management of patients with Stage II disease. Two courses are under cooperative study: (a) no treatment after lymphadenectomy, as in Stage I; (b) combination chemotherapy after lymphadenectomy (*Figure 1*). Those patients in the no-treatment group who develop stage III disease cross over to combined chemotherapy with cis-platinum, vinblastine and bleomycin (4-course programme). Since 1974, all but two of our patients with Stage II disease who progressed to Stage III have achieved complete remission with this 3-drug combination. Another new horizon is the potential for chemical cytoreduction of disseminated Stage III disease; persistent abdominal disease can be resected. It is the author's opinion that chemotherapy provides a safer, more extensive initial cytoreduction than the contrary approach of primary surgical cytoreduction and postoperative chemotherapy[13].

Serotesting for the β subunit of human chorionic gonadotrophin and for α-fetoprotein has been a helpful means of following patients with Stage II disease and for detecting tumour before it can be seen by any of the conventional radiological methods.

Although the future of retroperitoneal lymphadenectomy is still unclear and improvements in non-invasive staging will doubtless continue (serotesting for tumour-associated antigens, ultrasound, axial tomography and lymphangiography), it would seem unlikely that completely accurate staging can be obtained without surgical dissection and histological nodal examination. We have had recent experience with several patients in whom all these preoperative tests for metastases (including serotesting) were negative, yet they had evidence of multiple tumorous nodes on microscopic examination[14]. This suggests that the role of surgical staging with histological nodal study will remain central to the accurate definition of disease status and direction of therapy. Furthermore, in this disease, meticulous retroperitoneal surgery seems to influence survival positively.

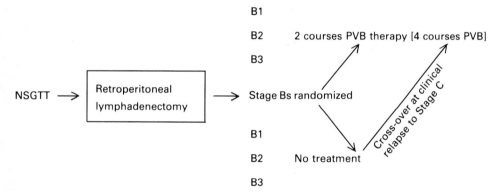

Figure 1 South Eastern (Cooperative) Cancer (Study) Group: Randomized trial, Stage B non-seminomatous germinal testicular tumour (NSGTT)

References

1. Cooper, J. F., Leadbetter, W. F., Chute, R. The thoracoabdominal approach for retroperitoneal gland dissection: its application to testis tumors. Surgery, Gynecology and Obstetrics 1950; 90: 486–496

2. Einhorn, L. H., Donohue, J. P. Improved chemotherapy in disseminated testicular cancer. Journal of Urology 1977; 117: 65–69

3. Busch, F. M., Sayegh, E. F. Roentgenographic visualization of human testicular lymphatics: a preliminary report. Journal of Urology 1963; 89: 106–110

4. Busch, F., Sayegh, E. S., Chenault, O. W. Some uses of lymphangiography in the management of testicular tumors. Journal of Urology 1965; 93: 490–495

5. Chiappa, S., Uslenghi, C., Bonadonna, G., Marano, P., Ravasi, G. Combined testicular and foot lymphangiography in testicular carcinomas. Surgery Gynecology and Obstetrics 1966; 123: 10–14

6. Chiappa, S., Uslenghi, C., Galli, G., Ravasi, G., Belladona, G. Lymphangiography and endolymphatic radiotherapy in testicular tumors. British Journal of Radiology 1966; 39: 498–512

7. Goldiner, P. L., Schweizer, O. The hazards of anesthesia and surgery in bleomycin-treated patients. Seminars in Oncology 1979; 6: 121–124

8. Donohue, J. P., Rowland, R. G. Complications of retroperitoneal lymph node dissection. Journal of Urology 1981; 125: 338–340

9. Donohue, J. P., Roth, L. M., Zachary, J. M., Rowland, R. G., Einhorn, L. H., Williams, S. G. Cytoreductive surgery for metastatic testis cancer: tissue analysis of retroperitoneal tumor masses after chemotherapy. Journal of Urology 1982; 127: 1111–1114

10. Donohue, J. P. Retroperitoneal lymphadenectomy: the anterior approach including bilateral suprarenal-hilar dissection. Urologic Clinics of North America 1977; 5: 509–521

11. Donohue, J. P., Einhorn, L. H., Williams, S. D. Is adjuvant chemotherapy following retroperitoneal lymph node dissection for non-seminomatous testis cancer necessary? Urologic Clinics of North America 1980; 7: 747–756

12. Williams, S. D., Einhorn, L. H., Donohue, J. P. High cure rate of Stage I or II testicular cancer with or without adjuvant therapy. Proceedings of the American Association for Cancer Research 1980; 21: 421 (abstract c-407)

13. Donohue, J. P., Einhorn, L. H., Williams, S. D. Cytoreductive surgery for metastatic testis cancer: considerations of timing and extent. Journal of Urology 1980; 123: 876–880

14. Rowland, R. G., Weisman, D., Williams, S. D., Einhorn, L. H., Klatte, E. C., Donohue, J. P. Accuracy of preoperative staging in Stages A and B non-seminomatous germ cell testis tumor. Journal of Urology 1982; 127: 718–720

15. Vurgrin, D., Cvitkovic, E., Whitmore, W. F., Jr, Golbey, R. B. Adjuvant chemotherapy in resected non-seminomatous germ cell tumors of testis: stages I and II. Seminars in Oncology 1979; 6: 94–98

Further reading

Donohue, J. P., Zachary, J. M., Maynard, B. Distribution of nodal metastases in non-seminomatous testis cancer. Journal of Urology 1982; 128: 315–320

Donohue, J. P., Einhorn, L. H., Perez, J. M. Improved management of non-seminomatous testicular tumors. Cancer 1978; 42: 2903–2908

Ferguson, L. R. J., Bergan, J. J., Conn, J., Jr. Yao, J. S. T. Spinal ischemia following abdominal aortic surgery. Annals of Surgery 1975; 181: 267–272

Fraley, E. E., Kedia, K., Markland, C. The role of radical operation in the management of non-seminomatous germinal tumors of the testicle in the adult. In: Varco, R. L., Delaney, J. P., eds. Controversy in surgery. Philadelphia: W. B. Saunders Company, 1976, 479–488

Patton, J. F., Mallis, N. Tumors of the testis. Journal of Urology 1959; 81: 457–461

Peckham, M. J., Barrett, A., McElwain, T. J., Hendry, W. P. Combined management of malignant teratoma of the testis. Lancet 1979; 2: 267–270

Ray, B., Hajdu, S. I., Whitmore, W. F., Jr. Distribution of retroperitoneal lymph node metastases in testicular germinal tumors. Cancer 1974; 33: 340–348

Scardino, P. T. Adjuvant chemotherapy is of value following retroperitoneal lymph node dissection for non-seminomatous testicular tumors. Urologic Clinics of North America, 1980; 7: 735–745

Skinner, D. G., Leadbetter, W. F. The surgical management of testis tumors. Journal of Urology 1971; 106: 84

Skinner, D. G. Non-seminomatous testis tumors: a plan of management based on 96 patients to improve survival in all stages by combined therapeutic modalities. Journal of Urology 1976; 115: 65–69

Staubitz, W. J., Early, K. S., Magoss, I. V., Murphy, G P. Surgical treatment of non-seminomatous germinal testis tumors. Cancer 1973; 32: 1206–1211

Van Buskirk, K. E., Young, J. G. The evolution of the bilateral antegrade retroperitoneal lymph node dissection in the treatment of testicular tumors. Military Medicine 1968; 133: 575

Whitmore, W. F., Jr. Treating germinal tumors of the adult testes. Contemporary Surgery 1975; 6(2): 17–21

Young, J. D., Jr. Retroperitoneal surgery. In: Glenn, J. F., Boyce, W. H., eds. Urologic surgery. 2nd ed. New York: Harper & Row, 1975; 848–858

Illustrations by Robert N. Lane

Surgery of the adrenal

W. Scott McDougal MD
Professor and Chairman, Division of Urology,
Vanderbilt University Medical Center, Nashville, Tennessee, USA

Anatomy and physiology

The adrenal glands are located in the retroperitoneum immediately cephalad and medial to the superior pole of both kidneys. They are surrounded by fatty tissues and engulfed by an extension of Gerota's fascia which also surrounds the corresponding kidney. The kidney is separated from the adrenal, however, by a few fibrous bands extending in an anterior and posterior direction between the leaves of Gerota's fascia.

1

The arterial supply to the adrenal is derived from three sources: the inferior phrenic artery, the aorta and the renal artery. Small veins within the substance of the adrenal join to form one central vein which, on the left, drains directly into the left renal vein and, on the right, into the posterolateral aspect of the vena cava.

The adrenal gland has two distinct parts: a cortex and a medulla, each of which is derived from separate and distinct tissues. The cortex during embryogenesis is derived from coelomic mesoderm at the level of the genital ridge. Histologically, the cortex has three parts: the zona glomerulosa, zona fasciculata and zona reticularis. The cortical cells are responsible for producing glucocorticoids, mineralocorticoids, androgens and oestrogens. The medulla is derived from neural crest tissue and synthesizes predominantly noradrenaline (norepinephrine) and modest quantities of adrenaline (epinephrine). Diseases of the adrenal generally present as manifestations of the hormone produced in excess.

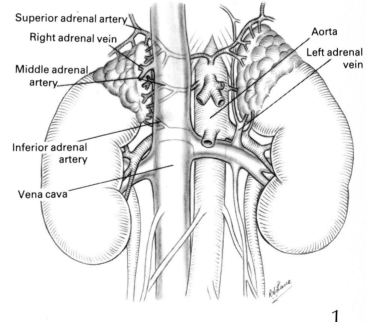

Superior adrenal artery
Right adrenal vein
Middle adrenal artery
Inferior adrenal artery
Vena cava
Aorta
Left adrenal vein

1

Diseases of the adrenal

Primary aldosteronism

Primary aldosteronism occurs when the adrenal is unresponsive to normal control mechanisms and produces aldosterone in excess. Aldosterone is synthesized within the zona glomerulosa of the adrenal cortex and acts on the distal renal tubule to increase sodium reabsorption and facilitate potassium secretion. Generally, this hormone is under renal control via the renin-angiotensin system. When primary aldosteronism occurs, the control system is abrogated and the adrenal is no longer responsive to the action of renin mediated through angiotensin. Thus, under normal circumstances various stimuli within the kidney, i.e. arteriolar hypotension or alterations in distal tubular sodium content, stimulate renin release which acts on an α_2 globulin to produce angiotensin I. Angiotensin I is a decapeptide which is acted upon by converting enzyme, a ubiquitously present enzyme, to cleave two amino acids from the molecule, thereby forming a vasoactive octapeptide, angiotensin II. Angiotensin II results in the production and release of aldosterone. Under circumstances of primary aldosteronism renin is not responsible for the increased level of aldosterone and therefore its absolute plasma value is suppressed.

Patients with the disease are generally between the ages of 30 and 50 years with a 2:1 predominance of females. The symptoms at the time of presentation may include one or all of the following: hypertension, muscle weakness, polyuria, headache, polydipsia, intermittent paralysis, muscle discomfort and fatigue. Laboratory examination reveals a hypochloraemic metabolic alkalosis, occasionally an abnormal glucose tolerance test, and occasionally hypernatremia and increased plasma volume. Rarely hyperchloraemia and hypomagnesemia may coexist[1]. Serum aldosterone and urinary aldosterone levels are elevated, while plasma renin levels are suppressed. More recent evidence indicates that the plasma aldosterone to plasma renin ratio is a better discriminator of primary aldosteronism. If the ratio exceeds 400, the patient invariably has primary aldosteronism, whereas if it is less than 200 primary aldosteronism is unlikely and the patient's hypertension is due to other causes. The test is particularly helpful since about 25 per cent of hypertensive patients have low-renin hypertension.

Primary aldosteronism is subclassified into four distinct types: aldosterone-producing adenoma; idiopathic hyperaldosteronism; indeterminate hyperaldosteronism; and glucocorticoid remedial hyperaldosteronism. Once the diagnosis of primary aldosteronism has been made, it is essential to subclassify the patient into one of the four types, since therapy is dependent upon the type of primary aldosteronism involved. Aldosterone-producing adenomas are the only form of primary hyperaldosteronism which respond to surgical therapy, and therefore it is critical that the surgeon be reasonably sure that this is the type he is dealing with before subjecting a patient to exploration. Aldosterone-producing adenomas are not suppressible either by saline infusion or by desoxycorticosterone-acetate (DOCA) administration. After infusing saline or administering DOCA, plasma aldosterone levels remain elevated. Moreover, when the patient changes from the supine to the upright position, plasma aldosterone levels fall.

Aldosterone-producing adenomas constitute about 60 per cent of the cases seen with primary aldosteronism. Idiopathic hyperaldosteronism constitutes the second major group, involving approximately 40 per cent of patients. Histologically, the adrenal glomerulosa is hyperplastic and these lesions also are non-suppressible with saline loading or DOCA administration. However, plasma aldosterone levels increase when the patient assumes the upright position. Indeterminate hyperaldosteronism is rare and is suppressible with DOCA and saline loading. Glucocorticoid remedial hyperaldosteronism is exceedingly rare and, although it is probably not suppressible, it is corrected by the administration of glucocorticoids. Since patients who have hyperplasia, i.e. idiopathic hyperaldosteronism, respond poorly to adrenalectomy, whereas those with aldosterone-producing adenomas are generally cured in well over 90 per cent of cases, and since these two constitute the bulk of lesions seen, it is important to differentiate between them. Both are non-suppressible; however, measurement of aldosterone in the supine and upright positions may help distinguish the two biochemically. Moreover, it has been shown that if the patient responds to spironolactone with a fall in blood pressure he is more likely to have an aldosterone-producing adenoma and, therefore, to respond to surgery.

Localization of the tumour is generally accomplished utilizing various diagnostic modalities. Initially, an intravenous pyelogram is obtained even though this rarely allows localization of the mass. Its importance lies in the fact that, should it become necessary during surgery to sacrifice the kidney due to complications of the procedure, one knows the status of the remaining kidney. Computerized axial tomography has been used extensively and, as the technology improves, lesions less than 1 cm may be diagnosed by this modality. Radionuclide imaging has been successful in localizing aldosterone-producing adenomas as small as 8 mm. Ultrasonography has also been successful in localizing these tumours, but is not generally useful unless the mass is large enough either to increase the size of the adrenal or significantly to distort its architecture. Finally, if all other methods fail, angiography may be used to localize the avascular adenoma by demonstrating displacement of vessels.

During angiography adrenal vein sampling is performed, at which time aldosterone production from each adrenal can be measured directly. It is important to note that owing to the relatively low flow in the adrenal vein, and the difficulty of cannulating the right adrenal vein, one should analyse the collections for an additional hormone other than the one being sought. For example, if one is interested in aldosterone levels, one should also measure cortisol or catecholamine levels. This allows one to have some confidence in the sample, since if the lesion is on the left and the aldosterone level obtained on the right is low one has no idea as to whether that collection is truly from the right adrenal vein or from the vena cava itself. If one also has a catecholamine or cortisol level which is markedly elevated and a low aldosterone level on the right one can be confident that the venous sample is indeed from the right adrenal vein. Retroperitoneal air insufflation and adrenal vein venography have been used in the past for diagnosis of adrenal masses, but because of their rate of complications and relatively low specificity most centres have abandoned these techniques in diagnosis.

SURGICAL THERAPY

Preoperatively, the patient's potassium losses and hypervolaemia must be corrected, in addition to the alkalosis. Generally, the patient is placed on spironolactone for several weeks prior to surgery and is given oral potassium supplements. The operative approach may be either anterior or posterior. However, if the lesion is localized the posterior approach is preferred by many.

Posterior approach

2

The incision is made over the 10th or 11th rib and angled cephalad for several centimetres as indicated

3

The rib is transected and a segment removed. A small portion (several centimetres) of the medial aspect of the adjacent cephalad rib may also be removed to facilitate exposure.

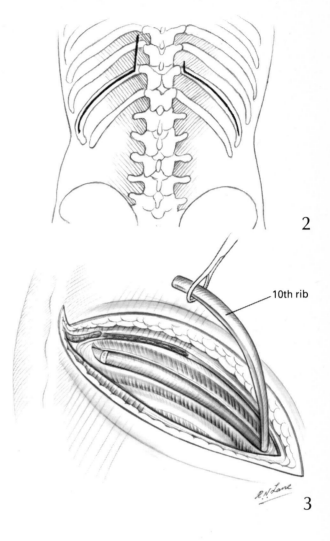

2

10th rib

3

4

The deep periosteum is incised, exposing the pleura and the retroperitoneal fat.

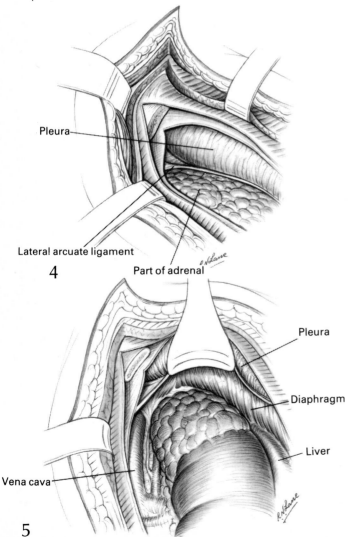

Pleura

Lateral arcuate ligament

Part of adrenal

4

Pleura

Diaphragm

Liver

Vena cava

5

5

The adrenal is exposed. This exposure can be facilitated by downward traction on the kidney.

Only in exceedingly rare cases is cortical tissue containing an aldosterone-producing adenoma found outside the adrenal cortex. Thus there is no need for an abdominal exploration. Postoperative complications are dependent to some degree upon the approach and are more common with the transabdominal approach. They include splenic lacerations, retroperitoneal bleeding, pneumothorax, and injury to the pancreas, liver or hepatic vein, to mention but a few.

Cushing's syndrome

Cushing's syndrome is due to an excess of glucocorticoid production. It may be due either to autonomous production of glucocorticoid by the adrenal or stimulated production through the action of adrenal corticotropic hormone (ACTH) or corticotropine-releasing factor (CRF). The clinical manifestations of the disease are moon face, truncal obesity, plethora, hirsutism, hypertension, osteoporosis, diabetes and psychosis. The syndrome is subdivided according to its aetiology: hyperplasia, adenoma, carcinoma. Seventy per cent of patients with Cushing's syndrome have bilateral adrenal hyperplasia. This is generally due to an increase in ACTH production or is a response to increased corticotropine-releasing factor. Twenty per cent of these patients have a chromophobe adenoma at the time of diagnosis of their disease or will develop one at a future date. Twenty to 25 per cent of patients with Cushing's syndrome have adrenal tumours, with adenomas being slightly more common than carcinomas. Finally, 5–10 per cent of patients have adrenal hyperplasia secondary to ectopically produced ACTH. The ectopic ACTH production is usually a result of oat cell pulmonary carcinomas, thymic tumours, or islet cell tumours of the pancreas. Laboratory evaluation reveals a loss of normal serum cortisol diurnal variation, increased circulating cortisol levels and increased urinary excretion of 17-hydroxysteroids. A more specific test for Cushing's syndrome is urinary free cortisol excretion, which is elevated in those having the disease.

It is important to determine the pathological type of the disease. This may be accomplished by means of several pharmacological tests. Low-dose dexamethasone suppression (dexamethasone 1 mg taken orally followed 12 hours later by a plasma cortisol level) reveals no suppression of the plasma cortisol in patients with Cushing's syndrome. This test is used as a screen to eliminate patients who do not have the disease. High-dose dexamethasone suppression tests consisting of dexamethasone 2 mg every 6 hours for several days, following which cortisol levels are determined each morning, will result in suppression of cortisol levels if hyperplasia is present, but levels will continue elevated and unsuppressed if the hypercorticism is due to adenoma, carcinoma or ectopic ACTH syndrome. The metapyrone test blocks 11 β-hydroxylation and therefore the biosynthesis of cortisol. Normally cortisol suppresses ACTH production. However, with metapyrone suppression, the feedback to the pituitary is blocked. In normal circumstances this results in an outpouring of ACTH and an increased biosynthesis by the adrenal which results in an elevated urinary excretion of 17-hydroxysteroids. In patients with hyperplasia, as well as normal patients, metapyrone results in an increased urinary excretion of 17-hydroxysteroids. If the patient has an adrenal neoplasm or ectopic ACTH syndrome there is no alteration in the urinary excretion of 17-hydroxysteroids. Finally, radioimmunoassay of ACTH, when elevated, indicates that the syndrome is due to ectopic ACTH or abnormalities of ACTH production and/or corticotropin-releasing factor. On the other hand, suppressed levels indicate an adenoma or carcinoma of the adrenal.

Studies used to locate the tumour are similar to those described for primary aldosteronism and include intravenous pyelography, radioisotope scanning[2], computerized axial tomography and angiography. Finally, roentgenograms of the sella turcica might suggest the diagnosis if a mass were noted in this area.

SURGICAL THERAPY

Patients who have tumours of the adrenal generally respond well to surgical removal and patients with hyperplasia also respond if they have failed on suppressive therapy. In the past an attempt has been made to perform a subtotal adrenalectomy on patients with bilateral hyperplasia so that lifetime steroid replacement would not be necessary. These operations have generally been unsuccessful, since Cushing's disease returns after some months as the remnant continues to produce excessive amounts of glucocorticoids. An attempt has been made to transplant the remnant adrenal tissue into the thigh using the saphenous vein as the drainage avenue. This has been successful in several cases and in one instance has been found to result in recurrence of the disease. Transplantation to the thigh, however, makes ablation of the remnant tissue relatively easy should the disease recur[3].

Other tumours of the adrenal cortex

Masses of the adrenal may be adenomatous in nature, in which case they may either be functional or non-functional. Functional tumours involving overproduction of glucocorticoids present with Cushing's syndrome as described above and those with overproduction of mineralocorticoids present with primary aldosteronism. Adenomas may also produce feminization or virilization or they may be non-functional. Cysts of the adrenal also present as masses and may be either parasitic, epithelial, endothelial, lymphangiomas or angiomas, or pseudocysts due to haemorrhagic complications. Masses may be carcinomatous in nature and these may be either functional or non-functional, much as the adenomas described above. Finally, myelolipomas of the adrenal have been described. These are benign masses generally discovered either incidentally or secondary to mass or pressure effects[4]. Half of the malignant masses of the adrenal produce sufficient hormone to present with symptoms indicative of an adrenal origin. Two-thirds of patients are female and virilization appears to be more common than feminization. Patients with these masses present with signs and symptoms of pain, abdominal mass, or various manifestations of the hormone production[5].

Non-functional cortical carcinomas are more prevalent in the male and usually present in the sixth decade[6]. Diagnosis involves the modalities described above – namely intravenous pyelography, computerized tomography, ultrasonography and radionuclide scanning. The latter, however, is somewhat less helpful in these patients since half will have tumours which are non-functional. Angiography completes the diagnostic sequence.

If the adrenal tumours are malignant therapy should be radical surgery with node dissection[7]. Usually the tumours should be approached with a thoracoabdominal incision so that adequate removal of the mass and all its surrounding contiguous structures may be accomplished. Generally, these tumours must be removed *en bloc* with the ipsilateral kidney, and therefore it is important to have a preoperative assessment of contralateral renal function. Even if the entire tumour cannot be removed it should be debulked, particularly if it is a hyperfunctioning, hormone-producing tumour. There have been reports where patients have lived many years after such therapy and, indeed, are easier to manage with suppressive medications. The prognosis for patients with carcinomas is exceedingly poor. The average survival is 1–2 years for the group as a whole and if the patient presents with metastases the average survival is 3–6 months. Adjuvant therapy is totally ineffective and radiotherapy has not achieved much benefit. Ortho, *p*'DDD has been used with some success.

Adenomas, cysts, cortical carcinoma and myelolipomas are generally difficult to differentiate from each other and therefore all are commonly subjected to extirpative surgery. These lesions are best approached transabdominally, or, more commonly, thoracoabdominally.

SURGICAL THERAPY

Thoracoabdominal and transabdominal approaches

6

A thoracoabdominal incision is made as described in the chapter on 'Surgical exposure of the kidney', pp. 21–33. The diaphragm is incised in a circumferential manner, thus exposing the retroperitoneum. The spleen on the left is mobilized medially and the left coronary ligament taken down. On the right the right coronary ligament is incised and the liver rotated medially. This affords excellent exposure of the adrenal.

7

The transabdominal approach and exposure of the left adrenal requires an incision in the gastrocolic ligament to expose the pancreas behind. An incision is made in the retroperitoneum, as depicted, immediately caudad to the lower border of the pancreas.

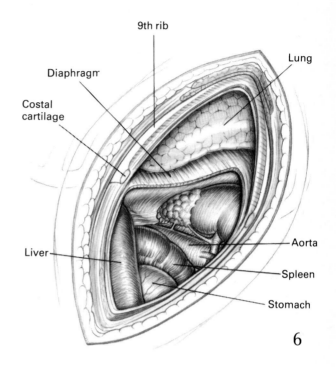

9th rib
Diaphragm
Costal cartilage
Lung
Liver
Aorta
Spleen
Stomach

6

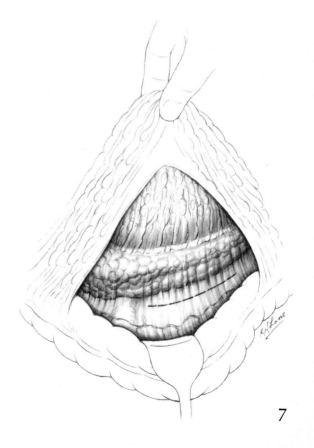

7

8

The transabdominal approach and exposure of the right adrenal requires an incision in the hepatocolic ligament.

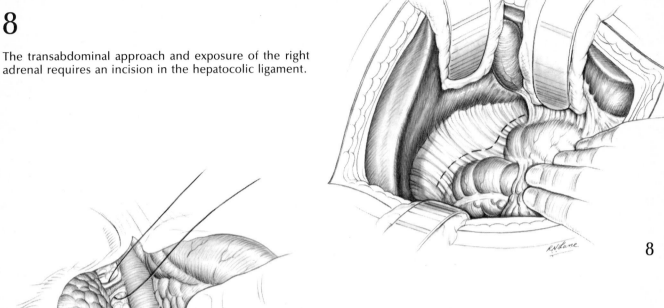

8

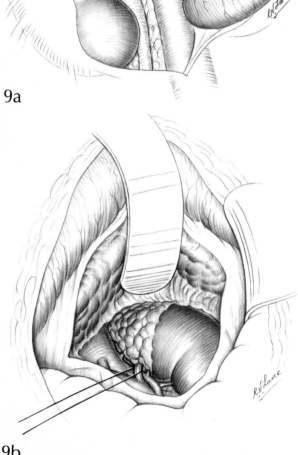

9a

9a & b

The superior pole of the right (or left) kidney is identified, thus exposing the inferior margin of the adrenal. Irrespective of the approach, the vein is isolated and ligated. Care must be exercised, for small adrenal veins as well as the central vein can be torn with ease from the vena cava on the right (a) and from the renal vein on the left (b), resulting in troublesome bleeding. Haemoclips are helpful in ligating small vessels which approach the gland as it is dissected free from surrounding tissue.

9b

Diseases of the medulla

There are four recognized tumours of the adrenal medulla: sympathicogonioma, neuroblastoma, ganglioneuroma and phaeochromocytoma. These tumours arise from a totipotential cell derived from the adrenal medulla. Sympathicogonioma is derived from a very immature cell form and is a highly malignant lesion. Generally, patients with this disease have an enlarged abdomen and metastatic lesions with ophthalmological signs and anaemia at the time of discovery. Approximately 80 per cent of cases occur in infancy and the disease is not generally found in patients older than 2½ years. It is a highly malignant, fatal lesion and should be treated aggressively with wide surgical extirpation.

Neuroblastoma is almost exclusively a disease of infancy and childhood. It differs from sympathicogonioma only in its somewhat greater maturity and the presence of some differentiating ganglion and phaeochrome cells. This disease metastasizes to bone in 30 per cent of cases, to regional lymph nodes in 26 per cent, to the liver in 20 per cent, to the skull or brain in 11 per cent, and to the lungs in 9 per cent of cases. It presents with a mass which is suprarenal in location and distorts the kidney rather than invading it. Fine calcifications are seen within the mass and one may find elevated urinary catecholamine or dopamine levels upon analysis. The differential diagnosis is usually between Wilms' tumour and neuroblastoma. Signs suggesting the latter include lack of destruction of the kidney, fine stippled calcifications within the mass, elevated catecholamine levels, finding the disease within the bone marrow, and site and location of distant metastases.

Ganglioneuromas usually occur in adults and are generally benign. They produce symptoms only by virtue of their size, and excision is curative.

In the adult 80–90 per cent of phaeochromocytomas are benign; 5–10 per cent in adults and 25 per cent in children are bilateral; 10 per cent in adults and 25 per cent in children are located extra-adrenally. Phaeochromocytomas are very vascular tumours and, as in all other lesions of the adrenal, the only valid criterion for determining malignancy is the presence of distant metastases. Symptoms at the time of presentation consist of hypertension (half with sustained hypertension and the other half with paroxysmal episodes), headache, palpitations, excessive perspiration, flushing, vomiting, abdominal pain and acute nervousness and anxiety. Laboratory examination reveals glucose intolerance and occasionally frank hyperglycaemia.

This disease may be associated with other endocrine and neuroendocrine disorders about 10 per cent of the time. It has a higher incidence of association with von Recklinghausen's neurofibromatosis, von Hippel-Lindau's disease and tuberous sclerosis. It may be part of the syndrome which includes medullary carcinoma of the thyroid and parathyroid gland tumours (Sipples syndrome). It may also be associated with other multiple endocrine adenopathies.

There is a frequent association of cholelithiasis with the disease. The tumour is found in the adrenal medulla 85 per cent of the time. Extra-adrenal locations include the organ of Zuckerkandl (located at the bifurcation of the aorta), along the periaortic region and along the perivertebral column in the thorax. Even more rarely, the tumour is found in the urinary bladder wall.

The diagnosis of adrenal phaeochromocytoma is made by serum and urinary determinations of the metabolites of catecholamines as well as by their direct measurement. Twenty-four-hour urines for vanilmandelic acid (VMA)[8], metanephrine and catecholamines are diagnostic in approximately 60–70 per cent of cases. Serum catecholamines are somewhat less likely to be diagnostic than urinary excretion. Because 30–40 per cent of cases are not diagnosed with initial screening procedures, other studies have been developed to aid in diagnosis. Provocative tests, including histamine, tyramine, and glucagon administration, are helpful in selected cases. They are risky in that they may produce uncontrolled malignant hypertension and cause considerable discomfort to the patient during administration. Glucagon stimulation, accompanied by 24-hour collections of urine for catechols, and serum catecholamine measurements have been touted recently for their success in the diagnosis of phaeochromocytoma. Phentolamine, an α-blocker, has also been used as a diagnostic procedure. However, it is relatively non-specific and may result in prolonged hypotension.

The clonidine suppression test has been used recently and shows considerable promise[9]. Since 5–10 per cent of patients with essential hypertension have symptoms suggestive of phaeochromocytoma and also have borderline increases in serum catecholamines, a diagnostic study is necessary to eliminate those without the disease. Clonidine suppression appears to have that specificity. Clonidine suppresses plasma noradrenaline (norepinephrine) levels by stimulating α-adrenergic receptors. Measurement of the plasma noradrenaline levels of patients with phaeochromocytoma reveals no suppression. However, patients without phaeochromocytoma who may be suspected of having the disease have suppressed noradrenaline levels after administration of clonidine.

It should also be noted that occasionally phaeochromocytoma is associated with fibromuscular dysplasia. Indeed, there have been several reports of renal artery lesions in conjunction with phaeochromocytoma. In the majority of instances the renal artery stenosis is secondary to mechanical compression by the phaeochromocytoma, but on rare occasions it may be due to fibromuscular dysplasia[10].

Radiological diagnoses include intravenous pyelography, ultrasonography and radionuclide scanning utilizing ^{131}I meta-iodobenzylguanidine[11]. Both localized and metastatic phaeochromocytomas can be diagnosed with this radionuclide. Finally, angiography may be definitive as well as provocative in the diagnosis of phaeochromocytoma. Preparation for angiography should include the use of α-adrenergic blockade (i.e. phenoxybenzamine) as well as β-blockade if cardiac arrhythmias or pulse rate abnormalities occur. Vena caval sampling for catecholamines may also be helpful in locating extra-adrenal tumours or localizing a small mass to the right or left adrenal. Computerized axial tomography may also be helpful. It is important to point out that not only should catecholamines be analysed in adrenal vein samples; glucocorticoids should also be analysed. As described above, this gives some assurance that one is sampling in the appropriate place and that the low value obtained on one side is due to suppression rather than the fact that the specimen has been obtained from an area other than the adrenal effluent.

Occasionally hypertension will have to be controlled preoperatively with a rapid acting drug, and this may be accomplished with phentolamine or sodium nitroprusside. Arrhythmias may need to be controlled with either propranalol or intermittent intravenous administration of lidocaine (lignocaine).

SURGICAL THERAPY

Preoperative preparation for surgery should include pharmacological blockade and restoration of plasma volume. Alpha-adrenergic blockage and blood pressure control are accomplished with phenoxybenzamine at a dose level generally between 40 and 100 mg per day. If, after adequate α-blockade, blood pressure is still difficult to control, α-methyltyrosine, an inhibitor of the biosynthesis of catecholamines, may prove successful. Following adequate control of blood pressure, plasma volume in 40–60 per cent of patients will require expansion with colloid or blood. Finally, several days prior to surgery a β-blocker such as propranolol is indicated, particularly if there are antecedent pulse or cardiac abnormalities. It should be noted that propranolol should never be given before adequate α-blockade has been established.

These patients should always be explored either thoracoabdominally or transabdominally (see *Illustrations 7, 8 and 9*), for adrenal medullary tissue occurs outside the confines of the adrenal in 10–15 per cent of cases of phaeochromocytoma[12]. Generally, if a large mass is localized to one side or another and it exceeds 10–15 cm in diameter, a thoracoabdominal incision is preferred (see *Illustration 6*). These masses should be approached carefully with an attempt to occlude the venous drainage before handling the lesion. It has been demonstrated repeatedly that handling the mass causes significant variations in the output of catecholamines, with marked changes in blood pressure. Care in dissecting the tumour and initial attention to occluding the venous outflow minimizes these complications. Finally, it should be noted that massive retroperitoneal haemorrhage may occur in the adrenal and generally indicates an adrenal tumour, commonly a phaeochromocytoma.

Complications

Complications of adrenal surgery include pneumothorax, pancreatic injuries, splenic injury, vena cava injury, adrenal vein injury, portal vein injury, hepatic vein injury, retroperitoneal haemorrhage and ventricular fibrillation. Postoperative complications include atalectasis, pneumonia, thrombophlebitis, wound infection, subdiaphragmatic abscess and adrenal insufficiency.

References

1. Conn, J. W., Knopf, R. F., Nesbit, R. M. Clinical characteristics of primary aldosteronism from an analysis of 145 cases. American Journal of Surgery 1964; 107: 159–172

2. Moses, D. C., Schteingart, D. E., Sturman, M. F., Beierwaltes, W. H., Ice, R. D. Efficacy of radiocholesterol imaging of the adrenal glands in Cushing's syndrome. Surgery, Gynecology and Obstetrics 1974; 139: 201–204

3. Hardy, J. D. Surgical management of Cushing's syndrome with emphasis on adrenal autotransplantation. Annals of Surgery 1978; 188: 290–307

4. Agyat, F., Fosslin, E., Kent, R., Hudson, H. C. Myelolipoma of the adrenal gland. Urology 1980; 16: 415–418

5. Hutter, A. M., Kayhoe, D. E. Adrenal cortical carcinoma: clinical features of 138 patients. American Journal of Medicine 1966; 41: 572

6. Shons, A. R., Gamble, W. G. Nonfunctioning carcinoma of the adrenal cortex. Surgery, Gynecology and Obstetrics 1974; 138: 705–709

7. Karakousis, C. P., Uribe, J., Moore, R. Adrenal adenocarcinomas: diagnosis and management. Journal of Surgical Oncology 1981; 16: 385–389

8. Farndon, J. R., Davidson, H. A., Johnston, I. D., Wells, S. A. Jr. VMA excretion in patients with pheochromocytoma. Annals of Surgery 1980; 191: 259–263

9. Bravo, E. L., Tarazi, R. C., Fouad, F. M., Vidt, D. G., Gifford, R. W. Clonidine-suppression test: a useful aid in the diagnosis of pheochromocytoma. New England Journal of Medicine 1981; 305: 623–626

10. DeMendonca, W. C., Espat, P. A. Pheochromocytoma associated with arterial fibromuscular dysplasia. American Journal of Clinical Pathology 1981; 75: 749–754

11. Sisson, J. C., Frager, M. S., Valk, T. W., et al. Scintigraphic localization of pheochromocytoma. New England Journal of Medicine 1981; 305: 12

12. Scott, H. W. Jr., Reynolds, V., Green, N., et al. Clinical experience with malignant pheochromocytomas. Surgery, Gynecology and Obstetrics 1982; 154: 801–818

Surgical exposure of the kidney

G. F. Murnaghan MD, ChM, FRCS(Ed.), FRCS, FRACS
Professor of Surgery, University of New South Wales;
Urological Surgeon to The Prince Henry and The Prince of Wales Hospitals;
Consultant Urologist The Royal South Sydney Hospital, Sydney
and The Royal Hospital for Women, Paddington, New South Wales, Australia

Preoperative

Preoperative assessment and preparation

Careful assessment of the patient's respiratory and cardiovascular systems is required before surgical exposure of the kidney is programmed. Retroperitoneal dissection, particularly through the loin, predisposes to respiratory complications and paralytic ileus. Smoking should be discontinued, chest physiotherapy should be used to ensure maximum ventilatory capacity and a control radiograph of the chest should be taken. Regular, adequate bowel action should be assured before operation as part of the routine preparation for general anaesthesia; the level of haemoglobin should be recorded and at least 2u of compatible blood should be available. The posture and range of lateral flexion in the dorsolumbar spine should be assessed and preoperative skin preparation should extend from the nipple line to the pubis and almost out to the opposite flank on both anterior and posterior aspects of the trunk. Representative and up-to-date radiographs should be chosen from the urological studies and illuminated for easy reference in the operating theatre.

Choice of incision

Choice of incision is influenced by the size, site and mobility of both the lesion and the kidney; by the age and build of the patient with respect to obesity, spinal mobility or curvature; and by the distance between the costal margin and the iliac crest in the midaxillary line where maximum width of the wound is usually obtained.

A standard approach to the kidney through the loin with a subcostal incision will give adequate exposure to a mobile kidney that is not enlarged and when a plain radiograph of the renal region shows that the 12th rib does not project below the midhilar level. The subcostal approach should be carefully considered whenever subsequent re-exposure of the kidney is likely to be required.

Exposure of a high, adherent or enlarged kidney can be significantly improved by resection of the 12th rib or the 11th rib if the 12th is underdeveloped. This transcostal approach is most useful when there has been previous exposure of the kidney by the subcostal route or when reconstructive renal surgery is contemplated.

Easier exposure of a large or fixed kidney with the particular need for access to the upper polar region or pedicle can be obtained without rib resection by a supracostal incision above the 11th rib or, less commonly, the 12th rib to give extrapleural and extraperitoneal exposure. Wide access may also be obtained through a Nagamatsu approach which extends the posterior end of a subcostal incision upwards in a paravertebral line to the 9th intercostal space to allow for resection of 2.5 cm segments of the posterior ends of the lower two or three ribs.

Similar wide exposure may be obtained by a transthor-

acic approach with a high transcostal or intercostal incision combined with an anterior abdominal extension of the wound to allow for simultaneous transperitoneal exploration and any concurrent lymph node dissection.

An anterior extraperitoneal approach to the kidney may be useful in infants and small children as an alternative to the limited exposure generally obtained through the lumbar incision in young patients. It provides direct but localized access to the lower renal pole, pelviureteric junction and upper ureter in all ages, but is particularly useful for the exposure of one or both kidneys in patients with severe cardiorespiratory limitations or with immobilizing disabilities such as osteoarthritis of the spine, scoliosis or kyphosis. Simultaneous exposure of both kidneys is best obtained through an extensive transverse or curved, muscle-cutting, upper abdominal approach with medial reflection of the organs and peritoneum overlying each kidney.

The operation

All illustrations show access to the right kidney; the posterior aspect of the wound is on the left.

1

Positioning the patient

For any lateral approach the patient lies on the opposite side, somewhat nearer to the operator on the operating table and with any segmented cushions replaced by a continuous sheet of thick sponge and with the kidney bridge just below the costal margin. The patient's back is maintained in the vertical plane by flexion of the lower knee and thigh whilst the upper thigh remains straight and is supported on a pillow. The upper arm is supported horizontally in a rest and is convenient for venous cannulation and monitoring of the blood pressure. The underneath arm is disposed in comfortable flexion with padded support. Rolling of the patient is then prevented by padded fixtures on the table and by a leather strap or broad band of adhesive strapping which crosses between the iliac crest and greater trochanter with firm attachment beneath the table top. Lateral flexion of the spine to open the costo-iliac space is obtained by a convenient combination or choice of sandbag in the opposite loin, elevation of the bridge and breaking of the table. The pelvis should be maintained in the vertical plane and it should be ensured that there is no embarrassment to cardiorespiratory function, that there has been no undue angulation of the spine and that the buttocks remain on the table. Anterior approach to the kidney is facilitated by localized support of the lower posterior chest and loin on one or both sides of the supine patient.

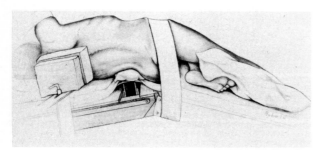

1

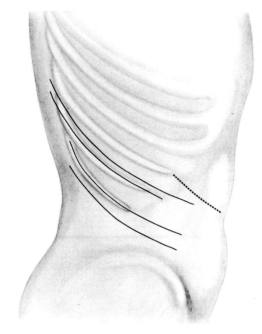

2

2 & 3

The incisions

The lines of skin incision for approach by the subcostal, the transcostal (12th rib), supracostal (11th rib) and thoracoabdominal (10th space) routes of exposure are illustrated. Incisions relating to ribs should curve downwards slightly in their abdominal extension to avoid damage to the neurovascular bundle from the rib above. The foreshortened skin incision for the anterior extraperitoneal exposure of the kidney is shown as a dotted line.

The muscular structures exposed are shown in *Illustration 3*.

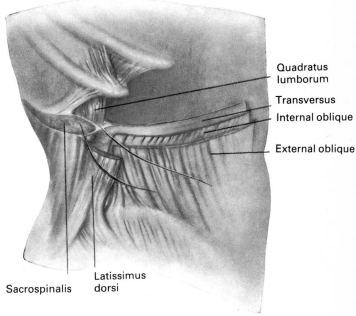

Quadratus lumborum

Transversus

Internal oblique

External oblique

Sacrospinalis   Latissimus dorsi

3

SUBCOSTAL APPROACH

4

The skin incision extends from the angle between the 12th rib and the outer border of the erector spinae muscles and passes forwards about 1 cm below and parallel to the rib and then to a point about 2 cm above and anterior to the anterior superior iliac spine. With careful haemostasis the fat and deep fascia are divided to expose the external oblique muscle in the anterior portion of the wound with latissimus dorsi muscle in the posterior portion. The next useful plane is entered by division of latissimus dorsi in the line of the incision to expose the posterior edge of the external oblique muscle and adjacent lumbodorsal fascia.

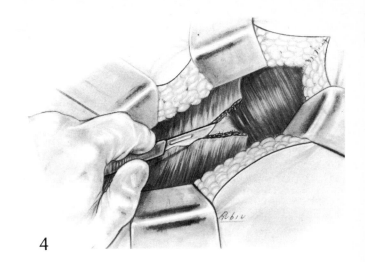

4

5

Division of superficial muscles

Posterior extension of the division of latissimus dorsi exposes the serratus posterior inferior, which is incised to expose the lateral edge of erector spinae beneath the lumbodorsal fascia. Division of the external oblique in the anterior portion of the wound allows for division of the internal oblique muscle from its posterior edge and forwards across the line of its fibres. Care must be taken to avoid the subcostal nerve which in thin patients may be seen crossing the wound beneath the lumbodorsal fascia, having left the 12th rib at about the junction between its middle and distal thirds.

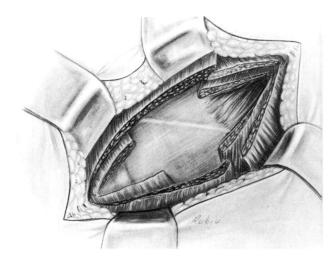

5

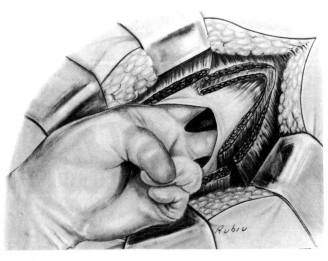

6

6

Division of lumbodorsal fascia

An incision is made into the lumbodorsal fascia in a somewhat more vertical direction than the main line of the incision so that the subcostal nerve is avoided. It can be recognized and dissected clear as the opening in the fascia is extended backwards as far as erector spinae. Blunt dissection forwards beneath the lumbodorsal fascia should proceed carefully to separate the parietal peritoneum from the deep layer of the transversus abdominis muscle, the fibres of which will separate as the fascial incision extends forwards. Careful haemostasis should be obtained and the subcostal neurovascular bundle may be retracted forwards or backwards to obtain the best access.

7

Exposure of the perinephric space

Retraction of the free edges of the lumbodorsal fascia allows for deep digital exploration of the posterior end of the wound and gentle gauze reflection forwards of the parietal peritoneum and extraperitoneal fatty tissue to expose the perirenal fascia. If the present exposure is considered to be inadequate, further upward retraction of the 12th rib will be facilitated by posterior extension of the incision of the anterior layer of the lumbodorsal fascia to include the external arcuate ligament, but any bleeding from subcostal vessels must be carefully controlled.

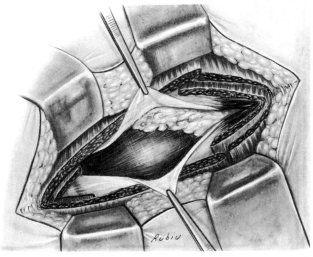

7

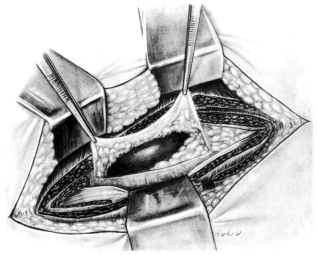

8

8

Incision of the perirenal fascia

A longitudinal cut with knife and then scissors is made through the perirenal fascia a short distance from and parallel to its reflection from the surface of the quadratus lumborum muscle. The anterior edge may be grasped in forceps and elevated to lift the perinephric fat to allow for gentle dissection and exposure of the capsular surface of the kidney.

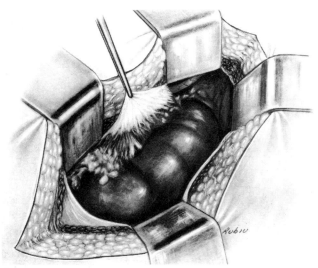

9

9

Exposure of the anterior surface and pedicle

Strong anterior retraction of the peritoneum will allow for continued forward dissection and elevation of the perirenal fascia, with displacement of the overlying abdominal organs. Gentle lateral traction on the kidney aids blunt dissection through the flimsy fascia to expose the pedicle in the hilum. In the presence of adhesions, the plane of the pedicle can more easily be entered after identification of the ureter, medial to the lower pole of the kidney, and by gentle upward dissection in the plane of the ureter and renal pelvis but with care to avoid segmental renal vessels.

10

Exposure of the posterior aspect

Recognition of the ureter near to the lower pole of the kidney is a useful guide into the plane of the renal pelvis. Access is facilitated by delivery of the lower pole of the kidney into the wound whilst the upper pole remains deep. Though the main pedicle usually lies anteriorly, all posterior dissection of the kidney should be careful and blunt in order not to jeopardize segmental renal vessels and ureteric blood supply.

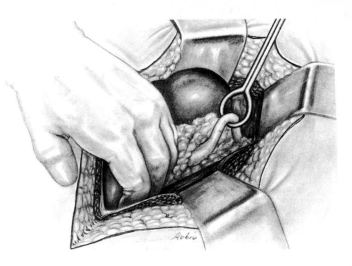

10

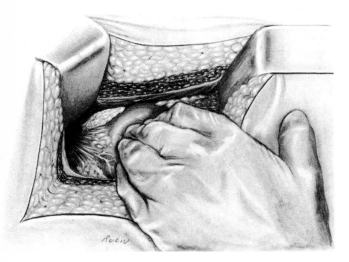

11

11

Exposure of the upper pole

Strong deep retraction of the posterior third of the wound rather than the posterior end of the incision, combined with downward and deep displacement of the kidney, will expose the upper renal pole and suprarenal gland. Strong fibrous brands intermingled with fat may adhere to the renal capsule and may contain quite large blood vessels.

TRANSCOSTAL APPROACH

12

Incision and exposure of rib

Accurate localization of the rib by palpation may be difficult until the skin, fat and superficial fascia have been divided. After subsequent identification a bold incision is made through the latissimus dorsi and serratus posterior inferior muscle onto the rib, which is steadied between fingertips placed in the 11th intercostal space and beneath the 12th rib. Incision should extend into the fascial attachments and periosteum of the outer surface of the rib with clearing of the external oblique muscle from the costal cartilage. Forward extension of the incision with division of the abdominal muscles is postponed until the rib has been resected.

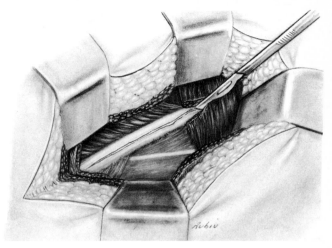

12

13

Excision of rib

The incised periosteum and its attachments on the outer surface of the rib are reflected to the upper and lower borders with a rougine or elevator. Safe and easy entry into the subperiosteal or extrapleural plane on the deep surface of the rib is obtained by careful passage of the rougine along the upper border of the rib from behind forwards and in the reverse direction along the lower rib border. This plane is carefully developed with a raspatory so that the rib is mobilized subperiosteally from the posterior angle to the costal cartilage. The posterior portion is divided with a costotome and the rib is elevated from its bed using a knife to divide the tip and margin of costal cartilage.

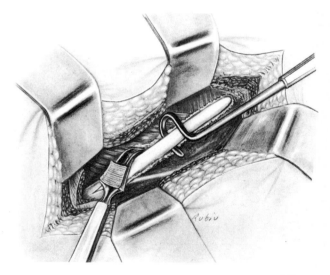

13

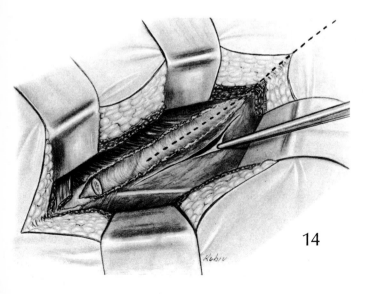

14

14

Division of abdominal muscles

The reflection of the pleura crosses deep to the periosteum of the rib bed. It may be difficult to identify and will restrict safe posterior extension of any incision through the rib bed into the extraperitoneal space. The subcostal neurovascular bundle should be identified as it leaves the lower margin of the rib bed beneath the lumbodorsal fascia. The fascia can be opened safely to avoid both the rib bed and the subcostal vessels and nerve, which can be dissected and displaced posteriorly to allow for easy access to the extraperitoneal space with forward extension of the incision into the abdominal wall muscles. This anterior dissection is similar to the subcostal approach as detailed in *Illustrations 5, 6* and *7.*

SUPRACOSTAL APPROACH

15

Mobilization of the rib

The skin incision extends along the whole length of the 11th rib and is deepened through the overlying muscle to expose but not incise the rib and is carried through the abdominal wall muscles for a short distance beyond the tip of the rib. The intercostal muscle is detached from the upper surface of the rib with a diathermy knife to leave the periosteum bare. A fingertip is inserted into the extrapleural space to protect the deep tissues as the extrapleural plane is developed. The supracostal release must extend posteriorly to allow for division of the posterior supracostal ligament so that the rib is free to rotate downwards at the costovertebral articulation.

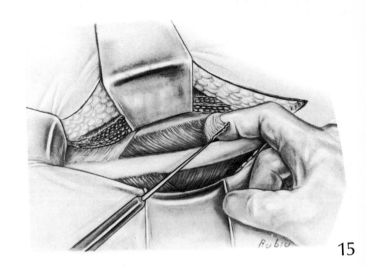

15

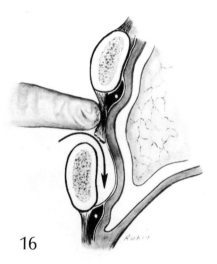

16

16

Release of the intercostal nerve

Incomplete division of the intercostal muscle leaves the innermost fibres intact so that they peel away from the rib with the extrapleural fascia as pressure is applied to the outside surface of the intercostal muscle. The extrapleural fascia splits along the lower border of the rib to enclose the intercostal nerve and the outer layer of fascia must be divided longitudinally with scissors in order to release the nerve and to allow for downward progression of the extrapleural dissection.

17

Division of the diaphragm

The diaphragm is divided as low down as possible to detach it from its origin but with preservation of its full length to facilitate closure. The 11th rib should retract downwards and backwards quite easily to give wide access to the subdiaphragmatic and retroperitoneal space. The peritoneum may be reflected forwards with concomitant fat to expose the perirenal fascia and suprarenal gland.

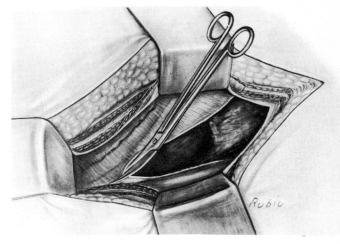

17

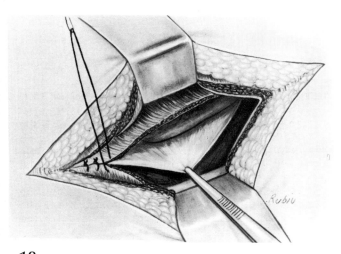

18

18

Closure of supracostal approach

The deeper closure with separation of the thoracic and abdominal compartments is accomplished by pulling the upper margin of the free edge of the incised diaphragm through the intercostal space so that it can be sutured to the intercostal muscles and to the muscles on the outer surface of the rib below, that is serratus posterior inferior posteriorly and latissimus dorsi anteriorly. Any pleural tear can also be approximated in these interrupted sutures after deliberate expansion of the lung by forced ventilation. The superficial muscles are closed in layers and any required drainage is effected through a separate stab incision below the subcostal nerve and 12th rib.

THORACOABDOMINAL APPROACH

19

Thoracotomy

Wide exposure of the kidney with easy access to the pedicle may be obtained by a transpleural approach through the bed of either the 10th or 11th ribs. The chosen rib is resected subperiosteally as described for the transcostal approach, with incision of overlying muscles including the latissimus dorsi, serratus posterior inferior posteriorly and some fibres of the external oblique muscle in the anterior portion of the wound. A similar exposure is afforded more easily by incision through the 9th or 10th intercostal space without rib resection. The superficial layers of muscle must be incised as far back as the lateral edge of the erector spinae.

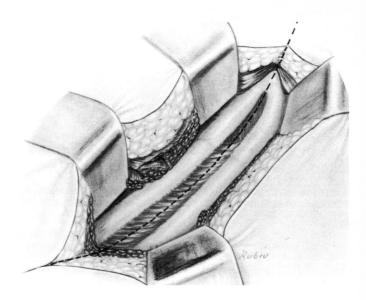

19

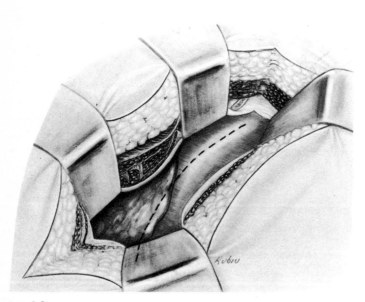

20

20

Exposure and incision of the diaphragm

Incision of the intercostal muscles, intercostal membrane, costal cartilage and underlying pleura exposes the lung, which collapses or is retracted to expose the diaphragm. The retroperitoneal space is then entered by division of the diaphragm and overlying pleura in the midportion of the wound. The diaphragmatic incision is then extended posteriorly towards the angle of the 12th rib so that adherent peritoneum may be dissected free from the undersurface of the diaphragm to allow for forward extension of the incision through diaphragm and the transversus abdominis muscle, which interdigitate. The wound is then extended forwards by incision of the abdominal wall muscles in a manner similar to the description for the anterior extraperitoneal approach (see Illustrations 21 and 22). The perinephric fascia is exposed by forward displacement of the subdiaphragmatic peritoneum and fat. The peritoneum may be incised in conjunction with the anterior extension of the thoracoabdominal approach to give extensive access to the abdomen.

ANTERIOR EXTRAPERITONEAL APPROACH

21

Exposure of the peritoneum

The skin incision extends from the tip of the 10th rib to cross the lateral edge of the rectus abdominis muscle in the direction of the umbilicus. The external and internal oblique muscles are divided across the line of their fibres and bundles of the transversus abdominis muscle are gently separated to enter the extraperitoneal plane. Finger or gauze dissection between the peritoneum and the transversalis fascia must be gentle but extensive. The peritoneum becomes more adherent to the posterior rectus sheath in the anterior portion of the wound. Both the anterior and posterior layers of the sheath of rectus abdominis can be incised over a short distance to improve access through this approach, which can also be combined with thoracotomy.

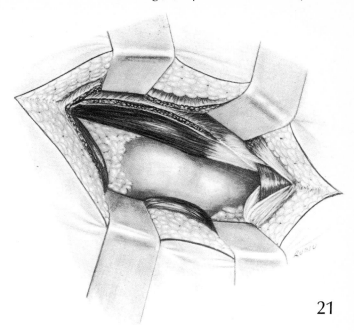

21

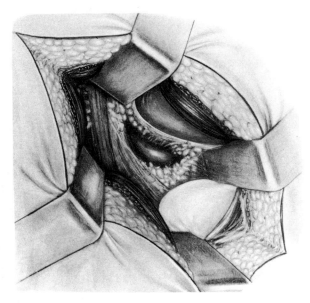

22

22

Retraction of the peritoneum

The extensive and lateral mobilization of the peritoneum allows it to be retracted medially so that the perinephric fascia is exposed on the stretch. The fascia is incised longitudinally, parallel to the renal axis and is mobilized medially with perinephic fat and peritoneum to expose the lower pole of the kidney, the pelviureteric junction and the upper spindle of the ureter.

RE-EXPOSURE OF THE KIDNEY

Most careful review of renal position and mobility and the nature of any previous renal surgery should precede the choice of incision for re-exposure. An alternative to the primary approach is usually desirable and the transcostal route is generally very much easier than direct surgery through the scar of a previous subcostal incision. Re-exploration is cautiously staged. Excessive tension in the parietes from lateral extension of the spine in the 'kidney position' must be avoided in order to prevent sudden splitting of any adherent kidney on the deep surface of the previous muscle closure as the incision is deepened and the wound edges separate. The extraperitoneal plane should be identified at the renal pole away from the major site of previous surgery. The peritoneum may be densely adherent on the lateral as well as the anterior aspects of the kidney and may be included in the scarring of previous drainage sites. Dissection may be started more easily around the upper ureter and a safe plane may be developed proximally to isolate the renal pedicle.

CLOSURE OF WOUNDS AFTER EXPOSURE OF KIDNEY

Despite careful haemostasis during surgery there is a tendency for serosanguinous oozing and there is sometimes risk of urinary leakage. Accordingly it is usually wise to institute drainage of the perinephric space with loose approximation of the perinephric fat and fascia around the drain using a few interrupted absorbable catgut sutures. Drains should be flexible and generally are more effective if corrugated rather than tubular in form. Gross drainage may be collected by surface applicator for measurement and analysis. Drains should be delivered in front of the midaxillary line where they can be included in muscular rather than fascial closure of the wound and will not cause added discomfort to the patient with change in lateral posture. Negligible drainage from the wound would encourage shortening of the drain by 2–3 cm each day and early removal from the retroperitoneal space discourages paralytic ileus.

In wound closure care should be taken to avoid suturing of intercostal or subcostal nerves. The initial deep sutures in the lumbodorsal fascia or rib bed should be placed at the posterior end of any loin wound before the bridge is lowered for the reduction of lateral spinal flexion to aid subsequent wound approximation. Wounds should be closed in separate muscle layers except when this is impracticable after re-exposure. Interrupted sutures of fine non-absorbable material are most dependable for the closure of clean wounds but this technique is time-consuming. Running sutures of 1/0 chromic catgut are a satisfactory alternative provided that independent interrupted sutures are placed on either side of any drain and in each muscle layer separately.

Diaphragmatic incisions must be securely approximated by a reinforced layer of interrupted horizontal mattress sutures of non-absorbable material other than silk. The parietal pleura and any periosteal bed of resected rib are carefully closed with a continuous suture of fine nylon before the parietal muscles are approximated with non-absorbable sutures. It is not necessary to approximate either the parietal pleura or the intercostal muscles in closing a thoracotomy through an intercostal space. The adjacent ribs are brought together and bound with interrupted ties of double 2/0 chromic catgut. The wound becomes airtight with approximation of the superficial muscles by a continuous suture of non-absorbable material. In closing the chest cavity care must be taken to re-expand the underlying lung and a soft intercostal catheter of size 32 Fr is inserted through a stab incision in the 8th intercostal space in the midaxillary line to provide for underwater sealed drainage.

The special technique for closure of the supracostal approach is shown in *Illustration 18*.

Postoperative care

Approaches to the kidney through the loin, lower thorax and retroperitoneal space predispose to pulmonary complications, tympanites and paralytic ileus. If the retroperitoneal dissection has been extensive and particularly in obese patients, oral fluids and food should be withheld and replaced by intravenous fluid and electrolyte therapy until there is evidence of adequate bowel tone. Chest physiotherapy with early mobilization of the patient, supported by analgesics and comfortable wound dressings, promote pulmonary expansion and avoid atelectasis.

Further reading

Nagamatsu, G. Dorsolumbar approach to the kidney and adrenal with osteoplastic flap. Journal of Urology 1950; 63: 569–577

Turner-Warwick, R. T. The supracostal approach to the renal area. British Journal of Urololgy 1965; 37: 671–672

Specialized surgical approaches to the kidney

Robert A. Riehle, Jr MD
Assistant Professor of Surgery (Urology), Cornell University Medical Center, New York;
Assistant Attending Surgeon, The New York Hospital, USA

E. Darracott Vaughan, Jr MD
James J. Colt Professor of Urology in Surgery, Cornell University Medical Center, New York;
Attending Surgeon-in-Charge, Division of Urology, The New York Hospital, USA

Introduction

Although the classic lumbar approach to the kidney continues to remain popular, specialized anterior and posterior incisions have been described and skilfully employed for renal surgery. The extraperitoneal flank exposure was historically devised as an avenue to drain infection from the perinephric spaces while avoiding peritoneal contamination. Recently, the more direct transabdominal exposure for extirpative or reconstructive surgery has been utilized widely. The dorsolumbar approach and the vertical posterior lumbotomy continue to be useful exposures for specific urological problems.

Preoperative

In addition to standard respiratory and cardiovascular evaluation, several preoperative points must be considered, regardless of the surgeon's choice of incision. First, gastrointestinal ileus often follows retroperitoneal surgery, and the patient should undergo mechanical bowel preparation, including cathartics and enemas, the day before surgery. Sympathetic denervation, as well as retroperitoneal drains and haematoma, cause a reflex ileus, and nasogastric decompression is indicated after major renal surgery. In those patients with decreased pulmonary reserve, a gastrostomy can be placed during the renal procedure, especially if the approach is transabdominal.

Secondly, preoperative pulmonary toilet is always advised, since the flank position for the dorsolumbar or posterior lumbotomy may cause pulmonary congestion and effusion in the most dependent pleural cavity. Diaphragmatic irritation during suprarenal dissection can often evoke a sympathetic ipsilateral pleural effusion.

Both the anterior transverse and the transcostal approaches cause postoperative respiratory splinting and decreased ventilation.

Thirdly, for dorsal lumbotomy or Nagamatsu exposure, the range of lateral flexion of the lumbar spine must be assessed before the patient is anaesthetized, since arthritis, spinal fusion or obesity may limit the exposure along the midaxillary line between the costal margin and iliac crest. Cervical spine mobility is important for an easy anaesthetic induction, and normal hip and knee range of motion allows more secure flank positioning.

Finally, preoperative hydration with saline-containing solutions prevents anaesthetic-induced hypotension. Expansion of the intravascular volume before surgery prepares the patient for the extravascular peripheral pooling which often accompanies the flank positioning. Antiembolic precautions require wrapping of the legs with pressure bandages from toes to mid-thigh, thus decreasing superficial venous pooling as well as providing cutaneous padding.

Choice of incision

As mentioned by previous authors[1, 2, 3], a surgeon must choose an incision only after considering the size and body habitus of the patient, the operative field to be exposed, and the type of surgery – extirpative or reconstructive – to be performed. The incision should provide easy exposure of the pathology with minimal retraction, and it should allow for extension should more radical surgery be indicated. It should avoid cutaneous nerves as well as major segmental vessels and minimize the division of muscle tissue. Obesity of the patient, axial skeletal hypomobility, angulation of the lower rib cage with a narrowed lumbar space, and previous surgical scars should be appraised before deciding on an incision.

The anterior approach

The anterior incisions depicted in this chapter can be utilized both for transperitoneal and extraperitoneal approaches. After induction of anaesthesia, a roll should be placed underneath the small of the patient's back to elevate the retroperitoneum. However, flexion of the table is discouraged, since this places the rectus muscles under tension and displaces the renal fossa away from the surgeon when the patient is in mild Trendelenburg position.

Alternatively, a sandbag may be placed under the ipsilateral sacroiliac joint to provide slight anterior rotation of the appropriate flank. The ipsilateral arm and shoulder can be placed in similar rotation on an arm-rest (Lyon's position) and some flexion is helpful.

THE ANTERIOR SUBCOSTAL APPROACH

1

Although frequently employed[4], the anterior transperitoneal approach to the kidney is certainly not the most direct. The costochondral angle limits cephalad retraction, and the intestines must be packed away prior to renal exposure. The incision, either a classic or modified Kocher (incision A), may be enlarged for better exposure by: (1) extension across the midline to the contralateral anterior rectus sheath, converting the exposure to an incomplete chevron; or (2) lateral extension through an intercostal space or through the rib bed after the subperiosteal resection of the 11th or 12th ribs. A transverse incision (incision D) is most frequently used for children. In adults, Lyon has described an incision[5] from the tip of the 12th rib to a point over the ipsilateral rectus muscle. Varying the angle of the incision alows for resection of the 11th or 12th rib if needed.

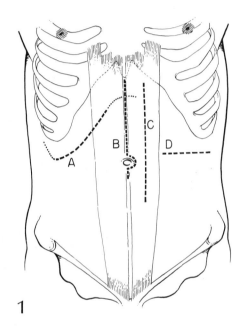

1

2

The incision is made briskly with the scalpel, two finger breadths below the costochondral arch. Subcutaneous fat is divided down to the anterior sheath medially and the external oblique aponeurosis laterally.

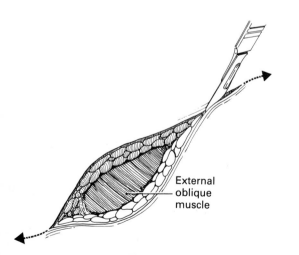

External oblique muscle

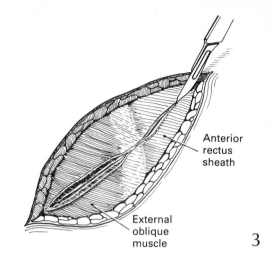

3

Anterior rectus sheath

External oblique muscle

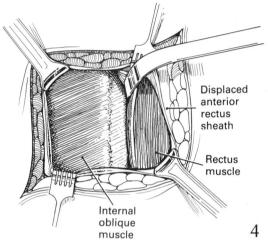

Displaced anterior rectus sheath

Rectus muscle

Internal oblique muscle

4

3 & 4

The rectus sheath is divided sharply, with care, to avoid the underlying rectus muscle, which is then pulled medially to expose the posterior sheath.

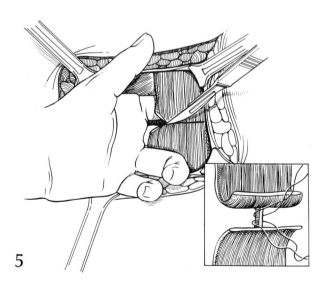

5

5

For better exposure the rectus may be divided after identifying and securing the epigastric vessels. Muscle division with cutting cautery is quite rapid and effective. To coagulate, the tip should be placed in the muscle before applying coagulation current, thus preventing recoil of the muscle.

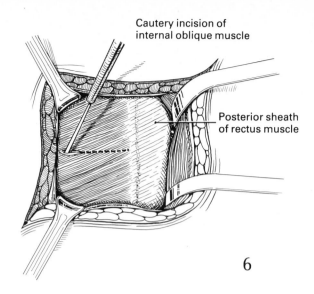

Cautery incision of
internal oblique muscle

Posterior sheath
of rectus muscle

6

6

The external and internal oblique are sharply divided using cutting cautery.

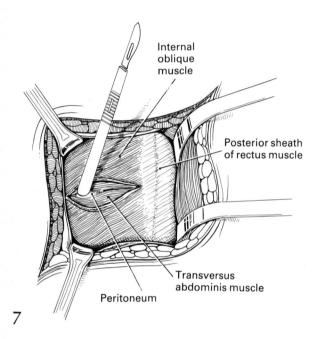

Internal
oblique
muscle

Posterior sheath
of rectus muscle

Transversus
abdominis muscle

Peritoneum

7

7

The transversus abdominis muscle is bluntly separated in the course of its fibres, revealing the peritoneum beneath. To facilitate later closure, the transversus should be gently dissected from the peritoneum using Metzenbaum scissors and a K-D dissector. This manoeuvre also allows more effective medial retraction of the peritoneal envelope and its contents.

8

The posterior rectus sheath is divided anterior to the peritoneal cavity. At this point the surgeon may enter the abdominal cavity or remain extraperitoneal.

If the approach is to be extraperitoneal, blunt dissection of the peritoneum from the transversus abdominis muscle and aponeurosis allows entrance to the retroperitoneal space laterally. The surgeon must proceed posterolaterally until he reaches the surface of the quadratus and psoas muscles. This plane will allow him to expose the posterior aspect of Gerota's fascia which is then incised in a vertical direction. A Deaver retractor is placed medially and gently reflects the peritoneum from the retroperitoneal kidney and vessels.

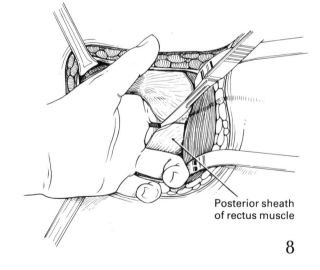

Posterior sheath
of rectus muscle

8

ANTERIOR PARAMEDIAN INCISION

The anterior paramedian incision (*see Illustration 1,* incision C), although slightly more tedious for the surgeon, has the advantage of allowing a strong closure with preservation of rectus muscle anatomy and function[6]. However, since the rectus is not divided, medial and lateral displacement of this muscle is limited, and this approach does not always provide the operator with the best exposure.

9 & 10

An anterior vertical incision is made approximately three finger breadths from the midline and deepened through subcutaneous tissue to the anterior rectus sheath, which is sharply incised.

11

The rectus muscle is separated from the anterior sheath using sharp and blunt dissection.

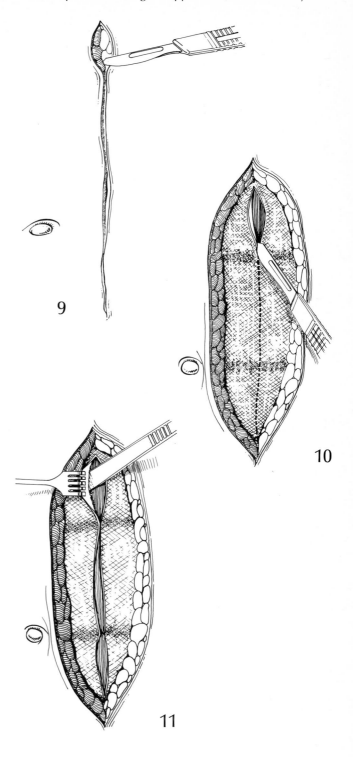

9

10

11

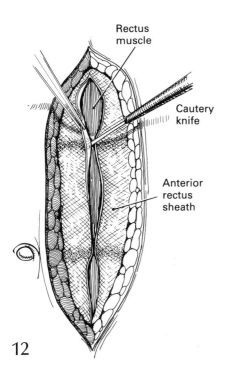

Rectus muscle

Cautery knife

Anterior rectus sheath

12

12

The tendinous bands between muscle and anterior sheath should be sharply divided with cautery since they often contain small vessels.

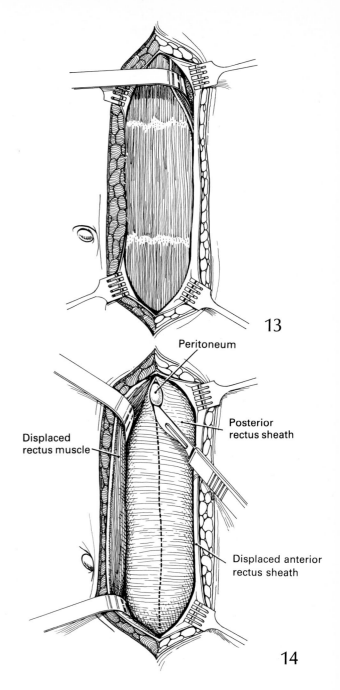

13

14

13 & 14

These tendinous bands do not attach to the rectus posteriorly and after retraction of the rectus medially, the posterior sheath, composed of the transversalis aponeurosis and posterior leaf of the internal oblique aponeurosis, is divided with care to identify the underlying peritoneum. At this point the surgeon may choose to remain extraperitoneal or to enter the peritoneal cavity.

Peritoneum

Displaced rectus muscle

Posterior rectus sheath

Displaced anterior rectus sheath

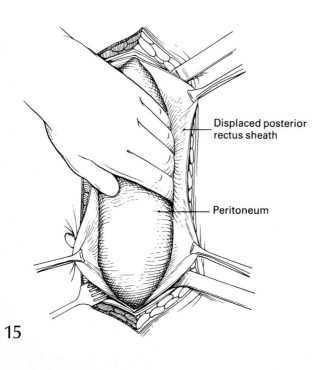

Displaced posterior rectus sheath

Peritoneum

15

15

To remain extraperitoneal, the peritoneum is bluntly and sharply dissected from the transversus abdominis muscle both superiorly and inferiorly. The peritoneum is usually adherent to the anterior abdominal wall at the lateral border of the posterior rectus sheath, and dissection here can be tedious. By entering the retroperitoneal plane cephalad under the diagram and inferiorly to the iliac crest, the peritoneal envelope and its contents are readily mobilized medially to expose the posterolateral surface of Gerota's fascia. Again, the surgeon must head posteriorly into the retroperitoneum before he can move medially towards the kidney.

THE ANTERIOR MIDLINE APPROACH

The standard midline incision (*see Illustration 1*, incision B) provides rapid access to the major vessels of the abdomen as well as control of the renal pedicles. This exposure is standard when operating for renal or abdominal trauma, since it affords access to the midportion of the retroperitoneum as well as the abdominal cavity. It is less advantageous for a large obese patient or a patient with an upper pole renal carcinoma. The midline approach is not acceptable for drainage of perinephric or paranephric infections since, in general, drainage of retroperitoneal infections should remain extraperitoneal. In the particular case of large infected polycystic kidneys, exploration may be anterior but drainage should be established posteriorly.

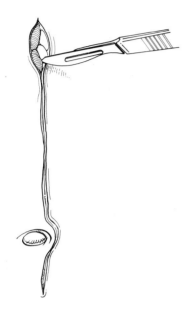

16

16

The midline incision should be made briskly from just below the xiphoid to just below the umbilicus and should reveal the linea alba of the rectus fascia with the first or second stroke of the scalpel. Care must be taken to circumscribe the umbilicus, and constant distraction of skin between the operator and his assistant will prevent bevelling this portion of the incision.

The scalpel should be allowed to float down through subcutaneous fat until it meets the resistance of the fascia. Subcutaneous bleeding vessels should be electrofulgurated. The intersection of fascial fibres identifies the linea alba.

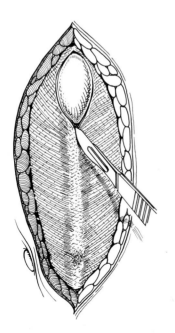

17

17

The linea alba is incised with the scalpel, revealing preperitoneal fat which varies in thickness and can be displaced from the midline by a thumb or retractor. The underlying peritoneum is elevated between forceps, incised and, after inserting a finger in the abdomen to check for adhesions, the remainder of the peritoneum is cut with Metzenbaum scissors. The ligamentum teres can be divided and the abdomen entered.

Once inside the abdomen, after exploration of the major organs and the bowel, the small bowel should be packed away using moist packs and the surgeon should palpate the retroperitoneal kidney, the renal hilum and the paraaortic and paracaval lymph nodes. The renal pedicle can be approached either directly through the posterior parietal peritoneum or after medial reflection of the colon. If the surgeon needs vascular control prior to dissecting the kidney, such as for heminephrectomy, renovascular reconstruction, renal trauma, or radical nephrectomy for tumour, he will choose to expose the renal pedicle first.

18

The right renal hilum may be approached most directly via a Kocher manoeuvre. The hepatic flexure of the transverse colon can be displaced superiorly or inferiorly depending on the colon's mesenteric length and the site of retroperitoneal attachment. Usually, as shown here, the colon can be displaced downwards by the assistant.

Incision lateral to the second portion of the duodenum reveals the anterior surface of the vena cava. Dissection at this point should remain directly on the anterior surface of the vena cava, posterior to the portal vein and anterior to the renal vein which enters the vena cava on the right lateral aspect. Care must be taken at this point to identify the following: the gonadal vein, which often has a slightly anterolateral insertion into the vena cava; accessory renal arteries which can run anterior to the vena cava; accessory polar renal veins. The right adrenal veins usually join the vena cava posterolaterally and 4–6 cm cephalad to the renal vein.

The renal artery itself may be found posterior to the renal vein along the vein's superior margin (inset). It may be isolated at this point or identified more medially as it passes between the vena cava and the aorta. After the hilar vessels have been dissected free, the line of Toldt along the right colon is sharply divided, freeing the lateral and superior colonic flexure ligaments. The hepatocolic ligament, which is slightly more developed laterally than medially, is usually divided using both blunt and sharp dissection. Freeing the lateral attachments first often makes the more medial dissection towards the vena cava easier. The colon is displaced inferiomedially, exposing the anterior Gerota's fascia. Care must be taken to separate the colonic mesentery from this perirenal fascia, since tumour invasion or collateral vessels can make this dissection tedious.

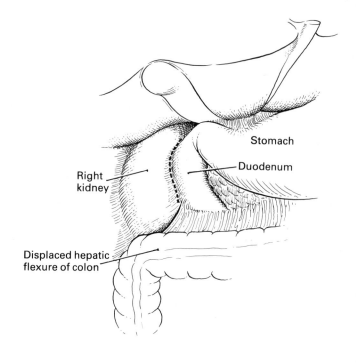

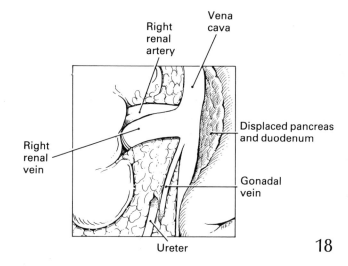

18

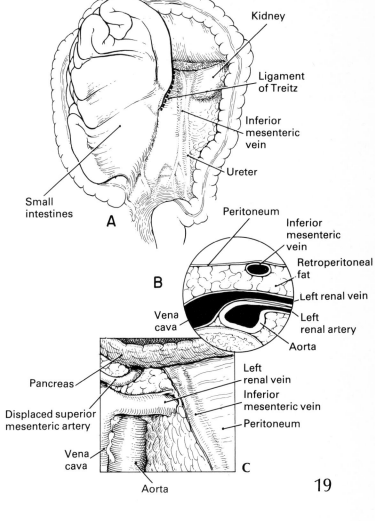

19

On the left side, a vertical incision is made in the posterior peritoneum just below the ligament of Treitz lateral to the fourth portion of the duodenum and medial to the inferior mesenteric vein. This incision will expose the anterior surface of the aorta. Dissection should proceed with care to preserve both the crossing left renal vein and the left gonadal artery which often assumes an anterior origin from the aorta (inset B). If the inferior mesenteric vein prevents cephalad exposure, it can be divided.

The superior mesenteric artery (inset C) should be identified as it takes origin from the anterior aorta slightly cephalad to the left renal artery. It should not be confused with the renal artery itself. Dissection should remain posterior to the pancreas and splenic vessels which run along the superior aspect of the back of the pancreas.

20

An alternative approach to the left hilum is through the lesser sac. The gastrocolic omentum is divided and the space anterior to the pancreas and posterior to the stomach is entered. The transverse colon is retracted inferiorly, and the posterior peritoneum inferior to the pancreas is incised. The left renal hilar vessels are isolated at this point in much the same manner as described above.

The left colon is then displaced medially and inferiorly and the splenocolic and renocolic ligaments are divided. Incision along the line of Toldt allows displacement of the colon from the anterior surface of Gerota's fascia. Again, care must be taken to enter the proper plane so that colonic mesenteric vessels are not injured.

On either the left or the right side the surgeon may choose to release the colon from its attachments first before isolating the vessels.

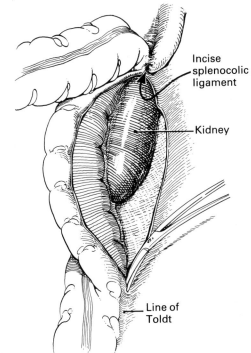

20

The dorsolumbar approach
(Nagamatsu[7])

This approach is a transthoracic extrapleural approach in which an osteoplastic flap of the three lowermost ribs is created, affording access to the subdiaphragmatic retroperitoneum. Although the thoracoabdominal approach is more popular today, this incision has the advantage of providing wide exposure without entering the pleural cavity[7].

The patient is positioned as for a standard flank approach with slight 15° anterior rotation. The ipsilateral arm must be supported. Once the patient is securely taped in position, the table may then be rotated anteriorly or posteriorly to accommodate the dorsal or lumbar portion.

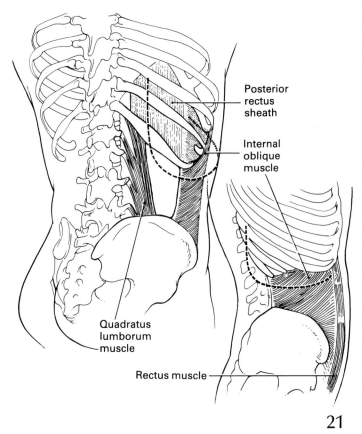

21

21

The vertical dorsal portion of the incision is started just below the 12th rib and sweeps upward medial to the angle of the ribs and slightly lateral to the sacrospinalis muscles until the 10th rib is reached. The anterior portion of the incision continues below the 12th rib and curves gently upwards, meeting the lateral rectus sheath at the level of the 10th rib.

22

The posterior portion of the incision is developed first, dividing the latissimus dorsi and posterior serratus over the lower ribs medial to the rib angle. Tendinous slips of the sacrospinalis are removed from this medial portion of the ribs to allow later rib motility.

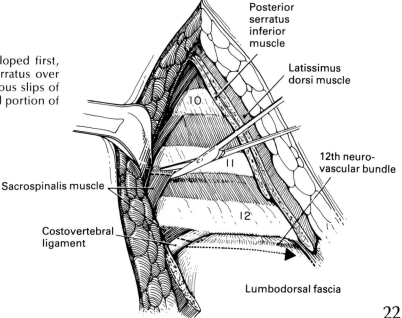

22

23

Swinging under the tip of the 12th rib, the external and internal obliques are sharply divided using scalpel or cautery. The 12th neurovascular bundle must be identified and preserved.

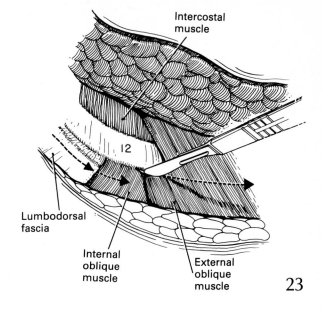

Intercostal muscle

Lumbodorsal fascia

Internal oblique muscle

External oblique muscle

12

23

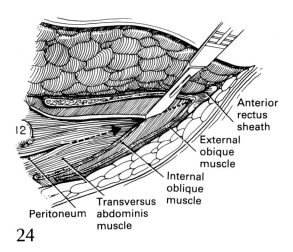

12

Anterior rectus sheath

External obique muscle

Internal oblique muscle

Peritoneum

Transversus abdominis muscle

24

24

Medially the fibres of the transversus abdominis are separated bluntly to reveal the underlying peritoneum. The peritoneum must be sharply dissected from the undersurface of the transversus abdominis to allow full retraction of the peritoneal envelope and its contents.

25

A 2 cm portion of the 11th and 12th rib medial to the angle is isolated subperiosteally using an Alexander periosteal elevator and a Doyen. These segments of rib are removed using the Guillotine rib resector. The pleura must be avoided here, and careful dissection of the periosteum from the posterior surface of the ribs will facilitate rib transection without threat to the pleura or neurovascular bundle. The rib resection must be performed medial to the rib angle to ensure proper thoracic wall mobility.

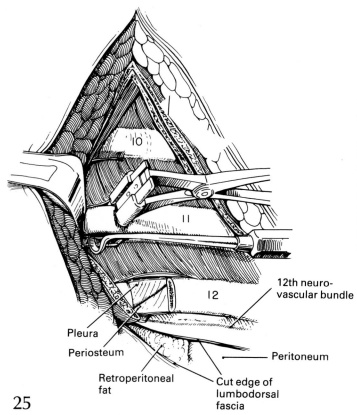

10

11

12

12th neuro-vascular bundle

Pleura

Periosteum

Retroperitoneal fat

Cut edge of lumbodorsal fascia

Peritoneum

25

26

The lumbodorsal fascia is divided, establishing access to the retroperitoneum. Dissecting along the undersurface of the fascia posterolaterally, the surgeon will encounter the quadratus lumborum and, more medially, the psoas muscles. During this dissection the lumbar portion of the iliohypogastric nerve may be visualized inferiorly and should be retracted with the lower portion of the incision. Note that the 11th and 12th intercostal bundles are not isolated or transected.

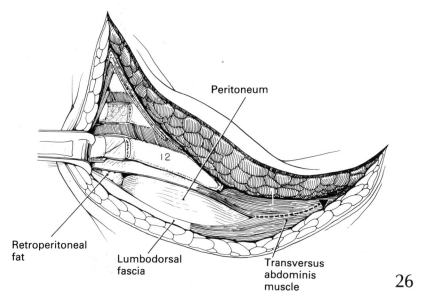

Peritoneum

Retroperitoneal fat

Lumbodorsal fascia

Transversus abdominis muscle

26

The final step to achieve osteoplastic mobility is division of the costovertebral ligament extending from the transverse vertebral process to the inferior aspect of the 12th rib (as in *Illustration 22*). This ligament should be divided 1 cm from the rib, allowing the diaphragm, ribs and overlying muscles to rotate up as a flap. Care must be taken to avoid the 12th intercostal bundle as it courses beneath this ligament. After dividing the ligament, each end should be tagged with a suture to facilitate later reapproximation.

27

After the placement of Deaver retractors, the peritoneal cavity is displaced medially and the retroperitoneum is well visualized. Elevation of the flap by the retractors tends to rotate the kidney and adrenal anteriorly, exposing the suprarenal area under the liver.

To close this incision, the costovertebral ligament must be realigned with permanent figure-of-eight sutures. This automatically restores the anatomical position of the chest wall flap.

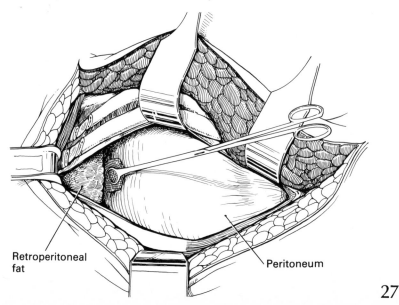

Retroperitoneal fat

Peritoneum

27

The posterior approach to the kidney

The advantage of the posterior approach is direct access to the kidney and renal pelvis without transecting major muscle groups. Although unfamiliar to surgeons in the United States, this retroperitonal approach has been employed in Europe extensively for pyeloplasty and pyelolithotomy as well as for renal biopsy[8]. Postoperative pain is diminished, since only aponeurotic attachments are divided, and the incidence of postoperative hernia or muscle denervation is minimal.

As recently described, the posterior approach is especially good for bilateral nephrectomies prior to transplantation when there have been previous transabdominal operations[9, 10].

For this bilateral approach the patient should be placed prone with mild flexion of the table, and with sandbags beneath the sternum and symphysis to allow full abdominal excursion. Thus two surgical teams can proceed simultaneously.

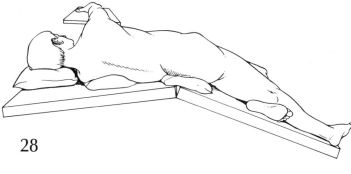

28

28

For a unilateral procedure, the patient is placed in a modified lumbar position with flexion and leg positioning as described above.

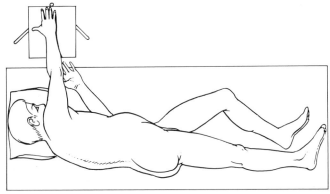

29

29

A slight anterior rotation of the torso is achieved by extending the ipsilateral arm over a padded Mayo stand with secure taping of the pelvis in a similar anterior rotation.

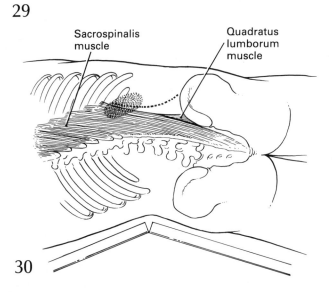

Sacrospinalis muscle

Quadratus lumborum muscle

30

30

The incision is made along the lateral edge of the sacrospinalis muscle, coursing from the inferior aspect of the 12th rib to the posterior superior iliac spine.

31

The subcutaneous fat is divided down to the aponeurosis of the latissimus dorsi. This well developed fascial layer is actually fused with the posterior layer of the lumbar fascia which is continuous with the aponeurosis of the transversus abdominis (see *Illustration 32*).

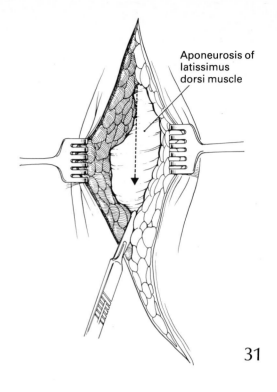

31

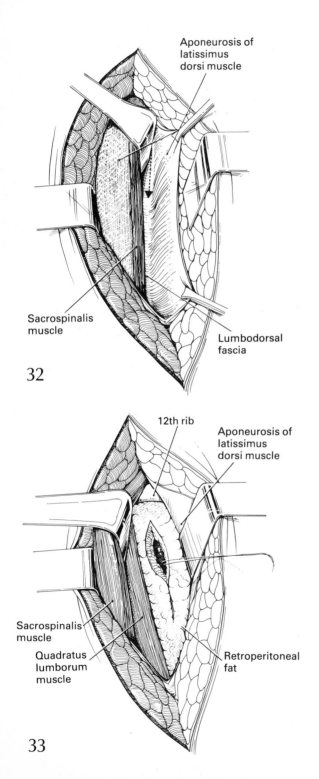

32

33

32

The latissimus aponeurosis is incised lateral to the sacrospinalis, which usually bulges through the incision. Superiorly, fibres of the latissimus dorsi and posterior serratus inferior may need to be divided since the aponeurosis is narrower in this area. This incision allows the sacrospinalis to be retracted medially and exposes the more anterior layer of the lumbar fascia which ensheaths the quadratus lumborum. Small bridging vessels should be cauterized. After elevating the lateral fascial edge, the slightly thinner anterior lumbar fascia (arrowed) should be incised lateral to the quadratus and 1–3 cm lateral to the tips of the vertebral transverse processes which can be easily palpated. During this incision, care must be taken to identify the lumbar portion of the iliohypogastric nerve which often crosses this area parallel to the 12th rib and deep to the anterior lumbar fascia.

33

After the quadratus lumborum is retracted medially and the iliohypogastric nerve retracted inferiorly, a self-retaining retractor may be placed in position. Gerota's fascia should be sharply incised in a vertical direction posteriorly near the quadratus to reveal the renal pelvis. Stay sutures should be placed in the renal pelvis prior to pyelotomy. The surgeon should remember that if he desires to locate the proximal ureter, his dissection should head medially along the psoas rather than into the perinephric fat. A sponge stick can be used at the superior aspect of the incision to elevate the lower pole of the kidney and place the ureter under slight stretch.

34

To provide more cephalad exposure, the costovertebral ligament between the transverse process and the inferior aspect of the 12th rib can be divided, allowing lateral and superior displacement of the rib itself. This manoeuvre will increase the surgeon's access to the upper pole. However, the 12th intercostal bundle which lies underneath this ligament must be avoided. Rarely the pleura may extend into this area. Note the use of a sponge stick to protect underlying structures.

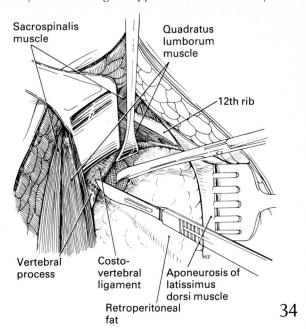

34

35

In summary, the posterior approach offers direct access to the posterior renal pelvis and proximal ureter. Appreciation of the anterior and posterior layers of the lumbar fascia aids the surgeon during his dissection. Occasionally, an areolar layer of the anterior lumbar fascia inserting anterior to the quadratus can be visualized.

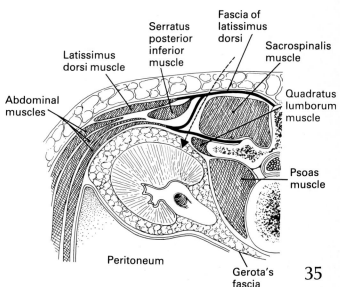

35

Acknowledgement

We should like to thank Dr George Nagamatsu who discussed with us the origins, executions and modifications of the dorsolumbar incision.

References

1. Lytton, B. Surgery of the kidney. In: Harrison, H. J., Gilles, R. F., Perlmutter, A. D., Stamey, P A., Walsh, P. C. Campbell's Urology, 4th ed., Vol. 3. Philadelphia: W. B. Saunders, 1979: 1993–2043

2. Roen, P. (ed.) Atlas of urologic surgery. New York: Appleton Century Crofts, 1967

3. Uson, A., Lattimer, J. Surgery of the kidney. In: Cooper, P., ed. The craft of surgery 2nd ed. Little Brown and Co., 1971: 1467–1495

4. Connor, W. T., van Buren, C. T., Floyd, M., Kahan, B. D. Anterior extraperitoneal donor nephrectomy. Journal of Urology 1981; 126: 443–447

5. Lyon, R. An anterior extraperitoneal incision for kidney surgery. Journal of Urology 1958; 79: 383–392

6. Tessler, A. N., Yavienco, F., Farcon, E. Paramedian extraperitoneal incision for total nephroureterectomy. Urology 1975; 5: 397–398

7. Nagamatsu, G. Dorso-lumbar approach to the kidney and adrenal with osteoplastic flaps. Journal of Urology 1950; 63: 569–577

8. Bensimon, H. Muscle protective incisions in renal surgery. Urology 1974; 4: 476

9. Bredael, J. J., Carson, C. C., Weineth, J. L. Bilateral nephrectomy by the posterior approach. European Urology 1980; 6: 251–254

10. Novick, A. Posterior surgical approach to the kidney and ureter. Journal of Urology 1980; 124: 192–195

Nephrostomy

W. Scott McDougal MD
Professor and Chairman, Department of Urology,
Vanderbilt University Medical Center, Nashville, Tennessee, USA

Introduction

Percutaneous nephrostomy performed under radiological control and internal ureteral stenting with the double J catheter have markedly reduced the frequency with which open nephrostomy must be performed. The latter provides an internal drainage route and is generally preferred when technically possible over nephrostomies which require an external appliance. There are situations, however, in which open nephrostomy is indicated, either as an adjunctive or as a primary procedure. Such circumstances might include drainage of the pelvis following ureteral pelvic junction repair, following renal stone surgery in which fragments cannot be completely removed, during exploration for trauma when associated duodenal, pancreatic or great vessel injuries occur concomitantly with significant ureteral or pelvic disruptions, following partial nephrectomy and following drainage of perinephric and intranephric abscesses. It may also be used as a primary procedure in rare circumstances where drainage of the kidney cannot be conveniently established by internal means.

There are two types of nephrostomy: single tube and loop nephrostomy. The latter has the advantage of two ports – an irrigation and drainage port. This is particularly useful for continuous irrigation for retained calculi.

Complications

Complications of the procedure include haemorrhage from the nephrotomy site, injury to the renal and/or great vessels, disruption of the ureteral-pelvic junction, calculus formation, pyelonephritis, perinephric abscess, sepsis, and duodenal, splenic and pancreatic injury.

The operations

Position of patient

The patient is placed in the lateral decubitus position with the table flexed as for a standard flank approach to the kidney.

SINGLE TUBE NEPHROSTOMY

The kidney is exposed and a small transverse pyelotomy made in the renal pelvis. The nephrostomy should be placed in the lower pole calyx and exit directly, in a straight line to the skin.

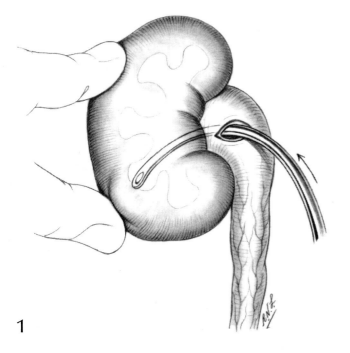

1

A transverse pyelotomy is made and a curved Randall stone forceps is gently passed into the inferior pole calyx.

1

2

A small incision is made in the parenchyma immediately over the stone forceps and it is pushed through the incision. A suture is looped through the Randall stone forceps and tied to a 16 Fr or 18 Fr Foley, Malecot or de Pezzer catheter. The catheter should be larger in size than the nephrotomy site in order to provide parenchymal tamponade.

The catheter is pulled into the renal pelvis, the loop suture cut and removed, and the balloon inflated if a Foley is used. If a Malecot or de Pezzer catheter is used, flanges must be maintained on stretch as they penetrate the renal parenchyma. The disadvantage of the latter catheters is that they cause considerable trauma upon their removal in the postoperative period.

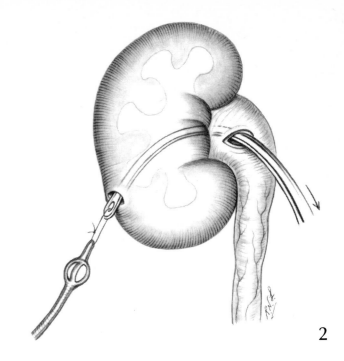

2

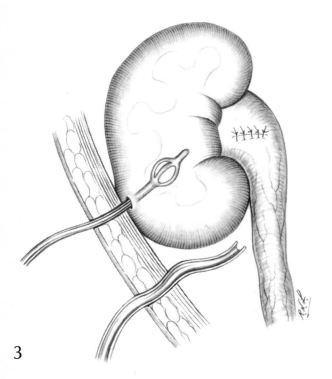

3

3

The pyelotomy is closed, the area drained, Gerota's fascia reapproximated and the nephrostomy tube brought out in a straight line to the skin.

The nephrostomy tube should be situated, if possible, in the anterior aspect of the flank so that the patient can change the catheter with some ease if necessary. The tube should also be secured to the skin with a non-resorbable suture. It should not be brought out through the incision, but rather through a separate stab wound. A straight course into the pelvis facilitates replacement of the catheter.

LOOP NEPHROSTOMY

4

In this instance the catheter is passed through the lower pole calyx and brought out through the pyelotomy incision. Randall stone forceps locate the midpole or upper pole calyx and a nephrotomy is performed immediately overlying the forceps. A suture is drawn back into the renal pelvis and tied to the end of the catheter issuing from the pyelotomy. By gentle traction on the suture the catheter is drawn into the pelvis and out of the middle pole calyx. It is important to note that multiple holes placed in the catheter must be positioned so that they lie within the confines of the renal pelvis. Perinephric extravasation of urine can occur when the holes in the side walls are dislodged and position themselves outside the pelvis.

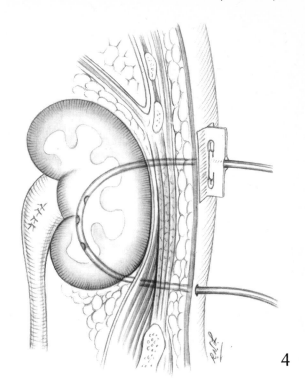

4

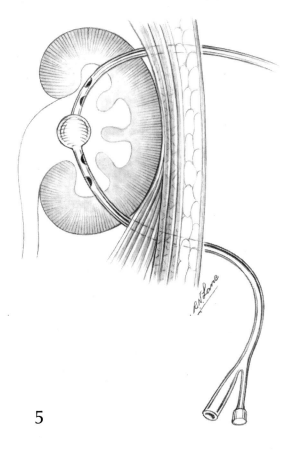

5

5

A loop nephrostomy tube with a balloon in the middle prevents inadvertent dislodgement of the catheter holes outside the confines of the renal pelvis. Some advocate suturing the kidney in a fixed position to the lateral flank side wall so that this distance is constantly maintained.

Penrose drains are placed in the base of the wound and the wound is closed in a standard manner.

Further reading

Brantley, R. G., Shirley, S. W. U-tube nephrostomy: an aid in the postoperative removal of retained stones. Journal of Urology 1974; 111: 7–8

Finney, R. P., Sharpe, J. R. Self-retaining loop nephrostomy. Journal of Urology 1977; 117: 638–640

Gillenwater, J. Y. Loop nephrostomy with the Cummings catheter. Journal of Urology 1977; 117: 641–642

Perinetti, E., Catalona, W. J., Manley, C. B., Geise, G., Fair, W. R. Percutaneous nephrostomy: indications, complications and clinical usefulness. Journal of Urology 1978; 120: 156–158

Illustrations by Robert N. Lane

Renal cysts

W. Scott McDougal MD
Professor and Chairman, Department of Urology,
Vanderbilt University Medical Center, Nashville, Tennessee, USA

Introduction

It is important to differentiate between solid and cystic renal masses, since the former are often cancerous and the latter usually benign. However, it is also necessary to differentiate between benign renal cystic masses and malignant cystic lesions. In the past, techniques for making this differentiation accurately were not available and many of these lesions required exploration and decortication in order to establish a diagnosis. With the advent of ultrasound and computerized axial tomography, the need to explore renal cysts has become increasingly remote. When the ultrasonogram reveals a perfectly round cyst wall, enhancement of the echoes posterior to the cyst and no intracavitary echoes, the cyst is benign and no exploration is necessary.

If these diagnostic criteria are not met, then further studies such as aspiration, with cytological and bio-chemical analysis of the fluid, and angiography are required. If the diagnosis is still in doubt, exploration is indicated to eliminate the possibility of cystic hyper-nephroma. On rare occasions exploration may also be required for benign solitary cysts. Large cysts which cause loin discomfort and which recur after aspiration, and central cysts which cause obstruction of the collecting system, may require open decortication. Complications of the procedure include parenchymal bleeding, urinary fistulae, perinephric abscesses and sepsis.

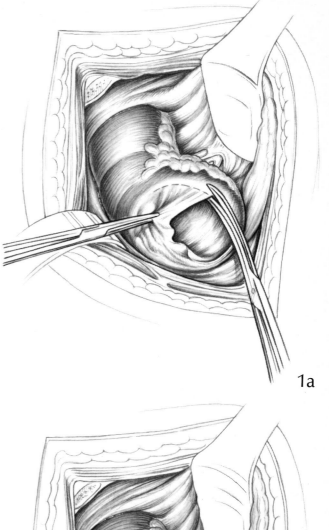

1a

1b

The operation

1a & b

Marsupialization of the cyst is performed as illustrated. The kidney is mobilized and the cyst identified. The cyst fluid is aspirated and sent to pathology for culture as well as cytological examination. The cyst wall is then removed (a) and haemostasis of its margins achieved with running suture of 4/0 chromic catgut (b). The area is drained and the wound closed in the standard manner.

Further reading

Hinman, F. Jr. Obstructive renal cysts. Journal of Urology 1978; 119: 681–683

Lingard, D. A., Lawson, T. L. Accuracy of ultrasound in predicting the nature of renal masses. Journal of Urology 1979; 122: 724–727

Pollack, H. M., Banner, M. P., Arger, P. H., Peters, J., Mulhern, C. B. Jr., Coleman, B. G. The accuracy of gray-scale renal ultrasonography in differentiating cystic neoplasms from benign cysts. Radiology 1982; 143: 741–745

Operative management of renal calculi

J. E. A. Wickham MS, FRCS
Director of the Academic Unit, Institute of Urology, University of London;
Senior Consultant Urological Surgeon, St Bartholomew's Hospital, London;
Consultant Surgeon, St Peter's Hospital Group, London, UK

Preoperative

Indications

Most renal stones with a diameter of less than 0.5 cm do not require operative removal from the kidney and, if mobile, will pass down the ureter spontaneously. Non-mobile stones lodged in a peripheral calyx may remain silently for many years and do not require operative removal, particularly in the older age groups.

Larger individual or multiple stones, including the staghorn or cast calculi, should, in general, be removed by operation. The principle reasons for removing these stones are:

1. to relieve recurrent renal pain – usually associated with the mobile stone;
2. to prevent recurrent urinary tract infection, seen particularly with phosphatic cast calculi;
3. to prevent loss of renal function produced by chronic intermittent calculous obstruction or sustained infection.

Preoperative preparation

Radiography

Intravenous urogram (IVU)   An adequate and recent IVU should be available to show the precise position of the stone or stones and to demonstrate the functional anatomy of the kidney.

Retrograde studies   If an excretion urogram does not demonstrate the intrarenal collecting system and ureter adequately, then retrograde ureteric pyelography should be performed. Most importantly, this is to exclude partial ureteric obstruction by further calculi below the kidney. Removal of renal calculi above an obstructed ureter will result in a persistent urinary fistula.

Plain abdominal X-ray   Immediately before operation this is mandatory with all stones, but particularly with the mobile calculus.

Tests of renal function

With severe bilateral stone disease or in the case of the solitary kidney, it is important to estimate renal functional capability with a 24-hour creatinine clearance test. Serum tests of renal function are inadequate. When severe depression of renal function is found, preoperative dialysis may be required to render the patient fit for surgery. Postoperative dialysis may be required to support the patient in the immediate postoperative period.

Renography

Differential isotope renography is often of value in assessing the comparative contribution of a particular kidney to overall renal function, for example a poorly functioning calculus-containing kidney with a normal contralateral organ might be better treated by nephrectomy than by nephrolithotomy. Conversely, when both kidneys show poor function, a conservative operative approach is indicated to preserve maximum overall function.

Metabolic screen

It is now totally inadequate to remove a renal stone without attempting to determine the aetiological cause of its formation. All stone patients should have:

1. duplicate serum calcium, phosphate, oxalate and protein estimates;

2. duplicate 24 hour urinary estimates of calcium, phosphate and oxalate;
3. serum uric acid;
4. spot test for cystine.

Any metabolic abnormality revealed from the tests should be vigorously treated to reduce stone recurrence rates after surgery to more acceptable levels.

Preoperative urinary culture

This should always be performed to identify any infecting organisms. If present, treatment of the infection should be started 24 hours before the operation with an appropriate antibiotic, usually ampicillin or gentamicin. This is particularly important for the avoidance of Gram-negative septicaemia which may be induced by the operative manipulation of an infected kidney.

Crossmatched blood

Crossmatched blood should always be available for any renal surgery. Two units are usually sufficient.

Hydration

Preoperative hydration of the patient is useful in maintaining a good urine flow, especially if ischaemic surgery is to be undertaken. One litre of intravenous dextrose saline given in the hour or two before operation is the best method.

Intraoperative radiology

When any renal stone surgery is performed, facilities should be available for taking contact X-ray films during the operation. It is most unwise to embark on this type of surgery without this ancillary aid.

Anaesthesia

General anaesthesia is required with endotracheal intubation and mechanical ventilation. Obese patients, when placed in the renal operative position, quite often become anoxic and hypercapnic with marked fall in blood pressure if not adequately ventilated.

There is no place for hypotensive anaesthesia in this type of surgery.

The operation

Exposure of the kidney using the lumbotomy incision

The kidney may be approached most easily through the classical loin incision, excising the anterior end of the twelfth rib (*see* chapter on 'Nephrolithotomy', pp. 84–93).

Alternatively, the kidney may be exposed, though with slightly more difficulty, through a posterior lumbotomy incision. This route, although requiring more operative care, undoubtedly results in a much smoother postoperative course with minimal morbidity.

1

Position of patient for the classical loin incision

The patient is placed on the operating table in the lateral position with the lumbar spine across the break. The upper arm is supported horizontally on a rest. The lower leg is flexed at the hip and knee to 90° and the upper leg is kept straight. Three small 'T'-piece rests are attached to blocks at the side of the table which is then tilted laterally so that the patient leans comfortably back on these rests. The table is broken until the lumbar spine just starts to flex laterally. Excessive lateral flexion can cause severe postoperative back pain in old people with osteoarthritis and should be avoided. It is quite often a good idea to insert a urethral catheter so that the anaesthetist may monitor urinary output during the operation.

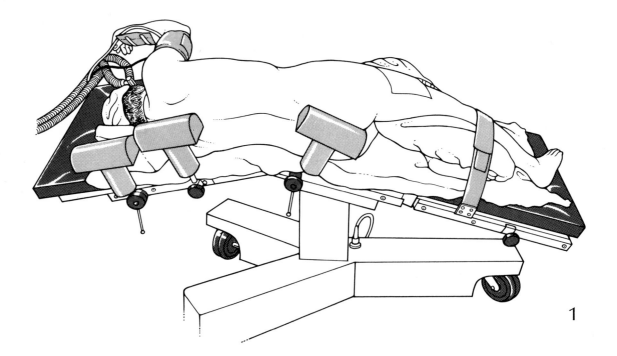

1

2

Position of patient for the lumbotomy incision

Here the patient is placed on the table in the classical prone oblique first-aid position for positioning of the unconscious patient. The lumbar spine is placed over the break and the table broken until spinal flexion just commences. The patient may be stabilized with the 'T' pieces or a length of 7.5 cm Elastoplast across the pelvis and buttocks.

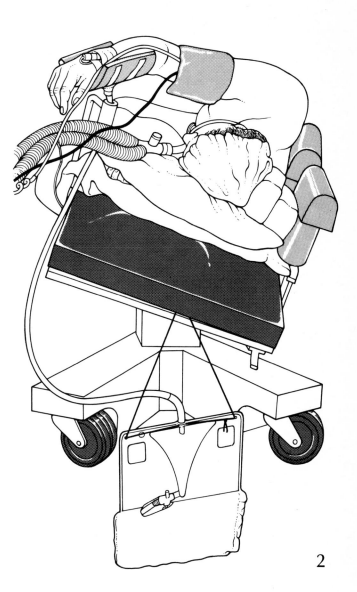

2

3

The skin incision is made vertically parallel and 2.5 cm lateral to the erector spinae muscle mass. It extends downwards and forwards for approximately 8 cm from the level of the twelfth rib almost to the iliac crest. The incision may be angled forward to parallel Langer's lines rather than the classical vertical lumbotomy which tends to lead to scar formation at the lower end on closure. The underlying subcutaneous fat is incised in the line of the incision to expose the fibres of the latissimus dorsi muscle. This muscle is incised in the line of its fibres to expose the underlying lumbar fascia and the twelfth rib covered by a small portion of serratus posterior.

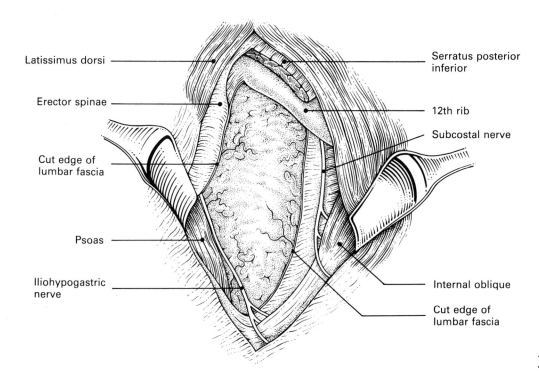

Latissimus dorsi

Erector spinae

Cut edge of
lumbar fascia

Psoas

Iliohypogastric
nerve

Serratus posterior
inferior

12th rib

Subcostal nerve

Internal oblique

Cut edge of
lumbar fascia

3

4

A 2.5 cm segment of the posterior end of the twelfth rib is removed with bone shears and the lumbar fascia arising from the lower border of the rib is divided in the line of the incision to expose the underlying perirenal fat. Care should be taken to preserve the subcostal nerve at the upper anterior end of the incision and the iliohypogastric nerve running just beneath the lumbar fascia posteriorly. The perirenal fat and fascia are then incised in the line of the incision to expose the kidney. The kidney is gently mobilized from the renal fossa and delivered into the wound.

Should greater exposure be desired, the incision may be enlarged upwards by excising a similar 2.5 cm segment from the posterior end of the eleventh or tenth rib if necessary, the pleura being gently mobilized away from the inner surface of the rib. The intercostal nerve should be retracted.

Very little muscle is transected in this incision and the patient can be mobilized early on the first postoperative day and can leave hospital within a week.

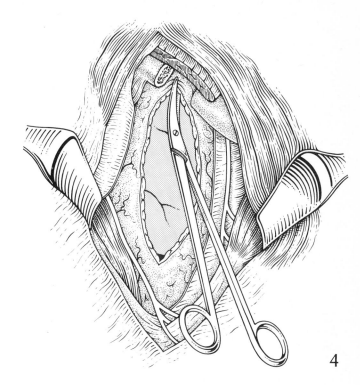

4

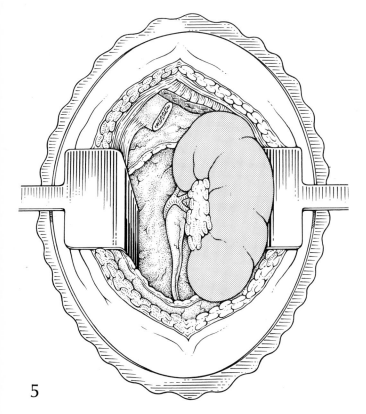

5

5

Retraction

With either the twelfth rib or the lumbotomy incision, exposure of the kidney is considerably facilitated by the use of a self-retaining ring retractor. The author's ring retractor with malleable adjustable blades is most useful (Leibinger, West Germany). A self-retaining twin-bladed retractor of the Finochietto or Pozzi bivalve type is satisfactory.

OPERATIONS AVAILABLE FOR THE REMOVAL OF RENAL STONES

1. Nephrectomy.
2. Pyelolithotomy: (a) simple; (b) extended.
3. Nephrolithotomy with vascular occlusion: (a) with short warm ischaemia or (b) with prolonged ischaemia utilizing hypothermic preservation (see pp. 84–93).
4. Percutaneous nephrolithotomy. It should be mandatory that all stones or stone fragments be removed during the definitive operation. This is particularly true of the infective phosphatic stone when residual fragments containing bacteria will perpetuate infection and lead to recurrent stone formation (see p. 93).

6

Nephrectomy

Nephrectomy is indicated when the renal substance has been so destroyed that significant function is unlikely to return after removal of stones. Obviously it must be established before operation that the contralateral kidney is able to support life.

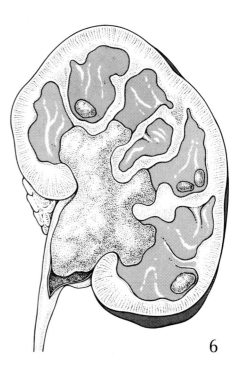

6

Pyelolithotomy

7

Simple pyelolithotomy

When a calculus lies within the renal pelvis the kidney may be rotated forward after exposure and the stone extracted directly through a small posterior vertical incision in the renal pelvis. If the pelvis is intrarenal, the renal substance must be elevated from the pelvis with a small retractor until sufficient exposure has been obtained to permit incision of the pelvis and removal of the stone. The incision in the pelvis is closed with interrupted 4/0 chromic catgut sutures. The wound is closed with 0 chromic catgut to the muscle layers and 3/0 nylon to the skin. A corrugated drain is placed down to the renal fossa.

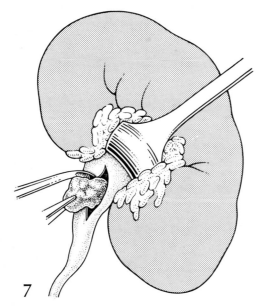

7

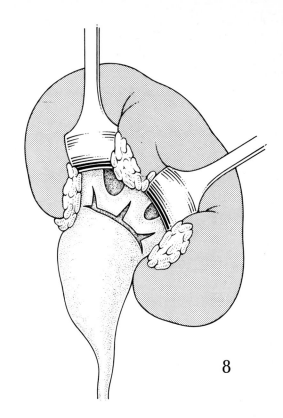

8

8 & 9

Extended pyelolithotomy

When stones lie within the pelvis and also within the major calyces it is often possible, particularly if there is hydronephrotic dilatation of the kidney, to use the technique described by Professor Gil-Vernet (*see* pp. 62–83). Here the relatively avascular plane between the wall of the collecting system and the renal parenchyma is exploited. By blunt dissection the parenchyma is gradually elevated from the pelvis and calyceal necks with small sinus retractors until both can be exposed sufficiently to permit incision and allow extraction of the contained calculus.

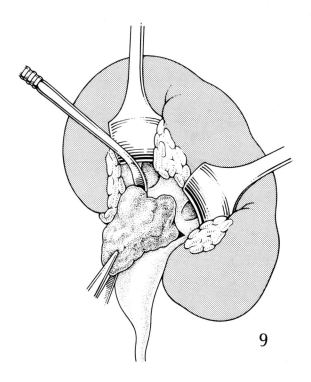

9

Extended pyelolithotomy

Jose Mª. Gil-Vernet
Department of Urology, University of Barcelona, Spain

Introduction

Surgery of renal lithiasis has improved in the past 20 years as a result of the following advances: (1) the discovery of an approach to the renal sinus leading to the development of intrasinusal surgery which allows the surgeon to remove calculi through the excretory tracts without damage to the renal parenchyma or its vessels; (2) the replacement of longitudinal pyelotomy by transverse pyelotomy* which is anatomically and physiologically more sound; (3) hypothermia, which allows prolonged operation without loss of renal function; (4) extracorporeal surgery and autotransplantation in special circumstances when conventional and conservative surgery are impossible; and (5) intraoperative X-ray, which produces a three-dimensional view of the kidney, thereby accurately locating a calculus in the renal space and reducing the likelihood of retained calculi.

* The term transverse pyelotomy is used in this chapter to mean that the incision is made perpendicular to the plane of the junction of the ureter and pelvis as shown in *Illustration 21*.

Principles

Experience has shown that all pyelotomies that extend to the parenchyma (Marion, Papin, Prather type), and particularly those in which an extensive nephrotomy is performed, jeopardize the vascular structures of the kidney and can result in a reduction in renal function. Surgery should be conservative and atraumatic[2,3]. Loss of any part of the parenchyma must be avoided and extraction of the calculi must be total. An effort must be made to avoid a nephrotomy, but if nephrotomy is unavoidable, it should be radial and minimal in extent. The guidelines for pyelotomy are as follows:

1. Preoperative radiographic exploration must be thorough and exhaustive, particularly with staghorn calculi.
2. The preferable surgical approach to the kidney is posterior vertical lumbotomy for simple lithiasis and the posterior lateral approach for complex lithiasis.
3. The renal sinus should be approached extracapsularly.
4. A transverse pyelotomy, intrasinusal enlarged pyelotomy or infundibulotomy is preferred.
5. The removal of staghorn calculi should be atraumatic.
6. Three-dimensional intraoperative X-ray control for the localization of residual calculi must be available.
7. A complementary minimal radial nephrotomy is employed only when pyelotomy fails to provide access to the calculus.
8. An axial nephrostomy is employed rarely.
9. Renal hypothermia in situ is used in exceptional cases when prolonged vascular compromise is necessary.
10. Extracorporeal renal surgery should be performed when relapsing lithiasis is associated with an obstructive lesion of the excretory tract not properly addressed by conventional surgery.

Indications

We perform pyelolithotomy for most forms of lithiasis and for all staghorn calculi. The absence of contrast elimination in an intravenous pyelogram, even in the most delayed films, must not be interpreted as an indication of irrecoverable renal function, nor must the preoperative confirmation of pyonephrosis mean that conservative surgery should be abandoned.

Pyelolithotomy is often required in patients with renal insufficiency when there are no contraindications. In non-obstructive cases of lithiasis we operate because the infection cannot be eradicated unless all calculi are removed. However, a urinary infection is very difficult to cure if the patient has advanced renal insufficiency, even if his urinary tracts are normal. If the renal insufficiency is terminal and irreversible, the patient can be a candidate for chronic dialysis or renal transplanation after all foci of infection have been removed.

Approach to the kidney

The kidney can be approached in two ways:

1. Posterior approach – lumbar or costolumbar and extraperitoneal. This is the approach most frequently used.
2. Anterior (abdominal or transthoracic) approach – paraperitoneal, transperitoneal or mixed. The anterior abdominal approach is less frequently used than the posterior approach; the transthoracic approach is rarely employed.

Preoperative radiographic exploration

The preoperative radiological study of the calculus includes a series of simple radiographic plates taken in the following planes: anteroposterior; obliques from different angles, to provide a profile of the calyces; and tomographs. The number and orientation on different planes of all the branches of the staghorn calculus and its possible articular surfaces can be studied from these plates as can the number and location of accessory calculi. Radiographic exploration is important not only to avoid leaving behind a fragment or free calculus, but also for establishing the force lines of the calculus, its branches, and the axis and direction in which the traction needs to be applied in order to remove the staghorn calculus successfully[4]. An intravenous pyelogram taken in the planes described above will make it possible to see the characteristics of the cavities where the calculi are lodged and the ducts through which they will eventually be removed.

POSTERIOR VERTICAL LUMBOTOMY

Indications

For simple renal and lumbar ureteral lithiasis, the posterior vertical lumbotomy is used routinely. It has no contraindications and can be used in very obese and kyphoscoliotic patients[5]. It is an atraumatic incision; sectioning only aponeurosis and leaving no muscle weakness. It affords excellent exposure of the renal pelvis and ureter with no need to free the kidney. Usually a patient who has had a calculus removed from the intra- or extrarenal pelvis through this incision and an associated transverse pyelotomy is discharged from hospital between the 3rd and 4th postoperative day. Because of the innocuous nature of this approach, we routinely perform a bilateral operation at the same sitting for bilateral lithiasis. The approach is also used for some simple pyelocalyceal calculi, including simple staghorn calculi. It does not present problems for obtaining intraoperative X-rays in the anteroposterior position. This incision is the most anatomical and direct approach to the renal hilum and results in the lowest morbidity. In complex renal lithiasis the preferred incision is posterolateral lumbotomy with resection of the 12th rib near its articulation, with detachment of the pleural cul-de-sac and sectioning of the insertion of the diaphragm. The extreme posterior extent of the lumbotomy is the key to good exposure of the hilar edge of the kidney.

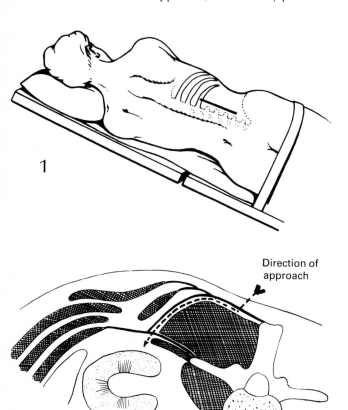

Direction of approach

The operation

1 & 2

The patient is placed in the lateral position without lumbar support and with the knees flexed toward the abdomen to suppress the physiological lordosis. The patient also can be placed in a prone position if there are no ventilation problems. The vertical incision is made in the middle of the mass of the sacrolumbar muscle and extends from the 12th rib to the posterosuperior iliac crest. The latissimus dorsi aponeurosis is sectioned and detached from the posterior surface of the sacrolumbar muscle. Then the external edge and the anterior surface of the muscle are freed until contact is made with the transverse processes. The posterior leaflet of the transversus aponeurosis, which is very thin and resembles mother-of-pearl, is thus exposed. It covers the quadratus lumborum muscle and is often crossed by the iliohypogastric nerve which can be pushed aside.

3, 4 & 5

This transversus aponeurosis is sectioned longitudinally, very close to its insertion on the transverse processes. The incision extends from the iliac crest to the inferior edge of the 12th rib, sectioning Henle's ligament but respecting the 12th intercostal muscle. At this level the superior edge of the transversus aponeurosis is lifted, and the external edge of the quadratus lumborum muscle is exposed and reflected towards the spine. The anterior leaflet of the transversus aponeurosis can now be seen. It is of very poor consistency, hardly perceptible and intimately united to the retrorenal tissues. The retrorenal tissues are seen entering the renal fossa. At this stage a self-retaining retractor with asymmetric branches is placed. Once the sacrolumbar and quadratus lumborum muscles are retracted, the kidney is rotated and its hilar edge presents perpendicular to the surgeon. The fat covering the posterior surface of the kidney is removed. The patient is placed head-down position and the kidney descends a few centimetres.

The operative field can be enlarged by removing, segment by segment, a few centimetres of the 12th rib. This facilitates the introduction of the contact plate for intraoperative X-rays. Closure is performed in two layers (transversus muscle aponeurosis and latissimus dorsi). Drains are placed prior to closure.

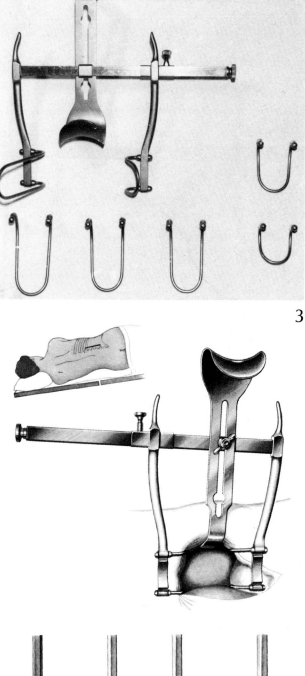

3

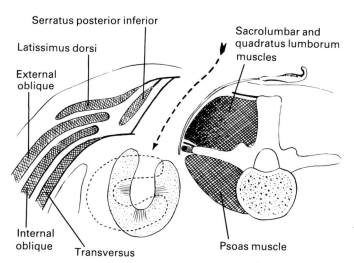

Serratus posterior inferior

Latissimus dorsi

External oblique

Sacrolumbar and quadratus lumborum muscles

Internal oblique

Transversus

Psoas muscle

5

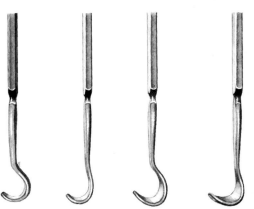

4

EXTRACAPSULAR APPROACH TO THE RENAL SINUS

Anatomical and surgical considerations

6a & b

In 1866 the term 'sinus renalis' was introduced by Henle, who described it as a rectangular cavity situated within the kidney, limited by two surfaces, anterior and posterior. Its external edge borders on the medulla in the parenchyma and its internal edge borders on the hilus. This sinus has a superior and an inferior extension, each containing one of the great calyces which are lined by the internal sheet of the fibrous capsule of the kidney. Although they may vary greatly, the average dimensions of the sinus are 5 cm vertically, 3 cm from the outside to the inside, and 2 cm from back to front. The sinus is an anatomically closed space, i.e. it is isolated from the retroperitoneal space.

The morphological characteristics of the internal or hilar renal edge (the hilar recess) are of great surgical importance. The hilus is usually in the shape of a vertically elongated oval fissure with an average height of 3.5 cm and an average width of 2.5 cm, but the shape and dimensions may vary among individuals. Very small, punctiform hili 1.5 cm in height and 1.2 cm in width can be observed in the malformed and anomalous kidney. Large hili 7 cm in height and 2.5 cm in width can be seen in elongated kidneys. The renal hilus is limited by two lips, one anterior and retracted and the other posterior and protruded. These join in the higher part to constitute the superior commissure and in the lower part to form the inferior commissure. The more recessed the sinus and the more open the hilus, the easier intrasinusal surgery will be.

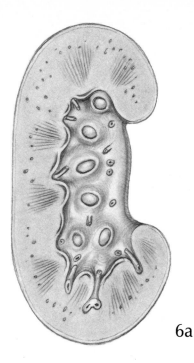

6a

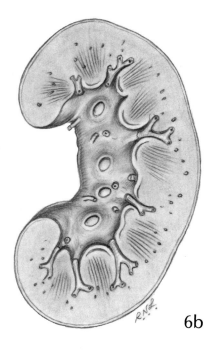

6b

7

The sinus is occupied by the intrarenal portion of the pelvis, the calyces, vessels, lymphatics and nerves. The space between the vessels, lymphatics and nerves and the pelvis and calyces is filled by fatty tissue which allows expansion and contraction of the calyces and pelvis within the sinus cavity. The sinus is elastic, allowing a significant amount of distension of the calyces, pelvis, and vessels by various pathological processes.

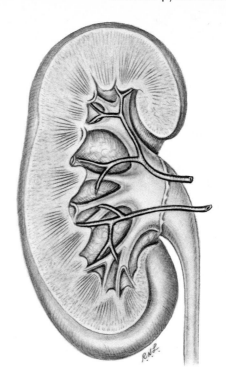

7

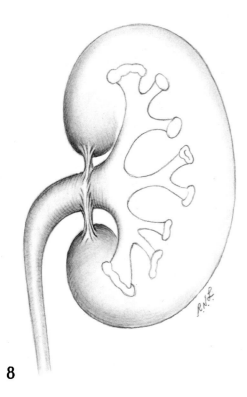

8

8

In 1981 Dise showed that at the hilus the fibrous capsule of the kidney sends out a bundle of dense fibres that surround and adhere to the extrarenal part of the pelvis, forming a capsular diaphragm. This closes the entrance to the sinus, isolating it from the retroperitoneal space and making it difficult to inspect.

9

The diaphragm can be cleared by blunt dissection without damaging any hilar or parenchymatous structures, even in cases with a strong sclerolipomatous inflammatory reaction. The surgeon can then penetrate the intrasinusal space and totally explore it without damaging the vessels, because the internal sheet of the fibrous capsule and the intrasinusal fatty tissue prevent close adherence between the parenchyma and the excretory ducts.

A knowledge of the anatomy of the retropyelic artery is useful when freeing the pelvis to avoid damage and for proper placement of the retractors to avoid prolonged compression. The retropyelic artery, which is usually not seen, branches off the main renal artery adjacent to the superior edge of the pelvis where it crosses behind it, sometimes on its extrahilar part and sometimes on its intrasinusal part. In the first case, when the artery passes slightly outside the posterior edge of the hilus, it is easily identified by palpation when freeing the pelvis. If the artery is covered by inflammatory tissue and the pelvis is the totally extrahilar type, there is a remote possibility of damaging the artery if the peripyelic shell is excessively resected, particularly at the level of the superior commissure. However, it is never necessary to enter the sinus space in cases with the extrahilar type of pelvis.

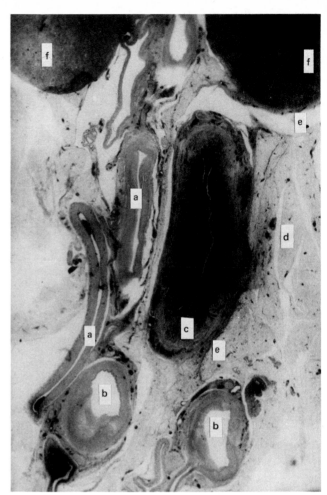

Microphotography of a sagittal cut at the hilus level: (a) veins; (b) arteries; (c) pelvis; (d) fatty tissue; (e) capsular diaphragm enclosing the pelvis; (f) renal parenchyma

9

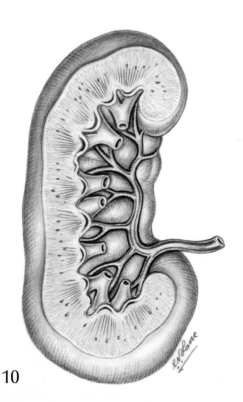

10

10

More commonly, the retropyelic artery runs through the interior of the renal sinus at a small or great distance (as illustrated) from the posterior edge of the hilus, and there is no danger of sectioning it. The extracapsular surgical approach to the renal sinus avoids the retropyelic artery, and therefore there is no possibility of damaging this artery or its branches.

Since 1960 we have performed more than 6000 intrasinusal pyelotomies, and only once did we section the retropyelic artery. A microsurgical anastomosis was performed at the sectioned ends and the operation for lithiasis was continued.

Operative technique

11

NORMAL SINUS

Approaching a normal sinus poses few problems. The pyeloureteral junction is identified and the peripyelic fat retracted toward the kidney using blunt-ended, curved scissors. The pelvic adventitia is separated from the peripyelic fat by blunt dissection. The scissors must be kept in close contact with the adventitia. When passing underneath the capsular diaphragm, the scissors are opened deliberately, breaking the circular diaphragm. One is now at the entrance to the sinus. A retractor is placed, encompassing the whole mass of peripyelic fat, the internal lip of the posterior edge of the kidney, and the retropyelic vessels. These tissues are retracted upwards without danger of tearing the parenchyma, which is protected by the capsule and the peripyelic fat. An open wet gauze is introduced until the sinus is totally filled; the gauze is removed and a second retractor of the same size or smaller is positioned. With both retractors, the posterior half of the kidney is firmly lifted, which makes the organ tilt, making visible the whole pelvis and the major calyces on its posterior surface. Performed correctly, this manoeuvre is completely bloodless.

THE PATHOLOGICAL SINUS

Easy exposure of the pelvis is not possible in pyelolithiasis, particularly with staghorns, because of the great amount of inflammation lithiasis causes around the kidney. The chronic inflammatory reaction of the perirenal fat is particularly intense at the hilus. The fat increases in density and quantity, forming a dense shell of sclerolipo-matous tissue (peripyelitis). It occurs equally on the anterior and posterior surfaces, and thus blocks the entrance to the hilus and to the sinus. Nevertheless, according to our observations, hilar perinephritis modifies the sinus fat very little.

12 & 13

The preferred procedure involves identifying the most superior and free part of the ureter and performing a retrograde dissection with blunt-ended scissors, detaching the sclerolipomatous tissue from the pelvis.

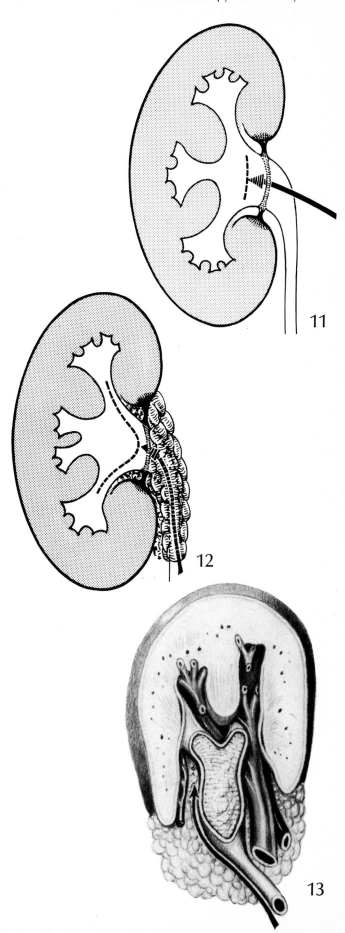

14

The retractor lifts the posterior edge of the hilus protected by the peripyelic fat and exposes the intrasinusal part of the pelvis and calyces. The arrow indicates the position in which the pelvis will be incised.

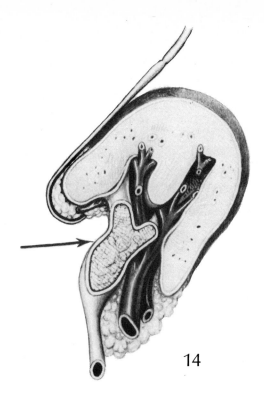

14

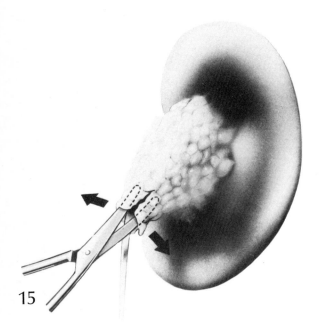

15

15

The fatty peripelvic tissue is dissected from the pelvis using scissor dissection. Spreading the scissors establishes the line of dissection.

16

The peripelvic fat is cut.

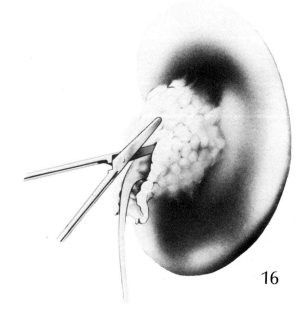

16

17

The scissors again are placed in the plane between the pelvis and fat and spread open, thus completely freeing the pelvis from surrounding fatty tissue.

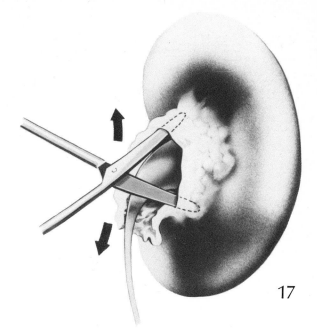

17

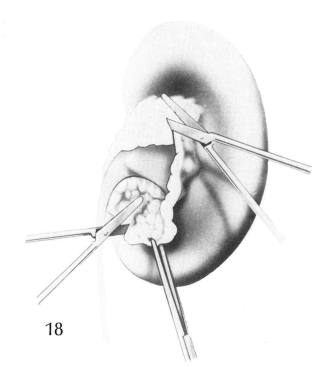

18

18

We advise freeing the posterior surface of the pelvis from the sclerosed shell that wraps it. This will create a better operating field and enhances free pyeloureteral peristalsis.

19

When resecting sclerosed tissue, one must stop a few millimeters before the posterior lip of the kidney to avoid sectioning the retropyelic vein and artery. The small strip of tissue also serves as a supporting point for the retractors to lift the renal edge. In general, two small retractors, one on the superior commissure and the other on the inferior commissure, are better than a single large one.

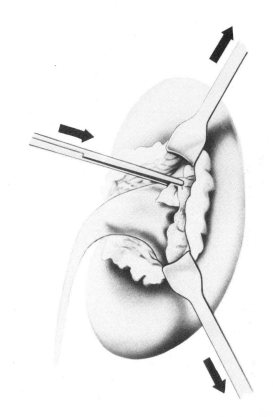

19

ENTERING THE RENAL SINUS

Instruments

20

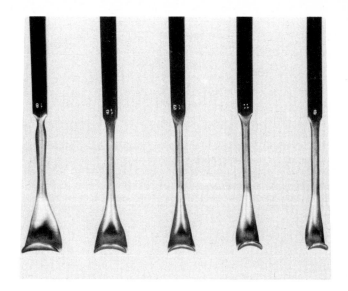

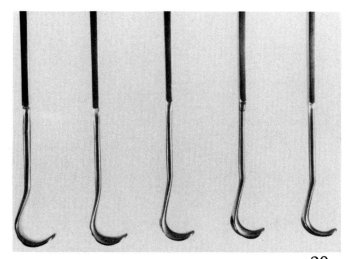

For this type of surgery it is essential, to use renal sinus retractors whose amplitude, curvature and depth conforms to the thickness of the posterior lip of the renal hilus. The edges are blunt, the handle long and rigid.

There are different sizes for the different morphological variants of the hilus for the adult as well as for the child. These retractors keep the kidney fixed and tilted, while simultaneously exposing it, and they also present the hilar edge perpendicular to the surgeon.

For the enlarged pyelotomy two narrow retractors are placed, one on the superior commissure and the other on the inferior. For the simple transverse pyelotomy a single, somewhat wider retractor is used.

If the operation is prolonged, it is advisable to loosen the retractors because they might compress the retropyelic vessels. Compression is manifested by a change in colour of an area on the posterior surface of the kidney. Frequently the retractor causing the compression is the one situated at the superior commissure at the level of the origin of the retropyelic artery. Compression may occur because of too vigorous traction by the assistant or because the rectractor is too small.

20

Transverse pyelotomy

The difficulty of performing a pyelotomy depends on anatomical and pathological considerations.

The shape, dimensions and situation of the pelvis relative to the renal parenchyma and the vessels vary. The small 'intrarenal' pelvis was impossible to approach before the intrasinusal approach was known. Closed or punctiform hili have also been a problem and intense sclerolipomatous reactions secondary to lithiasis increase the difficulties.

We favour transverse pyelotomy because it is the most anatomical and logical approach. The excretory tract consists of a system of spirals that run in different directions along the whole organ. This system of spiralled bundles adopts a different inclination according to the part of the excretory tract and at the superior end of the pelvis the bundles are almost circular.

21 & 22

Since the transverse incision is performed in the same direction as the pelvic musculature it does not alter the pyeloureteral physiology and avoids the danger of tearing towards the ureter. The incision must be performed at the middle part of the pelvis, far from the pyeloureteral junction. This permits one to see the entrance of the calyces and facilitates their exploration under visual or instrumental control.

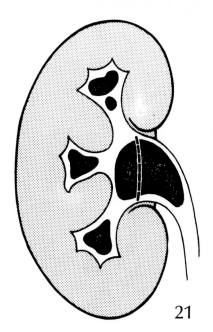

21

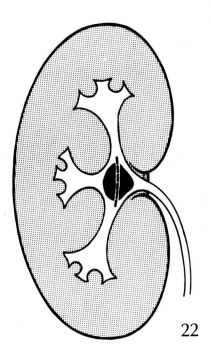

22

23

When the pelvis is of the extrahilar type, the pyelotomy incision must not be performed within the sinus.

Before suturing a pyelotomy it is essential to confirm that the ureter is not obstructed at any point in its entire length. A catheter is passed downwards through the incision checking the calibre of the junction at the same time. When the catheter is in the lumbar region 10–15 ml of normal saline are injected and must pass easily to the bladder.

The incision must be sutured with 6/0 catgut – a larger suture is not recommended. During suturing of a transverse incision there is less chance of tearing than with a longitudinal incision and the pelvic calibre is not decreased. Other advantages of transverse pyelotomy include the lack of stenosis of the pyeloureteral junction, and the shorter period of hospitalization. Experience accumulated during the past 15 years has shown that transverse pyelotomy has few complications, and that it is far superior to vertical pyelotomy.

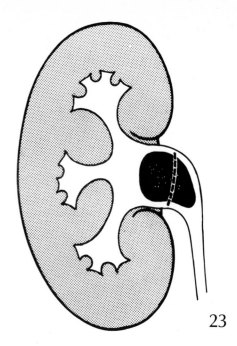

23

Infundibulotomy incision

24

When trying to remove a calyceal calculus of considerable size, we perform a longitudinal incision along the calyceal infundibulum. This infundibulotomy incision does not affect motility of the calyx, because this muscle sheath is longitudinal[2]. It does affect the musculus sphincter calycis and overcomes dysfunction of the calyceal muscle by serving as a sphincterotomy of the pyelocalyceal junction. The longitudinal incision of the calyx must not reach the fornix, because the retrocalyceal veins would then bleed making visibility difficult.

When the renal hilus is closed or very small, the calycotomy is difficult and not always possible. These are very rare cases in adults but more common in children. The calculus must be removed by means of an intrasinusal transverse pyelotomy which allows identification of the calyceal orifice, dilatation and introduction of forceps. A calyceal neck of small calibre is not sutured so that secondary epithelialization from its edges can occur, increasing the calibre and allowing emptying without difficulty.

24

Enlarged intrasinusal pyelotomy

25a, b & c

In staghorn calculi and in some cases of pyelocalyceal lithiasis, the ends of the transverse incision are extended towards the superior and inferior calyces. The incision is therefore longitudinal over the calyces, transverse over the pelvis, and far from the pyeloureteral junction. The final result is a pyeloinfundibulotomy, i.e. an enlarged intrasinusal pyelotomy[6]. This arched incision varies according to the morphology of the pelvis and the staghorn. The convexity of the incision must lie near the pyelic vertex of the calculus to allow it to be freed easily without danger of tearing, but as far as possible from the pyeloureteral junction.

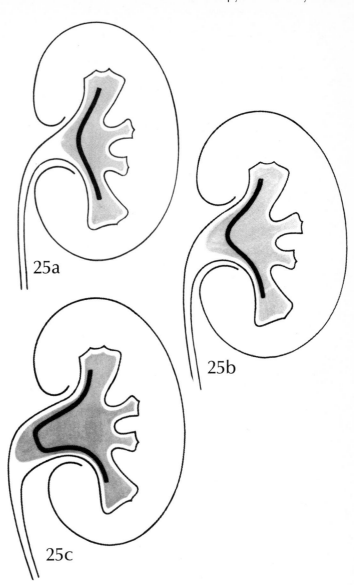

25a

25b

25c

26

The pyelic and infundibular incision is performed within the sinus with a small, fine scalpel and must be perpendicular to the tissues. Deepening of the incision is simple when the tissues are cut over the hard body of the calculus. The edges of the incision must not be clamped or used for placing traction sutures. Very fine atraumatic dissecting forceps are used to manipulate the edges during suturing.

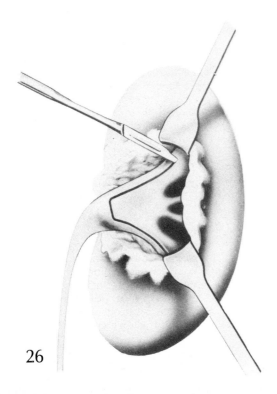

26

Removal of the staghorn

Detailed pre- and intraoperative X-ray studies (anteroposterior and obliques at different angles and projections) are necessary to localize the calculi and to study the lines of force of the calculus, so that traction can be applied in the correct axis and direction. Staghorn calculi *must never be wrenched out*. They must be gently mobilized from their fixation points and then gentle traction must be applied on two or more points to avoid fracture.

Basically, the staghorn always presents as a triangle within a cavity formed by the renal pelvis. The following considerations must be taken into account. First, the pelvic and infundibulocalyceal incision must allow the greatest possible access to the internal branches of the calyces to allow removal of all calculi. Second, damage caused by instruments to the mucosa must be avoided, and it is essential to use blunt instruments and to operate under visual control. The introduction of fingers must be avoided, and in those calyces which are not visible the infundibulum should be gently dilated with forceps. Third, damage to the renal parenchyma must be avoided. This is the key point in intrasinusal surgery.

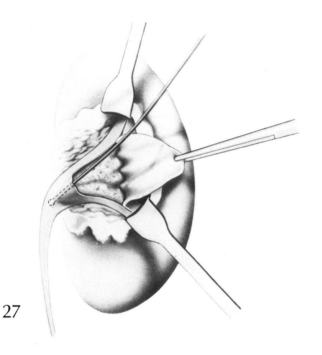

27

27

Once the pyelotomy incision has been enlarged, the apex of the calculus is delivered. This is an easy manoeuvre that must be done with a malleable stiletto, mobilizing the lateral and inferior surfaces of the vertex of the calculus with respect to the incision of the pelvis.

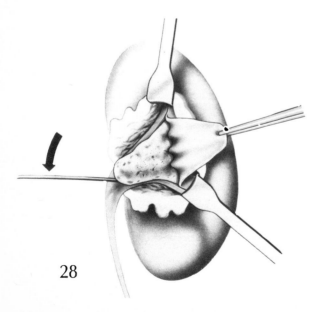

28

28

Delivery of the apex exposes 60–70 per cent of the calculus.

29

Another branch of the calculus is now delivered. This is a very delicate manoeuvre. Using all the data obtained by X-ray studies, one must attempt to remove the branch that seems most mobile and shortest. At this stage it is important always to pull along the 'mobilization axes' of the calculus and to take into consideration the 'free spaces' in the collecting system that allow partial mobilization of the calculus and exteriorization of one of its embedded branches. If the exteriorization of the second branch is particularly difficult, the neck of the calyceal infundibulus, which is the more rigid segment, must be dilated by gently opening very fine, long, curved mosquito forceps. After mobilization and exteriorization of the second branch, the remaining calculus follows easily.

When the above manoeuvres are impossible, it is preferable to break the calculus to avoid damaging the intrarenal excretory tracts of the parenchyma. This must be done carefully; the branch that holds the calculus and is most difficult to remove is broken. Afterwards, the infundibular neck which contains the retained calculus is dilated or incised to facilitate its complete removal.

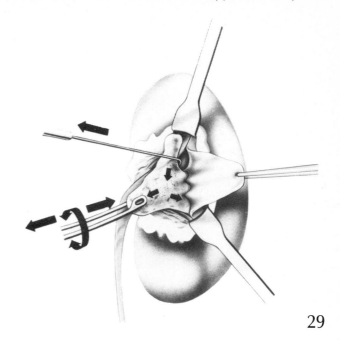

29

Remaining calyceal calculi

After revoval of the body and principal branches of the staghorn, three-dimensional X-rays of the kidney are performed. *Intraoperative X-ray control is absolutely necessary*. If this is not available, it is preferable not to operate because complete removal of the calculus cannot be assured.

30

When the number and location of the remaining calculi have been established, a systematic search by areas is begun. The finger must not be introduced to check and localize a calculus or fragment. Exploration must be done using a malleable stiletto with a small rounded end. This communicates to the hand of the surgeon the sensation of rubbing against a foreign body.

Visual examination is frequently incomplete, particularly in the middle calyceal group. These calyces are difficult to visualize because their infundibulae empty at right angles to the plane of the transverse pyelotomy.

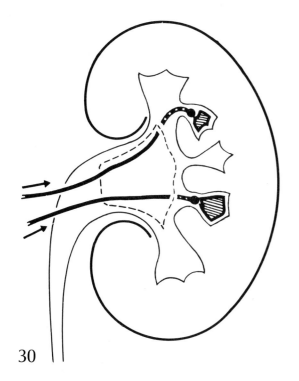

30

31

If the calculus is larger than the infundibulum through which it must be removed, the infundibulum is dilated. This manoeuvre must be performed gently to avoid a discrete haemorrhage that can block vision. If haemorrhage does occur, the calyx is packed while other calculi are sought and removed.

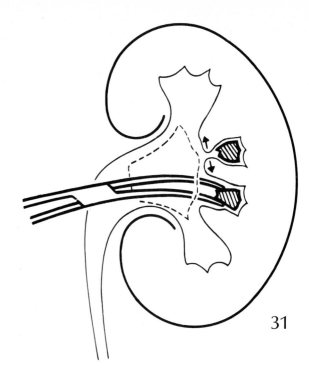

31

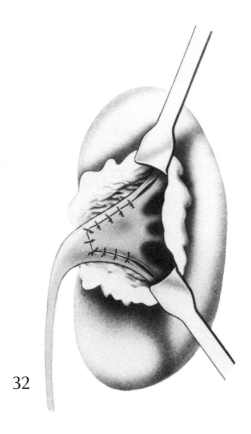

32

32

When total removal has been achieved, the pelvic segment, but not the calyceal segment, is sutured.

33

Once the retractors are removed, the posterior lip of the kidney covers the enlarged pyelotomy.

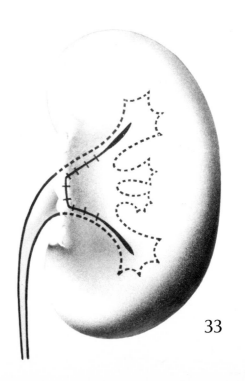

33

Complementary nephrotomies

Our experience has shown that the vast majority of staghorn calculi (75 per cent) can be totally removed through the enlarged intrasinusal pyelotomy. Nevertheless, in some cases (25 per cent) the enlarged pyelotomy must be complemented by one or more *small* nephrotomies when:

1. There is a very large calyceal cavity, full of calculi and with a thin parenchyma.

2. A large calculus is within a calyx with a long and narrow infundibulus.

3. A calculus is located in an ectopic calyx.

Nephrotomy is a complementary measure to the enlarged pyelotomy procedure and is always used as a last resort. Nephrotomies must be minimal, radial, and fall upon the peripheral area of the lithiasic calyx. Because the parenchyma is thinner here, damage to nephrons is minimized and the section of interlobar arteries is avoided. The length of these incisions must be equivalent to the thickness of the calculus to be removed. However, if the calculus is large and the parenchyma not too thin, it is preferable to fragment the calculus, which can be exactly localized by three-dimensional X-rays, so that it can be removed through a small nephrotomy.

If the parenchyma is of normal thickness, prior to each small nephrotomy the renal artery is clamped with a small, very soft, bulldog clamp covered in rubber to avoid damaging the artery. Clamping must not exceed 7–9 minutes – enough time to remove the calculus, explore and wash the calyceal cavity, and suture the nephrotomy. Clamping can be repeated as many times as necessary if the intervals in which circulation is restored are the same as the ischaemic time, providing the kidney does not show signs of vasospasm. To prevent renal damage, a normal blood volume must be maintained and traction on the pedicle must be avoided, particularly when the kidney is exteriorized to obtain X-rays. However, with the contact minichassis now available, it is not necessary to place the kidney on excessive traction.

In those infrequent cases in which there is great arborization of calyces, an intrarenal pelvis or a very closed renal hilus, cases in which there have been reoperations, or when the need for multiple nephrotomies over a thick parenchyma is foreseen, it is advisable to give mannitol or frusemide (furosemide) 30 minutes prior to clamping. The osmotic diuresis possibly has some protective effect upon the kidney against ischaemia. Nevertheless, hypothermia is unquestionably the safest way to preserve the renal function when exceptional circumstances necessitate prolonged renal ischaemia. This occurs in some 3–4 per cent of operations on staghorn calculi.

In complicated lithiasis accompanied by renal insufficiency, there are always cavities where the parenchyma is very thin and in some areas laminar. In these cases the renal artery must not be clamped for two reasons: (1) the nephrotomy bleeds only slightly, and therefore does not interfere with the view of the cavity; and (2) the pyelonephritic kidney is more sensitive to anoxia and tolerates even short periods of ischaemia poorly.

The renal cavities must be washed out with normal saline (37°C). The washing must be atraumatic and must be done in each of the calyces, including the non-lithiasic ones, because mucoprotein matter not detected by X-rays can dwell in them. The pressure used for the wash-outs must be low; otherwise, lesions similar to those obtained with high pressure retrograde ureteropyelography can be produced, and calyceal, lymphatic, venous and interstitial reflux may be caused, leading to acute pyelonephritis. When the renal artery is clamped, with no peripheral resistance, the reflux caused by the wash-out is more harmful to the kidney. At the end of the wash-out a final X-ray must be performed. These small nephrotomies are sutured with 5/0 catgut. A lumbotomy must never be closed without making sure that all calculi have been removed.

Nephrostomy

In general we are against urinary decompression when dealing with renal or ureteric calculi. However, we make an exception to this rule when dealing with certain staghorn calculi.

34

In large, sclerosed, sometimes non-reducible intrarenal cavities that have contained a friable staghorn and mucroprotein matter with persistent infection, especially by *B. proteus*, we perform an axial nephrostomy[7] with a small multiperforated Silastic tube. After the first 5–6 days, when an intravenous pyelogram reveals the absence of leakage from the collecting system, the tube is connected to an antibiotic solution to which the urine culture is sensitive for 2–3 days. The pressure must be no greater than 20 cmH$_2$O. This is very efficient as a local treatment of infection and for washing out bacteria, casts, cellular detritus, fibrin, etc. Frequently, we get a negative urine culture. It would be dangerous and absurd to use the nephrostomy to 'dissolve' residual calculi.

Before closing the lumbotomy, the whole operating field must be washed generously with 3–4 litres of normal saline. This is particularly useful if the urine is infected.

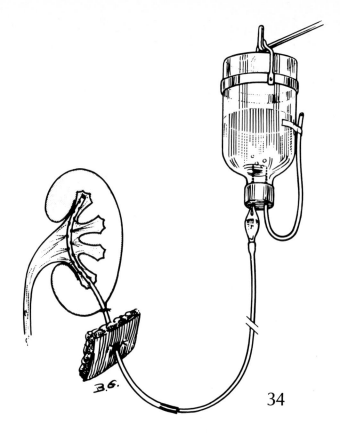

34

Reoperations

Although residual calculi should theoretically not be a problem, they do occur and reoperation is then necessary. The main problems in reoperation involve the surgical approach to the kidney and the pyelotomy.

If the patient has been operated on through a posterovertical lumbotomy, the disposition of the anatomical planes will not vary. On reaching the renal cell, a small area adhering to the deep planes is found corresponding precisely to the place where the renal pelvis is found, the only structure dissected during the first operation. If the patient presents with a classic lumbotomy scar, care must be taken not to damage the kidney, which can be attached to the superficial plane. The old incision can be crossed to reach a retroperitoneal anatomical plane with no scars; from this point previously operated areas can be entered.

If the sinus space was not entered or if the pyelotomy was extrahilar in the first operation, there will be no problem in proceeding extracapsularly to reach the sinus. However, if an intrasinusal pyelolithotomy was performed in the first operation, then it will be very difficult or almost impossible to proceed in the same way because of the firm adhesions formed between the posterior wall of the pelvis and the internal sheet of the kidney's fibrous capsule. The sinus can be reached using a manoeuvre similar to that used in the first operation by entering through the anterior and inferior surfaces of the pelvis in which the detachment plane is unscarred. From there, by dissecting on the pelvis, its posterior surface can be reached. Some resistance is found here, making it necessary to use scissors.

Renal hypothermia in lithiasis

Without doubt, hypothermia is a formidable resource that has made possible the development of extensive renal surgery. Nevertheless in the field of lithiasis, it is indicated only in exceptional circumstances.

There are two basic methods for producing hypothermia in the lithiasic kidney: superficially by external refrigeration; and by internal perfusion. We prefer to use a combination of both methods, initially perfusing the kidney to produce hypothermia, followed by saline irrigation to maintain renal cooling.

35

To avoid damaging the renal artery, we have designed an atraumatic needle, very curved, with a very short bevel and a stop 5 mm from the tip. The mouthpiece is connected to the bottle containing the perfusion fluid.

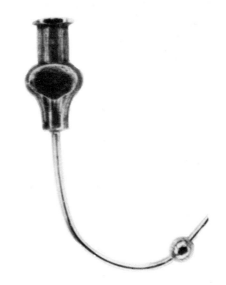

35

36

Once the kidney is freed and its pedicle dissected a clamp covered with foam-rubber is placed at the level of the ureter. The artery is punctured while it is pulsating to avoid perforation or damage to the opposite wall.

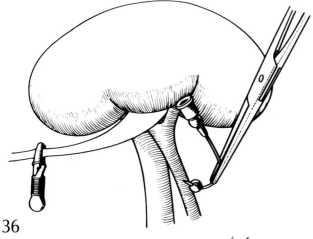

36

37

A soft bulldog clamp is then placed proximal to the needle. A bulldog clamp is placed on the vein and a small venotomy is made on its inferior edge, through which the perfusion fluid will exit.

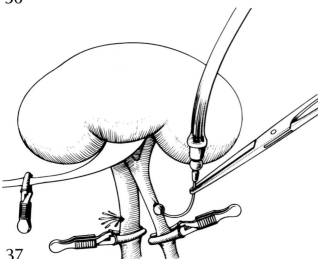

37

38

After 300 ml of Collins' solution at 4°C has been infused, the needle is removed and the venotomy closed. Sometimes it is necessary to place a suture on the orifice of the arterial puncture.

From this point, the renal surface is refrigerated by irrigating it continuously with normal saline at 4°C. This irrigation does not disturb the surgeon, and the cold ischaemia can be maintained for hours with good preservation of renal function and without the danger of thrombosis or red cell sludging. Irrigation also has the advantage that, because the renal parenchyma remains free of blood, its thickness is diminished, facilitating entrance to the sinus cavity and localization of the calculi by palpation. Exceptionally clear intraoperative X-ray images are also ensured.

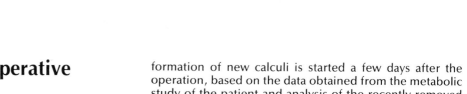
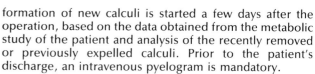

38

Pre-, intra- and postoperative evaluation

The regulation of fluids requires full evaluation of the patient. From a nephrological viewpoint it is necessary to know the patient's blood pressure, urine output for 24 hours, and the following laboratory data: creatinine clearance, plasma electrolytes, blood acid-base balance, and culture/sensitivity of the urine. If the patient is hypertensive, the hypertension treatment is continued until the moment of the operation. If there is a urine infection, we give the appropriate antibiotic, in doses adjusted to the renal function, 2 days prior to the operation and 3 days afterwards. Altered electrolytes and acid-base balance is corrected by conservative means preoperatively if this is possible. If the alterations are severe, such as in advanced renal insufficiency, the patient is prepared by dialysis.

During the immediate postoperative period and while the patient is incapable of adequate intake, solutions are administered intravenously according to the hydration state and the urinary and other losses; we prefer not to use diuretics but adjust the fluid intake, taking care when renal insufficiency in advanced. Urine and exudates from the drains are cultured repeatedly, but after the first 3 postoperative days we do not give antibiotics unless the patient presents signs of systemic infection. Once the urinary catheters have been removed we try to resolve the urinary infection by administering the appropriate antibiotic, although eradication can be difficult if the urinary tracts are not normal or are not free of calculi and/or if renal function is defective. Treatment to prevent the

formation of new calculi is started a few days after the operation, based on the data obtained from the metabolic study of the patient and analysis of the recently removed or previously expelled calculi. Prior to the patient's discharge, an intravenous pyelogram is mandatory.

Complications

The removal of calculi through the excretory tracts does not require the administration of blood or clamping of the renal artery. Operative haemorrhage, if it occurs, is always of minor importance provided it is stopped by gentle manual compression of the kidney for a few minutes. Prolonged urine drainage has occurred in 6 per cent of our staghorn cases. We have not seen permanent fistulae, late haemorrhages, secondary narrowing of the pyeloureteral junction, or hypertension. Infection of the wound and haematomas have occurred with the same frequency as in other lumbotomies, although recently we have seen a significant reduction in infection and serum collection since we have been irrigating the operating field copiously with normal saline. The only important postoperative haemorrhagic complication was noticed in 2 of the cases in which small complementary nephrotomies were necessary.

Intrasinusal surgery has no mortality. After 20 years of experience in intrasinusal surgery we have reached the conclusion that this surgery is the least traumatic of all the recommended operations for the removal of renal calculi. The latest advances in intraoperative X-ray control consolidate and reinforce the efficiency of this method.

References

1. Marshall, V. F. Complete longitudinal nephrolithotomy. Surgical procedures. (Warner-Chilcott), June 1966

2. Gil-Vernet, J. Mª. New surgical concepts in removing renal calculi. Urologia Internationalis 1965; 20:255–288

3. Truc, E., Grasset, D. Lithiase rénale. Encyclopédie méd Chir. 1960; 9:5

4. Gil-Vernet, J. Mª. La cirugiá intrasinusal de los cálculos coraliformes. Rapport XVᵉCong. Soc. Inter. Urologia. Tokio 1970; 1:11

5. Gil-Vernet, J. Mª. La lombotomie verticale posterieure: considerations a propos de 366 cas. Acta Urologica Belgica 1964; 32:391–400

6. Gil-Vernet, J. Mª. Las voies d'abord du bassinet et des calices dans la chirurgie de la lithiase rénale. Progrès de la Medicine, 479 Editions Medicales. Paris: Flammarion

7. Gil-Vernet, J. Mª. Minimum nephrostomy. Urology 1977; 9:620–623

Illustrations by Philip Wilson

Nephrolithotomy

J. E. A. Wickham MS, FRCS
Director of the Academic Unit, Institute of Urology, University of London;
Senior Consultant Urological Surgeon, St Bartholomew's Hospital, London;
Consultant Surgeon, St Peter's Hospital Group, London, UK

Introduction

When peripheral renal stones cannot be removed by extended pyelolithotomy, then incision of the renal parenchyma is required to evacuate stones from the calyces. Incision of the parenchyma is also often required for the extraction of large branched staghorn stones.

PREPARATION FOR NEPHROLITHOTOMY

The vascularity of the kidney is so considerable that even a modest incision of the parenchyma can produce significant haemorrhage. It is therefore strongly advised that prior to nephrolithotomy either the renal artery or, occasionally, the whole renal pedicle be occluded.

Ischaemic nephrolithotomy can be performed in two ways.

With short warm ischaemia

When only one calyceal stone is to be extracted, it is often sufficient to occlude the renal artery, incise the parenchyma radially, extract the calculus and suture the nephrotomy. It is, however, important that the period of renal artery occlusion during this manoeuvre does not exceed 15 minutes or deterioration of renal function will occur.

With prolonged ischaemia

When multiple calculi or a large staghorn calculus require extraction, multiple nephrotomies may be necessary to remove all stones. Here an ischaemic period of up to 2 hours may be required for complete clearance and renal function will necessarily deteriorate unless some form of protective technique is used. The two principal methods of protection are renal hypothermia and the use of inosine.

Hypothermia

Hypothermia may be achieved by various methods. Cold solutions may be injected directly into the renal artery or the kidney may be much more simply cooled by the application of ice or cooling coils to the renal parenchyma.

1

Ice slush cooling   After arterial clamping the renal fossa is packed with a sterile slush ice for about 10 minutes to lower the temperature of the kidney to 5°C. Alternatively the kidney may be surrounded by ice water contained in a plastic bag[1]. When adequate cooling has been achieved, the slush or water is removed and incision of the parenchyma is performed as necessary.

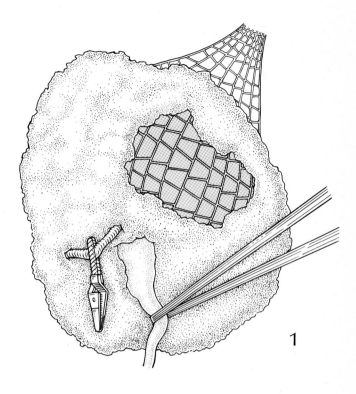

1

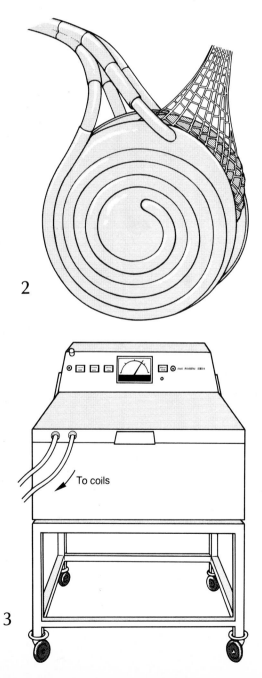

2

3

To coils

2 & 3

Heat exchanger coils with external coolant reservoir   A more sophisticated technique is to surround the kidney after arterial occlusion with two small plastic heat exchanger coils. Coolant solution can be pumped through the coils from an external reservoir until a renal core temperature of 15°C is obtained. The coils are then removed and the parenchyma can be incised as necessary to extract any stones. Cooling initially takes about 8 minutes and reapplication of the coils is simple if further cooling is required after 35–40 minutes.

In both techniques the core temperature of the kidney is measured by an indwelling telethermometer probe.

4 & 5

Inosine

The basic nucleotide inosine has been shown to have protective value in renal ischaemia. Injection of 2.0 g of inosine (Trophicardyl) either directly into the renal artery or into a peripheral renal vein about 5 minutes prior to clamping the renal artery can give up to 1 hour's functional protection, which is usually an adequate period for dealing with a normal staghorn calculus. This method makes a good substitute for regional hypothermia and does not entail any apparatus or the preparation of sterile crushed ice. It is strongly emphasized that the ischaemia time should not exceed 1 hour.

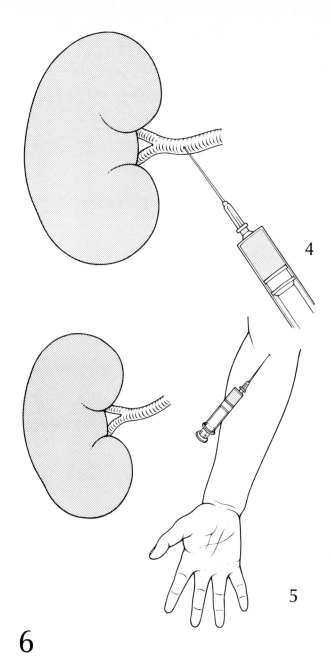

4

5

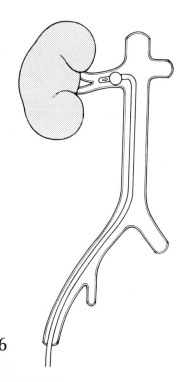

6

6

Intra-arterial perfusion of the kidney using a Schwann Ganz catheter[2]

In this technique a fine balloon catheter is passed by way of the femoral artery through the aorta and into the renal artery of the kidney to be operated on. Once *in situ* the balloon of the catheter is inflated to occlude the renal circulation. Through the second channel distal to the balloon the renal parenchyma can then either be perfused with cold saline or with inosine to achieve functional protection. Once the operative procedure has been completed the catheter is deflated and removed.

This is a very sophisticated technique but does require coordination with the radiologist.

THE OPERATIONS

Exposure of the kidney

The kidney is exposed either through the classical loin incision, excising the anterior end of the twelvth rib, or by the posterior lumbotomy incision (*see* chapter on 'Operative management of renal calculi', pp.54–61).

Mobilization

The kidney is mobilized from the surrounding perinephric fat. Dense fibrous adhesions may require division if the kidney has been infected. To stabilize and hold the organ it is helpful to pass a Netelast bandage sling over the mobilized kidney, using a nylon tape drawstring to fit the Netelast gently, but not too tightly, around the pedicle. The kidney can then be held easily by the assistant without damage to the parenchyma. The renal vessels are exposed together with the pelvis and upper ureter. A thin rubber sling is passed around the renal artery and a second around the ureter. Pelvic calculi or the pelvic portion of a cast calculus is then extracted through a pyelotomy incision.

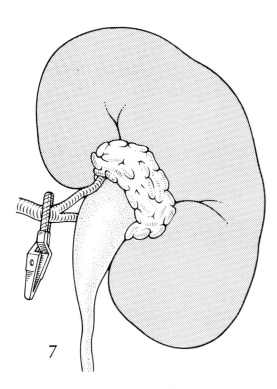

7

7

Occlusion of renal artery

A small bulldog clamp is then placed across the renal artery. Very occasionally, if the vessels are deeply fibrosed, a whole pedicle clamp (not shown) may be applied.

SINGLE NEPHROTOMY FOR SOLITARY CALYCEAL CALCULUS

When only one peripheral stone is to be removed, a short period of warm ischaemia of up to 15 minutes is usually sufficient. Any nephrotomy should be made radially and parallel to the intrarenal vessels.

TECHNIQUES FOR MULTIPLE PERIPHERAL STONES OR THE LARGE STAGHORN CALCULUS

When a number of calyces need exploration and the ischaemia time is necessarily prolonged, some form of renal protection must be utilized, as discussed earlier. The two principal methods of calculus extraction are the Boyce anatrophic procedure and the Wickham multiple nephrotomy technique.

The Boyce anatrophic procedure

8

This technique depends upon the exploitation of the plane between the arterial territories of the anterior posterior branches of the renal artery. The plane is delineated as follows. The kidney is mobilized and the renal artery and main branch arteries exposed. A small bulldog clamp is placed on the posterior branch of the renal artery and 10 ml of methylene blue injected intravenously. The dye circulates to the kidney and stains the anterior portion of the kidney blue, leaving the posterior portion uncoloured. The line of demarcation is clearly marked with coloured ink and then the whole renal artery is clamped and the kidney buried in crushed ice until the core temperature has reached the required level.

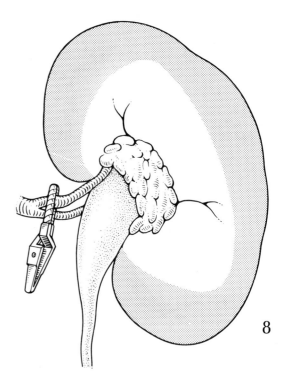

8

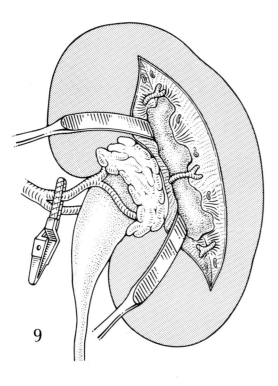

9

9

The convexity of the kidney is then incised down the line of demarcation between the arterial territories, until the collecting system is reached.

10

The pelvic portion of the calculus and the contained calyceal elements can then be removed directly from the collecting system.

The longitudinal nephrotomy is sutured carefully, paying particular attention to ligation of large intrarenal veins.

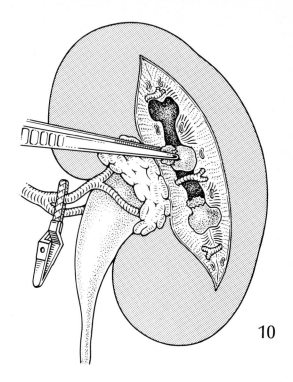

10

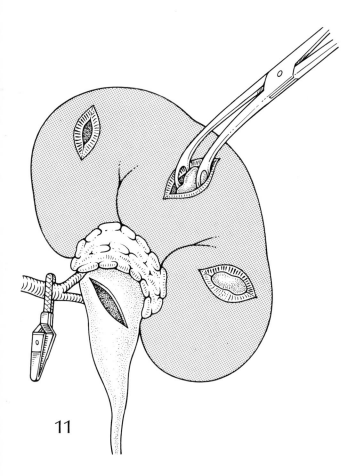

11

Technique of multiple radial nephrotomy (Wickham)

11

Here the pelvic portion of the calculus is removed through a pyelostomy incision and then the renal artery is clamped. Regional hypothermia is induced and when the renal core temperature has reached 15°C multiple radial dissection nephrotomies are made into the parenchyma over the calyces occupied by calculi. Great care is taken during dissection to avoid the small branches of the intralobar arteries passing to the peripheral cortex. These can usually be identified and retracted en route to the calyx. All calculi are removed under direct vision.

12

Irrigation

Pressure irrigation of the collecting system with pre-cooled saline at about 10°C is then carried out. Saline is delivered through a sterile drip extension tube at high pressure by compressing bags of sterile intravenous saline with a Fenwall bag compressor. A malleable antrum cannula attached to the drip tubing forms an ideal irrigating instrument. Alternatively, saline may be pumped at a slightly higher pressure from a mechanical irrigator such as a Lavajet.

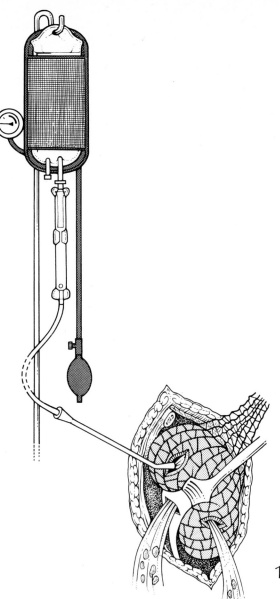

12

13

X-Ray localization

Liga clips are now placed on the Netelast suspensory bandage in a random pattern. A small contact X-ray film is placed behind the kidney and an X-ray exposure made with a portable X-ray machine. A sterilizable metallic cone which can be attached by the surgeon to the X-ray unit is a useful adjunct.

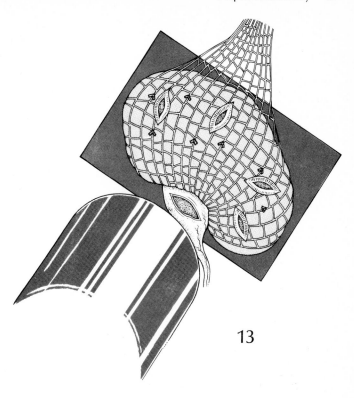

13

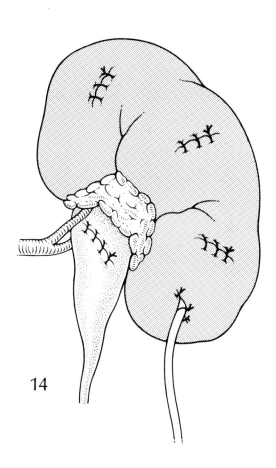

14

14

Closure of nephrotomies

When all the calculus is extracted the nephrotomies are closed by simple suture of the renal capsule, including a 2–3 mm bite of underlying parenchyma. Chromic catgut (4/0) is used. A 10 or 12 Fr nephrostomy tube is inserted through the lower calyx to allow drainage of blood from the intrarenal collecting system for the avoidance of clot colic. The arterial clamp is removed and a corrugated drain is placed down to the renal fossa. The wound is closed in layers, using 0 or 1 chromic catgut with 3/0 monofilament nylon to the skin.

15 & 16

COAGULATION PYELOLITHOTOMY

Occasionally when multiple small fragments of stone lie diffusely within the collecting system, it may be possible to inject a fibrin type of coagulum into the collecting system by way of a needle inserted into the renal pelvis. The coagulum solidifies within the renal collecting system, entrapping the small fragments of calculus, which may then be removed through a single pyelotomy. The coagulum mixture must be pre-prepared in two separate syringes so that coagulation does not occur until the mixture has reached the inside of the renal collecting system. The first syringe has a 25 ml capacity and contains 20 ml of thrombocyte-enriched plasma plus 5 ml of human fibrinogen. The second, 5 ml capacity syringe contains 1 ml of thrombin plus 4 ml of calcium chloride. Both syringes are connected to a small butterfly cannula through a 'Y' piece and the solutions are injected simultaneously. The ureter must be occluded below the renal pelvis. A longitudinal pyelostomy is made and the fibrin coagulum removed.

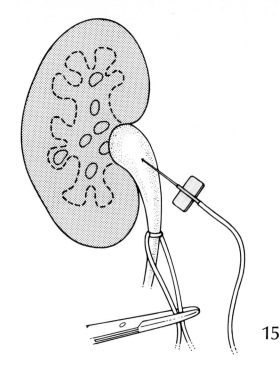

15

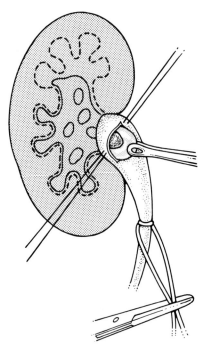

16

17

PERCUTANEOUS RENAL SURGERY

In the last two years the technique of endoscopic percutaneous surgery has rapidly developed. A fine Teflon-sheathed needle is passed into the kidney. Once the collecting system is penetrated the needle is removed and a fine angiographic guide-wire is passed down the retained sheath. Graduated plastic dilators are passed over the guide-wire to dilate a suitable track to 26 Fr. Once the track is established, a small plastic tube (Amplatz) is passed over the last graduated dilator. Endoscopes may be passed down this plastic conduit into the interior of the kidney. By means of both solid rod and flexible nephroscopes the entire interior of the kidney becomes accessible to direct vision. The stones contained in the collecting system may be visualized and removed by small alligator forceps or baskets. Larger stones may be fragmented by ultrasound or electrohydraulic disintegrators.

It is felt at the time of writing that this technique will rapidly supersede the older methods of open operative nephrolithotomy described above.

Finally it should be mentioned that with the development of the Dornier extracorporeal shock-wave stone disintegrator, all methods of open renal surgery may rapidly become obsolete.

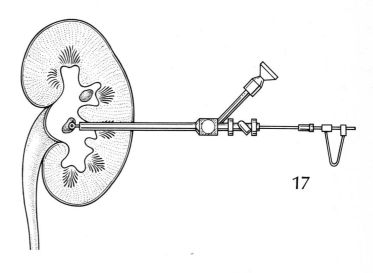

17

References

1. Graves, F. T. Renal hypothermia: an aid to partial nephrectomy. British Journal of Surgery 1963; 50:362–367

2. Marberger, M., Gunther, R., Mayer, E. J., Wiestler, M. A simple method for *in situ* presentation of the ischaemic kidney during renal surgery. Investigative Urology 1976; 14:191–193

Further reading

Wickham, J. E. A. ed. Urinary calculous disease. Edinburgh: Churchill Livingstone, 1979

Wickham, J. E. A. ed. Intrarenal surgery. Edinburgh: Churchill Livingstone, 1984

Wickman, J. E. A., Miller, R. A. eds. Percutaneous renal surgery. Edinburgh: Churchill Livingstone, 1983

Percutaneous renal pelvic and ureteral surgery

W. Scott McDougal MD
Professor and Chairman Department of Urology; Vanderbilt University School of Medicine, Nashville, Tennessee

Introduction

With the advent of extracorporeal shock wave lithotripsy the role that percutaneous endoscopic pelvic stone manipulation will play in the future management of renal stone disease is uncertain. In any event it seems clear that in selected cases it will continue to be a useful procedure. The advantage of this technique over open surgery is that it can be performed through a smaller incision with less morbidity. The disadvantages are that direct control of bleeding may be difficult and access to some stones or lesions, particularly those located in a middle pole calyx, can be difficult. The procedure should not be performed in patients with an active infection of the urinary tract or with a bleeding diathesis.

The procedure

1 & 2

Renal calyceal anatomy

There are four to twelve calyces in each kidney. Those located in the upper and lower poles are often compound and project directly to their respective poles. The remainder are arranged in an anterior and a posterior row (see *illustration 1*). Those in the anterior row form an angle of 70° to the frontal plane and are the calyces which are seen laterally on the anteroposterior view of an intravenous urogram (see *illustration 2*). The posterior calyces form an angle of 20° with the frontal plane and are those seen medially on the urogram. It is important to locate accurately the calyx in which the calculus or lesion resides for proper placement of the percutaneous nephrostomy and subsequent location of the calculus endoscopically.

Percutaneous nephrostomy

The nephrostomy can be made at the time of stone manipulation or the day before, depending on the preference of the surgeon. Placement and immediate dilatation with stone manipulation can be performed under one anaesthetic and is less likely to result in an infected urinary tract before surgery. To perform percutaneous nephrostomy the renal pelvis must be located. This may be accomplished by four methods: (1) by the use of ultrasound, (2) with the aid of an intravenous contrast, (3) by placement of a ureteral catheter with retrograde injection of contrast and (4) by direct injection of contrast through a thin needle inserted into the renal pelvis under fluoroscopic guidance.

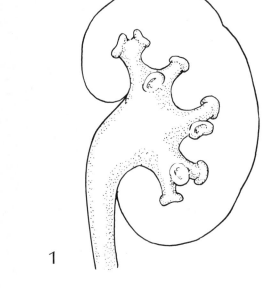

1

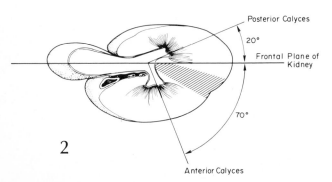

Posterior Calyces

20°

Frontal Plane of Kidney

70°

2

Anterior Calyces

3

The kidney is usually punctured through the infundibulum of the lower or middle calyx of the posterior row, provided the stone can be reached through this route. This area is preferred since it can be approached from beneath the 12th rib and most parts of the collecting system can be visualized when the endoscope enters from this area. To perform the puncture the patient is placed in the prone position and tilted up 30° on the side of the kidney to be entered. The posterior calyces thus project vertically, allowing direct access to them. The opacified system is punctured, a guide wire placed down the ureter and the tract dilated. A second guide wire or safety wire is inserted and dilatation continued over the first wire with coaxial dilators or a balloon dilator. The tract is dilated to 24–26 Fr.

It is most important to emphasize the need for two guide wires. Following dilatation placement of the sheath through which the endoscope will enter the renal pelvis requires removal of one of the guide wires. Thereafter, should the sheath become dislodged, one still has a means of finding the renal pelvis using the second guide wire.

Endoscopic manipulation

With the tract dilated a sheath is passed through it into the renal pelvis and the endoscopic instrument is introduced. A craniotomy drape or one which will catch the irrigant is placed about the wound so that the excess irrigant can be collected without draining over the patient, the table and the floor. Stones are grasped and removed or, if too large, they may be broken mechanically with ultrasound or electrohydraulically with shock waves. The irrigant used is usually normal (physiological) saline, but this may need to be modified if electrohydraulic shock wave lithotripsy is preferred. When stones are fragmented care must be taken not to lose fragments down the ureter. This may be prevented by placing a Fogerty balloon catheter up the ureter to occlude the ureteropelvic junction before breaking the stones. Renal pelvic and upper ureteral stones may be approached with this technique. At the termination of the procedure a 14 Fr Malecot nephrostomy is left in place for 4–5 days. Before its removal a nephrostogram is performed to ensure that all fragments have been removed and that fluid can move freely from renal pelvis to bladder.

Chemolysis of calculi

Should retained fragments be discovered on the nephrostogram the renal pelvis may be irrigated with a

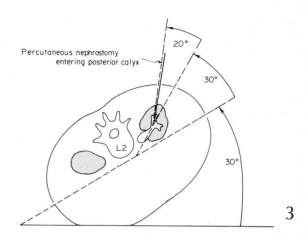

Percutaneous nephrostomy
entering posterior calyx

20°

30°

30°

L2

3

solution formulated to dissolve the stone. Continuous irrigation may be obtained by placing a second percutaneous nephrostomy tube in the renal pelvis or by passing a ureteral catheter cystoscopically into the renal pelvis. Uric acid stones are treated with sodium bicarbonate or tromethamine solution, cystine stones with sodium bicarbonate, tromethamine or acetylcysteine, struvite stones with Suby's solution G, appatite stones with hemiacidrin and calcium oxalate stones with ethylenediaminetetracetic acid (EDTA).

Complications

Complications of this procedure include bleeding, renal pelvic and ureteral disruption, sepsis, fluid overload from excessive irrigant absorption, loss of the kidney, perirenal fibrosis and injury to the lung, colon, spleen and liver. In most series significant complications resulting in serious mobidity occur in less than 5% of cases.

Further reading

Marberger, M. Disintegration of renal and ureteral calculi with ultrasound. Urologic Clinics of North America 1983; 10: 729–242

Smith, A. D., Lee, W. L. Introduction to endourology: percutaneous nephrostomy and ureteral stents. AUA Update Series 1984; 3: 5

Anatrophic nephrolithotomy

Lloyd H. Harrison MD, FACS
Professor of Surgery (Urology), Section of Urology, Bowman Gray School of Medicine
of Wake Forest University, Winston-Salem, North Carolina, USA

Jonathan C. Boyd MD
Fellow in Urology, Section of Urology, Bowman Gray School of Medicine
of Wake Forest University, Winston-Salem, North Carolina, USA

Introduction

Anatrophic segmental surgery is based upon renal arterial anatomy. Its goals are to preserve renal function by avoiding damage to renal segmental arteries, to remove existing calculi and to improve drainage. Because the kidney is divided into segments by its arterial blood supply with no major collaterals between segments, the surgeon may gain entrance to the pelvis and calyces by placing the nephrotomy between the posterior and anterior segments of the kidney with little damage to the parenchyma[1]. In context, the term anatrophic means to 'prevent atrophy, prevent a waste of tissue'. The nephrotomy allows wide exposure of the collecting system and facilitates plastic reconstruction. Better understanding of renal ischaemia and hypothermia plus the addition of microsurgical instruments, microsutures and new antimicrobial agents, has established anatrophic nephrolithotomy as the procedure of choice in those patients with branched or multiple renal calculi with infundibular stenosis[2]. Individuals with small intrarenal pelves or pelves scarred from previous surgery are also excellent candidates for this procedure[3].

Extensive preoperative genitourinary and metabolic workups are necessary to rule out anatomical and metabolic abnormalities which predispose the patient to stone disease[4]. Included in this profile are X-ray identification of number and site of stones, evaluation of renal function, a thorough cardiovascular examination and an anaesthesia consultation. Preoperative antibiotics and steroids (methylprednisolone 15 mg/kg) are given[5].

The operation

After induction of general endotracheal anaesthesia, the patient is placed in the flank position. Some surgeons prefer to tape the patient before elevating the kidney rest and flexion of the table. Others tape after the table is positioned. However, taping first draws the skin edges apart after the incision is made and exposure is much improved.

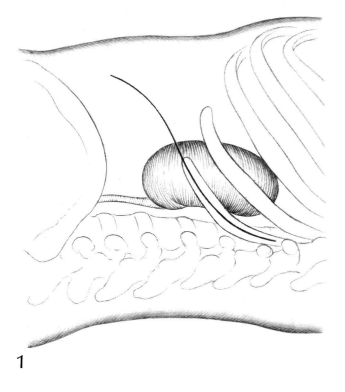

1

Skin incision

1

A generous 12th rib incision is made from the lateral margins of the rectus to the paraspinal muscles. The rib is resected far posteriorly at its angle. The medial aspect of the incision should not trail inferiorly as it does in the routine hockey-stick position. It should terminate perpendicularly to the rectus muscle, more superiorly. The incision is opened further in a standard fashion, taking care to avoid the pleura. Gerota's fascia is opened on its posterolateral aspect with extreme care taken by the surgeon to preserve this layer[6].

Mobilization

The kidney is fully mobilized from the perinephric fat with the exception of the region of the pelvis and proximal ureter. This improves the accuracy of subsequent intraoperative X-rays[7], clarifies segmental demarcation, and protects the collateral blood supply to the proximal ureter and renal pelvis. This procedure is time-consuming, particularly in reoperation or in cases of chronic pyelonephritis. The surgeon should be prepared to spend several hours at this stage. Wide umbilical tapes are placed about the kidney to provide elevation and to aid in renal arterial dissection.

Identification of posterior segment

2

The posterior segmental artery can usually be identified by its course and calibre. It is normally the first branch of the main renal artery.

With the kidney retracted upward, the renal artery is first palpated from the superior aspect of the renal sinus to the aorta, then dissected near its origin. This should be outside any perirenal inflammation caused by stone disease, not far from the aorta. One must search for accessory vessels, particularly if the vessels found appear inappropriately small. Only enough dissection should be done to allow identification and clamping. Too vigorous dissection will cause vasospasm.

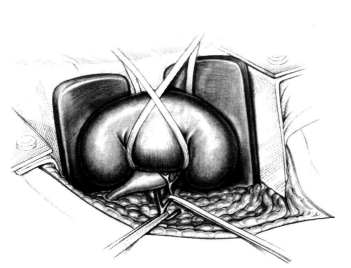

2

3

To verify identification of the posterior segmental artery, the branch may be temporarily occluded with a disposable bulldog clamp which will cause immediate blanching in the posterior renal segment. Repetition of this manoeuvre with peripheral injection of 10–20 ml of methylene blue will demarcate the posterior segmental anatrophic line. The entire line should then be drawn on the surface of the kidney with methylene blue. Or a radiopaque marker from a gauze sponge can be sewn to the capsule following this delineation. This will aid in positioning the nephrotomy incision.

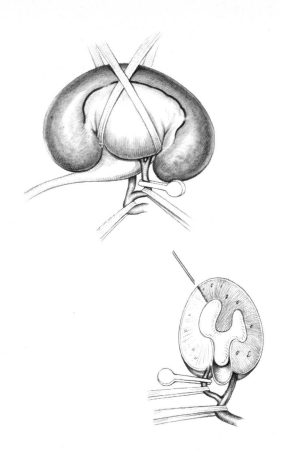

3

4

X-rays

Following full mobilization and elevation as decribed, posterior-anterior films should be taken on the table of the kidney. Using two overlapping small cassettes, the surgeon can ensure that the whole kidney is visualized. The marker overlying the anatrophic line can be seen in this example. In this case, a nephrotomy of nearly the entire posterior segment was necessary to extract all the stones.

4

5

Renal ischaemia and hypothermia

Ten minutes after intravenous administration of mannitol 25 g, the renal artery should be clamped[8]. The kidney is then separated from surrounding structures by the placement of gauze packing and a rubber dam. This step also helps to avoid cooling of the patient's body. Ice slush (Ringer's lactate) is then packed about the kidney[9].

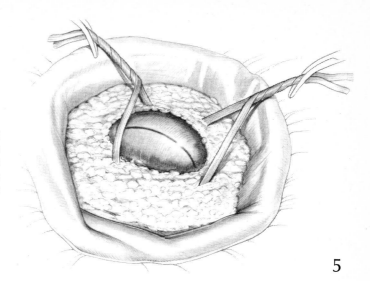

5

Nephrotomy incisions

Magnifying loupes and microinstruments should be utilized at this point. An incision is made along the previously identified line between the posterior and anterior segments, using the scalpel on the capsule only. Blunt dissection should be done with the scalpel handle or spatula to enlarge the nephrotomy. For those stones involving the posterior calyces, the parenchyma is dissected toward the anterior aspect of the posterior calyces. If the calculus involves the posterior calyces and the pelvis, the dissection should extend to the intersection of the renal pelvis and the posterior calyces of the renal pelvis. If the anterior calyces are involved, the dissection from the anatrophic line to the renal pelvis is slightly more anterior. Dissection is carried along the sites of all involved calyces. A longitudinal midpelvic incision is made and the calyces containing stones are opened through their infundibula[6].

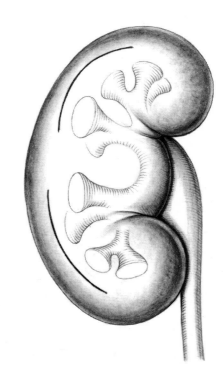

6

If the pelvis is bifid and there are calculi in each segment, the surgeon must use caution to avoid the anterior and superior segmental arteries which frequently run through the bifurcation. Separate incisions should be made for exploration of each pelvis.

6

7

The anatrophic line should be mapped to its inferior termination if a large pelvis stone is located in a lower pole calyx.

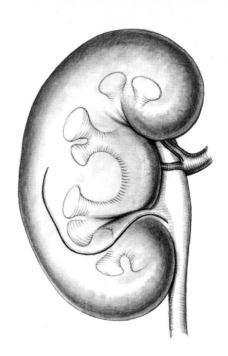

7

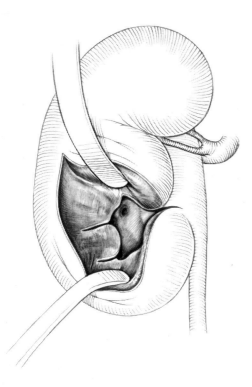

8

8

Dissection of the renal pelvis can be continued under the parenchyma, with division of the parenchyma if extension is necessary, cutting through the infundibula of the calyces as in the other nephrotomies[5].

After opening all the affected regions, stone removal is accomplished with nerve hooks, drum elevators, brain spatulas or any instruments which are comfortable in the surgeon's hand. Repeat X-rays are needed to ensure that all stones and stone fragments are extracted. The ice should be removed temporarily from around the kidney in order to improve the quality of the X-rays. If there are many stones or fragments, a stent should be placed from the renal pelvis to the urinary bladder early in the procedure to avoid the possibility of debris dropping down the ureter.

Plastic reconstruction of calyces

Often renal calculus disease will cause anatomical changes in the collecting system. Infundibular stenosis is a frequent occurrence and the two recommended methods for correcting this problem are calycoplasty and calyrrhaphy.

9, 10 & 11

Calycoplasty joins the two adjacent stenotic infundibulae, forming one large calyx. Stay sutures of 6/0 Prolene are placed midway between the two calyces above the collecting system. Using microsurgical technique, 7/0 Dexon (double-armed with knots tied outside the collecting system) is run from deep within the pelvis to the initial, more superficial pelviotomy. This is sewn doubly as the first tie should halve the double-arm suture.

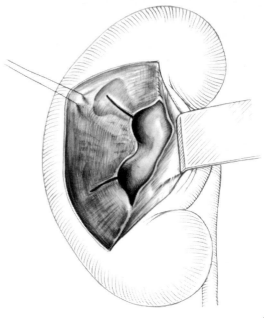

9

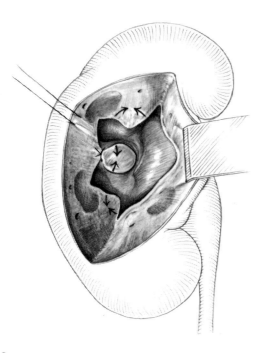

10

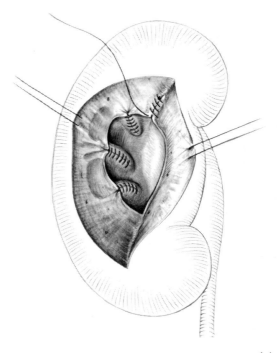

11

12

Calyrrhaphy is simply the horizontal closure of a vertical incision (i.e. the Heineke-Mikulicz procedure). The infundibulum is shortened and widened. There is usually enough atrophy around the diseased calyx to allow for any distortion caused by bringing the infundibulum lining to the renal pelvis.

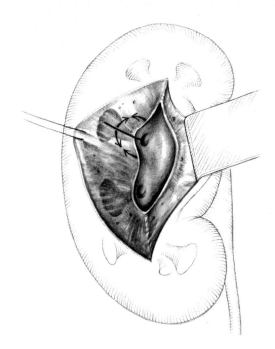

12

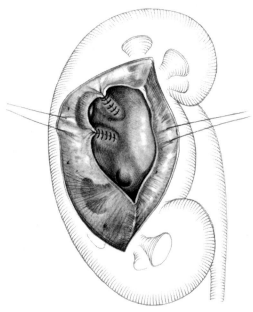

13

13

The calyceal infundibulum is sutured to the muscularis and epithelium of the renal pelvis, taking care to suture only the epithelium and muscularis. The interlobar arteries lie adjacent to the infundibulae and are easily damaged.

Closure of nephrotomy

After repairing all calyces a 14 Silastic stent is advanced from the renal pelvis to the bladder and left indwelling. The renal pelvis is closed with a 7/0 Dexon running suture. The parenchyma is closely observed for open venous channels and the capsule closed with a running 4/0 chromic suture[8].

Icepacks, and the renal artery clamp are removed. There should be prompt return of colour and turgor to the renal parenchyma with minimal bleeding from the nephrotomy. If there is brisk, bright red bleeding, the renal artery must be reclamped, the nephrotomy opened after cooling again and the offending artery tied. Nephrostomy or pyelostomy tubes are not recommended. A ½ inch (2.5 cm) soft rubber drain is left in the renal fossa and brought out through a low posterior stab wound. It is usually removed within 72 hours. Gerota's fascia is reapproximated as well as possible. However, if none exists, omentum through a peritoneotomy can be used to wrap the kidney[6]. The flank is closed in separate layers in standard fashion.

References

1. Boyce, W. H. Renal calculi. In: Glenn, J. F., Boyce, W. H., eds. Urologic surgery, 2nd ed. New York: Harper & Row, 1975, 169–189

2. Boyce, W. H., Harrison, L. H. Complications of renal stone surgery. In: Smith, R. B., Skinner, D. G., eds. Complications of urologic surgery. Philadelphia: W. B. Saunders, 1976, 87–105

3. Resnick, M. I. Evaluation and management of infectious stones. Urologic Clinics of North America 1981; 8: 265–276

4. Pitts, G. W., Resnick, M. I. Urinary stone formation, patient evaluation and management. Urologic Clinics of North America 1980; 7: 45–58

5. Harrison, L. H. Anatrophic nephrolithotomy: update 1978. In: Bonney, W. W., ed. AUA Courses, Vol. 1. Baltimore: William and Wilkins, 1979, 1–23

6. Harrison, L. H., Nordan, J. M. Anatrophic nephrotomy for removal of renal calculi. Urologic Clinics of North America 1974; 1: 333–344

7. Boyce, W. H. The localization of intrarenal calculi during surgery. Journal of Urology 1977; 118: 152

8. Smith, M. J. V., Boyce, W. H. Anatrophic nephrotomy and plastic calyrrhaphy. Transactions of the American Association of Genito-Urinary Surgeons 1967; 59: 18–24

9. Metzner, P. J., Boyce, W. H. Simplified renal hypothermia: an adjunct to conservative renal surgery. British Journal of Urology 1972; 44: 76–85

Illustrations by Robert N. Lane

Coagulum pyelolithotomy

Lloyd H. Harrison   MD, FACS
Professor of Surgery (Urology), Section of Urology, Bowman Gray School of Medicine
of Wake Forest University, Winston-Salem, North Carolina, USA

Jonathan C. Boyd   MD
Fellow in Urology, Section of Urology, Bowman Gray School of Medicine
of Wake Forest University, Winston-Salem, North Carolina, USA

Introduction

Coagulum pyelolithotomy, first described by Dees in 1943[1], is indicated for the removal of multiple, small, free stones. It is particularly useful for small stones and dilated pelves with open infundibulae. The procedure is not suitable for pelves with infundibular stenosis or small renal pelves which cannot be mobilized[1].

Early clots were formed from the injection of pooled human fibrogen and clotting globulin. Later, bovine fibrogen and topical thrombin were introduced. Trials were made with fresh frozen plasma as the fibrogen source but tensile strength was found to be inadequate. Cryoprecipitate as a fibrin source began experimental trial in 1977. The optimum ratio to form a slow clot was found to be 1 ml of cryoprecipitate to 2 units of thrombin to 1 mg of calcium chloride[2]. The material should be warmed to body temperature before mixing and injecting[3].

The operation

Preoperative metabolic and genitourinary workups should be done. Any infection should be treated preoperatively.

The standard flank approach is used and the pelvis and ureter are mobilized from the surrounding tissues. The ureter is temporarily occluded, the renal pelvis aspirated with a syringe and the volume noted. The pelvis is remeasured with injections of normal saline. The correct volume of cryoprecipitate, thrombin and calcium chloride can be calculated more easily utilizing a published chart[2]. The thrombin and calcium chloride can be mixed together at leisure. However, with the addition of cryoprecipitate, the coagulum forms within 15 s.

1

After mixing, the solution should be rapidly injected into the renal pelvis. The coagulum is formed within 45 s and pyelotomy should be delayed for 3 min.

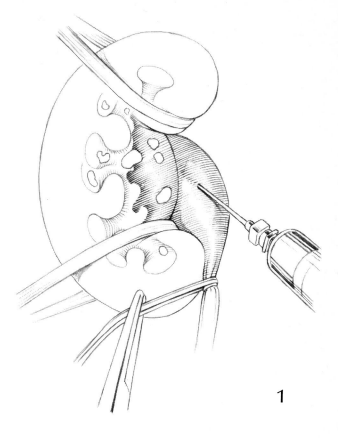

1

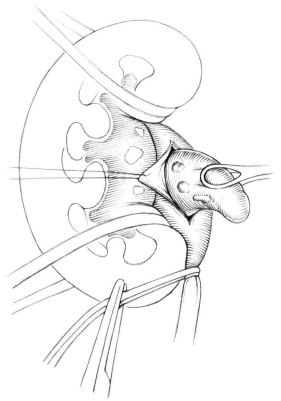

2

2

A pyelotomy is made and the coagulum easily teased from the renal pelvis and calyces. Since the clot is friable, good exposure and lack of tension is necessary to remove all the clots without rupture.

The clot is then inspected for stones and the pelvis irrigated and checked for retained coagulum. If there is any question of retained calculi, the coagulum should be X-rayed and comparison should be made with the preoperative X-rays[3]. Occasionally, intraoperative films of the kidney may be necessary to locate residual stones.

Ureteral occlusion is released and the pyelotomy is closed in the standard manner; Gerota's fascia is reapproximated. A drain is left in the renal fossa and brought up through a separate wound. The flank is then closed.

Complications

Following the report of a fatal complication[4], there has been much concern about the quantity of thrombin injected[5]. Mixing the thrombin, cryoprecipitate and calcium chloride *ex vivo* prior to injection limits the amount of thrombin which could possibly be absorbed. Circulating normal levels of antithrombin, as well as the high pelvic pressure needed to extravasate this material, ensure a natural defence against pulmonary embolus. The dog models would suggest that there is very little chance for a significant amount of thrombin to extravasate with low concentrations of thrombin in normal pressures needed for filling.

Coagulum can be formed without any thrombin[6]. The tissue thromboplastin is adequate to form a clot. However, the tensile strength and the time for coagulation make this a less acceptable method of clot formation.

Retained coagulum does not form a nidus for new stone development since urokinase will dissolve the fibrin clot.

References

1. Dees, J. E., Anderson, E. E. Coagulum pyelolithotomy. Urologic Clinics of North America 1981; 8: 313–317

2. Fischer, C. P., Sonda, L. P., Diokno, A. C. Use of cryoprecipitate coagulum in extracting renal calculi. Urology 1980; 15: 6–13

3. Fischer, C. P., Sonda, L. P., Diokno. A. C. Further experience with cryoprecipitate coagulum in renal calculus surgery: a review of 60 cases. Journal of Urology 1981; 126: 432–436

4. Pence, J. R., Airhart, R. A., Novicki, D. E., Williams, J. L., Ehler, W. J. Pulmonary emboli associated with coagulum pyelolithotomy. Journal of Urology 1982; 127: 572–573

5. Burns, J. R., Finlayson, B. Coagulum pyelolithotomy: tensile strength of coagula as a function of variables. Urology 1982; 19: 381–385

6. Kalash, S. S., Young, J. D., Harne, G. Modification of cryoprecipitate coagulum pyelolithotomy technique, Urology 1982; 19: 467–471

Illustrations by Michael J. Courtney

Partial nephrectomy and heminephrectomy

J. C. Christoffersen MD, MA
Professor of Surgery and Director of Urology, Bispebjerg Hospital, Copenhagen, Denmark

Introduction

In the present context partial nephrectomy is the operation by which a segment is excised from an anatomically normal kidney while heminephrectomy is the method by which one half of a double kidney is removed or, more rarely, one half of a horseshoe kidney. The two types of surgery differ in that the vascular supply must be more carefully assessed prior to partial nephrectomy in order to preserve the supply to the remaining part of the kidney, whereas such assessment is less important in the case of heminephrectomy since the two renal elements are in the main individually supplied and are in addition provided with two renal pelves which never communicate.

Indications

The main indication for partial nephrectomy is the presence of calculi in the lower pole of the kidney, especially if the lower calyces are dilated. The operation may also be of benefit in other cases of nephrolithiasis, for instance in the presence of multiple stone or minor coralliform calculi. A localized, infective focus, whether specific (tuberculous) or non-specific (carbuncle), may be an indication, though not as often now that antibiotic control has become more efficient. Tumour formation in a solitary kidney is a rare but definite indication. Cysts may be managed by way of partial nephrectomy, but excision of the cyst will usually be sufficient.

Partial nephrectomy may be indicated in cases of renal rupture and it should be noted that in conservative treatment of large hydronephroses it is often useful to remove a dilated, poorly functioning lower pole of the kidney.

Heminephrectomy is indicated in the presence of tumour formation, hydronephrosis, infection, or stone in one part of the double kidney. Furthermore, it is indicated in the presence of an ectopically ending ureter from a double kidney manifesting itself as incontinence.

Diffuse pyelonephritic change affecting the entire kidney is a specific contraindication.

Special investigations and equipment

Renal angiography may occasionally be of value, though it is rarely essential except in the case of a tumour in a solitary kidney.

If the intrarenal intervention is expected to be of long duration it may be of value to have equipment by which the kidney can be cooled while a clamp is employed for compression of the renal pedicle. This technique is described in the chapter on 'Nephrolithotomy' pp. 84–93.

The operations

PARTIAL NEPHRECTOMY

1

Exposure

The approach is from the loin as for nephrectomy (*see* p. 111). Through a wide incision the kidney is mobilized and the pedicle dissected free. The ureter is disengaged and marked. The hilar vessels, and also the vessels to the segment to be excised, are dissected free. By compression of these vessels, and on the basis of the line of demarcation which appears, it will be possible to determine the scope of the resection to be done. The vessels are then ligated. A soft clamp is applied to the remaining part of the pedicle so that it will be possible to accomplish the resection without bleeding. Manual compression of the parenchyma at a site above the line of resection will occasionally be sufficient. If the intrarenal procedure is expected to last more than 10–12 min, the clamp may be slackened or the compression discontinued for a short time while the kidney is perfused with blood.

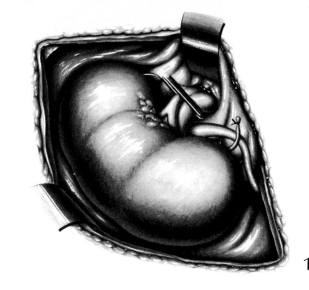

1

2

Incision

Partial nephrectomy can be performed with either a wedge-shaped or a transverse excision. The former method is preferred since it facilitates haemostasis and the closure of the cut surfaces. In this way the fibrous capsule need not be disengaged. A sharp incision into the parenchyma is made immediately above the line of demarcation or occasionally at a site indicated by the pathological process or by the findings obtained by preoperative investigation. If a transverse incision is to be used, the renal capsule should first be opened over the pole and reflected from the segment to be excised.

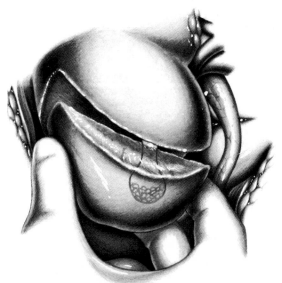

2

3

Excision

When the incision measures a few millimetres, traction is exerted on the circumcised renal segment and blunt or sharp dissection is then continued obliquely towards the neck of the calyx, which should be the last structure to be cut. Then the renal pelvis should be opened to the extent required.

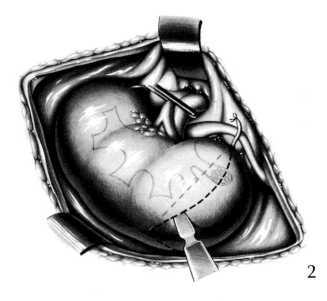

3

4

Haemostasis

After completion of the intrarenal intervention, compression of the pedicle or parenchyma is discontinued and definitive haemostasis established by ligation or stitching of the arteries and veins using 3/0 catgut. If major branches of the artery or vein have been by accident cut tangentially during the procedure they must be sutured while compression is re-established for a short time. Oozing is of minor importance since it stops as soon as the cut surfaces are closed.

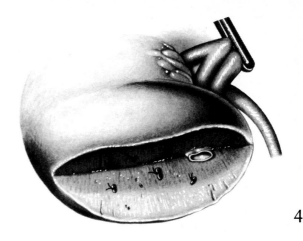

4

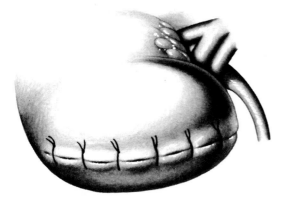

5

5

Closure of the pelvis

The neck of the calyx and incisions, if any, extending into the pelvis are closed by continuous catgut 3/0 suture on an atraumatic needle.

6

Closure of the parenchyma

The cut surfaces are closed by deep sutures, using 2/0 catgut. Coaption of the surfaces is usually easy and mattress sutures should be avoided as they give rise to marginal necrosis. If a transverse guillotine cut has been used for the incision, fat or muscle tissue may be sutured to the surfaces of the resection before the latter is covered by the fibrous capsule which was previously everted from the pole of the kidney.

The kidney is then replaced in the fossa. If it is very mobile it may be stabilized by tightening the fatty capsule into the form of a cushion below the resected pole and if necessary by attaching it to the fascia of the psoas muscle. Drainage is accomplished by means of a corrugated rubber drain.

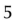

6

7

PARTIAL NEPHRECTOMY: RESECTION OF THE UPPER POLE

This requires that the vessels are dissected free more carefully than would be necessary in the case of the lower pole. A blind cut may involve an injury to the descending branch of the posterior segmental artery, which may thus compromise the vascular supply of large parts of the kidney to be preserved.

Resection of the middle part of the kidney is rarely indicated and most authors advise against it. Preliminary ligature of the segmental arterial branches is hardly ever possible and there is a large venous plexus in the hilum. Both these factors complicate the establishment of haemostasis and deep controlling sutures may compromise the vascular supply to the adjacent segment.

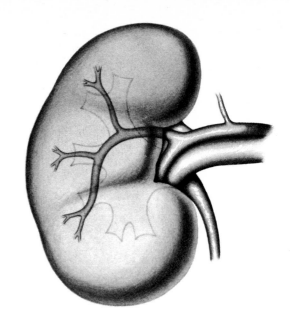

7

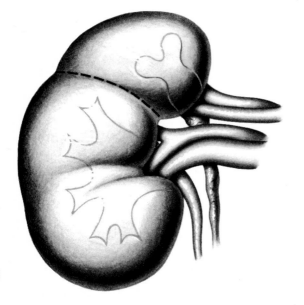

8

8

HEMINEPHRECTOMY

This operation is generally easier to perform than partial nephrectomy as the pelves of the two renal segments are always separated and they usually have separate vascular supplies. Furthermore, the transition between the two segments is often evident from the pathological process affecting one of them. If not, the line of demarcation will at least become more distinct as soon as the vessels have been ligated. The connecting bridge of tissue where the incision is made should not contain the calyx from either pelvis.

During isolation and cutting the ureter from the affected segment, care must be taken to ensure that the vessels to the unaffected segment are not injured. Delicate dissection may be necessary at this point.

Postoperative care

The drain can be removed on the 3rd day if there is no urinary leakage or bleeding. Leakage practically always stops after a few days. Secondary haemorrhage may be serious enough to demand intervention, and, if it is necessary, a further resection at a higher level will be the operation of choice. If this is not possible, nephrectomy may be inevitable.

Further reading

Bischoff, P. F. The surgical treatment of solitary kidney. Urologia internationalis 1969; 24: 527–550

Coleman, C. H., Wilkerington, R. A review of 117 partial nephrectomies. Journal of Urology 1979; 122: 11–13

Culp, O. S., Hendricks, E. D. Potentialities of partial nephrectomy. In: Whitehead, E. D., Ed. Current operative urology. Maryland: Harper and Row, 1975: 28–48

Marshall, V. R., Singh, M., Tresidder, G. C., Blandy, J. P. Place of partial nephrectomy in management of renal calyceal calculi. British Journal of Urology 1975; 47: 759–764

Pedersen, J. F. Partial nephrectomy for nephrolithiasis. Scandinavian Journal of Urology and Nefrology 1971; 5: 171–176

Puigvert, A. Partial nephrectomy for renal tumor: 21 cases. European Urology 1976; 2: 70–78

Rose, M. B., Follows, O. J. Partial nephrectomy for stone-disease. British Journal of Urology 1977; 49: 605–610

Illustrations by Daniel S. Beisel

Simple nephrectomy

Thomas J. Rohner, Jr MD
Professor of Surgery (Urology), Chief, Division of Urology, Pennsylvania State University
College of Medicine and The Milton S. Hershey Medical Center, Hershey, Pennsylvania, USA

Introduction

The first deliberate nephrectomy was carried out by Professor Gustav Simon of Heidelberg, Germany, in 1869. Simon's patient had a complicated left ureterocutaneous fistula caused by ureteral avulsion during resection of an ovarian tumour 18 months earlier. After four unsuccessful attempts at closing the fistula, Simon considered removal of the kidney. At that time it had not been shown that a kidney could be surgically removed and the opposite kidney provide adequate renal function. After carrying out successful unilateral nephrectomies in several dogs, Simon removed the patient's kidney using an extraperitoneal approach with a good eventual result. An interesting account of Simon's experience is provided by Thorwald[1].

General considerations

Simple nephrectomy involves removal of the kidney and upper ureter without removing the perinephric fat or Gerota's fascia. It is generally performed through a subcostal or anterior 12th rib extraperitoneal flank incision. The choice of incision depends on the position of the kidney.

Preoperative indications

Simple nephrectomy is often done for poorly or non-functioning kidneys due to ureteropelvic junction or ureteral obstruction, calculus disease, chronic pyelonephritis, infection, ureteral fistula, vascular disease or late trauma. The decision to carry out nephrectomy indicates that reconstructive efforts to preserve the kidney have been considered and deemed either unreasonable or inappropriate or that the function of the kidney is so poor that further reconstructive procedures are not justified. Simple nephrectomy using an extraperitoneal approach is particularly applicable when it is considered likely that infection is present and one wants to avoid contamination of the peritoneal cavity.

In the past, simple nephrectomy using an extraperitoneal flank approach was used for resection of renal adenocarcinomas. It has been shown that 13–30 per cent of renal adenocarcinomas will extend through the renal capsule into the perinephric fat, and for this reason radical nephrectomy, involving removal of the kidney with surrounding perinephric fat and Gerota's fascia, should provide superior local tumour control[2]. The preferred transabdominal approach to renal tumours provides easier and earlier access to the vascular pedicle. A transperitoneal approach is also recommended for acute trauma and renal injuries within the first 72 hours so that early control of the renal vessels can be gained and associated intra-abdominal injuries can be ruled out.

Preoperative preparation

One unit of blood should be typed and crossed. The procedure is best carried out under general endotracheal anaesthesia in the full flank position. The patient's pulmonary status should be assessed. A specific antibiotic for positive urine cultures should be given 2 hours before surgery. Proper patient informed consent should include discussion of the general hazards related to major surgical procedures and those possible complications peculiar to nephrectomy, including haemorrhage, colon or duodenum injury, and pleural injury with pneumothorax.

The operation

1

After induction of general endotracheal anaesthesia in the supine position, the patient is placed in the lateral decubitus position with kidney bar raised and the operating table flexed so that the upward exposed flank is nearly parallel to the floor. The bottom leg is flexed, with a pillow placed between the knees. Depending on the position of the kidney, either a subcostal or anterior 12th rib incision with resection of the distal portion of the 12th rib is made.

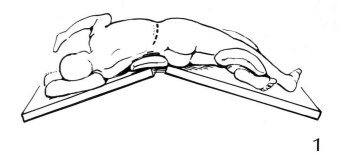

2

After the external and internal oblique muscles are sharply incised, the transversus muscle and lumbodorsal fascia at the posterior extent of the incision is bluntly opened with a Kelly clamp and the retroperitoneal space entered. Blunt finger dissection is carried anteriorly to split the transversus muscle in the direction of its fibres.

Particular attention should be paid to the 12th thoracic intercostal nerve, which lies between the transversus and internal oblique muscles. This nerve should be identified and retracted posteriorly, but not divided, to avoid postoperative abdominal muscle relaxation. The peritoneum is bluntly pushed forward to avoid entering it. Gerota's fascia is identified and the lateral aspect is grasped with smooth forceps and incised, exposing the pale yellow perinephric fat.

Mobilization of the kidney is best done using blunt finger dissection. Dense fibrous bands or fat adherent to the renal capsule is sharply divided, using scissor dissection. The lower pole is mobilized first, followed by the anterior and posterior kidney surfaces. If the kidney has been obstructed and is hydronephrotic, trocar suction can be used to empty the collecting system. This will result in a smaller kidney and will greatly improve surgical exposure.

The upper ureter is identified, divided between clamps and ligated. This manoeuvre permits easier retraction of the kidney and the ureter can be followed to the hilum.

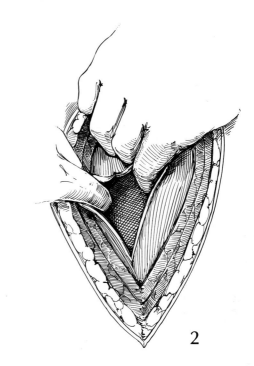

The significant event during nephrectomy is the identification and secure ligation of the renal artery and vein. More than a single renal artery occurs in 25 per cent of individuals and, accompanied by a vein, often supplies the lower or upper pole of the kidney. While freeing the lower pole of the kidney, the possibility of accessory vessels should be kept in mind so that inadvertent avulsion with haemorrhage does not occur. Resistance encountered during blunt finger dissection should be considered a vascular structure and divided between ligatures or clips before division.

The main renal artery and vein in the hilum can be approached either anteriorly or posteriorly. The artery should always be ligated first to minimize vascular congestion and bleeding. It should be remembered that the renal vein lies anterior to the artery, and for this reason the posterior approach has the advantage of providing access to the artery without having to retract the overlying vein. Individual ligation of the artery and vein is more secure and preferable to mass ligation of the pedicle. Arteriovenous fistula is uncommon but has been noted as a complication following mass pedicle ligation.

3

A right-angled clamp is useful in freeing up and passing ties around the artery, following which it is triply ligated in continuity and divided between the distal two ties.

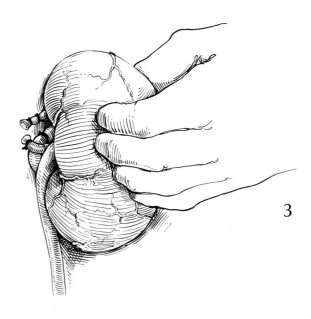

3

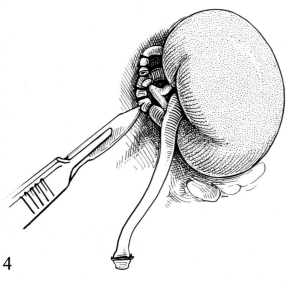

4

4

The vein is then similarly triply ligated and divided.

If extensive perinephric inflammatory disease has been present or several previous kidney operations have been done, the hilum and renal vessels may be encased in thick fibrous tissue, making individual vessel identification and ligation very difficult. In this situation the use of mass pedicle ligation can be considered[3].

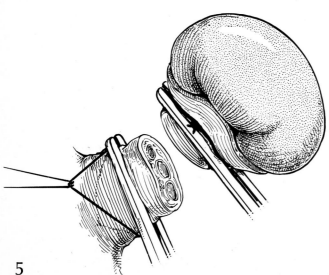

5

5

The renal pedicle, including the artery and vein, is thinned as much as possible and ideally three pedicle clamps are placed across the renal vesels and the pedicle divided between the two distal clamps. Most often only enough pedicle can be mobilized to accommodate two clamps. The pedicle is then ligated proximally using 0 silk ties, loosening the clamps, and then reapplying them after the ties are snugged down.

6

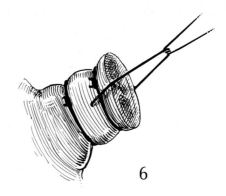

6

It is important to maintain control of the pedicle and one should be able to reapply the clamps immediately should bleeding occur. A suture ligature between the two proximal ties can be used for added security.

In the presence of gross infection No. 1 chromic catgut should be used to ligate all vessels. The use of non-absorbable suture material in this situation may result in a persistent draining fistula or sinus tract.

Sudden haemorrhage during the course of gaining control or tying the renal vessels should be dealt with by direct finger or surgical sponge compression while efforts are organized to deal with the bleeding. These efforts include setting up a second suction line and being certain 5/0 vascular suture material and non-crushing vascular clamps are available. It is also appropriate to inform the anaesthetist of the presence of uncontrolled bleeding and make certain either that blood is available for transfusion or arrange for further blood to be typed and crossed. Blind clamping is to be condemned, since further vascular injury can occur or injury to other structures close to the renal vessels, especially the duodenum, vena cava or colon.

If, during the course of nephrectomy, dense adhesions are encountered binding the renal capsule to the perinephric fat, the surgeon may find an easier plane of dissection between the renal parenchyma and capsule than between the capsule and perinephric fat. In that event, one may continue using the subscapular technique of nephrectomy (see chapter on 'Subcapsular nephrectomy', pp. 116–118).

Another technique to be remembered when one encounters dense adhesions and fibrosis involving the peritoneum and renal pedicle is to extend the incision medially, open the peritoneum and either reflect the colon medially to gain control of the renal artery and vein lateral to the colon, or incise the peritoneum medial to the colon and identify and isolate the renal vessels even more proximally[4]. This area has usually not been exposed during previous urological procedures.

In the distant past, opening the peritoneal cavity during the course of nephrectomy in the presence of gross infection was a serious problem, with fatal peritonitis often resulting. With appropriate antibiotic therapy and reapproximation of the peritoneum, this is now very uncommon, although an extraperitoneal approach is still preferred for simple nephrectomy.

Mobilization of the upper pole is generally done after dividing the renal vessels. This is best done using blunt finger dissection and staying close to the upper renal pole to avoid removing or injuring the adrenal. If the adrenal is torn, haemostasis can usually be achieved either by suture ligation of the torn edge using a running locking 4/0 chromic suture or large haemostatic clips placed along the avulsed edge.

After the kidney is removed, the renal fossa is fully exposed and can be inspected carefully for bleeding. Either suture ligatures or haemostatic clips can be used to achieve haemostasis. We always drain the renal fossa for 24 hours, using a Penrose drain led out from the posterior extent of the wound. Any hypotensive episode or unexplained tachycardia in the immediate postoperative period can then be evaluated, with significant bleeding from the renal fossa unlikely if the drain is dry.

After haemostasis has been achieved, the pleura at the posterior extent of the wound should be inspected for injury. It may be helpful to fill the incision with saline to detect any bubbling as a result of a small pleural tear. If a pleural opening is seen, it should be sutured with a running locking 2/0 chromic suture with the lung expanded as the final suture is tied down. It is important to obtain an upright chest X-ray in the recovery room, with the patient in the sitting position, to detect pneumothorax. If significant pneumothorax is present, an anterior chest tube should be inserted and placed on waterseal suction until the lung has re-expanded.

The wound is closed using a running locking 0 chromic suture to close the transversus layer. Interrupted 0 chromic sutures are used to approximate the internal and external oblique layers individually. The subcutaneous tissue is approximated using interrupted 3/0 plain catgut sutures and either skin sutures or clips used for skin closure. In the paediatric patient we generally use a subcuticular 4/0 chromic suture to minimize scar formation.

References

1. Thorwald, J. Century of the surgeon. New York: Pantheon Books, 1957: 180–199

2. Skinner, D. G., Vermillion, C. D., Colvin, R. B. The surgical management of renal cell carcinoma. Journal of Urology 1972; 107: 705–710

3. Hinman, F. Nephrectomy. Surgery, Gynecology and Obstetrics 1927; 45: 347–358

4. Scott, R. F., Jr, Selzman, H. M. Complications of nephrectomy: review of 450 patients and a description of a modification of the transperitoneal approach. Journal of Urology 1966; 95: 307–312

Illustrations by Daniel S. Beisel

Subcapsular nephrectomy

Thomas J. Rohner, Jr MD
Professor of Surgery (Urology), Chief, Division of Urology, Pennsylvania State University
College of Medicine and The Milton S. Hershey Medical Center, Hershey, Pennsylvania, USA

Joseph R. Drago MD
Associate Professor of Surgery (Urology), Pennsylvania State University
College of Medicine and The Milton S. Hershey Medical Center, Hershey, Pennsylvania, USA

Introduction

The technique of subcapsular nephrectomy was first described by LeForte in 1880. Early this century simple nephrectomy was most often carried out using large pedicle clamps, with an operative mortality of 10–25 per cent[3]. Major difficulties included haemorrhage encountered during ligation of the pedicle and injury to adjacent bowel or vena cava. These complications were especially likely to occur in the presence of perirenal inflammation and fibrosis, which tend to make exposure and isolation of the pedicle difficult. Subcapsular nephrectomy became a frequently used method[2,3] and was described as a standard procedure in several texts[4]. However, in recent years it has rarely been required. This is probably because effective antibiotics and earlier conservative surgical procedures have reduced the need for simple nephrectomy for inflammatory disease.

General considerations

The subcapsular technique of simple nephrectomy is not a preoperatively planned approach to nephrectomy, but rather an expedient way to complete a nephrectomy when one encounters marked fibrosis involving the perinephric space, with dense adhesions between the perinephric fat and renal capsule. While attempting to develop the proper and usual plane of dissection between the perinephric fat and renal capsule, the surgeon may find that he is stripping the capsule from the kidney. If continued efforts to develop a plane of dissection outside the capsule are difficult, the surgeon can proceed with subcapsular mobilization of the kidney and nephrectomy. This technique is most useful when carrying out simple nephrectomy in patients with pyohydronephrosis or chronic renal inflammatory disease associated with calculi, post-trauma or several previous surgical procedures involving the kidney. It is clearly contraindicated in patients with renal tumours. The preoperative indications and preparation are thus the same as for simple nephrectomy (see p. 112).

The operation

The kidney is approached through a subcostal or anterior 12th rib extraperitoneal incision. If a previous flank scar is present, the skin scar should be excised and the incision carefully carried through the old incision using sharp knife dissection. The posterior extent of the incision should be developed first to avoid entering the peritoneum or injuring underlying bowel. As the incision is carried through the previous scar, a finger should be introduced posteriorly and an attempt made to develop the perinephric space bluntly. The incision can then be extended anteriorly, with two fingers elevating the old incision and pushing the peritoneum and bowel out of the way. If it is ascertained that the kidney itself is directly underneath and adherent to the old incision, it may be best to extend the incision further anteriorly than the old incision and enter a new, previously unoperated area. Entering the peritoneum and approaching the renal pedicle transperitoneally is another technique that may be helpful in the presence of dense perinephric adhesions.

In finding and developing the proper and usual plane of extracapsular dissection between the perinephric fat and renal capsule, dense adhesions may be encountered. The surgeon may find the renal capsule torn and the exploring finger may enter the renal capsule. It is at this point that a subcapsular nephrectomy should be considered.

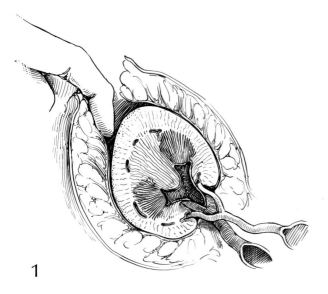

1

1

If it is decided to proceed with subcapsular nephrectomy, continued blunt finger dissection is done gently to free the parenchyma from the overlying capsule. The blunt separation of renal parenchyma from the capsule must be done carefully to avoid tearing the parenchyma, which will result in significant bleeding.

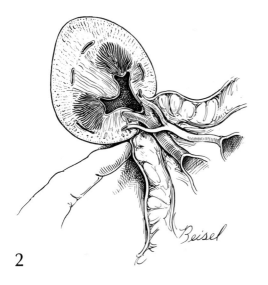

2

2

After the kidney has been fully mobilized within the capsule to the hilum, the renal vessels can be dealt with. It must be remembered that the capsule is adherent at the hilar area and the vessels lie in the renal sinus outside the capsule; that is, the capsule will be between the dissecting finger and the renal vessels.

Once the hilum is reached, the capsule is carefully incised in a circular fashion to expose the vascular pedicle. It is generally best to incise the capsule posteriorly to expose the vessels, since the renal artery lies posterior to the renal vein. First the artery and then the vein should be triply ligated in continuity and divided.

3 & 4

Often, individual vessel ligation will be difficult because of surrounding fibrosis, and in this situation an alternative technique is to excise the majority of the capsule with scissors and actually incorporate the hilar portion of the capsule with the renal vessels within pedicle clamps.

If the capsule is incised posteriorly in the hilar area and the renal artery ligated, it is possible that only the posterior branch of the artery has been ligated and divided. One should use a right-angled clamp and forceps to seek an additional artery or main renal artery before ligating and dividing the renal vein.

All vessels should be triply ligated in continuity with silk before being divided. If gross infection is present, No. 1 chromic ties should be used. After the renal vessels have been secured, excess capsule can be sharply excised and removed to minimize postoperative infection.

After removal of the kidney, the renal fossa should be carefully inspected for haemostasis. The incision is closed using a running locking suture for the transversus layer with interrupted 0 chromic sutures used to approximate the internal and external oblique layers. If a previous incision has been opened, the usual three anatomical layers will be obliterated. In this event, a single-layer closure with interrupted No. 1 chromic suture material is used. Two large 2.5 cm (1 inch) Penrose drains should be led out from the posterior extent of the incision, kept in place for several days and only removed when drainage ceases.

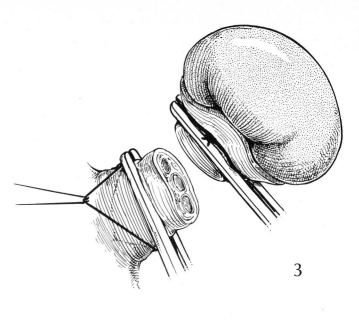

3

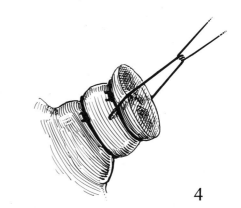

4

References

1. Mathé, C. P. Evaluation of different types of nephrectomy: review of 247 cases. Journal of Urology 1945; 53: 85–96

2. Kittredge, W. E., Fridge, J. C. Subcapsular nephrectomy: comparison of 53 cases with 385 classic nephrectomies. Journal of the American Medical Association 1958; 168: 758–760

3. Kimbrough, J. C., Morse, W. H. Subcapsular nephrectomy. Surgery, Gynecology and Obstetrics 1953; 96: 235–239

4. Young, H. H., Davis, D. M. Young's practice of urology, Vol II. Philadelphia: W. B. Saunders, 1926: 282

Illustrations by Geoff Lyth after M. Mackay

Radical nephrectomy

C. J. Robson MD, FRCS (Can.), FACS
Professor of Urological Surgery, University of Toronto;
Head, Division of Urological Surgery, Toronto General Hospital;
Consultant Urologist, Sunnybrook Hospital,
Hospital for Sick Children and Women's College Hospital, Toronto, Canada

Preoperative

Indications

Radical nephrectomy by definition is the removal *en bloc* of the kidney, the perinephric fat overlying Gerota's fascia, the posterior parietal peritoneum and the adrenal gland. The lymph nodes from the crus of the diaphragm to the bifurcation of the great vessel on the ipsilateral side are also removed, together with the nodes behind, in front and medial to that great vessel. Where possible this is done in continuity with the nephrectomy but in the case of a large tumour the kidney may have to be removed prior to lymph gland dissection because of its size. The prime indication for this type of nephrectomy is adenocarcinoma of the kidney, where the perinephric fat is shown to be involved in 42 per cent of cases, the adrenal in 6 per cent and the lymph nodes in 23 per cent. This operative procedure has also been used in cases of carcinoma of the renal pelvis and nephroblastoma, although with advances in chemotherapy the necessity for dissection of the lymphatic drainage field in the latter case is questionable.

Special contraindications

There have been many case reports of spontaneous disappearance of secondaries from adenocarcinoma of the kidney after removal of the primary; however, the advisability of doing a radical nephrectomy in the presence of multiple known secondaries is questionable. A radical nephrectomy is probably justifiable where a solitary secondary in one lobe of the lung is resectable, because surgery offers the only hope of cure in these cases.

Preoperative preparation

These cases should be staged as completely as possible preoperatively and the preparation should consist of the following.

(*1*) Assessment of the contralateral renal function by a selective creatinine clearance or an isotope study. (*2*) Complete skeletal survey and scan using Technetium-99m. (*3*) CT scan of abdomen and chest. It is now generally accepted that computerized tomography studies of the abdomen give more information than any other single modality or combination. Not only will they show the lines of cleavage or lack of such between the kidney and the surrounding structures e.g. posterior abdominal muscles, liver, spleen etc., but will also show enlarged lymph nodes and involvement of the inferior vena cava when present. CT studies of the lungs are particularly important to pick up early pulmonary metastases and are to be preferred to full lung tomograms. (*4*) Angiography. Although recently there have been papers which have pointed out that angiography was no longer a necessary investigation in these cases, we do not agree with this because one of the most important factors in the improved prognosis of renal cell carcinoma with the thoracoabdominal approach, is the early localization and interruption of the arterial blood supply to the kidney. This is best shown by a flush-type of aortogram which will show the numbers and the location of the artery thus allowing complete avascularization before manipulation of the tumour growth. The coeliac axis should be catheterized also in an attempt to demonstrate the presence or absence of liver metastases. A vena cavagram should also be done in order to demonstrate the involvement of tumour thrombi with the renal vein and/or the cava, and its extent. (*5*) Liver function studies. In about 10 per cent of cases certain liver function tests, e.g. α_2-globulin, alkaline phosphase and prothrombin time, are elevated. Their return to normal levels following nephrectomy is a good prognostic sign, whereas their re-elevation at a later date gives a very poor prognosis.

The operation

Exposure of the kidney

The surgical approach, by whatever route, should allow the surgeon to (a) occlude the renal vessels at a very early stage of the procedure; (b) remove the kidney, together with the overlying peritoneum, Gerota's fascia and the perinephric fat capsule intact; (c) permit access to the lymphatics from the crus of the diaphragm to the pelvic brim. We have routinely used the thoracoabdominal approach through the bed of the 9th or 10th rib except where there has been previous chest disease or where respiratory reserve is low. In such cases we have used a supra-T10 extrapleural approach or, for small tumours in the lower pole, the transperitoneal route.

1

Exposure of renal vessels

The dissection commences on the lateral side of the ascending or descending colon which is routinely displaced towards the midline by the tumour. On the right side the duodenum is also mobilized using the Kocher procedure. The line of dissection is then carried down along the medial aspect of the great vessel of the side involved until the renal vein and renal artery are located. On the left side the superior mesenteric artery must be carefully avoided because it may be displaced by a very large tumour and may be mistaken for the renal artery.

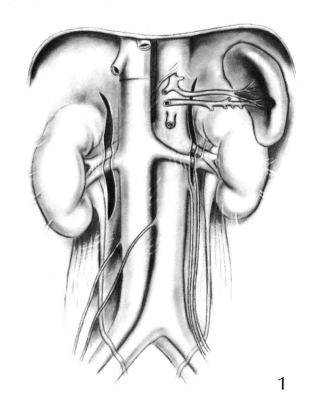

1

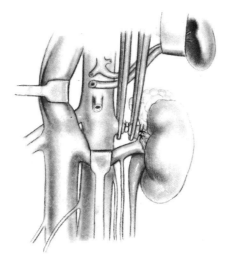

2

2

Clamping of the renal vessels

The renal artery should be occluded prior to the vein wherever possible. This minimizes tumour emboli due to handling of the kidney and change of haemodynamics which result from clamping the vein primarily. This can usually be facilitated by gentle retraction of the renal vein using a long eyelid retractor. A second such instrument may be used to retract the vena cava.

3

This composite drawing shows the left renal vein and the gonadal vein being occluded after the renal artery has been divided. One way of dealing with a thrombus which has involved the vena cava is shown on the right side. After the renal artery has been divided, a Satinsky clamp may be used to occlude the vena cava partially, thus allowing the renal vein and cava to be opened and the tumour-thrombus removed. An alternative method is to occlude the vena cava above and below by vessel clamps and to occlude the opposite renal vein and the lumbar veins draining into that segment of the cava. The cava may then be opened in a longitudinal fashion and the thrombus removed. It is usually free and rarely involves the wall of the cava. The opening in the cava should then be closed using a running waxed silk 6/0 arterial suture.

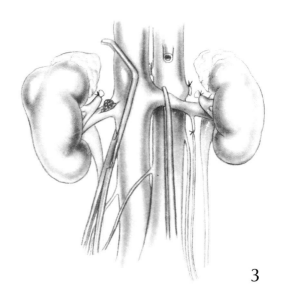

3

Removal of the kidney

The dissection then proceeds, keeping Gerota's fascia intact. Superiorly, the adrenal is included and the blood supply is easily managed using small plastic clips. The ureter is divided in the usual manner and ligated.

4

Node dissection

Node dissection should extend from the crus of the diaphragm to the bifurcation of the aorta on the left and to the inferior end of the vena cava on the right. Lymphatics should be removed in continuity from the lateral side of the great vessel, behind the involved great vessel and between the two great vessels. Lumbar veins may be ligated and divided with impunity but it is wise not to divide more than three lumbar arteries in continuity. Again, large retractors, such as the type shown, are of great use in retracting the vessels. allowing as clean a dissection as possible. On the left side the inferior mesenteric artery may be divided with impunity but this should be done close enough to the aorta to allow the collateral circulation to take over. The operative site has not been drained routinely and where the pleura has been opened, as in the case of a thoracoabdominal incision, the author has not drained the chest unless there were numerous pleural adhesions in the dissection.

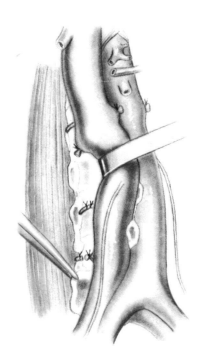

4

Further reading

de Kernion, J. B. Lymphadenectomy for renal cell carcinoma. Urology Clinics of North America, 1980; 7

Peters, P. C., Brown, G. L. The role of lymphadenectomy in the management of renal cell carcinoma. Urology Clinics of North America, 1980; 7

Robson, C. J., Churchill, B. M., Anderson, W. The results of radical nephrectomy for renal cell carcinoma. Journal of Urology, 1969; 101:297–301

Skinner, D. G., de Kernion, J. B. Clinical manifestations and treatment of renal parenchymal tumours. In: Skinner D. C., de Kernion J. B. eds. Genitourinary cancer. Philadelphia: W. B. Saunders, 1978:127

Renal cell cancer with extension into vena cava

John A. Libertino MD
Director of Transplantation, Department of Urology;
Vice Chairman, Division of Surgery, Lahey Clinic Medical Center, Burlington, Massachusetts, USA

Introduction

1

Intracaval tumour thrombus is often a manifestation of advanced renal cell carcinoma. Infrequently it is associated with carcinoma of the adrenal gland and Wilms' tumour. Adenocarcinoma of the kidney involves the inferior vena cava in approximately 5 per cent of patients undergoing surgical treatment for this tumour. The tumour may extend as a small thrombus in the inferior vena cava or as an extensive thrombus into the right atrium. A recent classification of extension of the tumour into the vena cava is shown. Extended survival can be achieved after surgical removal of the vena caval thrombus when distant metastasis is not present and when the perirenal fat and regional nodes are free of tumour.

The diagnosis of vena caval extension should be considered in patients who have a renal tumour, oedema of the lower extremity, varicocele, dilated superficial abdominal veins, albuminuria, recent history of pulmonary embolism, right atrial mass, or perihilar mass associated with a non-functioning kidney seen on intravenous pyelography. These patients should be evaluated preoperatively by intravenous pyelography, computed tomography, aortography, selective renal angiography and inferior venacavography. Occasionally it is necessary to study the inferior vena cava with an injection of contrast material from below and above to determine the exact length of vena caval involvement.

This is clearly indicated in patients who have complete occlusion of the vena cava. In addition to superior venacavography, a right heart study may be warranted in patients who have complete occlusion of the inferior vena cava. Preoperative studies must delineate the proximal and distal limits of involvement of the vena cava to determine the most appropriate surgical approach.

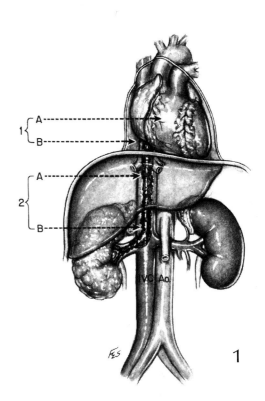

Vena caval thrombus classification
1. Supradiaphragmatic
   A Intracardiac
   B Intrapericardial

2. Infradiaphragmatic
   A Suprahepatic veins
   B Infrahepatic veins

Surgical anatomy

2

Knowledge of the venous drainage of the kidneys and adrenal glands is essential in planning the operative procedure. The right kidney has very little in the way of collateral venous drainage. This is in contrast to the left kidney, which has drainage through the adrenal, lumbar and gonadal vessels. The right kidney has no communication with the gonadal or lumbar systems. This takes on surgical significance when resection of the vena cava is contemplated in conjunction with left radical nephrectomy. It is necessary, then, for the surgeon to create venous outflow for the right kidney by hooking a segment of saphenous vein either from the right renal vein to the vena cava above the point of resection or into the portal vein. This improvisation is usually not necessary on the left side because of the excellent drainage of the left kidney through the lumbar, gonadal and adrenal venous runoff.

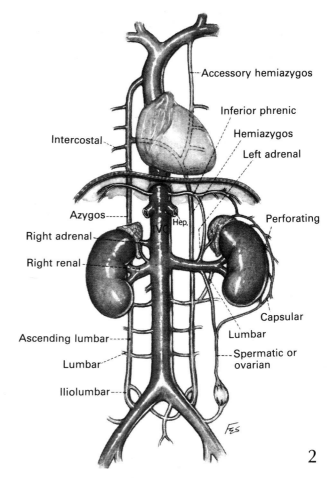

2

Venous system of renal area (schematic)

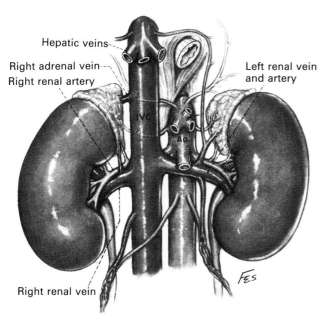

3

3

This is the normal anatomical situation of the inferior vena cava from the renal hilum to the level of the hepatic veins.

4

The relationship of the liver, right triangular ligament, coronary ligament and left triangular ligament to the inferior vena cava is seen here. Also shown is the relationship between the inferior vena cava and the hepatic veins.

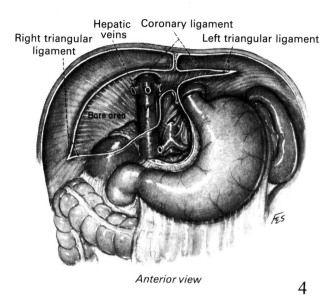

Anterior view

4

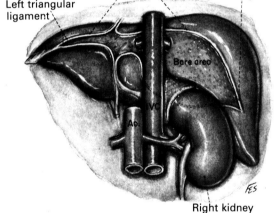

Posterior view

5

5

The same anatomical region as above is viewed here from the posterior aspect. It is necessary to know these anatomical relationships to carry out the intended Langenbeck manoeuvre.

The operation

6

Regardless of whether the tumour arises in the right or left kidney or adrenal gland, we believe this procedure is best carried out through a right 8th or 9th intercostal thoracoabdominal incision. This is primarily a vena caval operation, and this incision provides the best exposure and control of the vena cava. For left-sided renal tumours, it is simple to extend the incision across the midline to remove the left kidney.

In creating this incision, we outline the entire incision but initially open the abdominal portion of the incision to assess operability. During the abdominal exploration it is essential to rule out the presence of hepatic metastases, invasion of the mesocolon, the presence of involved perihilar nodes, or extension of the tumour into the posterior abdominal musculature. The presence of any of these conditions precludes an extensive vena caval procedure as the patient has a poor prognosis. When the abdominal exploration proves that the vena caval procedure is not contraindicated, the thoracic portion of the incision is opened.

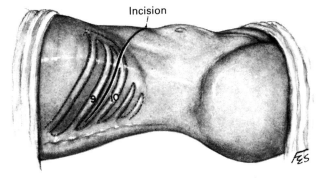

6

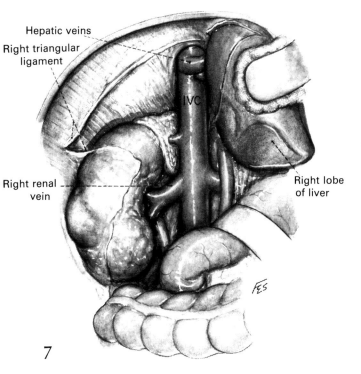

7

7

Most of these tumours which extend into the vena cava arise in the right kidney. Initially the right colon is mobilized from the hepatic flexure along the small bowel mesentery to the ligament of Treitz. The duodenum and head of the pancreas are mobilized by the Kocher manoeuvre. Control of the renal pedicle is achieved with vessel loops placed about the renal artery and vein. At this point the right triangular ligament is divided and the liver is rotated medially like the page of a book. With careful dissection, the major and minor hepatic veins are mobilized. Usually one or two minor hepatic veins are encountered and these can be ligated without difficulty.

8a & b

Before the vena cava itself is mobilized, a DeWeese clip is placed above the tumour thrombus to obviate the possibility of a tumour pulmonary embolus. This clip, which is left in place until the operative procedure is completed, is removed or placed below the left renal vein if the patient has the propensity for the development of pulmonary emboli.

Once the DeWeese clip is secured, umbilical tapes are placed about the vena cava above and below the tumour thrombus and around the left renal vein. The right renal artery is ligated and divided. It is occasionaly necessary to put a microvascular bulldog clamp on the left renal artery as the left renal vein and vena cava are about to be occluded. The need for this is determined by the collateral venous outflow. The Roumel tourniquets are cinched down and the inferior vena cava is opened. The tumour thrombus is extracted as shown (b). Usually this tumour thrombus does not invade the wall of the vena cava except for the region around the ostium of the right renal vein.

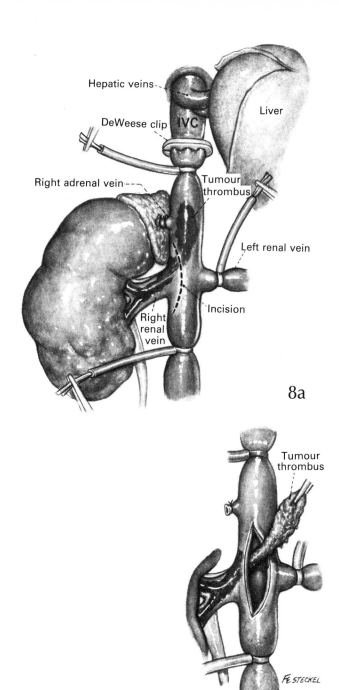

8a

8b

9a & b

Partial cavectomy is carried out by encircling the ostium of the renal vein to ensure that a good cuff of vena cava is removed with the ostium of the renal vein. The venacavotomy is closed with a continuous 5/0 Surgilene suture (b). The Roumel tourniquets on the left renal vein and inferior vena cava are loosened and the microvascular bulldog clamp is removed from the left renal artery.

If the tumour extends above the level of the hepatic veins or is in the intrapericardial portion of the vena cava, the DeWeese clip must be placed at this level. In addition, it may be necessary to place a Fogarty clamp on the porta hepatis to control the arterial inflow to the liver and also across the major hepatic veins to prevent back bleeding when the venacavotomy is created.

When the tumour thrombus extends into the supra-diaphragmatic vena cava, the operative approach is determined by the presence or absence of intra-atrial tumour. When an intra-atrial tumour has not grown, a DeWeese clip is placed about the intrapericardial inferior vena cava and the tumour thrombus is extracted from below the diaphragm using the method already described. Cardiopulmonary bypass is not needed in this situation.

The presence of macroscopic tumour within the right atrium indicates the need for cardiopulmonary bypass with atriotomy. In these patients a Chevron incision combined with median sternotomy provides the best exposure. Cardiopulmonary bypass is not performed until the entire kidney has been mobilized and is attached only by the renal vein. To avoid excessive bleeding, this portion of the procedure must be carried out before the systemic heparinization required for cardiopulmonary bypass.

For cardiopulmonary bypass the heart is cannulated, with the arterial return placed in the ascending aorta and the venous drainage cannulas placed in the superior vena cava and right common femoral vein. Bypass is then instituted. The right atrium is opened and the intra-atrial portion of the tumour is removed. Attention is then directed to the infradiaphragmatic portion of the procedure. After complete removal of the tumour thrombus, the atriotomy and vena cava are sequentially closed and the patient is removed from cardiopulmonary bypass.

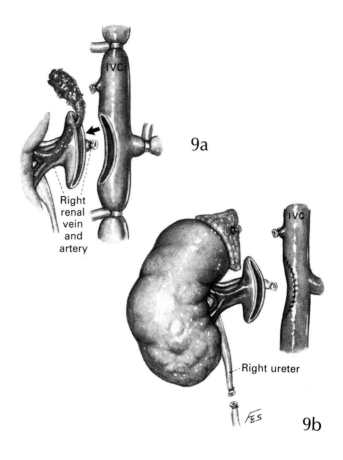

Further reading

Schefft, P., Novick, A. C., Straffon, R. A., Stewart, B. H. Surgery for renal cell carcinoma extending into the inferior vena cava. Journal of Urology, 1978; 120: 28–31

DeWeese, M. S., Hunter Jr, D. C. A vena cava filter for the prevention of pulmonary embolism. Archives of Surgery, 1963; 86: 852–868

Radical nephroureterectomy

Thomas J. Rohner, Jr MD
Professor of Surgery (Urology), Chief, Division of Urology, Pennsylvania State University
College of Medicine and The Milton S. Hershey Medical Center, Hershey, Pennsylvania, USA

Joseph R. Drago MD
Associate Professor of Surgery (Urology), Pennsylvania State University,
College of Medicine and The Milton S. Hershey Medical Center, Hershey, Pennsylvania, USA

Introduction

Total nephroureterectomy was first described and carried out as a planned procedure by Howard Kelly at Johns Hopkins in 1893 for tuberculous stricture of the distal ureter and non-functioning kidney. It is notable that Kelly was unable to remove the distal ureter because of severe periureteral fibrosis. In 1921 Beer provided indications for nephroureterectomy and emphasized the importance of removing the kidney and entire ureter as a single intact specimen. Since then several workers have further documented the need to remove the entire distal ureter, including the intramural portion and a bladder cuff, to prevent local recurrence of urothelial tumours. Reservitz[1] has written an excellent historical review of nephroureterectomy.

Today radical nephroureterectomy includes resection as a single specimen: the kidney, surrounding perinephric fat, Gerota's fascia and the entire ureter, including the intramural ureter and a cuff of bladder surrounding the ureteral orifice. Total nephroureterectomy includes removal of the kidney and ureter without removal of Gerota's fascia and the perinephric fat. The procedure can be and is generally done extraperitoneally through one or two incisions. The survival of patients with transitional cell carcinoma of the ureter or renal pelvis following nephroureterectomy is directly related to the grade and stage of the tumour[2]. There is no clear evidence that a transperitoneal approach or more radical operative procedure offers any therapeutic advantage to the patient.

Preoperative

Indications

Radical nephroureterectomy is primarily indicated for transitional cell tumours arising in the renal collecting system or ureter. It is designed to accomplish two purposes. First, it provides for wide surgical resection of the tumour. Secondly, by removing the entire ipsilateral upper tract, it eliminates the possibility of either recurrent or new transitional cell tumour growth in the collecting system or remaining ureteral stump. The chance of subsequent tumour developing in a remaining portion of the ureter or collecting system is at least 25–30 per cent and is related to the presence of epithelial dysplasia or carcinoma *in situ* in the specimen and the length of ureter remaining[3]. Total nephroureterectomy is also appropriate for those patients with non-functioning kidneys and dilated ureters due to benign causes such as vesicoureteral reflux, impacted distal ureteral calculus, distal ureteral stricture or ureterocele. It often involves patients in the paediatric or young adult age groups.

Diagnosis

It is important to stress that the ultimate success of this operation, when done for urothelial cancer, is complete tumour removal without tumour spillage. For this reason, appropriate preoperative diagnostic studies are important to differentiate and distinguish between calculi and transitional cell tumour. These studies will generally include cystoscopy with retrograde ureteral or renal pelvic washings or brushings for cytology and/or fluoroscopic or plain tomographic evaluation of filling defects in the renal pelvis or calyces. If these studies are inconclusive and a non-opaque uric acid stone is suspected, a trial of urinary alkalinization with sodium bicarbonate for 3–4 weeks is appropriate. If the filling defect persists and a tumour remains highly suspect, radical nephroureterectomy should be done. We do not believe the diagnosis should be confirmed at the time of nephroureterectomy by opening the renal pelvis or carrying out intraoperative nephroscopy, except under unusual circumstances such as a solitary kidney. It is virtually impossible not to spill tumour cells during these procedures, regardless of precautions taken.

Preoperative preparation

This procedure is best carried out under general endotracheal anaesthesia. Two units of whole blood should be typed and cross-matched and preoperative antibiotics are indicated.

The operation

1a & b

Radical nephroureterectomy can be carried out using either a single-incision (a) or two-incision (b) approach. The major advantage of the single incision[4] is that it requires less operating time by eliminating the need to reposition and redrape the patient which is required with the two-incision approach. The major disadvantage of the single incision is that operative exposure of the midureter is best, with poorer exposure at both the upper and lower ends where the best exposure is needed. Access to the renal vessels and the nephrectomy portion of the operation is generally the more compromised portion of the procedure by the one-incision approach. The single incision is best used when initial exploration of the lower or midureter discloses a tumour and the need for nephroureterectomy is recognized, at which point the incision can be extended both superiorly and inferiorly.

The two-incision approach includes mobilization of the kidney and upper ureter through a standard 12th rib flank incision with the patient in the lateral decubitus position, and then, with the patient repositioned in the supine position, a lower-quadrant modified Cherney incision is made to remove the entire specimen including the distal ureter. This approach yields smaller abdominal scars and is especially preferred for paediatric and young patients requiring nephroureterectomy for benign disease. It is also a clear choice for obese patients with high kidneys.

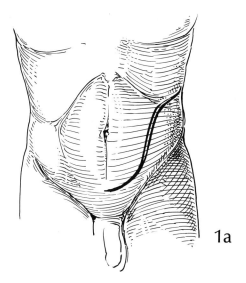

1a

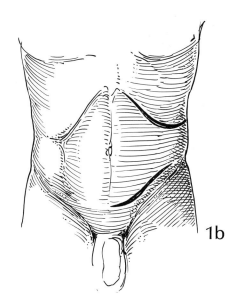

1b

SINGLE-INCISION APPROACH

2

This approach, facilitated by elevating the involved flank to 30°, is made with the operating table slightly flexed and a sandbag placed under the ipsilateral flank to hyperextend the abdomen.

A curved S-shaped skin incision is made from the tip of the 12th rib and carried medial to the anterior superior spine and then to the midline of the abdomen two fingerbreadths above the symphysis. The rectus sheath should be incised just beyond the midline but it is usually not necessary to divide the rectus muscle or aponeurosis. If added medial exposure is necessary to gain access to the bladder, the rectus muscles are separated in the midline and the prevesical space exposed.

The external and internal oblique aponeuroses are incised and the transversus muscle divided. It is easiest to enter the retroperitoneal space just below the anterior superior spine and bluntly retract the peritoneum. After the retroperitoneal space is identified and entered, the peritoneum and its contents are bluntly mobilized and the entire incision is opened by sharp division of all muscle layers.

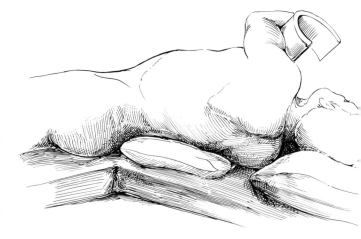

2

3

This extensive incision allows one to reflect the kidney within Gerota's fascia and the perinephric fat laterally to gain exposure of the renal pedicle, using primarily blunt finger dissection.

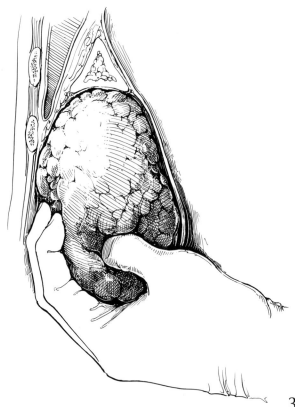

3

4

Attention is directed to the renal vein, which lies anterior to the renal artery. After careful blunt dissection of the vein and ligation and division of its tributaries, including the left gonadal vein and the inferior adrenal vein, the renal vein is elevated using a vein retractor. The renal artery posterior to it is identified, triply ligated in continuity and transected.

The renal vein is then doubly ligated and divided. The lateral aspect of Gerota's fascia is mobilized primarily using blunt finger dissection. Any adherent vessels are divided sharply with scissors between haemostatic clips.

Sharp scissor dissection is used to divide and enter Gerota's fascia at the level of the upper renal pole and blunt finger dissection again used to fully mobilize the upper pole of the kidney. Further blunt finger dissection is used to mobilize the medial and posterior aspect of the kidney. Any resistance encountered to blunt finger dissection is usually due to fibrous bands or minor blood vessels. These should be clipped doubly before being divided.

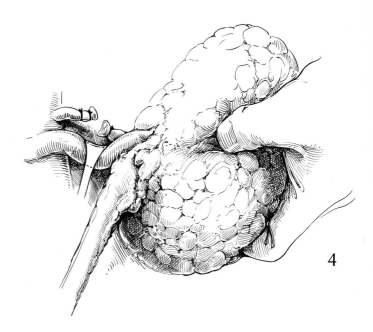

4

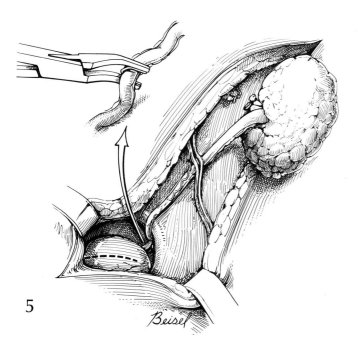

5

5

After division of the major vessels and mobilization of the kidney within Gerota's fascia, the ureter remains intact and is bluntly freed distally. A large Deaver or Willauer retractor is useful to retract the abdominal wall and peritoneal contents to provide exposure of the ureter. It is important to divide small blood vessels supplying the ureter between haemostatic clips to prevent troublesome bleeding. The ureter is mobilized using both sharp and blunt dissection to its most distal extent. The superior vesical artery crosses the ureter just above the point where the ureter enters the bladder. The superior vesical artery should be identified, ligated in continuity and divided. After freeing the ureter to the intramural portion, a large haemostatic clip is placed across the ureter to prevent any tumour dissemination along the ureter.

We prefer to remove the intramural ureter and bladder cuff by opening the bladder and incising the bladder cuff from within the bladder. Extravesical techniques to remove the distal ureter and bladder cuff have been described, but in our experience these provide poor exposure of the area and often result in incomplete removal of the distal ureter and bladder. The intramural ureter and bladder cuff are best removed by making a transverse bladder incision and placing surgical sponges and Deaver retractors in the bladder to visualize both ureteral orifices.

6

A 3/0 chromic suture is used to close the ureteral orifice and provide a means of gentle countertraction. Sharp knife dissection is used to incise the mucosa surrounding the orifice.

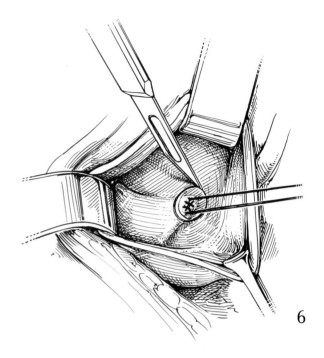

6

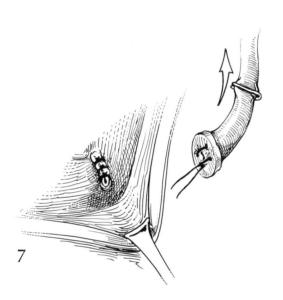

7

7

Sharp and blunt scissor dissection is used to free up the intravesical and intramural segment of the ureter, and this is then passed to the outside behind the bladder. Interrupted 2/0 chromic sutures are placed intravesically to close the muscle hiatus where the ureter has been resected. The cystotomy is closed using a full-thickness running locking 2/0 chromic suture.

After removal of the entire kidney and ureteral specimen, a 1-inch Penrose drain is placed in the renal fossa and led out from the lateral extent of the incision. A second Penrose drain is placed at the bladder base and brought out through a stab wound inferior to the incision. The entire incision is closed using interrupted non-absorbable sutures. A 20 Fr Foley catheter is left in place for 7–10 days. The upper Penrose drain is removed the day following surgery; the lower Penrose drain is removed on day 4 unless urinary drainage is present, in which case it is left in place until it is dry.

TWO-INCISION APPROACH

The patient is placed in the lateral decubitus position with the kidney bar raised and the table flexed. The skin incision is carried over the bed of the 12th rib and the rib identified. A scalpel is used to incise the periosteum and the anterior third of the 12th rib is resected using periosteal elevators and Doyen retractors. The rib is then removed and the bed of the 12th rib incised, with the incision carried medially to incise the external and internal oblique muscles and transversus fascia (see chapter on 'Surgical exposure of the kidney', pp. 21–32). The kidney, surrounded by the perirenal fat and Gerota's fascia, is freed bluntly. Attention is directed to the renal vessels which are identified and ligated in continuity and divided. After division of the renal vessels, the kidney is mobilized bluntly. The ureter is then bluntly freed distally as far as possible through the flank incision, but not divided. A large Deaver retractor in the inferior extent of the wound is helpful in obtaining maximal mobilization of the ureter through this upper incision. It is important to divide vessels supplying the ureter between haemostatic clips. The kidney and upper ureter are then left in a deep inferior position in the wound and the flank incision closed after careful inspection to be certain haemostasis is complete. A Penrose drain is led out through the posterior extent of the wound (and generally removed the day following surgery).

The surgical instruments are now moved away from the sterile operative field. The patient is placed in the supine position and draped after the skin has been prepared. A lower-quadrant modified Cherney curved incision is carried out from the anterior superior spine to the midline, approximately two fingerbreadths above the symphysis pubis. The external and internal oblique muscles are divided and the transversalis fascia is divided. The incision is extended to include the rectus fascia. The rectus muscles are retracted medially but not divided. The retroperitoneal space is entered bluntly and the ureter identified. The ureter is mobilized bluntly with its vessels divided between haemostatic clips. The kidney and previously mobilized upper ureter are brought into this lower incision. From this point on, the distal ureter and bladder cuff are removed, using the intravesical approach in a similar fashion as described for the single-incision approach, including the use of a large haemostatic clip across the ureter to prevent distal tumour dissemination.

References

1. Reservitz, G. B. A historic review of nephroureterectomy. Surgery, Gynecology and Obstetrics 1967; 125: 853–858

2. Bloom, N. A., Vidone, R. A., Lytton, B. Primary carcinoma of the ureter: a report of 102 new cases. Journal of Urology 1970; 103: 590–598

3. Strong, D. W., Pearse, H. D., Tank, E. S., Jr., Hodges, C. V. The ureteral stump after nephroureterectomy. Journal of Urology 1976; 115: 654–655

4. Culp, O. S. Anterior nephroureterectomy: advantages and limitations of a single incision. Journal of Urology 1961; 85: 193–198

Extracorporeal renal surgery

Andrew C. Novick   MD
Chief, Renal Transplant Service, Department of Urology,
Cleveland Clinic Foundation, Cleveland, Ohio, USA

Introduction

Transfer of a kidney from one site to another in the same patient evolved as a logical extension of the field of renal allotransplantation. The first successful autotransplant was performed in 1962 by Hardy[1] in a patient whose ureter had been severely damaged by previous aortic surgery: in 1963, Woodruff[2] achieved the first successful autotransplant for renovascular hypertension. Effective methods of renal preservation and microvascular surgical techniques subsequently resulted in the advent of extracorporeal renal surgery for complex renal disorders. In 1967, Ota[3] reported the first successful extracorporeal renal arterial repair combined with autotransplantation in a patient with renovascular hypertension. A wave of enthusiasm for this approach followed, and many other cases were reported employing varying methods of renal preservation and surgical repair. As increasing experience was gained, more specific indications and contraindications were defined, and renal bench surgery with autotransplantation is now the treatment of choice for selected patients with complicated upper urinary tract disorders.

General considerations

In general, renal bench surgery should be considered when its use will improve the likelihood of a good result, or when *in situ* techniques cannot be performed safely. The current indications for this approach include complicated renovascular disorders, bilateral or solitary renal neoplasms and advanced nephrolithiasis. The advantages of performing extracorporeal repair of the kidney include optimum exposure and illumination, a bloodless surgical field, greater protection of the kidney from ischaemia, more facile employment of microvascular techniques and optical magnification and diminished risk of tumour spillage in cases of carcinoma.

In patients undergoing renal bench surgery, preoperative renal and pelvic arteriography should be performed to define renal arterial anatomy, to ensure relatively disease-free iliac vessels for autotransplantation and, in patients with branch renal artery disease, to evaluate the hypogastric artery and its branches as a reconstructive graft. Autotransplantation of kidneys involved with severe renal parenchymal and/or small vessel disease should be avoided. Such kidneys generally flush poorly following their removal, often leading to irreversible ischaemic damage and nonfunction postoperatively. In patients with bacteriuria, organism-specific parenteral antibiotic therapy is initiated 48 hours preoperatively.

The operations

1

Most extracorporeal renal operations are performed through an anterior subcostal transperitoneal incision to remove the kidney, combined with a separate lower-quadrant, transverse semilunar incision for autotransplantation. Alternatively, in non-obese patients, a single midline incision extending from the xiphoid to the symphysis pubis may be used.

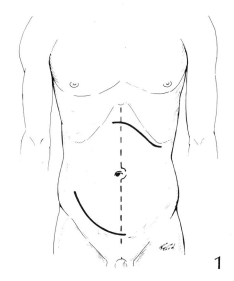

1

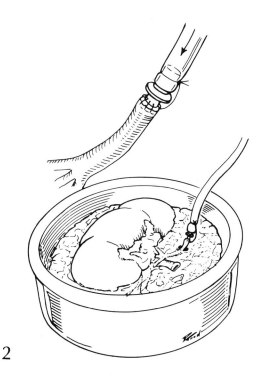

2

2

Immediately following its removal, the kidney is flushed with 500 ml of chilled Collins intracellular electrolyte solution and is then submerged in a basin of ice slush saline to maintain hypothermia. The extracorporeal operation is completed under ice slush surface hypothermia and, if there has been minimal warm renal ischaemia, the kidney can safely be preserved in this manner for many more hours than are needed to perform even the most complex renal repair[4]. In performing renal bench surgery, we have found it cumbersome to work on the abdominal wall with the ureter attached. It is generally preferable to divide the ureter and place the kidney on a separate workbench. This provides better exposure for the extracorporeal operation, facilitates the performance of X-rays and nephroscopy, and allows a second surgical team to prepare the iliac fossa simultaneously. This approach is also justified by the low incidence of complications following ureteroneocystostomy in renal allotransplantation[5]. The vascular techniques for performing autotransplantation of the kidney are identical to those employed in renal allotransplantation, which is discussed in the chapter on 'Renal transplantation', pp. 201–212.

RENOVASCULAR DISEASE

The greatest experience in extracorporeal renal surgery has been gained in the management of complicated renovascular disorders such as preparation of donor kidneys for allotransplantation with anomalous vessels (*see* chapter on 'Renal transplantation', pp. 201–212; and extensive branch renal artery lesions that cannot be repaired *in situ*[3,6–10]. Most branch renal artery lesions are caused by fibrous diseases which occur in young patients and often progress with nonoperative management. Hypertension in these cases is generally difficult to control and revascularization is indicated both to preserve renal function and to minimize the need for long-term antihypertensive therapy[11]. Renal artery aneurysms also frequently involve arterial branches since these are typically located at the bifurcation of the main renal artery. Aneurysmectomy is indicated when these are the cause of significant hypertension, or to obviate the risk of rupture associated with absent or incomplete calcification, size greater than 2 cm, or pregnancy[12]. Renal arteriovenous malformations and traumatic injuries to the vascular pedicle of the kidney are rare indications for revascularization[13,14]. It is distinctly uncommon for atherosclerosis to involve branches of the renal artery.

Extracorporeal branch arterial repair and autotransplantation are indicated primarily when preoperative arteriography with oblique views indicate intrarenal extension of renovascular disease. Removing and flushing the kidney causes it to contract in size, thereby enabling more peripheral dissection in the renal sinus for mobilization of distal arterial branches. In patients with dissecting fibrous lesions, partially calcified aneurysms, or prior renovascular operations, the diseased renal vessels are also more difficult to mobilize *in situ* because of intense surrounding fibrotic reaction and adherence to adjacent hilar structures. Some of these cases are more safely and effectively managed with extracorporeal revascularization.

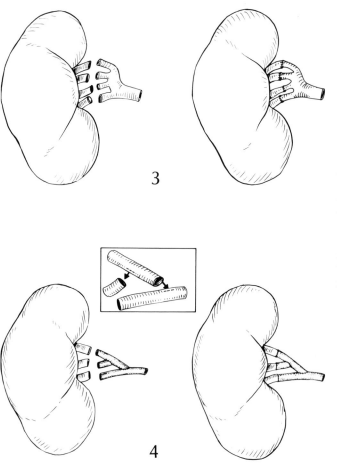

3

4

3 & 4

The most commonly employed method for extracorporeal branch renal artery reconstruction involves procurement and/or fashioning of a branched autogenous vascular graft. This technique permits separate end-to-end microvascular anastomosis of each graft branch to a distal renal arterial branch. A hypogastric (internal iliac) arterial graft is the preferred material for vascular reconstruction since this vessel can be obtained intact with two or more of its branches. When atherosclerotic degeneration precludes use of the hypogastric artery, a long segment of saphenous vein can be harvested and, employing sequential end-to-side microvascular anastomoses, a branched graft can be fashioned from this vessel.

5

Branched grafts of the hypogastric artery and saphenous vein may occasionally prove too large in calibre for anastomosis to small secondary or tertiary arterial branches. In these cases, the inferior epigastric artery provides an excellent alternative free graft for extracorporeal microvascular repair[15]. This artery measures 1.5–2.0 mm in diameter, is rarely diseased, and coapts nicely in calibre and thickness to small renal artery branches. The inferior epigastric artery can also be employed as a branched graft, either by itself or in conjunction with a segment of saphenous vein.

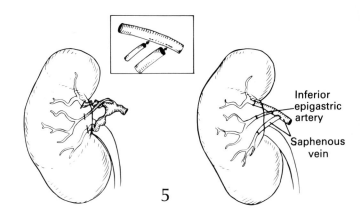

Inferior epigastric artery

Saphenous vein

5

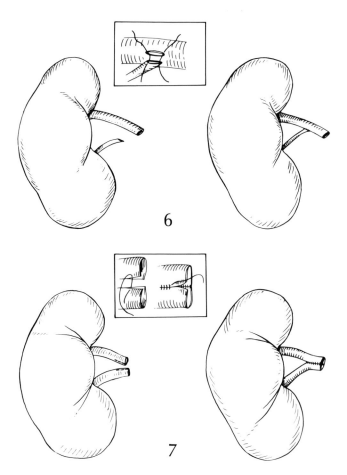

6

7

6 & 7

Although use of a branched autogenous vascular graft provides a simple, versatile, and effective method for branch arterial reconstruction, other techniques are occasionally preferable. In some patients with localized segmental intrarenal branch lesions there may be other arterial branches which are either uninvolved or have more proximally located vascular disease. Such branches with longer disease-free distal segments may be anastomosed end-to-side either into a larger arterial branch or into the reconstructive vascular graft. Occasionally two distal disease-free arterial branches of similar diameter are found adjacent to one another. When this occurs, the two adjacent branches can be conjoined and then anastomosed end-to-end to a single limb of the branched graft.

8 & 9

Renal artery aneurysms have a highly variable presentation, and the method of extracorporeal repair will be determined by whether renovascular involvement is focal or diffuse. If the renal artery wall at the base of an aneurysm is intact, aneurysmectomy with either primary closure or patch angioplasty can be performed. Aneurysms with short focal involvement of renal artery branches may also be simply resected with end-to-end branch reanastomosis. In other cases, with more diffuse vascular disease, aneurysmectomy and revascularization with a branched autogenous graft will be indicated.

Occasionally multiple renal veins are encountered during performance of bench surgery on the kidney. These are less common than multiple renal arteries and occur more frequently in the right kidney. Small renal veins can be simply ligated without risk. When double renal veins of approximately equal size are present, both of these must be preserved to avoid increased intrarenal venous pressure after revascularization. In this situation, extracorporeal venous reconstruction is generally performed with a conjoined anastomosis of the two veins.

These extracorporeal renovascular operations are all performed with the kidney preserved by surface hypothermia in a basin of ice slush saline and employing microvascular instruments, 7/0 to 9/0 suture material and optical magnification. During dissection and mobilization of the renal vessels, care is taken not to interfere with ureteral or pelvic blood supply. While revascularizing multiple arterial branches, one must anticipate the position that the various branches will assume in relation to one another upon completion of the repair. Individual branch anastomoses are then performed with careful attention to avoid subsequent malrotation, angulation or tension.

When extracorporeal repair has been completed, prior to autotransplantation, the kidney is placed on the hypothermic pulsatile perfusion unit. With the perfusion pressure set at the patient's systolic pressure, any arterial anastomotic leaks can be readily identified and controlled. Another useful adjunct is to instill 2 ml of indigo carmine into the arterial cannula: if this is evenly distributed throughout the perfused kidney, patency of all branch anastomoses is verified.

These microvascular reconstructive techniques are technically simple, allow for repair with autogenous tissue grafts, and they involve anastomosis of vessels which are similar in calibre and thickness. In all cases, extracorporeal repair leads to fashioning of a single main renal artery so that autotransplantation may be performed with one arterial anastomosis *in situ* and no increase in the critical revascularization time. Postoperative urethral catheter drainage of the bladder is maintained. However, surgical drains are generally not employed in these cases.

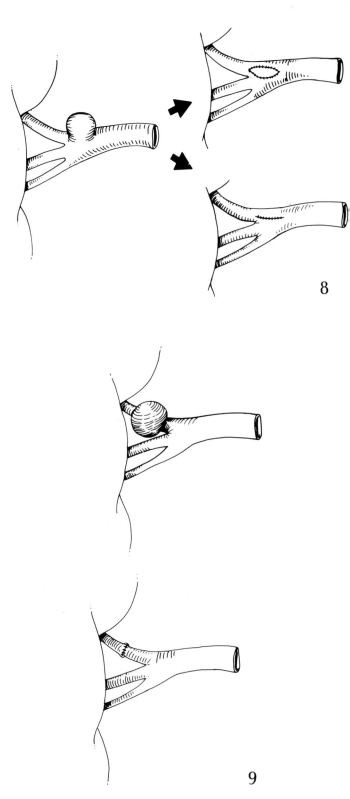

8

9

RENAL TUMOURS

In patients with bilateral synchronous renal malignancies or carcinoma in a solitary kidney, partial nephrectomy represents the primary curative form of treatment[16, 17]. In most cases, this operation can be performed satisfactorily *in situ*: only those patients with large, centrally located renal carcinomas, Wilms' Tumour or transitional-cell renal pelvic tumours will be candidates for extracorporeal partial nephrectomy and autotransplantation[18, 19]. This approach is best reserved for patients with no metastatic disease wherein surgical therapy is undertaken to achieve complete tumour excision. Renal bench surgery offers the advantage of more accurate delineation and removal of the tumour-bearing portion of the kidney with maximal conservation of uninvolved parenchyma. One study has also shown that postoperative local tumour recurrence is less common following extracorporeal partial nephrectomy than when this operation is performed *in situ*[16].

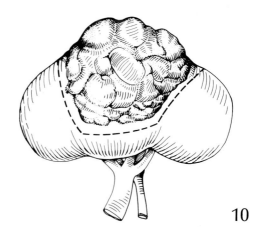

10

10, 11 & 12

Extracorporeal excision of the tumour is performed following *en bloc* radical nephrectomy and regional lymphadenectomy, with the flushed kidney in ice slush saline. These operations may be particularly complicated. Since complete tumour excision may compromise the normal ureteral blood supply, it is best to leave the ureter attached to preserve its inferior collateral vascular supply where possible. When this is done, the ureter must be occluded temporarily to prevent retrograde blood flow to the kidney and rewarming during the extracorporeal operation. Care must also be taken while moving the kidney not to rotate it and risk an obstructive torsion of the ureter. Although the ureter may follow a redundant course to the bladder after autotransplantation, normal ureteral peristalsis will provide effective drainage of urine from the kidney. The flushed kidney is first divested of all perinephric fat in order to appreciate the full extent of the neoplasm. Since such tumours are generally centrally located, dissection is begun in the renal hilus and carried out to the periphery of the kidney. Major arterial and venous channels directed toward the neoplasm are secured and divided, while those vessels supplying uninvolved renal parenchyma are preserved. The overlying capsule and parenchyma are progressively incised to preserve a 2 cm margin of normal renal tissue around the tumour. Microvascular techniques and optical magnification are invaluable aids to securing transected blood vessels and closing the collecting system, generally with interrupted 4/0 or 5/0 chromic sutures.

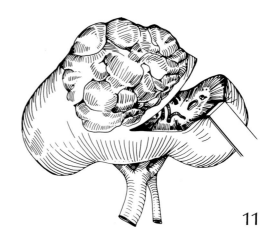

11

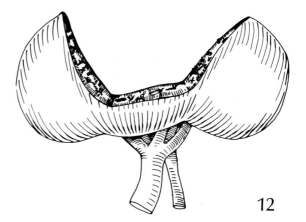

12

13

After completing the resection, tumour-free margins may be verified by frozen sections and/or extracorporeal arteriography. If arteriography is done, iothalamate should be employed rather than diatrazoate contrast material since the latter may crystallize at low temperatures. The kidney should also be reflushed immediately further to obviate toxicity of contrast agents or their cold-induced precipitation[20]. The renal remnant is placed on the pulsatile perfusion unit to assess pressure-flow relationships and to facilitate identification and suture ligation of remaining potential bleeding points. At this stage, the kidney is perfused alternately via the renal artery and vein to ensure both arterial and venous haemostasis. Since the perfusate lacks clotting capacity, there may continue to be some parenchymal oozing which can safely be ignored.

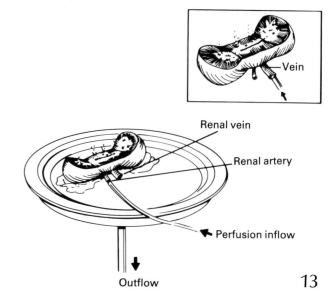

Vein

Renal vein

Renal artery

Perfusion inflow

Outflow   13

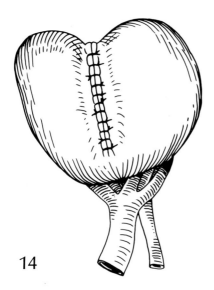

14

14

If possible, the defect created by the partial nephrectomy is closed by suturing the kidney upon itself further to ensure a watertight repair. Following autotransplantation, a Penrose drain is positioned extraperitoneally in the iliac fossa away from the vascular anastomotic sites. When removal of the neoplasm has necessitated extensive hilar dissection of vessels supplying the renal pelvis or ureter, a nephrostomy tube is left indwelling for postoperative drainage.

ADVANCED NEPHROLITHIASIS

The vast majority of patients undergoing surgical therapy for renal calculus disease can be managed satisfactorily with *in situ* anatrophic nephrolithotomy or extended pyelolithotomy. However, in selected patients with advanced nephrolithiasis and failed prior surgical therapy, renal bench surgery and autotransplantation provide the best method for achieving complete stone removal and unobstructed drainage from the upper urinary tract. The indications for this approach in patients with renal calculus disease are: (*1*) recurrent nephrolithiasis with stenosis of the renal pelvis and/or ureter[6]; (*2*) recurrent obstructing ureteral calculi and intractable colic[21]; and (*3*) selected patients with recurrent staghorn calculi, particularly in a solitary kidney[22]. For patients in the first two categories it is often possible to remove the calculi with standard *in situ* methods. The rationale for removing the kidney in these cases is to perform autotransplantation and thereby ensure unobstructed drainage of urine and/or recurrent calculi from the upper urinary tract to the bladder.

Specific advantages of renal bench surgery in patients with stone disease include the superiority of extracorporeal radiography for detection of retained calculi, facilitation of nephroscopy and the ability to extract difficult stones under direct fluoroscopic visualization. In reoperative cases with extensive perihilar fibrosis, the ureter and renal pelvis can be dissected meticulously while preserving their blood supply and avoiding injury to major arterial or venous channels. Also, since the removed flushed kidney contracts in size, more peripheral intrasinusoidal exposure is possible for performing extended pyelolithotomy. This may obviate the need for nephrotomy incisions that would otherwise be required to achieve complete stone removal *in situ*. Preservation of the removed flushed kidney is achieved with surface hypothermia. Pulsatile perfusion in these cases is unnecessary and carries the risk of bacteria and/or tiny stone fragments entering the perfusate and being disseminated into the renal circulation.

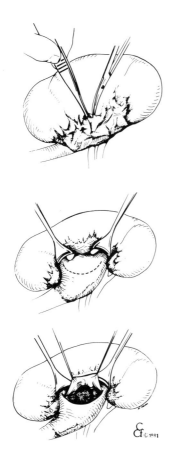

15

The extracorporeal operation begins with mobilization of the renal pelvis and infundibula posteriorly, extending well into the renal sinus. There may be considerable perihilar fibrosis, and meticulous microsurgical dissection is performed to avoid injury to either the collecting system or adjacent renal vessels. The exposure provided by this intrasinusoidal approach is excellent and allows most calculi to be removed with an extended pyelotomy incision. Nephroscopy is a valuable adjunct for locating and removing retained calculi. Direct extraction under fluoroscopy is also available for stones which are small and difficult to find. To preserve renal parenchyma, nephrotomy incisions are reserved for calyceal stones which cannot be removed through a pyelotomy because of severe impaction or a stenotic infundibulum. In the latter case, repair of the intrarenal collecting system is done, as described by Smith and Boyce[23], to ensure unobstructed drainage. One can also inject several millilitres of indigo carmine into renal artery branches to demarcate clearly the most appropriate line for intersegmental incisions into the renal parenchyma. Plain X-rays of the kidney are essential to ensure complete removal of all calculi prior to autotransplantation.

15

16

Following the renal bench operation there are several methods for restoring urinary continuity. Ureteroneocystostomy is the preferred technique when there is an adequate length of unobstructed proximal ureter. In some cases where extensive fibrotic obstruction of the upper ureter is present, the stricture areas are resected and the proximal ureter or renal pelvis is anastomosed to the lower, disease-free ureter. In patients with recurrent renal colic, the entire ureter is resected and pyelovesicostomy is performed by fashioning a Boari bladder flap over a 22 Fr catheter for anastomosis to the renal pelvis. This facilitates passage of subsequent calculi directly to the bladder. Following autotransplantation a Penrose drain is positioned in the iliac fossa and a urethral catheter is left in the bladder. Nephrostomy drainage is employed in selected cases where extensive upper urinary tract reconstruction has been performed.

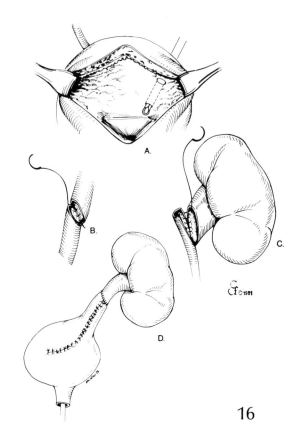

16

Postoperative care

Within the first 24 hours postoperatively, a technetium renal scan is obtained to verify perfusion of the autotransplanted kidney. Subsequent radioisotope monitoring is performed with ^{131}I orthoiodohippurate, which provides a functional assessment of the autograft. In the absence of postoperative vasomotor nephropathy, this scan will show prompt uptake, early excretion and complete clearance of isotope from the graft. Urethral catheter drainage of the bladder is maintained for one week postoperatively. Patients are then instructed to void at least every 2 hours and the Penrose drain, if present, is gradually removed over the next 48 hours. When a nephrostomy tube has been employed, a gravity nephrostogram is performed prior to its removal to document free flow into the bladder without extravasation. Prior to the patient's discharge from hospital, digital subtraction angiography of the pelvis is obtained following intravenous administration of 30 ml of contrast material[24]. This provides an excellent noninvasive method for evaluating main arterial patency of the autograft. In patients undergoing extracorporeal branch renal artery reconstruction, conventional pelvic arteriography is performed to evaluate more accurately the intrarenal microvascular anastomoses. A standard intravenous pyelogram is obtained 6 weeks postoperatively to ensure unobstructed urinary drainage from the autograft.

Acknowledgement

Illustrations 3–11 are reproduced from Novick[25].

References

1. Hardy, J. D. High ureteral injuries: management by autotransplantation of the kidney. Journal of the American Medical Association 1963; 184: 97–101

2. Woodruff, M. F. A., Doig, A., Donald, K. W., Nolan, B. Renal autotransplantation. Lancet 1966; 1: 433

3. Ota, K., Mori, S., Awane, Y., Ueno, A. *Ex situ* repair of renal artery for renovascular hypertension. Archives of Surgery 1967; 94: 370–373

4. Novick, A. C., Magnusson, M. O. Extracorporeal and *in situ* renal preservation. In: Novick, A. C., Straffon, R. A., eds. Vascular problems in urologic surgery. Philadelphia, London: W. B. Saunders, 1982: 73–81

5. Novick, A. C., Braun, W. E., Magnusson, M. A., Stowe, N. Current status of renal transplantation at the Cleveland clinic. Journal of Urology 1979; 122: 433–437

6. Gil-Vernet, J. M., Casalps, A., Revert, L., Andreu, J., Carretero, P., Figuls, J. Extracorporeal renal surgery. Workbench surgery. Urology 1975; 5: 444–451

7. Lawson, R. K., Hodges, C. V. Extracorporeal renal artery repair and autotransplantation. Urology 1974; 4: 532–539

8. Lim, R. C., Eastman, A. B., Blaisdell, F. W. Renal autotransplantation. Adjunct to repair of renal vascular lesions. Archives of Surgery 1972; 105: 847–852

9. Novick, A. C., Straffon, R. A., Stewart, B. H. Surgical management of branch renal artery disease. *In situ* versus extracorporeal methods of repair. Journal of Urology 1979; 123: 311–316

10. Salvatierra, O., Olcott, C., Stoney, R. J. *Ex vivo* renal artery reconstruction using perfusion preservation. Journal of Urology 1978; 119: 16–19

11. Novick, A. C., Stewart, B. H. Surgical treatment of renovascular hypertension. Current Problems in Surgery 1979; 16: 1–74

12. Poutasse, E. F. Renal artery aneurysms. Journal of Urology 1975; 113: 443–449

13. Pfeffermann, R. A., Kate, S., Shapiro, A., Durst, A. L. Successful repair of combined renal pedicle injury: a new application of the *ex vivo* 'Bench' technique. Israel Journal of Medical Science 1980; 16: 724–728

14. Gutman, F. M., Homsy, Y., Schmidt, E. Avulsion injury to the renal pedicle: successful autotransplantation after bench surgery. Journal of Trauma 1978; 18: 469–471

15. Novick, A. C. Use of inferior epigastric artery for extracorporeal microvascular branch renal artery reconstruction. Surgery 1981; 89: 513–517

16. Jacobs, S. C., Berg, S. E., Lawson, R. K. Synchronous bilateral renal cancer: total surgical excision. Cancer 1980; 46: 2341–2345

17. Novick, A. C., Stewart, B. H., Straffon, R. A., Banowsky, L. H. Partial nephrectomy in the treatment of adenocarcinoma. Journal of Urology 1977; 118: 932–936

18. Novick, A. C., Stewart, B. H., Straffon, R. A. Extracorporeal renal surgery and autotransplantation: indications, techniques and results. Journal of Urology 1980; 123: 806–811

19. Pettersson, S., Brynger, H., Johansson, S., Nilson, A. E. Extracorporeal surgery and autotransplantation for carcinoma of the pelvis and ureter. Scandinavian Journal of Urology and Nephrology 1979; 13: 89–93

20. Alfidi, R. J., Magnusson, M. O. Arteriography during perfusion preservation of kidneys. American Journal of Radium Therapy and Nuclear Medicine 1972; 114: 690–695

21. Olsson, C. A., Idelson, B. Renal autotransplantation for recurrent renal colic. Journal of Urology 1980; 123: 467–474

22. Andersen, O. S., Clark, S. S., Marlett, M. M., Jonasson, O. Treatment of extensive renal calculi with extracorporeal surgery and autotransplantation. Urology 1976; 7: 465–469

23. Smith, M. J. V., Boyce, W. H. Anatrophic nephrotomy and plastic calyrhaphy. Journal of Urology 1968; 99: 521–527

24. Meaney, T. F., *et al*. Digital subtraction angiography of the human cardiovascular system. American Journal of Radium Therapy and Nuclear Medicine 1980; 135: 1153–1160

25. Novick, A. C. Renal bench surgery. In: Glenn, J., ed. Urologic Surgery, 3rd ed. New York: Lippincott, 1983: 137–147

Renal biopsy

T. M. Barratt MB, FRCP
Consultant Paediatric Nephrologist, Hospital for Sick Children, Great Ormond Street, London;
Professor of Paediatric Nephrology, Institute of Child Health, London, UK

Introduction

The introduction of percutaneous renal biopsy in 1951 by Iversen and Brun[1], its widespread application in adults[2] and its use in children[3-5] have led to a new understanding of renal pathology, particularly in the field of glomerulonephritis. Considerable skill, which may only be achieved by continued experience, is required for both the safe collection and reliable interpretation of renal biopsy material. For this reason, the technique should be restricted to centres which undertake at least 25 renal biopsies a year and which have the services of a pathologist with an informed interest in the histology of renal disease.

Many investigators use the Silverman needle. It is essential to have Franklin's modification[2], in which the pointed tip of each hollowed prong is filled with silver solder, obviating the need for rotation of the needle. The instrument has been further modified for children by White[6]. A particular improvement of this model is the use of aluminium alloy to reduce the weight, and the length of the biopsy may also be adjusted. These needles have a limited life and should be discarded after some 10 to 20 biopsies. Great care is required during cleaning so that the inner prongs are not distorted. Good results are also obtained with a disposable modification, the Vim Tru-Cut[7]. Beginners find the technique easier to learn with this needle than with the standard Silverman model, and it is

this equipment which appears in the illustrations below. The disposable model may in fact be reused after ethylene oxide sterilization.

The safety of the procedure and the quality of the biopsy are much improved if the kidney is located during the procedure by fluoroscopy using an image intensifier[8], and adequate tissue should be obtained by these techniques in at least 95 per cent of cases. Alternatively, the biopsy needle may be guided by ultrasound, which gives a better indication of the depth of the kidney. This technique is more suitable for cases in which renal function is poor and urographic visualization therefore unsatisfactory.

It is not appropriate to specify precisely the indications for renal biopsy; as information accumulates on the various forms of glomerulonephritis, so the need for histological definition of the lesion in each individual patient varies. It is unwise to attempt percutaneous renal biopsy in a solitary functioning kidney or in an individual with a haemorrhagic diathesis. Hypertension should be controlled before biopsy, and the risks are increased in the uraemic state. A urogram or isotope scan should be obtained before the biopsy and bleeding time, clotting time and platelet counts checked. The blood group should be ascertained, and blood cross-matched beforehand. Informed consent must be obtained.

The operation

1

Local anaesthesia with sedation is satisfactory in most cases, although in younger or particularly apprehensive children general anaesthesia may be preferable. The patient lies prone on an X-ray table with a radiolucent cushion under the abdomen. An intravenous injection of contrast medium is given and the kidneys located on the television screen during the nephrographic phase 2–3 min later. The biopsy site is selected in the lower pole about 1 cm from the margin of the kidney. A small skin incision is made and the biopsy needle inserted with the central needle covered by the outer sheath. It is safer if the patient does not breath while the needle is advanced into the kidney. The tip of the needle should just penetrate the renal capsule – this can be felt more easily with the standard Silverman needle than with the sharper disposable model – and its position is then checked fluoroscopically. If the needle is in the kidney, its tip will move exactly synchronously with the renal shadow during respiratory excursions.

2

The central needle is advanced into the kidney.

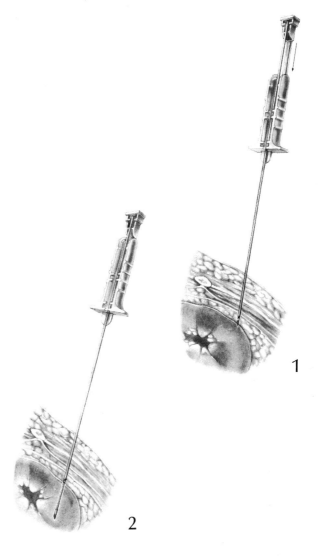

1

2

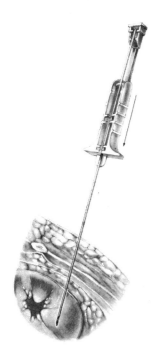

3

3

The top of the needle is then held still while the outer sheath is advanced downwards to cut the biopsy tissue. This manoeuvre is the most difficult of the whole procedure: a common error is to withdraw the central needle rather than to advance the outer sheath, or to fail to cover the needle with the outer sheath before withdrawal from the kidney. The latter results in traumatizing the biopsy specimen and tearing the kidney, with an increased risk of haemorrhage. Only one kidney should be biopsied and not more than three attempts at biopsy of this kidney should be permitted at one session.

It is worth observing that the manufacturer's package insert recommends a slightly different technique for the disposable needle: the needle covered by the outer sheath is inserted into the kidney to the full intended depth of the biopsy, which is then cut out by withdrawal and readvancement of the sheath while the central needle is held still. The author has tried both methods and prefers the version illustrated.

Postoperative care

After biopsy the patient should remain in bed for 24 hours. The pulse and blood pressure should be observed regularly and a high fluid intake maintained.

The most common complication is haemorrhage, either retroperitoneal or into the urinary tract, where it may cause clot colic. In experienced centres the incidence of haemorrhage requiring transfusion is low, somewhat less than 1 per cent[8]. Occasional cases of infarction of the kidney have been described, necessitating nephrectomy[9], and in Kark's survey[7] the mortality was 0.07 per cent. Intrarenal arteriovenous fistulae have been reported following needle biopsy[10], and may sometimes be suspected by the detection of a bruit over the affected kidney. In some instances these fistulae have regressed spontaneously. They should therefore be managed conservatively but may occasionally require embolization. There is no doubt that the incidence of complications is lower in experienced hands.

SPECIMEN HANDLING

It is an advantage to have a dissecting microscope available in the biopsy room so that the presence of glomeruli may be ascertained immediately. The biopsy specimen requires special handling and the pathologist should always be consulted beforehand. For light microscopy the tissue should immediately be placed in special fixatives. The sections should be cut 2μm or less thick and several histological stains are required. The presence of immunoglobulin, complement or fibrinogen in glomeruli may be demonstrated by immunofluorescence using fluorescin-conjugated antisera. For this purpose, snap-frozen biopsy material is usually required. Further diagnostic information may be obtained by electron microscopy, or by light microscopic examination of ultrathin sections of tissue embedded in epoxy resin, as for electron microscopy[11]. The range of techniques required for the complete examination of renal biopsy specimens is wide, and renal biopsy should not be performed in centres without access to these methods.

References

1. Iverson, P., Brun, C. Aspiration biopsy of kidney. American Journal of medicine 1951; 11: 324–330

2. Kark, R. M., Muehrcke, R. C. Biopsy of kidney in prone position. Lancet 1954; 1: 1047–1049

3. Vernier, R. L., Forquhar, M. G., Brunson, J. G., Good, R. A. Chronic renal disease in children. Correlation of clinical findings with morphologic characteristics seen by light and electron microscopy. American Journal of Diseases of Children 1958; 96: 306

4. Dodge, W. F., Daeschner, C. W., Brennan, J. C., Rosenberg, H. S., Travis, L. B., Hopps, H. C. Percutaneous renal biopsy in children. 1. General considerations. Pediatrics 1962; 30: 287–296

5. White, R. H. R. Observations on percutaneous renal biopsy in children. Archives of Diseases in Childhood 1963; 38: 260–266

6. White, R. H. R. A modified Silverman biopsy needle for use in children. Lancet 1962; 1: 673

7. Kark, R. M. Renal Biopsy. Journal of the American Medical Association 1968; 205: 220–226

8. Edelmann, C. M., Greifer, I. A modified technique for percutaneous needle biopsy of the kidney. Journal of Pediatrics 1967; 70: 81–86

9. Muecke, E. C., Marshall, V. F., eds. Conferences in paediatric urology. Baltimore: Williams and Wilkins Co, 1965: 48

10. De Beukelaer, M. M., Schreiber, M. H., Dodge, W. F., Travis, L. B. Intrarenal arteriovenous fistulas following needle biopsy of the kidney. Journal of Pediatrics 1971; 78: 266–272

11. Eastham, W. N., Essex, W. B. Use of tissues embedded in epoxy resin for routine histological examination of renal biopsies. Journal of Clinical Pathology 1969; 22: 99–106

Illustrations by Susan I. Klug

Renal ectopia
Pelvic kidney, crossed fused ectopia, horseshoe kidney

George W. Kaplan   MD, FACS, FAAP
Clinical Professor of Surgery/Urology, School of Medicine, University of California, San Diego;
Chief of Pediatric Urology, University of California, San Diego;
Senior Staff, Children's Hospital and Health Center, San Diego, California, USA

William A. Brock   MD, FACS, FAAP
Associate Clinical Professor of Surgery/Urology, School of Medicine, University of California, San Diego;
Chief of Urology, Children's Hospital and Health Center, San Diego, California, USA

Introduction

An ectopic kidney is one that does not occupy its normal lumbar position because of a developmental abnormality of fusion or ascent. The kidneys normally lie at a higher retroperitoneal level than their embryological site of origin within the true pelvis. As 'ascent' occurs, each kidney undergoes medial rotation on its vertical axis, obtaining its blood supply from adjacent vessels – the middle sacral, external iliac and common iliac arteries, and finally, the aorta. The exact aetiology of fusion or position anomalies is not known and may include fusion of the two nephrogenic cords, origin of two kidneys from a single nephrogenic cord, aberrant vasculature or abnormal ureteric buds.

The majority of ectopic or fused kidneys are clinically asymptomatic. If ascent does not occur normally, however, the resulting abnormality of position or rotation of the kidney, the anomalous origin and course of the vasculature to the ectopic kidney, or the unusual course of the ureter draining an ectopic kidney may result in a much higher incidence of impaired ureteropelvic junction drainage. Thus, nephrectomy of the severely hydronephrotic half of a horseshoe kidney, pyeloplasty or pyelolithotomy are the procedures performed most commonly on ectopic or fused kidneys.

Thorough preoperative knowledge of the anatomy of the collecting systems and the number and location of the renal vessels is critical in the surgical management of the fused or ectopic kidney. In addition, because of the high incidence of contralateral renal anomalies (including absence) and associated gynaecological disorders, the status of the entire genitourinary system must be ascertained before treatment.

Intravenous pyelography with tomography, supplemented by retrograde ureteropyelograms as needed, will usually suffice to delineate the anatomy of the collecting system. The most important feature affecting surgery of the horseshoe kidney or the fused kidney, however, is the anomalous vasculature. This usually will require angiography before surgery to prevent intraoperative catastrophe or loss of otherwise salvageable renal parenchyma.

Anatomy

1

Simple ectopic kidneys

The ectopic kidney is usually differentiated from the ptotic kidney by the fact that a short ureter and retroperitoneal vascular fixation preclude placement of the ectopic kidney in its normal position[1]. In contrast, the thoracic kidney has a ureter which is generally longer than normal. The *simple ectopic kidney* lies on the same side of the midline as it normally would but in a position inferior or superior to its usual location adjacent to the second lumbar vertebra, i.e. thoracic, lumbar or pelvic. The ureter of the simple ectopic kidney enters the bladder on the same side as the ectopic kidney. The simple pelvic kidney lies anterior to the sacrum below the aortic bifurcation. The simple lumbar kidney is found opposite the sacral promontory anterior to the iliac vessels[2, 3]. The simple ectopic kidney is found in either the lumbar or pelvic positions with equal frequency (approximately 1 in 850 urological admissions or 1 in 920 autopsies)[4]. The ectopic pelvic or lumbar kidney is usually smaller than normal with an anteriorly located irregular pelvis which may drain extrarenal calyces.

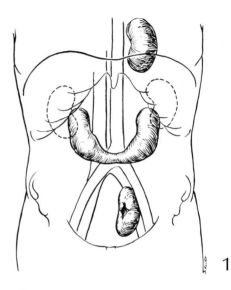

1

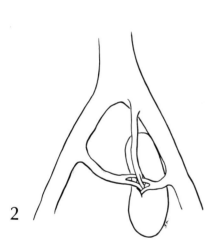

2

2

Vasculature

The vasculature to the pelvic or lumbar kidney is variable: arteries may arise from the aorta, the common iliac artery, the external iliac artery, the internal iliac artery, the inferior mesenteric artery or the median sacral arteries[1, 5]. Usually there are several individual major vessels supplying various segments of the pelvic or lumbar kidney. The blood supply may arise from the major vessels in the area in which the ectopic kidney finally comes to lie, or, in some cases of crossed ectopia, it may arise from the side of origin and cross over with the kidney. Because of the variability and multiplicity of the blood supply to ectopic kidneys, angiography is a most useful preoperative aid.

3

Crossed ectopic kidneys

In addition to simple ectopia, an ectopic kidney may be 'crossed', in which case it lies across the midline from its normal position and may or may not be fused with its contralateral mate. In crossed fused or unfused ectopia the ureter draining the ectopic kidney crosses the midline to enter the bladder on the normal side. Crossed ectopia with fusion occurs once in every 1000 urological admissions; crossed ectopia without fusion occurs once in every 2200 urological admissions. The left kidney more frequently crosses over to the right side (3:2 ratio) and lies inferior to the normally positioned kidney[4]. Ninety-five per cent of all crossed fused ectopic kidneys exhibit this unilateral inferior ectopic configuration. As can be seen from *Illustration 3*, the renal pelvis can be oriented in a variety of directions with anteromedial orientation occurring most commonly. The blood supply is variable and may arise from the side of origin of the crossed ectopic kidney or from the vessels in the area of the kidney's final position. The number of vessels to the kidney also varies widely. The vasculature to the contralateral normal kidney is anomalous in a high percentage of cases[6].

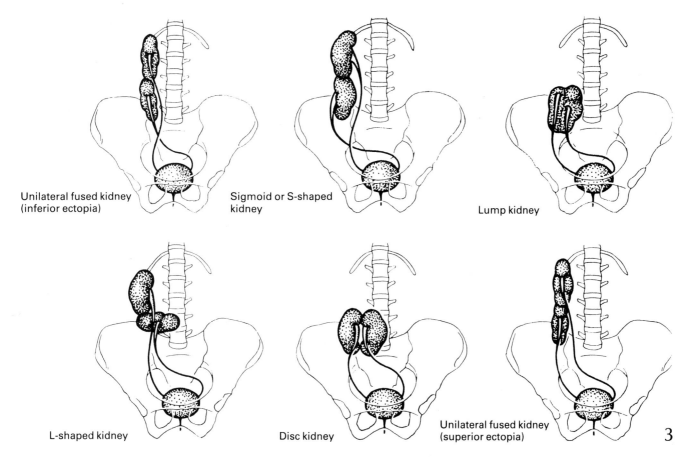

Unilateral fused kidney
(inferior ectopia)

Sigmoid or S-shaped
kidney

Lump kidney

L-shaped kidney

Disc kidney

Unilateral fused kidney
(superior ectopia)

3

(Reproduced from McDonald, J. H., McClelland, D. S. American Journal of Surgery 1957; 93: 995–1002)

4

Thoracic kidneys

The thoracic kidney is rare. It was encountered in only 2 of 15 919 autopsies[7]. The majority of thoracic kidneys are left-sided and function normally[8]. The major significance of the thoracic kidney lies in the differential diagnosis of a posterior mediastinal or thoracic mass[9]. Most thoracic kidneys are infradiaphragmatic and not within the pleural cavity. They are usually separated from the pleural cavity by a thin membranous segment of diaphragm. The anatomical features of the thoracic kidney include: (1) rotational anomaly about the long axis of the kidney; (2) medial deviation of the lower pole of the kidney; and (3) a long ureter. The renal vessels have been reported to arise from their normal position or from a position slightly higher on the aorta than normal[10].

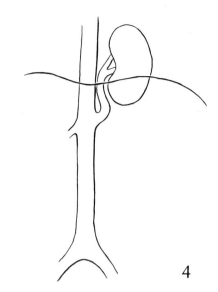

4

5

Horseshoe kidneys

The horseshoe kidney is the most common form of renal fusion anomaly and occurs second only to ureteral duplication as an upper urinary tract variant. Horseshoe kidneys are found once in every 400–500 births[11]. The horseshoe kidney is located at the level of the 3rd or 4th lumbar vertebra with its isthmus or point of fusion lying astride the vertebral column. The fact that 89–99 per cent of horseshoe kidneys are fused at their lower poles accounts for the characteristic medial deviation of the lower poles of the kidney seen on intravenous urography[12, 13]. The isthmus is usually composed of functioning renal parenchyma of variable thickness but may be represented by a simple fibrous strand. It usually lies anterior to the great vessels but has rarely been reported to lie between or posterior to them[12]. The renal pelves are often anteriorly placed, in which case the ureters cross over the anterior surface of the isthmus to which they may be bound closely. High insertion of the ureter into the renal pelvis is a common finding. If the pelves are laterally rotated, the ureters may be widely separated. If the fusion between the lower poles is to one side (lateral fusion) rather than midline (midline fusion) there is a greater likelihood that one of the pelvicalyceal systems will drain tissue that extends across the midline and a higher incidence of associated hydronephrosis[14]. Preoperative definition of the situation by retrograde pyelography or intraoperative recognition of the anatomy is quite important if division of the isthmus is to be undertaken without leaving behind an undrained segment of renal tissue and collecting system.

The blood supply of the horseshoe kidney is variable and may be asymmetrical. Graves has reported the basic

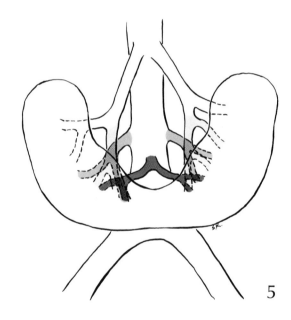

5

patterns of blood supply to the horseshoe kidney[5, 15]. A single main renal artery may supply each half of the horseshoe kidney with subsequent branches supplying the upper, middle and lower segments. Alternatively, the lower segments may be supplied by separate arteries arising directly from the aorta or as a single common stem vessel which then divides to enter the lower segments. Vessels to the lower segment may also arise inferiorly from the area of the aortic bifurcation or from the common iliac arteries. The most frequent of these patterns are shown.

6

Blood supply to the isthmus

The renal isthmus may be supplied by branches from the lower segment or more commonly by vessels arising from the aortic bifurcation and entering posteriorly as unilateral or bilateral single or multiple vessels. These posterior and inferior vessels may occur in addition to other vessels supplying the isthmus from above. Occasionally they will arise from the common iliac vessels or rarely from the hypogastric or middle sacral arteries. Indeed, in rare instances, the entire blood supply to both renal segments of the horseshoe kidney may enter through the isthmus. Intraoperative knowledge of the arterial anatomy is critical to successful surgery in the area of the isthmus (removal of one-half of horseshoe kidney or symphysiotomy). Preoperative angiography coupled with meticulous dissection in this area and direct intra-arterial injection of indigo carmine is often necessary to prevent unnecessary haemorrhage as well as inadvertent devascularization of the renal parenchyma that is to remain behind.

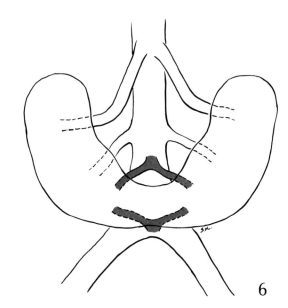

6

Treatment of horseshoe kidney

The majority of cases of fusion anomalies or renal ectopia are asymptomatic and require no treatment. However, the combination of rotational abnormality of the renal pelvis and the anomalous course of the ureter anterior to renal parenchyma means that hydronephrosis is a significant occurrence. Because of the poor drainage, renal calculi are commonly found. Approximately 25 per cent of horseshoe kidneys will require some form of surgical treatment[11, 15, 16]. The operation performed most commonly in the past has been removal of one-half of the fused or horseshoe kidney. Pyelolithotomy and pyeloplasty have been the procedures most commonly employed when nephrectomy is not necessary[4, 5, 15, 16]. The operative approach for these three procedures is to a large part determined by the position and degree of renal fusion as well as by the accompanying disease[4].

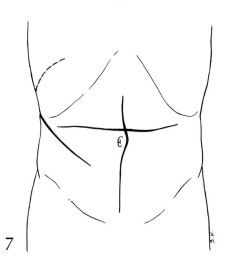

7

7

Choice of incision

In cases of crossed ectopia or simple lumbar ectopia, in which the renal mass lies above the sacral promontory, the standard extraperitoneal flank incision or lower quandrant Gibson incision may be employed. Both of these incisions may be extended toward or across the midline as necessary during the procedure. Lateralized incisions such as these may prove limiting during the operation, as the isthmus may not be well exposed initially or may drop from view (and control) if it is divided. A transverse or midline transperitoneal incision affords excellent exposure and access to the deep pelvic kidney or the fused renal mass that lies at or below the sacral promontory. This is especially useful when isthmic dissection will be necessary as it allows for better definition of the vascular anatomy as well as control of both halves of the isthmus after division.

Because of the high incidence of contralateral renal abnormality when a pelvic kidney is present, it is necessary to define the presence and normality of the contralateral kidney. Unknowing removal of a solitary pelvic kidney is a disaster that has faced some surgeons in the past.

8

Flank incision and exposure

The patient is placed in the lateral decubitus position as for standard flank surgery or, if the renal mass is low enough, the patient may be placed supine with the side of incision elevated on towels and the upper torso twisted medially. Because of the generally lower position of the fused renal mass, a standard flank incision can be started laterally at or below the tip of the 12 rib. More superiorly placed incisions will limit exposure and require greater degrees of inferomedial extension. Once the skin has been divided, we prefer to use the pure cutting current of the electrosurgical unit for division of the underlying external and internal oblique muscles. In dividing the internal oblique muscle in the line of the skin incision, care must be taken to avoid injury to the subcostal nerves which run beneath it and above the transversus abdominus muscle. After exposure of the transversus abdominus it is bluntly entered at the most lateral extent of the incision, taking care to avoid entry into the peritoneal cavity. In children, the peritoneum may extend further laterally and posteriorly than in adults so that the surgeon must use caution to avoid celiotomy. The peritoneum is then bluntly swept off the posterior surface of the transversus abdominus with the finger tip or a Kütner (peanut) dissector in a medial direction. After the peritoneum has been completely swept medially, the transversus abdominus muscle is bluntly or sharply divided, exposing the kidney. A self-retaining Balfour retractor or several Deaver retractors placed over moistened gauze pads provide adequate exposure of the

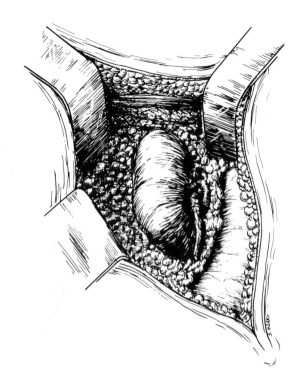

8

kidney. There is often a paucity of perinephric fat surrounding fused or ectopic kidneys and Gerota's fascia may be absent. The adrenal gland, since it has a different embryological origin, is not necessarily situated astride the upper pole of an ectopic or fused kidney.

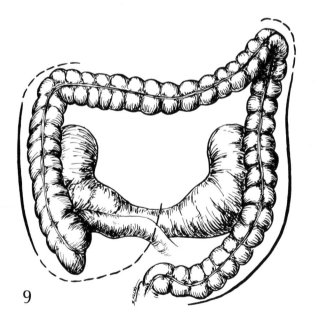

9

9

Transabdominal incision

For a midline or transverse transabdominal (transperitoneal) incision, the patient is placed in the supine position. If the midline incision is employed, the linea alba is divided and care is taken to avoid injury to underlying intestine – especially if there are adhesions from previous surgery. The transverse abdominal incision should be placed a short distance above the umbilicus and should extend from at least the midclavicular line on either side. The ends of the incision may be gently sloped in a chevron fashion to avoid the margins of the lower costal cartilage and to allow more secure wound closure. Once the peritoneal cavity has been entered, the intestines are packed superiorly and a self-retaining ring retractor is placed. Depending on the site and type of disease, the posterior peritoneum may be incised along an avascular plane lateral to the right or left colon.

10

Transperitoneal exposure of right kidney

On the right side, the incision can be extended in a reverse 'J' fashion back up the root of the small bowel mesentery toward the renal isthmus or mass. The caecum and ascending colon are retracted medially, exposing the fused kidney. Care must be taken to identify and avoid injury to the inferior mesenteric artery which runs down the anterior surface of the fused kidney. The origin of the inferior mesenteric artery is generally the anatomical reason that the fused poles of the horseshoe kidney have been unable to ascend normally. Because of the probability of anomalous vasculature, care must be exercised in exposure of the isthmus. At this point, the disease can be studied and final decision regarding surgical treatment made.

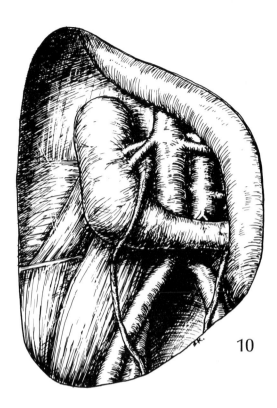

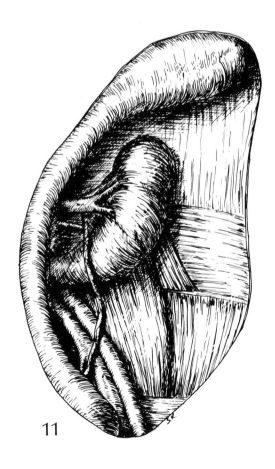

11

Transperitoneal exposure of left kidney

When the affected structures lie primarily to the left side of the isthmus of the horseshoe kidney, the retroperitoneum is entered by incising the left pericolic gutter and reflecting the posterior parietal peritoneum medially. It may be necessary to take down the splenic flexure to obtain adequate peritoneal mobilization towards the isthmus. A combined approach utilizing the left pericolic incision plus dissection of the posterior parietal peritoneum along the root of the small bowel mesentery, as on the right, may be necessary to expose the isthmus clearly. It may even be possible to expose the left half of the horseshoe kidney by extending the right-sided 'J' incision further cephalomedially across the isthmus.

12

Transection of the isthmus of the horseshoe kidney

Since the operation performed most commonly on the horseshoe kidney is removal of one-half of the fused kidney for hydronephrosis, it will usually be necessary to divide the isthmus at some point in this procedure. Whether it is necessary to divide the isthmus and fix the lower pole of the remaining kidney laterally at the time of pyelolithotomy or pyeloplasty to improve drainage is uncertain at present[12, 13, 16]. We approach these situations individually and have found in many instances that vascular fixation of the two halves of the horseshoe kidney precludes lateral nephropexy, despite symphysiotomy. If, however, a bulky isthmus appears to be impeding drainage despite pyeloplasty and freedom of ureteral attachments from the anterior surface of the isthmus, we will attempt to divide the isthmus and rotate the lower poles laterally.

Unfortunately, a convenient midline location does not necessarily correspond to the actual line of demarcation of the two renal halves. In instances of lateral fusion of the kidneys, the pelviocalyceal system of one side may actually cross the midline. This may be suggested by preoperative radiography or intraoperative findings. Division of the isthmus must be performed at the line of demarcation to avoid leaving residual undrained parenchyma and calyces that may lead to urinary fistula formation or parenchymal haemorrhage. Mobilization of the isthmus before division is helpful. After any anteriorly located renal arteries are identified and isolated with Silastic vessel loops, dissection is begun along the inferior border of the isthmus, lifting the isthmus up and away from the aorta while searching for posteriorly placed vessels. When these have been located, an arterial line of demarcation should be established. Temporary occlusion

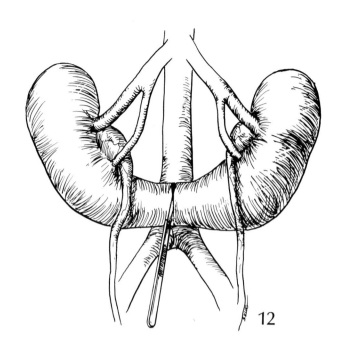

12

of the vessels with atraumatic vascular clamps (bulldog clips) with direct injection of indigo carmine into the arteries in question may be helpful. It must be remembered that the entire blood supply to both renal segments can enter through the isthmus. Once the point of division has been selected, the overlying renal capsule is incised sharply down to, but not into, the underlying parenchyma. The capsule is then gently stripped back 2–3 cm on either side of the incision, care being taken not to injure it as it will be used in closing the renal stump after symphysiotomy. The back edge of a knife is then used to divide the isthmus bluntly in a guillotine fashion.

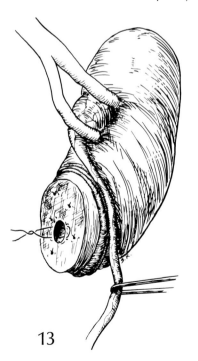

13

13

Bleeding vessels can be suture-ligated with fine 4/0 or 5/0 chromic catgut figure-of-eight sutures on a tapered needle. Occasionally, spot electrocoagulation with the current at a high setting will stop small troublesome bleeding points. If possible (i.e. with the isthmus well mobilized) manual compression of the cut edge between an assistant's thumb and forefinger will minimize blood loss while haemostasis is being attained. A careful search must be made for any contralateral calyceal system remaining with the normal kidney and it should be removed. If the calyceal system of the remaining normal kidney was entered, it must be closed with a watertight running suture of 5/0 chromic catgut swaged onto a small reverse taper urological needle. If a nephrostomy tube is to be left in this half of the horseshoe kidney, meticulous closure may not be necessary.

14

After isthmus transection has been completed and residual calyceal tissue handled appropriately, evenly spaced interrupted horizontal mattress sutures of 3/0 chromic catgut swaged onto a large tapered or blunt-ended curved needle are placed 1 cm back from the cut edge to compress it. Tying the sutures over free fat pads obtained from surrounding tissue or over plugs of oxidized cellulose gauze (Gelfoam) helps to keep the sutures from pulling through the renal parenchyma. Care must be taken not to use excessive pressure in tying down these sutures.

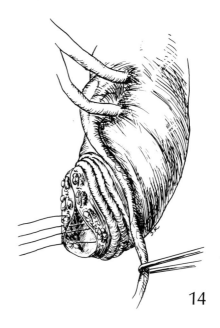

14

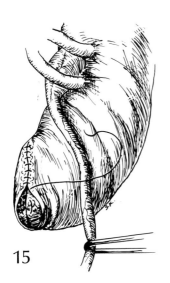

15

15

The previously reflected renal capsule is then closed over the renal stump with a running fine chromic catgut suture. If the capsule has a tendency to tear and macerate, a running horizontal mattress stitch is helpful.

Pyeloplasty

16

When ureteropelvic junction obstruction is encountered in a horseshoe kidney, the anteriorly malrotated renal pelvis and high take-off of the ureter tend to lend themselves well to performance of a Y–V type pyeloplasty. The surgical approach is determined by the position of the kidneys, the side of the obstruction and any need to perform simultaneous bilateral operations. Once the renal pelvis has been identified and vessels in the area secured and retracted away from the site of pyeloplasty, an inverted Y-shaped incision is mapped out on the inferior surface of the renal pelvis. Silk 4/0 stay sutures are used to mark the limits of the 'Y' and maintain future orientation. The base leg of the inverted 'Y' (AB) should extend several centimetres down the posterior surface of the ureter – well past the ureteropelvic junction. Using fine angled (Pott's) dissecting scissors, flap BC is then created, to be advanced into the resultant opening of the ureter along AB, completing the Y–V plasty. A Silastic vessel loop placed around the ureter often helps maintain gentle traction for exposure.

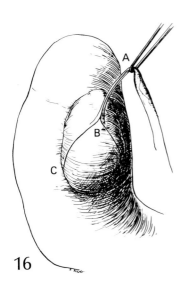

16

17 & 18

After all the preliminary incisions have been made the renal pelvic flap BC is advanced down the ureter to point A and tested for undue tension. Points A and B are then united with two fine 5/0 chromic catgut sutures; one suture is placed on either side of the apex to be run back up the renal pelvis to point C. We use a running, locking suture for this repair, but an interrupted repair can be performed as well. Before the pyeloplasty is completed a decision regarding the use of a ureteral stent and nephrostomy tube must be made. If the repair has technically gone well and the renal parenchyma appears reasonable, tube drainage or stents are not used. A Penrose drain is placed to the site of repair and follows a retroperitoneal course to exit through a lateral stab wound. If tube drainage is considered necessary, both a ureteral stent (a 5 or 8 Fr feeding tube) across the anastomoses as well as a nephrostomy tube are used. Both tubes then exit through the renal parenchyma retroperitoneally. At 10 days the stent is removed and the nephrostomy tube clamped. If there is good transport across the ureteropelvic junction as determined fluoroscopically or by the finding of minimal residual urine, the nephrostomy tube is removed a day later. Glenn[11] has suggested that lateral nephropexy of the involved segment of the horseshoe kidney is necessary at the time of pyeloplasty to improve drainage. This requires division of the isthmus and, as discussed earlier, may be impossible to perform because of vascular fixation of the kidneys[12, 17]. After completion of the pyeloplasty, the posterior peritoneum over the horseshoe kidney is closed and the wound is closed in a standard fashion.

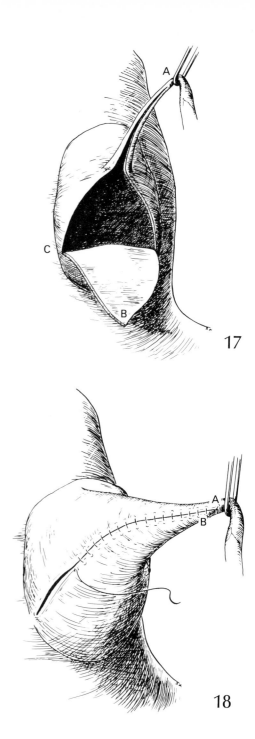

17

18

Treatment of crossed fused ectopia

19 & 20

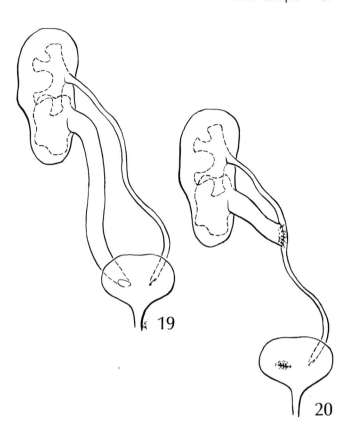

The most commonly encountered form of crossed ectopia is the inferior, unilateral fused variety in which the ectopic kidney (more often the left kidney) is fused to the lower pole of its contralateral mate. The unusual need for upper tract surgery on the rarely encountered crossed fused ectopic kidney, as well as the wide variability of the vascular supply and type of fusion, precludes making any general recommendations regarding surgical treatment. At times, the abnormality can be handled in a manner similar to cases of renal and ureteral duplication. Because of interdigitation of the collecting systems of the two halves of the crossed fused ectopic kidney, however, this approach may be impossible. In that situation, ureteroureterostomy would be preferable to drain the abnormal segment into the normal ureter. A transperitoneal approach is favoured to allow adequate exposure of the fused mass and its vascular supply. The presence of this anomaly has been associated with such a marked increase in lower tract problems – especially reflux – that screening all children with ectopic or horseshoe kidneys is recommended by some surgeons for this condition[2, 18, 19].

References

1. Ward, J. N., Nathanson, B., Draper, J. W. The pelvic kidney. Journal of Urology 1965; 94: 36–39

2. Malek, R. S., Kelalis, P. P., Burke, E. C. Ectopic kidney in children and frequency of association with other malformations. Mayo Clinic Proceedings 1971; 46: 461–467

3. Perlmutter, A. D., Retik, A. B., Bauer, S. B. Anomalies of the upper urinary tract. In: Harrison, J. H., Gittes, R. F., Perlmutter, A. D., Stamey, T. A., Walsh, P. C., eds. Campbell's urology, Vol. 2. 4th ed. Philadelphia: Saunders, 1979: 1309–1398

4. Abeshouse, B. S., Bhisitkul, I. Crossed renal ectopia with and without fusion. Urology International 1959; 9: 63–91

5. Graves, F. T. The arterial anatomy of the congenitally abnormal kidney. British Journal of Surgery 1969; 56: 533–541

6. Rubinstein, Z. J., Hertz, M., Shahin, N., Deutsch, V. Crossed renal ectopia: angiographic findings in six cases. American Journal of Roentgenology 1976; 126: 1035–1038

7. Campbell, M. F. Anomalies of the kidney. In: Campbell, M. F. ed. Urology, Vol. 2. 2nd ed. Philadelphia: Saunders, 1963: 1539–1617

8. Merimsky, E., Firstater, M. Ectopic thoracic kidney. British Journal of Urology 1978; 50: 282

9. Moazzenzadeh, A. R., Khodadadian, P., Potter, R. T. The intrathoracic kidney. Journal of Thoracic and Cardiovascular Surgery 1977; 73: 480–482

10. Ang, A. H., Chan, W. F. Ectopic thoracic kidney. Journal of Urology 1972; 108: 211–212

11. Glenn, J. F. Analysis of 51 patients with horseshoe kidneys. New England Journal of Medicine 1959; 261: 684–687

12. Dajani, A. M. Horseshoe kidney: a review of twenty-nine cases. British Journal of Urology 1966; 38: 388–402

13. Pitts, W. R., Jr., Muecke, E. C. Horseshoe kidneys: a 40-year experience. Journal of Urology 1975; 113: 743–746

14. Cook, W. A., Stephens, F. D. Fused kidneys: morphologic study and theory of embryogenesis. Birth Defects: Original Article Series 1977; 13: 327–340

15. Boatman, D. L., Cornell, S. H., Kölln, C. P. The arterial supply of horseshoe kidneys. American Journal of Roentgenology 1971; 113: 447–451

16. Culp, O. S., Winterringer, J. R. Surgical treatment of horseshoe kidney: comparison of results after various types of operations. Journal of Urology 1955; 73: 747–756

17. Kilpatrick, F. R. Horseshoe kidneys. Proceedings of the Royal Society of Medicine 1967; 60: 433–438

18. Kelalis, P. P., Malek, R. S., Segura, J. W. Observations on renal ectopia and fusion in children. Journal of Urology 1973; 110: 588–592

19. Hendren, W. H., Donahoe, P. K., Pfister, R. C. Crossed renal ectopia in children. Urology 1976; 7: 135–144

Surgery of genitourinary tuberculosis

J. G. Gow MD, ChM, FRCS
Consultant Urologist, Emeritus, Liverpool AHA (Teaching), UK

Introduction

Surgery still has an important role to play in the management of genitourinary tuberculosis, but it must always be considered in conjunction with other forms of treatment, never alone.

The diagnosis of the disease is confirmed by the isolation of M. tuberculosis from urine, and the success or failure of treatment depends on the expertise used to detect the organism. All drugs, including those used for treating non-specific organisms, especially kanamycin, gentamicin, chloromycetin and tetracycline, should be stopped for at least a week before specimens are collected. At least 3, preferably 6, consecutive early morning specimens should be sent for culture. Every specimen should be treated separately and bacteriological examination of the urine carried out as soon as possible after voiding. It is customary in many centres to store the specimens until all are collected, but this is not recommended, as cases with infected urine will be missed. With advances in artificial culture techniques, guinea-pig inoculation tests are only required in very special cases.

The presence of acid-fast bacilli in direct smears should not be accepted as confirmation of genitourinary tuberculosis. Treatment with antituberculous drugs must not be commenced until a positive culture has been obtained or there is unequivocal clinical and radiological evidence of the disease.

Investigations

Radiology

A high-dose intravenous pyelogram is essential in all suspected cases of genitourinary tuberculosis. This technique has been a major advance in the investigation of renal disease and has made retrograde pyelography a very infrequent investigation. Tomograms combined with high-dose urography may give more precise information in difficult cases, and dynamic studies using the image intensifier are invaluable in assessing the severity of strictures at the pelviureteric and ureterovesical junctions.

Retrograde pyelography

Retrograde pyelography is seldom necessary but it may give valuable information if there is any suggestion of a stricture in the ureter, particularly at the lower end. A bulb catheter, e.g. Braasch or Chevassu, is used and the investigation carried out under the control of the image intensifier.

Cystoscopy

This investigation should be carried out under a general anaesthetic, especially if the bladder symptoms are severe and the bladder capacity small. At the first cystoscopy the bladder is inspected during the filling phase. If a small bladder is over-distended, bleeding will occur, making a good view impossible. The disease in the bladder always starts around a ureteric orifice. The appearances vary from simple inflammation to bullous oedema, granulations and superficial ulceration. A biopsy is not recommended as lesions in the bladder are secondary to renal tuberculosis, and, if the bladder is affected, tubercle bacilli will always be found in the urine. A biopsy, however, is suggested for bladder lesions, either ulcers or tubercles, which are seen some distance from a normal ureteric orifice: these lesions are never due to tuberculosis if both ureteric orifices are normal, and they may be carcinoma *in situ*.

Chemotherapy

Genitourinary tuberculosis is a local manifestation of a general infection and consequently all methods of treatment must be directed towards complete eradication of the disease, not just the local lesion. For many years streptomycin, isoniazid and para-aminosalicylic acid have been the standard first-line drugs. These drugs, however,

have many disadvantages, the most important being the length of time they have to be taken and, in the case of streptomycin, necessity of parenteral administration. Following the discovery of rifampicin, extensive clinical trials with short courses of treatment were carried out with excellent results and it was only a matter of time before a course of chemotherapy of short duration became standard practice. All these trials were carried out on patients suffering from pulmonary tuberculosis, but there is no reason why genitourinary lesions should not respond just as well or even better. The number of tubercle bacilli is smaller in renal lesions, tissue penetration is excellent and the drugs are excreted in high concentration in the urine.

If short courses are to be effective, combinations of the most bactericidal drugs should be used. The three drugs that fit into this category are rifampicin, isoniazid and pyrazinamide. A satisfactory regimen is:

rifampicin 600 mg	taken daily for 2 months,
isoniazid 300 mg	last thing at night
pyrazinamide 1.5 mg	

This regimen should be followed by:

rifampicin 900 mg	taken 3 times a week in divided
isoniazid 600 mg	doses for a further 2 months

This course therefore lasts 4 months in all, and will control any case of genitourinary tuberculosis. If the disease is very acute, streptomycin 1 g daily can be added to the rifampicin, isoniazid and pyrazinamide for the first 2 months.

The drug dosages are not calculated according to body weight as the suggested doses give excellent results irrespective of the weight of the patient. Patients should be monitored every week on both these regimens and liver fuction tests should be carried out as there is a small risk of liver damage. Also the urine is inspected since only if it turns orange, is the patient taken the rifampicin.

Follow-up investigations

Once it has been accepted that any surgical treatment required will be carried out during the first 2 months of the 4-month course of chemotherapy, a short follow-up period can be recommended. Ideally 6 consecutive early morning specimens of urine should be examined at the end of the course and again after a further 6 months. If all the specimens are sterile the patient is discharged but advised to report again immediately should any urinary symptoms recur.

Patients who have renal calcification on discharge are advised to report annually for a straight abdominal X-ray to exclude any increase in size of the calcification. Patients who have had an enterocystoplasty are seen at 6-monthly intervals. At these follow-up reviews high-dose excretion urograms are taken to assess renal function and residual urine. In this type of case the follow-up routine is continued for 5 or more years.

Surgery

Just as there has been a critical reappraisal of the conventional methods of chemotherapeutic treatment, so in surgery many traditional ideas are being challenged.

For some time it has been customary to advocate that surgery for active tuberculosis is unnecessary except in a very few cases. Many authorities have stated that, provided chemotherapy is adequate, the disease can be contained. However, bearing in mind that tuberculosis affects all parts of the body and that short courses of treatment are now widely accepted, surgical treatment, when indicated, should be undertaken during the first 2 months of intensive triple therapy. The antituberculous drugs can kill small foci of disease which may persist in other parts of the body.

Surgical treatment can be divided into two types:

1. Excision of diseased tissue: nephrectomy, partial nephrectomy, cavernotomy, epididymectomy.
2. Reconstructive surgery: ureteric stricture, enterocysto-plasty, urethral strictures.

EXCISION OF DISEASED TISSUE

Nephrectomy

The indications for nephrectomy are as follows:

1. A non-fuctioning kidney with or without calcification.
2. Extensive disease involving the whole of the kidney, together with superimposed secondary infection.
3. Small kidney with very little function, calcification and a pelviureteric obstruction causing intermittent and often severe renal pain.
4. Coexisting renal carcinoma. This is a rare combination which has been reported, and if selective arteriography suggests the double disorder a nephrectomy should be carried out.

If renal tuberculosis coexists with hypertension, nephrectomy should not be performed merely to improve the hypertension. Of those that show an initial fall in blood pressure, 40 per cent deteriorate later. The indications for nephrectomy are the same irrespective of the presence or absence of hypertension. It is never necessary to carry out a complete removal of the ureter as, once the source of infection has been removed, modern chemotherapy controls any residual infection in the ureteric stump. A length of ureter is removed with the kidney. It is wise not to attempt to remove too much because if the ureter breaks it may be difficult to find the stump. If this is left without a ligature a fistula may result. An anterior transverse incision is not recommended for the nephrectomy because of the difficulties encountered in removing a kidney destroyed by long-standing tuberculous disease and surrounded by dense adhesions.

Complications are rare, although occasionally invasion by secondary organisms causes a postoperative discharge. Prolonged treatment with the appropriate antibiotic controls the infection.

Partial nephrectomy

Partial nephrectomy is only rarely required. The main indication is an infection in an area of kidney containing calcified material which is not responding to treatment and in which the calcification is slowly increasing in size. It should never be carried out for a local uncalcified lesion. With modern chemotherapy such areas can always be managed without surgery. Cooling of the kidney is rarely necessary. Only the renal artery should be occluded and the clamp is released periodically during the resection. Sometimes a single large vessel supplies the area of the kidney to be removed. This can be ligated separately, making dissection of the main renal artery unnecessary. The cut calyceal stem should be sutured carefully with 4/0 Dexon and all bleeding in the renal parenchyma controlled with an under-run suture. The two main complications are urinary leak and haematuria. Both of these usually subside spontaneously, but occasionally secondary nephrectomy may be required. (For the illustrated technique of heminephrectomy *see* chapter on 'Partial nephrectomy and heminephrectomy', pp. 107–111).

Cavernotomy

Cavernotomy or deroofing of a tuberculous renal abscess is no longer recommended in the surgical treatment of tuberculosis. With modern sophisticated radiological techniques, the contents can be aspirated under the image intensifier and the cavity filled with a combination of 5 per cent isoniazid and 1 per cent rifampicin. With this regimen there have been no complications and the patient is spared surgical treatment.

Technique

If cavernotomy or deroofing is unavoidable the roof of the abscess is excised at the level of the kidney substance and the edge is oversewn with a running suture to guarantee haemostasis. The wound is closed without drainage. However, using an image intensifier to identify the position of the needle, it is possible to aspirate cavities on the rare occasion when surgical intervention is indicated. The only possible indication for surgery is a walled-off abscess which does not communicate with a calyx and which slowly increases in size, causing symptoms of renal discomfort. Calcification in the wall may or may not be present. Cavernotomy should never be carried out if there is any communcation with a calyx. Urinary fistula is the only postoperative complication, but this is rare.

Epididymectomy

The incidence of tuberculous epididymitis is decreasing but epididymectomy is still required on rare occasions when there is a caseating abscess which has not responded to chemotherapy. Involvement of the testis is uncommon and orchidectomy is required in only 5 per cent of cases. Prophylactic vasectomy of the contralateral vas should never be carried out if there is no palpable involvement of the epididymis. Chemotherapy will always control occult foci, and many patients with unilateral epididymitis have fathered children. The only complication is testicular atrophy, which occurs in about 6 per cent of cases. It is confined to the severe type of case in which the whole of the epididymis is involved and where there is difficulty in dissecting the globus major from the vascular pedicle. If the lesion is firm and fibrotic and there is no improvement after the 3-month intensive course of chemotherapy, the differential diagnosis of tumour should be considered. Cases of seminoma of the epididymis have been reported with the presence of tubercle bacilli in the urine. Excision will confirm the diagnosis. (For the illustrated technique of epididymectomy see chapter on 'Epididymectomy', pp. 669–671).

RECONSTRUCTIVE SURGERY

The ureter

Strictures occur at the pelviureteric junction, the middle third of the ureter and the ureterovesical junction. Occasionally the whole ureter is stenosed.

Pelviureteric junction

It is rare to find a kidney destroyed by gross renal disease without coincidental obstruction at the pelviureteric junction. All too often, by the time the patient presents for treatment the combination of acute renal tuberculosis and pelviureteric obstruction has caused irreversible renal damage. Consequently strictures at this level are seldom seen. However, once they are diagnosed they should be corrected as soon as possible, but not more than 3 or 4 weeks after commencing intensive antituberculous chemotherapy. The presence of active infection is no contraindication to surgery. The Anderson-Hynes procedure has proved a very satisfactory method but the Culp technique can also be used and gives equally good results (see chapter on 'Surgical correction of congenital ureteropelvic junction obstruction', pp. 255–267).

Now that Silastic tubing is available, a splint of this material should be placed through the anastomosis and brought out through a separate incision at least 10 cm down the ureter. In addition, a pyelostomy is essential: not only does it drain the kidney but it also allows the instillation of a mixture of 5 per cent isoniazid and 1 per cent rifampicin into the pelvicalyceal system. The ureteric splint should be removed in 2 weeks and the pyelostomy drain after 2–3 weeks. Complications are: a urinary leak, which usually heals spontaneously but may persist, making nephrectomy necessary; and progression of the disease which may necessitate removal of the kidney (extremely rare if modern chemotherapeutic agents are correctly used).

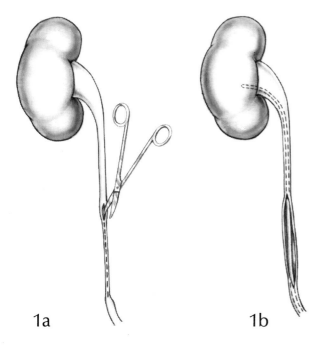

1a

1b

1a & b

Middle third of the ureter

Strictures at this level are very rarely seen. The only satisfactory method of treatment is by the Davis intubated ureterotomy. The midureteral stricture is incised throughout its length, the incision extending into normal ureter proximally and distally. Provided there is some residual mucous membrane in continuity the ureter should reform over a Silastic tube which is left in the lumen for a minimum of 4–6 weeks. The tube is passed up the ureter into the pelvis of the kidney and can be brought out distally either onto the skin or through the urethra. The latter method is satisfactory since it is carried out through a cystoscope passed at the same time as the ureterotomy is performed. Recurrent stricture must be a complication, but so far results of the reported cases treated by this technique have been satisfactory.

Lower end of the ureter

Strictures at the lower end of the ureter are found in about 5 per cent of patients. The management can either be medical, by dilatation or by surgery.

Medical

It has been suggested that conservative management is wholly justified and that, by the judicious use of corticosteroids in conjunction with adequate chemotherapy, a high percentage of ureteric strictures can be treated without surgery. Therefore, corticosteroids should be commenced immediately when any obstructive lesion is demonstrated. This concept is open to serious criticism: it is likely that in many of these patients the obstructions are due to oedema, which will disappear once the infection is under control. In the author's experience this often happens. A more satisfactory regimen is to give the most active bactericidal drug combination available (rifampicin, isoniazid and pyrazinamide) for 8 weeks and monitor progress at weekly intervals. If there is no improvement after 3 weeks, corticosteroids are added to this regimen in the form of prednisolone (20 mg 3 times a day). This may seem a high dose, but the rifampicin increases the excretion of cortisol, so that double the normal dose of prednisolone has to be given to achieve a similar effect. The combined treatment is continued for a further month. The same monitoring programme is adopted every week; if the stricture has not improved at the end of this time, surgical relief is carried out.

Dilatation

Dilatation is suggested as an initial procedure in many cases. It is sometimes difficult to negotiate the stricture but if the treatment is successful the stricture can be dilated up to about size 8 using a Braasch dilator. The dilatation must be repeated every 2 weeks at first, but the intervals will gradually become longer. If this fails, surgical treatment will be necessary. The indications for this method are becoming less frequent.

2, 3 & 4

Surgery

The indications for surgical intervention are an obstruction of the lower ureter leading to upper tract dilatation and impaired renal function. The diagnosis is confirmed by serial pyelography and an attempt is made to assess the length of the stricture using an image intensifer, as this is important in planning the best surgical procedure. If the stricture is short and the ureter dilated, an antireflux reimplantation is carried out. If, however, there is excessive ureteric dilatation the ureter must be tailored so that at least 5 cm of the narrowed ureter lie in the submucous tunnel with the suture line placed against the muscle. Complications are a urinary leak and a recurrence of reflux which may require reimplantation.

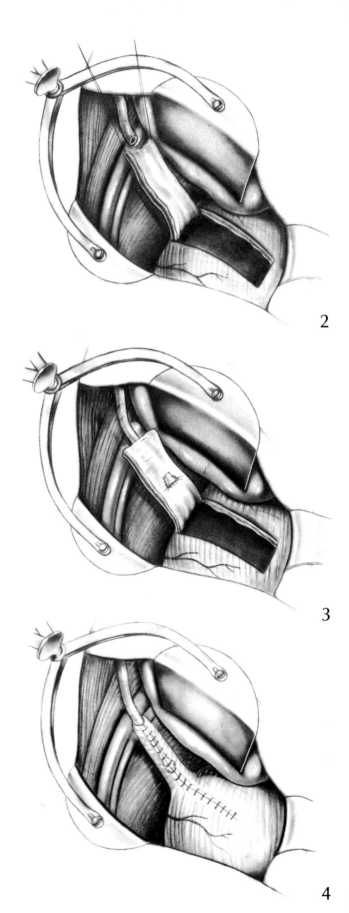

2

3

4

Enterocystoplasty

Enterocystoplasty now has an established place in the treatment of tuberculous cystitis. At first the ileum was used for this procedure but was found to be unsatisfactory. Now the choice lies between the colon and the caecum. The caecum has some advantages, but these are marginal. It is best used in cases with ureteric reflux, when the ureter can be implanted into the terminal ileum. Reflux is prevented by the combination of the ileocaecal valve and a reflux-preventing anastomosis of the ureter into the ileum. Active inflammation is no contraindication to enterocystoplasty when there are severe urinary symptoms with a bladder capacity of less than 100 ml. Bladder neck obstruction must be excluded in all cases, and a micturating cystourethrogram is an essential investigation. If bladder neck obstruction is present, any patient needing an enterocystoplasty should have a bladder neck resection either before or at the same time as the enterocystoplasty.

Technique

There are certain points which should be emphasized. Bladder remnants must be as large as possible. The anastomosis between the caecum and the bladder should be as wide as can be obtained, since the caecal reservoir is essentially passive during voiding. It only has a pressure of between 12 and 16 cm H_2O, so that during the caecal voiding phase excretion is largely achieved by abdominal straining.

If the ureter has to be anastomosed to the terminal ileum, this part of the operation should always be carried out before the caecum is anastomosed to the bladder. Otherwise, technical difficulties may be formidable.

Finally, it is always wise to wrap a layer of omentum around the anastomosis of the caecum to the bladder, both posteriorly and anteriorly, and the anastomosis should always be tested by introducing 200–300 ml of fluid into the bladder and caecum to ensure that there are no leaks. (For the illustrated technique see chapter on 'Cytoplasty', pp. 335–344).

The complications are incontinence and enuresis, urinary tract infection and urinary leak. Bladder pressure studies before surgery may guide the surgeon as to the advisability of reconstructive bladder surgery. It is usually advisable to avoid an enterocystoplasty in the presence of enuresis or previous history of psychotic disturbance.

Urinary tract infections are controlled by the appropriate antibiotic and are often symptomless. Urinary leaks are rare if a two-layer closure is performed and the anastomosis covered by omentum. They should all heal spontaneously with continuous bladder drainage.

Urinary diversion

Urinary diversion by ureterocolic anastomosis, ileal or colonic conduit or cutaneous ureterostomy has very little place in the contemporary management of genitourinary tuberculosis. There is only one indication for these procedures and that is where the patient has complete incontinence which is not improved with antituberculous chemotherapy, and where bladder pressure studies have shown that the sphincter mechanism has been so damaged that there is no possibility of improvement. In this case, enterocystoplasty should not be performed but a urinary diversion carried out. The best method is an ileal urinary conduit. (For the illustrated technique see chapter on 'Ileal conduit diversion', pp. 273–281).

Urethral stricture

Urethral stricture is a rare complication of genitourinary tuberculosis, but it is still seen from time to time. It is always due to long-standing disease which is usually inactive by the time the stricture develops. The management is the same as for any other inflammatory stricture of the urethra.

Conclusion

The management of genitourinary tuberculosis has changed considerably in the last few years owing to the introduction of the short-course regimens of bactericidal drugs. It should be possible to supervise these cases in the same way as other infections of the urinary tract. This disease no longer demands special treatment and management, but has joined the mainstream of surgery where its supervision will be the responsibility of practising urologists and surgeons.

Illustrations by Janis Kay AtLee

Surgery for renal and perirenal infections

Robert C. Flanigan MD
Assistant Professor of Surgery (Urology),
University of Kentucky Medical Center, Lexington, Kentucky, USA

Surgical anatomy

1a & b

A knowledge of renal and perirenal anatomy is essential in understanding the treatment of renal and perirenal infections. The true renal capsule is closely applied to the surface of the kidney by penetrating nephrocapsular capillaries and lymphatics. Outside its capsule the kidney is surrounded by abundant perirenal (perinephric) fat, which is in turn confined within a perinephric (Gerota's) fascia. Although there are conflicting opinions as to the anatomical arrangement of Gerota's fascia, it is well known that perinephric abscesses do not spread to the contralateral side, suggesting that the perinephric spaces are not connected in the midline.

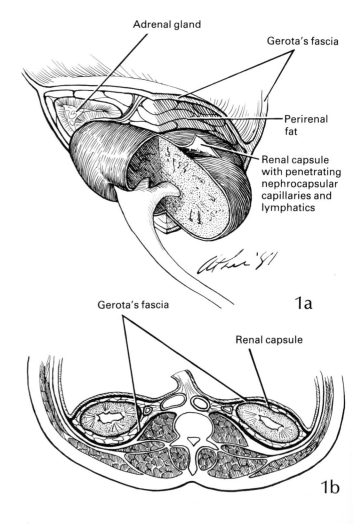

Adrenal gland

Gerota's fascia

Perirenal fat

Renal capsule with penetrating nephrocapsular capillaries and lymphatics

1a

Gerota's fascia

Renal capsule

1b

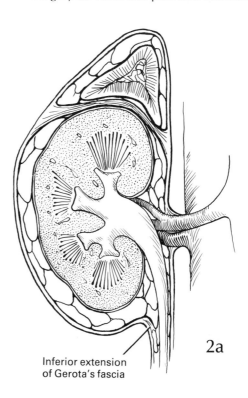

Inferior extension
of Gerota's fascia

2a

2a & b

Inferiorly, the perinephric fascia fuses weakly around the ureter allowing perirenal infections to course down into the periureteral fat. Cranially, firm fibrils extending from the renal capsule to the perinephric fascia become particularly dense, forming the duodenorenal ligament on the right and the splenorenal ligament on the left.

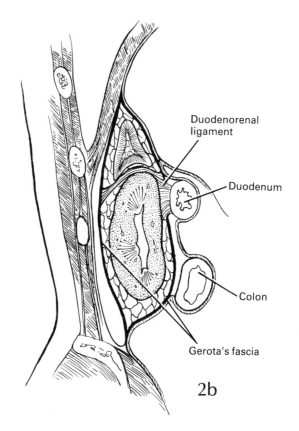

Duodenorenal
ligament

Duodenum

Colon

Gerota's fascia

2b

The operations

SUBCOSTAL, FLANK APPROACH

3

Position of patient

The anaesthetized patient is placed in a lateral position after insertion of an endotracheal tube and positioned so that the tip of the 12th rib lies directly over the kidney rest. The bottom leg is then flexed to 90° and the top leg remains straight for maintenance of stability. An axillary roll is placed below the axilla to prevent compression of the axillary nerves and vasculature and a pillow is generally placed between the knees. Careful positioning of the patient is important not only for optimal surgical exposure but also to preclude serious complications secondary to axillary injury. At this point, the kidney rest is raised slowly and the table is flexed with careful monitoring of the patient's blood pressure. This position is generally well tolerated but can result in decreased venous return by compression of the inferior vena cava and the dependent position of the lower extremities. In addition, if often limits excursion of the lung on the dependent side.

4

The incision extends from the lateral border of the sacrospinalis muscle, where it crosses the inferior edge of the 12th rib, along the lower border of the rib and onto the anterior abdominal wall. The medial end of the incision is generally carried downwards onto the abdomen to avoid damage to the subcostal nerve. The latissimus dorsi muscle, which passes upward from the lumbodorsal fascia over the chest wall and inserts on the humerus, is divided in the posterior aspect of the wound. This exposes the posterior edge of the external oblique muscle.

5

The external oblique and serratus posterior muscles are then divided. This exposes the lumbodorsal fascia at a point where it gives rise to the internal oblique and transversus abdominis muscles.

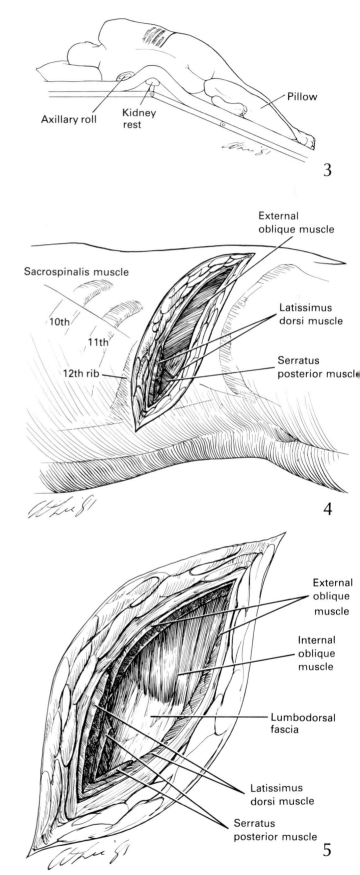

6

After the lumbodorsal fascia is incised, fingers are used to peel the peritoneal reflection off the undersurface in the anterior direction thus allowing division of the internal oblique and transversus abdominis muscles without damage to the underlying peritoneal structures. The subcostal neurovascular bundle should be identified as it courses downwards between the internal oblique and transversus abdominis muscles. This neurovascular bundle can be mobilized by incising the fascial sheath that surrounds it and can be displaced safely to one side of the wound. Similarly, fingers are used to sweep pleura and diaphragmatic attachments posteriorly off the lumbodorsal fascia, allowing posterior extension of the incision. Visualization of pleura during respiration will allow for precise, sharp division of the diaphragmatic attachments and avoid unnecessary pleural injury.

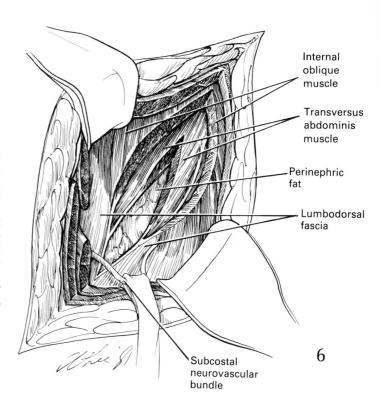

Internal oblique muscle

Transversus abdominis muscle

Perinephric fat

Lumbodorsal fascia

Subcostal neurovascular bundle

6

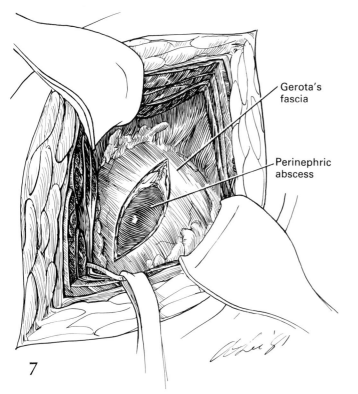

Gerota's fascia

Perinephric abscess

7

7

At this point an incision is made in Gerota's fascia, over the posterior aspect of the kidney, and the perinephric space is entered. If the perinephric abscess is to be drained, this can be done either through the posterior aspect of this incision, or, as the author prefers, through a separate stab wound. It is important to place the drains posteriorly and dependently to facilitate drainage.

LUMBAR APPROACH (POSTERIOR LUMBOTOMY)

8

Although this approach is used frequently for removal of small kidneys at the time of bilateral nephrectomy in patients with chronic renal failure, or for posterior approach to the adrenal glands, it can also be used for surgical treatment of renal and perirenal infections. The advantages associated with this incision are that it provides a direct approach to the renal and perirenal spaces avoiding division of muscles, thus decreasing postoperative pain and improving wound closure strength. The major disadvantage is limited access to the renal hilum. If nephrectomy or stone removal is contemplated in the treatment of perinephric abscess, an incision through the 11th or 12th rib is preferred by the author, as this allows for easier approach to the renal pedicle and pelvis.

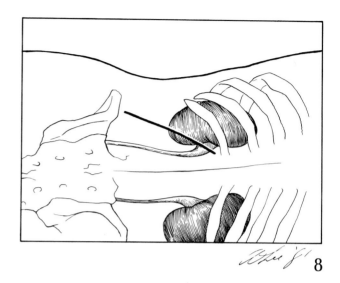

8

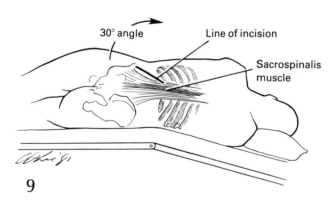

9

9

The patient is placed in a lateral position and rotated approximately 30° anteriorly with the tip of the 12th rib over the break in the table. A sandbag is placed between the abdomen and the table. This serves further to support the abdomen and to push the kidneys posteriorly. The table is then slightly flexed. If access to both kidneys is required, the patient can be placed in the prone position. It is essential that the patient is supported over the sternum and pubis so that there is free excursion of the anterior abdominal wall to facilitate respiration and venous return. The incision is made from the lateral border of the sacrospinalis muscle where it crosses the 12th rib down to a point lateral to where the sacrospinalis muscle meets the iliac crest.

10

The lumbodorsal fascia is incised in the direction of the incision and the sacrospinalis and quadratus lumborum muscles are retracted medially.

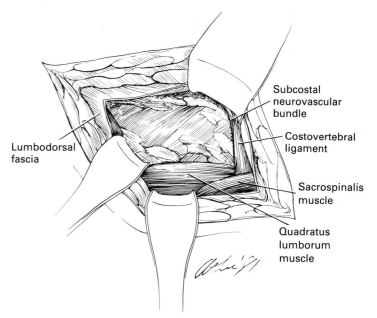

Subcostal neurovascular bundle

Costovertebral ligament

Lumbodorsal fascia

Sacrospinalis muscle

Quadratus lumborum muscle

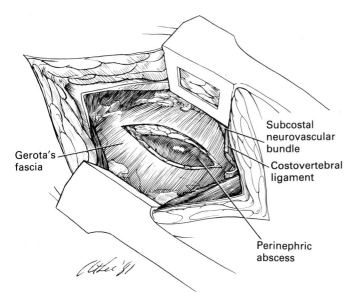

Gerota's fascia

Subcostal neurovascular bundle

Costovertebral ligament

Perinephric abscess

11

Gerota's fascia is incised in the direction of the incision and the perinephric space is entered. If greater exposure is necessary, the costovertebral ligament to the 12th rib may be incised in the upper aspect of the wound. Care must be taken to avoid damage to the subcostal neurovascular bundle which lies immediately below or anterior to the costovertebral ligament. Once the ligament is divided, the rib can be retracted cephalad. We find that a Finochietto retractor maintains excellent exposure of the kidney.

12a–d

PERCUTANEOUS APPROACH

Percutaneous drainage of perinephric abscesses may be useful as a temporary measure to convert a septic, emergent clinical situation to a non-septic, non-emergent one. Indeed, some centres have suggested that serial dilatation of the tract and insertion of a large catheter may serve as definitive treatment for perinephric abscess.

The procedure we favour involves entering the abscess cavity with a trochar and sheath (*a*), removal of the trochar and insertion of a guide-wire through the sheath (*b*), removal of the sheath and passage of a pigtail drainage catheter over the guide-wire (*c*), and finally removal of the guide-wire (*d*). The pigtail catheter is also secured to the skin with a suture and is placed to gravity drainage. Irrigation of the catheter may be necessary after institution of antibiotic coverage.

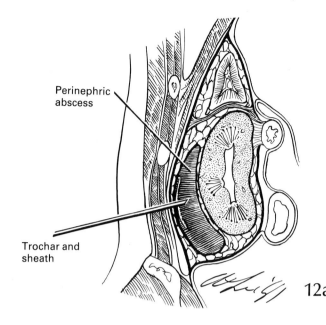

Perinephric abscess

Trochar and sheath

12a

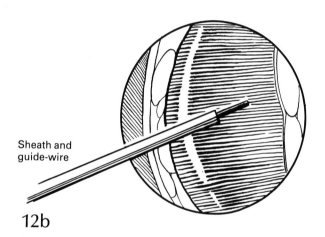

Sheath and guide-wire

12b

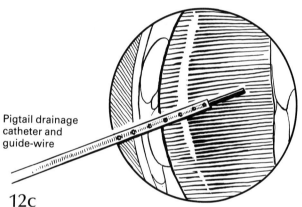

Pigtail drainage catheter and guide-wire

12c

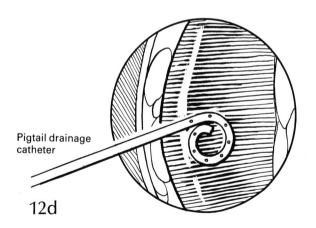

Pigtail drainage catheter

12d

References

1. Timmons, J. W., Perlmutter, A. D. Renal abscess: a changing concept. Journal of Urology 1976; 115: 299–301

2. Thorley, J. D., Jones, S. R., Sanford, J. P. Perinephric abscess. Medicine 1974; 53: 441–451

3. Jimenez, J. F., Lopez Pacios, A., Llamazares, G., Conejero, J., Sole-Balcells, F. Treatment of pyonephrosis: a comparative study. Journal of Urology 1978; 120: 287–289

4. Malgieri, J. J., Kursh, E. D., Persky, L. The changing clinicopathological pattern of abscesses in or adjacent to the kidney. Journal of Urology 1977; 118: 230–232

5. Segura, J. W., Kelalis, P. P. Localized renal parenchymal infections in children. Journal of Urology 1973; 109: 1029–1032

6. Brush, R. III, Gooneratne, N. S., Rittenberg, G. M., Rous, S. N. Gallium-67 scanning and conservative treatment in acute inflammatory lesions of the renal cortex. Journal of Urology 1979; 121: 232–235

7. Caldamone, A. A., Frank, I. N. Percutaneous aspiration in the treatment of renal abscess. Journal of Urology 1980; 123: 92–93

Illustrations by Freda Wadsworth and T. Bell

Renal artery reconstruction

Charles Rob   MC, MD, MChir, FRCS
Professor of Surgery, Uniformed Services,
University of the Health Sciences, Bethesda, Maryland, USA

Introduction

Renal artery stenosis is now a well established although relatively infrequent cause of renal hypertension. The most common causes of renal artery stenosis are atheroma and fibromuscular hyperplasia. While external bands may cause obstruction, these may be associated with intrinsic arterial disease; therefore should a band appear to be the cause of obstruction, the flow rate should be checked after division as a supplementary reconstruction may be needed.

The disease may be unilateral or bilateral but when it is bilateral it is rarely symmetrical so that there are usually functional differences between the two kidneys.

Evidence of the disease may rarely be given by an episode of pain in the loin (due to a small embolus) and suspicion of renal artery stenosis in a hypertensive patient may be aroused by the finding of a murmur on auscultation just above and to one side of the umbilicus or posteriorly over the renal artery. The majority of cases are, however, discovered from the hypertensive population after screening tests, the most important being the intravenous pyelogram and renogram. The pyelogram may show reduced size of the affected kidney, delayed excretion and increased contrast density in the later films. There may also be some evidence of collateral vessels shown by notching of the pelvis and ureter. The [131]I Hippuran renogram shows a delayed peak and an impaired second phase and usually an impaired third phase.

Definitive diagnosis

Renal arteriography

Selective catheterization and injection of the renal arteries exactly defines the anatomy of the disease but the apparent radiological obstruction may be disproportionate to the functional ischaemia. A plaque of atheroma on the anterior or posterior wall will be much less evident than a concentric narrowing or a plaque on the superior or posterior wall. The florid lesions of fibromuscular hyperplasias are easily seen but the finer intimal proliferations of this disease may only be detected after critical examination, particularly in the distal vessels.

Renin level

While peripheral vein renins may be useful in excluding hyperaldosteronism they are not particularly helpful in the diagnosis of renal artery stenosis. The ratio between the renal vein renin on both sides may however be helpful, a ratio of 1.5:1 or more being strongly suggestive of renal artery obstruction.

Treatment

Atheromatous lesions, although apparently solitary, are usually evidence of widespread disease and a significant reduction in life expectancy from other lesions such as coronary and cerebral artery disease can be expected. It is usually better to treat these patients medically in the first instance and to reserve surgery for the more severe cases which fail to respond to medical treatment. Fibroplasia tends on the other hand to have a good prognosis. It is most common in young females, and surgical treatment may be contemplated at an early stage providing the lesion is anatomically suitable. Arterial reconstruction is preferable to nephrectomy but the latter procedure may be indicated in poor risk patients or those with widespread disease of the peripheral arteries. Some type of bypass procedure or transluminal balloon dilatation is the usual method of reconstruction but thromboendarterectomy may sometimes be of value in atheromatous lesions.

The operation

1

The incision

An anterior incision is far preferable to a posterior renal exposure as it gives much better exposure and control of the vessels. The incision may be either paramedian or a transverse upper abdominal incision. The latter is favoured in most instances as it gives an extremely good exposure and good healing with a very low incidence of hernia. The incision is about 2.5–3.8 cm above the umbilicus, the exact height depending upon the build of the patient and the subcostal angle. It is extended to the costal margin on the affected side and can be further extended into a thoracoabdominal incision should greater exposure be required. In many patients of a favourable build the incision need only go a little beyond the midline but in more difficult cases or in bilateral lesions it should extend from one costal margin to the other. Both rectus abdominus muscles with their sheaths and linea alba are divided, as are the internal and external oblique muscles together with the transversus abdominis. The peritoneum is opened throughout the length of the incision and the ligamentum teres divided just above the umbilicus.

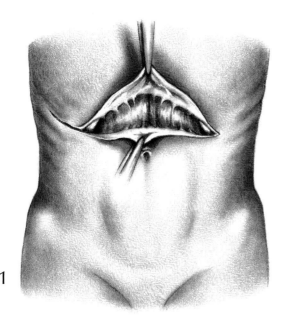

1

Exposure of kidneys, renal arteries and aorta

2

Right renal artery

After a full abdominal exploration the right renal artery is exposed by incising the posterior peritoneum lateral to the second part of the duodenum so that the head of the pancreas and duodenum can be retracted to the left, the liver upwards and the hepatic flexure of the colon downwards. It is usually necessary to pass a tape around the vena cava and the right renal vein before exposing the artery deep to the renal vein.

The stenosis, even if fibromuscular, may lie deep to the vena cava and an atheromatous stenosis will lie medially behind the vena cava. Palpation of the artery may give obvious evidence of the stenosis but on some occasions, particularly in fibromuscular hyperplasia lesions, there may be very little macroscopic evidence of a very florid radiological obstruction. Auscultation of the artery with a sterile ultrasound probe and/or pressure and flow measurements may occasionally help.

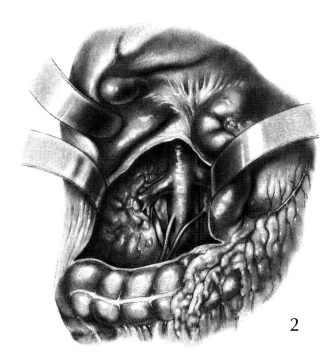

2

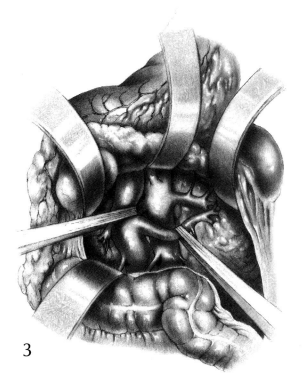

3

3

Left renal artery and aorta

The left renal artery is exposed by dividing the peritoneum along the lateral side of the descending colon and lateral to the splenic flexure so that the splenic flexure and descending colon can be retracted medially. The tail of the pancreas is seen in the upper part of the incision and if use of the splenic artery is contemplated it may be helpful to expose it at this stage. Small pancreatic branches of this artery may be found running into the pancreas. It is important to isolate and ligate these because if divided accidentally, they may bleed profusely. The left renal artery may be more easily exposed back to the aorta after taping the left renal vein.

The aorta is mobilized with care. It is usually necessary to divide at least one pair of lumbar arteries and often two pairs; otherwise they may be torn during aortic clamping. The lower border of the superior mesenteric artery is identified and if a bypass graft is to be taken from the lower part of the aorta the inferior mesenteric artery may also need identification.

AORTA-TO-RENAL ARTERY BYPASS

A bypass graft is usually the method of choice on the right side and may also be needed on the left if the splenic artery is unsuitable for use. A saphenous vein graft has the advantage of using autogenous tissue and its long-term results are excellent. Although the ovarian or testicular vein may appear suitable the tensile strength of these vessels is not as great as that of the saphenous vein. Their use carries the risk of rupture, and should be avoided.

4

Isolation of the saphenous vein

A longitudinal incision is made in the leg starting at the upper end of the saphenous vein about 3.8 cm below and lateral to the pubic tubercle (A). The vein is exposed and its branches ligated carefully with fine silk ligatures before being divided. It is advisable to remove a length about 1½ times longer than is thought necessary so that there is adequate length to select a suitable place for a tension-free anastomosis. Care is taken to mark the distal end (B) which must be anastomosed to the aorta so that the direction of blood flow conforms with the arrangement of the valves.

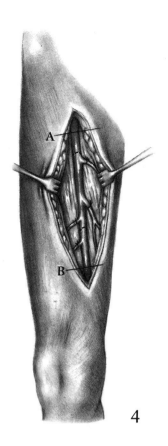

4

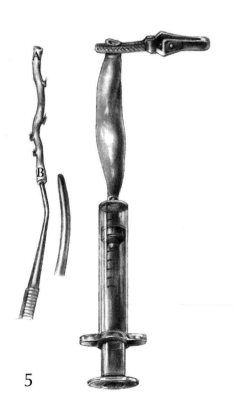

5

5

The vein contracts markedly on removal and it is essential to dilate it moderately before making the anastomosis. This can be done initially with a small probe or Hegar's dilator. It is then possible to dilate it hydrostatically with saline using a syringe with one end of the vein clamped. It must not be overdilated; this can damage the vein.

6

Anastomosis of vein to aorta

The aorta is clamped transversely above and below the area selected for anastomosis. This should be a relatively disease-free part of the aorta and there seems to be no disadvantage in running the graft obliquely upwards from the lower aorta or, even, in some instances where the aorta is grossly diseased, using the common iliac artery. An oval window is cut in the aorta to match the obliquely cut distal end of the vein graft to give as long a suture line as possible. A suture of 6/0 Prolene is used. On completion of this suture line the renal end of the vein graft is clamped and blood allowed to distend the graft so that the optimum length for anastomosis to the distal renal can be chosen with the vein under arterial pressure.

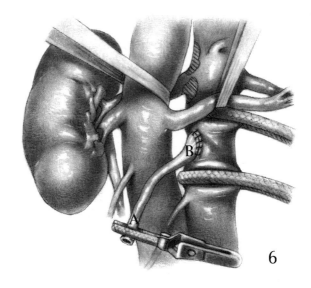

6

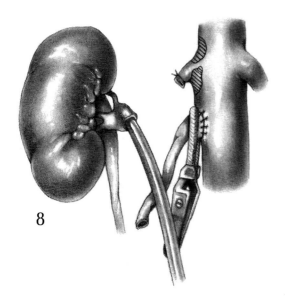

7

Anastomosis of vein to distal artery

7

When the length is decided the bulldog clamp is moved from the end (A) (*see Illustration 6*) of the vein graft to the other end so that the vein is clamped flush with the aorta. The renal artery is then divided, its proximal end being ligated securely and the distal end is turned up for anastomosis. There is often a considerable back-flow from capsular collaterals so that the distal artery or its terminal branches must be clamped. The alternative is to anastomose the vein graft to the side of the renal artery. This is technically more difficult.

8

In cases of fibromuscular hyperplasia if there is any narrowing of the distal arteries these may be dilated at this stage using a metal dilator.

8

9

An end-to-end anastomosis is then made with 7/0 Prolene making an oblique suture line. On removing the clamps the vein takes up a natural curve in front of the vena cava.

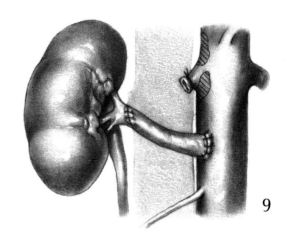

9

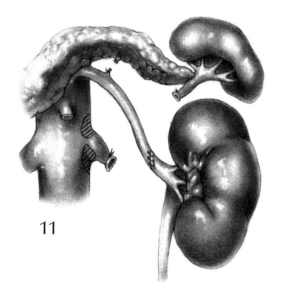

10

10

Use of plastic prosthesis

A plastic prosthesis may be used instead of a vein graft but this is thought in most centres to have a greater risk of long-term failure. If a plastic prosthesis is used it is advisable to do the distal anastomosis first as there is no great problem in selecting the correct length. Furthermore, the greater rigidity of the plastic material may lead to tearing of the thin distal arterial wall if there is any degree of post-stenotic dilation should this suture line be done when the aortic end is fixed in position.

11

Splenorenal anastomosis

On the left side if the splenic artery is healthy it may be used in a similar way for anastomosis to the distal renal artery.

11

THROMBOENDARTERECTOMY

This operation is suitable for some cases of atheromatous obstruction where the disease is localized. It should be noted that although the obstruction may appear radiologically to be within the renal artery, it starts as a plaque in the aorta and should be approached from the aorta.

12 & 13

The facility of this operation often depends upon the exact relationship of the left renal vein crossing the aorta and the position of the two renal arteries. The aorta is exposed and cross-clamped above and below the renal arteries. In some cases it may be possible to place the upper clamp obliquely to allow blood to continue flowing through the contralateral kidney. The aorta is then incised, usually through an oblique incision and the atheromatous plaque around the renal artery ostium is dissected away. It is usually possible to pull any obstructing plaque from the renal artery but if there is any doubt as to whether the distal part of the removal is clear then the renal artery may need to be opened. The incision is then closed with 6/0 Prolene suture.

If the disease is bilateral or if there is any residual aortic plaque which may later obstruct the opposite side then the direction of the upper clamp can be reversed and a similar procedure carried out on the opposite side. The closure can be performed with a Dacron patch if necessary.

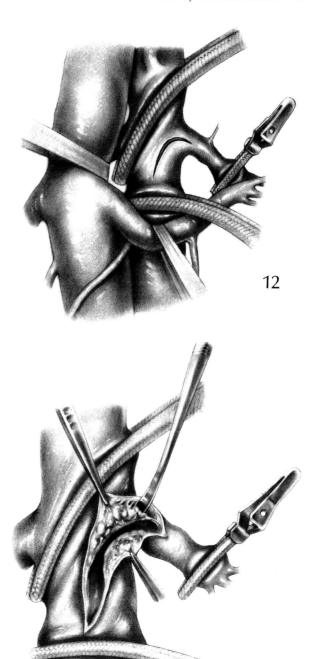

12

13

14

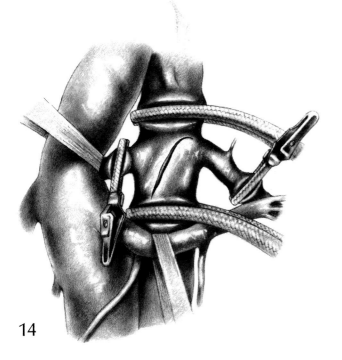

14

An alternative procedure is to cross-clamp the aorta above both renal arteries but if this is done care must be taken to complete the procedure within 30 min to avoid ischaemic renal damage. It is wise to give an intravenous infusion of mannitol before removing the clamps to lessen the risk of oliguria.

ALTERNATIVE PROCEDURES

15

Common iliac artery to renal artery

In young children any renal artery reconstruction must allow for growth. On the left side this is relatively easy using the splenic artery and interrupted sutures but can present a problem on the right side. In such young children with a healthy lower-limb vasculature the common iliac artery can be divided proximal to its division and swung up to anastomose to the renal artery using a long oblique suture line with interrupted sutures. A good collateral circulation to the leg very rapidly develops and this procedure produces no disability although it use must clearly be restricted to young children with a healthy circulation. Should there be any doubt about the circulation to the lower limb then a vein graft or prosthesis could be used to bridge the gap between aorta and distal common iliac artery.

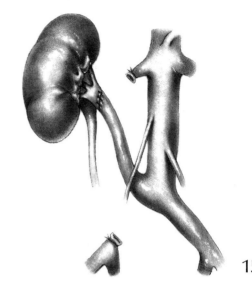

15

16

Internal iliac artery graft

In some instances of fibromuscular hyperplasia the disease may extend into the proximal part of the renal arteries, making dilation impossible, and necessitating a branched replacement. A free internal iliac artery segment may be used for this replacement. Its main divisions are anastomosed to two renal artery branches and any further branch can be anastomosed to the side of the graft. The main trunk is anastomosed to the aorta. As with a plastic prosthesis it may be easier to perform the distal anastomosis before the aortic end. Such a reconstruction can usually be done satisfactorily within a safe ischaemia time, particularly as there is some protection against ischaemic damage by the collateral capsular circulation. However, if prolonged ischaemia is necessary for a difficult technical reconstruction the kidney can be removed, perfused and cooled and then replaced as an autograft, anastomosed to the iliac vessel (see chapter on 'Extracorporeal renal surgery', pp. 134–143).

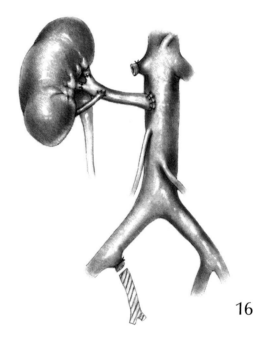

16

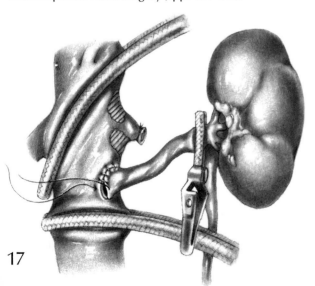

17

17

Reimplantation of the renal artery to the aorta

This procedure may often seem tempting on consideration of the radiological appearance. In practice, however, it is rarely possible to obtain an adequate length of renal artery to anastomose to the most suitable healthy portion of the aorta without producing undue tension or angulation.

BALLOON CATHETER DILATATION OF THE RENAL ARTERIES

18

Atherosclerotic stenosis of the renal artery can be corrected by balloon dilatation using the technique introduced by Dotter and Judkins[1] and modified into its present form by Gruntzig and Hopff[2]. This technique may give good results when the stenosis involves the main stem of the renal artery but the results have been unsatisfactory with a high recurrence rate if the plaque or atheroma involves the origin of the renal artery from the abdominal aorta.

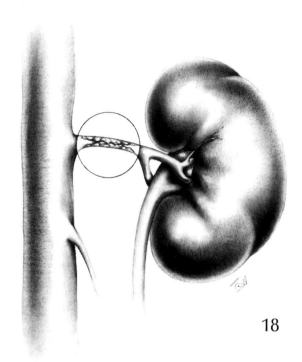

18

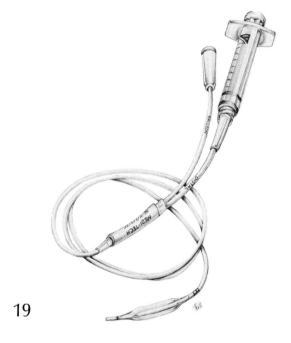

19

19 & 20

The balloon catheter, mounted on a guide-wire, is introduced into the common femoral artery and threaded up the iliac arteries into the aorta. Because the diameter of the apparatus is greater than that of the conventional Seldinger angiography catheter, the puncture in the wall of the femoral artery is larger. This necessitates arterial compression for at least 20 min followed by observation for 8 hours or more so that a haematoma does not develop.

The balloon catheter is then introduced into the renal artery and passed completely through the arterial stenosis. It is important that the balloon covers the whole area of arterial stenosis so that the dilatation can be complete in a longitudinal direction.

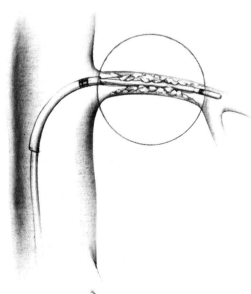

20

21

The balloon is inflated and the atherosclerotic stricture is dilated. This requires a pressure of 404–606 kPa (4–6 atm) which is introduced into the balloon through the second lumen of the double-lumen balloon catheter.

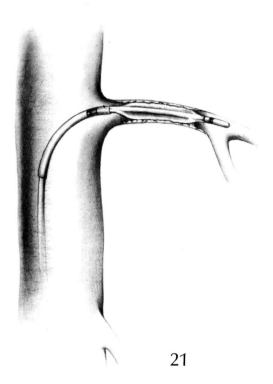

21

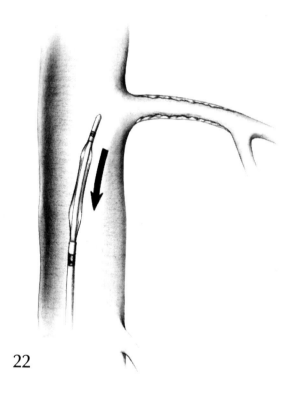

22

22

The balloon is deflated and the catheter withdrawn a short distance. A small amount of contrast is injected to confirm that a satisfactory dilatation of the stricture has been achieved. The balloon catheter is then withdrawn into the abdominal aorta and out through the original puncture site in the common femoral artery.

NEPHRECTOMY OR PARTIAL NEPHRECTOMY

This is the simpliest operation and may be the procedure of choice in patients whose general condition is poor; it is also indicated when a conservative arterial reconstruction has failed. In most patients an arterial reconstruction operation is the best treatment because the kidney on the affected side may be the better kidney after a normal blood flow has been restored, having been protected by the arterial stenosis from secondary hypertensive changes.

Postoperative care

Prophylactic measures

Ischaemic renal damage

The risk of ischaemic damage is slight as these procedures can usually be done well within the safe ischaemia time limit. The tolerance of the kidney beyond a renal artery stenosis is also probably significantly greater than normal in view of the considerable collateral circulation through capsular and other vessels as evidenced by the brisk backflow from the distal end of the artery. However, if prolongation of the ischaemic period beyond 30 min is necessary it is wise to give an infusion of mannitol intravenously before releasing the clamps.

Paralytic ileus

Because of the extensive retroperitoneal dissection performed in operations for stenosis of the renal arteries it is essential to take prophylactic measures against paralytic ileus. Gastric suction and intravenous fluid replacement should be used until the patient has good bowel sounds and is passing flatus.

Anticoagulant drugs

Anticoagulant drugs are used after balloon dilatation but not after the other procedures in the immediate postoperative period because of the danger of haemorrage.

Blood pressure

The fall in blood pressure in successful cases usually occurs slowly after operation and it is often months before it returns completely to normal and secondary hypertensive changes regress. Severe hypertensive retinopathy is seen to revert to almost normal within 3 months after an operation for reconstruction of the renal artery. Occasionally there may be a more precipitate fall of blood pressure in which case a careful search should be made for the usual causes such as haemorrhage, lung infection, acute gastric dilation or gram-negative bacteraemia before assuming that such a fall is due to an overswing following correction of the renin-angiotensin stimulus.

References

1. Dotter, C. T., Judkins, M. D. Transluminal treatment of atherosclerotic obstruction: description of a new technique and a preliminary report of its application. Circulation 1964; 30: 654–670

2. Gruntzig, A., Hopff, H. Perkutane Rekanalisatsion chronischer arterieller Verschlüsse mit einem neven Dilatationskatheter: Modifikation der Dotter-Technik. Deutsche Medizinische Wochenschrift 1974; 99: 2502–2510

Further reading

Belzer, F. O., Salvetierra, O., Perloff, D., Grausz, H. Surgical correction of advanced fibromuscular hyperplasia of the renal arteries. Surgery 1974; 75: 31–37

Foster, J. H., Maxwell, M. H., Franklin, S. S., et al. Renovascular occlusive disease: results of operative treatment. Journal of the American Medical Association 1975; 231: 1043–1048

Gruntzig, A., Vetter, W., Meier, B., Kuhlman, U., Lütolf, U., Siegenthaler, W. Treatment of renovascular hypertension with percutaneous transluminal dilatation of a renal artery stenosis. Lancet 1978; 1: 801–803

Najarian, J. S., Ascher, N. L. Renovascular hypertension in children and adolescents. Advances in vascular surgery. Chicago: Year Book 1982: 427–433

Rob, C. G., Frank, I. N. Renal artery occlusive disease with hypertension. In: Hardy, J. D., (ed) Hardy's textbook of surgery. Philadelphia: Lippincott 1983: 888–893

Stoney, R. J., Lusby, R. J. Renovascular hypertension in adults. In: Advances in vascular surgery. Chicago: Year Book, 1983: 421–426

Illustrations by Robert N. Lane

Traumatic injuries of the kidney

W. Scott McDougal MD
Professor and Chairman, Department of Urology;
Vanderbilt University Medical Center, Nashville, Tennessee, USA

Introduction

Renal injury occurs with a frequency of approximately 2 per 100 000 of the population and is most commonly encountered in men in their 20s and 30s. Blunt trauma is responsible for two-thirds of the cases, while penetrating trauma accounts for the remainder. Only about 7 per cent of patients with penetrating abdominal wounds, however, have injuries involving the kidneys.

The protection afforded the kidney by the ribcage, vertebral column and investing fascia accounts for the relatively low incidence of injury in the adult. However, despite this protection, the kidney is the organ most frequently injured in children as a result of blunt abdominal trauma. The lack of perinephric fat in children (which serves to buffer the kidney from blunt injury) probably accounts for the difference in incidence between children and adults. In addition, pre-existing renal disease may also contribute to the higher incidence of renal injury in children since one-fifth of children with renal trauma have pre-existing renal abnormalities. Renal injuries, blunt or penetrating, are commonly associated with other injuries. Indeed, renal trauma is often unsuspected, since the associated injury is usually recognized initially and may obscure the signs and symptoms of renal injury. Associated injuries are more commonly found in penetrating trauma than in blunt injury. The organs most often injured in descending order of frequency are the liver, lungs, spleen, small bowel, stomach, pancreas, duodenum and diaphragm.

Signs and symptoms

Signs and symptoms of renal injury may be protean. However, those most commonly encountered include haematuria, tenderness or ecchymosis over the flank, a flank mass, and entrance or exit wounds on the skin overlying the renal fossa. Although 80–90 per cent of patients with renal injury present with haematuria, many patients are found to have urine free from blood cells. Indeed, patients with renal pedicle injuries invariably have a normal urine analysis. Because many of the signs and symptoms are not specific for renal injury, a high index of suspicion must be maintained when evaluating the trauma patient if these injuries are not to be missed.

Diagnosis

Roentgenography is generally the first aid employed in confirming a diagnosis of suspected renal injury. The studies are obtained in a logical progression beginning with the plain film or KUB. Unfortunately, in only about 15 per cent of cases does the KUB suggest the diagnosis.

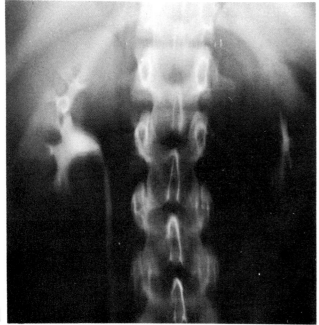

Nephrotomogram of a fractured left kidney. Notice the poor concentration of the dye and the lack of clarity of the renal border

Renal injury is suggested by fractures of overlying ribs or vertebral bodies, obliteration of the psoas outline, blurring of the kidney outline and displacement of loops of bowel away from the renal fossa.

1

Nephrotomography

Following the KUB, an infusion or high-dose intravenous pyelogram with nephrotomography is obtained. This investigation has a diagnostic accuracy of about 95 per cent. An injury is suggested by a lack of or delay in visualization, extravasation of contrast, lack of continuous renal outline, an enlarged renal shadow, or radiolucent areas within the confines of the kidney.

Infusion pyelography provides the patient with a large osmotic load and may contribute to haemodynamic instability if it is administered to an inadequately resuscitated patient. Seizures and further aggravation of the shocked state due to loss of fluid, because of the osmotic diuresis, can occur. Moreover, the dye may precipitate acute renal failure if administered to the unstable trauma patient. Therefore, it is necessary to resuscitate the trauma victim properly prior to performing an infusion pyelogram.

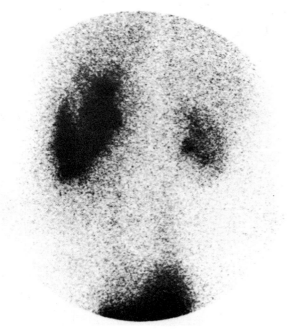

2

Renal scans

Renal scans have also been successfully employed in the initial diagnosis of renal injury and have the advantage of neither exacerbating haemodynamic instability nor causing acute renal failure in the inadequately resuscitated patient. Technetium 99m glucoheptonate is the radionuclide usually employed. Pedicle injuries or segmental arterial injuries may be diagnosed by a lack of tracer flow to the kidney or to a part of it. Parenchymal fractures may also be demonstrated provided the defect is large and the parenchymal tissue is separated by more than 1 cm. Unfortunately, the inability to obtain scans in most hospitals on an emergency basis limits their usefulness in the initial evaluation. However, they are of considerable help in following the renal injury over the long term.

Renal scan of a patient with traumatic disruption of the right lower pole and renal pelvis. Notice the extravasation of the radionuclide

3a & b

Ultrasonography

Ultrasonography is perhaps the most significant recent advance in the diagnosis and management of renal injury. With its use, the frequency with which renal angiograms must be obtained has been considerably reduced. This modality is particularly useful in the diagnosis of subcapsular haematomas, confirming the integrity of renal parenchyma when the entire renal outline cannot be visualized by pyelography and confirming the location of a kidney which does not visualize on infusion pyelography.

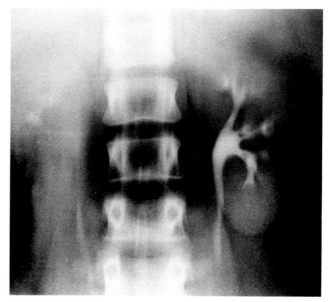

3a

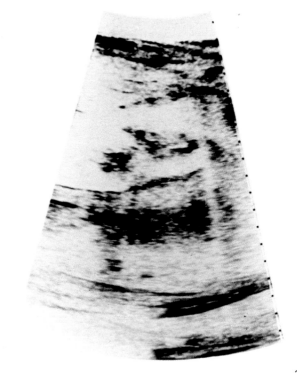

3b

(a) Nephrotomogram of a patient who sustained a traumatic injury to the right kidney. Notice the obscured inferior pole of the right kidney. (b) Ultrasonogram demonstrating a subcapsular haematoma of the inferior pole of the right kidney

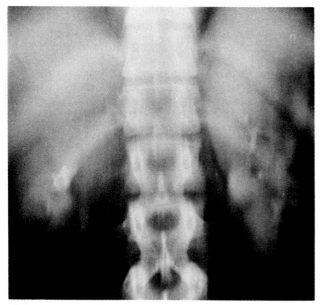

4a

(a) Nephrotomogram of a patient who sustained blunt trauma to the right flank. Notice the poor filling of the inferior calyces. (b) Computerized axial tomograph. Notice the extensive haematoma formation on the lateral border of the right kidney

4a & b

Computerized axial tomography

Computerized axial tomography, obtained routinely in patients suspected of having substantial abdominal trauma, has recently been advocated. Initial reports suggest that this is an excellent modality for determining the presence and extent of renal injury. With the intravenous injection of a radiocontrast agent, parenchymal injuries as well as collecting system injuries can be diagnosed with a high degree of accuracy.

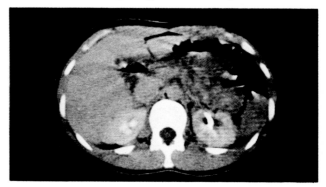

4b

5

Angiography

The above diagnostic procedures select a group of patients who are candidates for angiography. Those who should have an angiogram are: those suspected of having a renal pedicle injury; individuals in whom major fractures or separation of renal fragments are suspected and in whom, if confirmed, an operation will be performed; and those who have persistent haematuria or in whom continued bleeding occurs. It is also helpful, usually later in the patient's post-traumatic course, for documenting an arteriovenous fistula.

When extravasation of contrast is extensive, documentation of the size and location of the collecting system injury is best obtained by retrograde pyelography. Indeed, children who sustain acute hyperextension injuries in whom a renal injury is suspected may have disruptions of the ureteropelvic junction and should have a retrograde pyelogram if the intravenous pyelogram does not indicate continuity between the renal pelvis and the proximal ureter.

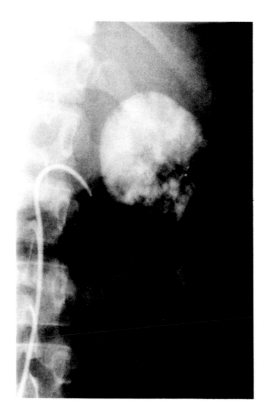

5

Renal angiogram demonstrating extensive fracture of the left kidney (same case as Illustration 1)

Classification of injuries

6a–e

Renal injuries are classified into one of five groups depending on their severity and location: (a) contusions; (b) lacerations; (c) fractures; (d) pedicle injuries; and (e) pelvic injuries.

Contusions

Renal contusions account for approximately 85 per cent of kidney injuries. They are usually due to blunt trauma and include subcapsular haematomas and minor cortical lacerations. Patients commonly present with flank pain and microscopic haematuria. The latter may persist for a week or more. The intravenous pyelogram is often suggestive when a portion of the renal outline cannot be clearly defined (see Illustration 3a). However, frequently the intravenous pyelogram is normal and a diagnosis can only be made by ultrasonography (see Illustration 3b) or angiography. Clearly, the latter is not indicated in these patients and the non-invasive ultrasonogram is the diagnostic procedure of choice. These patients are treated conservatively with bedrest until the gross haematuria clears; their activity is limited until the microscopic haematuria abates.

Lacerations

Lacerations which extend deep within the parenchyma of the kidney account for somewhat less than 10 per cent of all renal injuries. The treatment of this group remains controversial since there are advocates of both conservative and operative treatment. Those suggesting conservative treatment note that the incidence of nephrectomy in this group is less when non-operative treatment is employed initially than if there is immediate surgical intervention. Moreover, delayed complications in a conservatively treated group are reportedly minimal. They include: delayed rupture of the kidney, persistent haematuria, perinephric abscess, renin-mediated hypertension and arteriovenous fistulae.

Those arguing for immediate exploration, debridement and suture of the laceration with drainage of the wounds suggest that the complications of conservative management are for the most part eliminated and that better preservation of renal function is achieved. A prospective study is required to settle this issue.

Diagnosis of lacerations is generally made by infusion pyelography with the aid of ultrasonography. If these two modalities do not clearly indicate the extent of the lesion, angiography is indicated.

Fractures

Fractures involve multiple portions of the kidney in which segments of the parenchyma are not in continuity with the remaining kidney as a whole. The diagnosis of this injury is made by intravenous pyelography, ultrasonography and, finally, angiography.

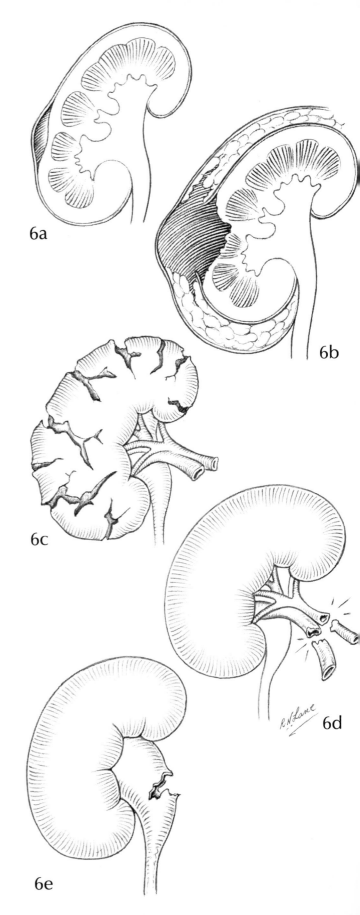

6a

6b

6c

6d

6e

Pedicle injuries

Vascular injuries of the pedicle occur as a result of deceleration-type injury and less frequently as a consequence of blunt or penetrating injuries. When they are due to the latter, associated intra-abdominal injuries involving either the duodenum and/or pancreas often make *in situ* repair difficult. In these circumstances, the kidney should be removed, and, if the patient's stability permits, autotransplanted to the pelvis (*see* chapter on 'Renal transplantation', pp. 201–212).

An arterial repair adjacent to a major injury of the pancreas or duodenum is fraught with postoperative complications and a very high mortality rate. Less commonly, pedicle injuries are unassociated with multiple injuries and the patient's stability allows for *in situ* repair. These injuries are usually of a deceleration type and involve intimal tears which occur approximately 1 cm from the origin of the renal artery from the aorta. The diagnosis is suspected on intravenous pyelography in which there is marked delay or non-visualization of the kidney. Renal scans may also indicate lack of perfusion of the kidney and angiography is diagnostic. Initial vascular control is absolutely mandatory and therefore these lesions are approached through the abdomen, gaining vessel control before exposing the kidney.

Renal pelvic injuries

Injuries of the collecting system of the kidney are diagnosed by noting extravasated dye on the intravenous pyelogram; their extent is confirmed by retrograde pyelography. If the extravasation is minimal, retrograde pyelography is generally not indicated and the patient may be treated expectantly. On the other hand, if a major laceration is suspected, retrograde pyelography confirms the extent. If there are no other associated injuries, a ureteral catheter may be left in place and this may be all that is necessary. On the other hand, if there is extensive loss of pelvic tissue, then immediate exploration, drainage and repair of the devitalized pelvis is necessary (*see Illustrations 8a–d*). It is important to remember that acute hyperextension injury in a child may result in disruption of the ureteral pelvic junction. Retrograde pyelography is diagnostic in these patients.

Surgical technique

7

Patients who require immediate exploration of the kidney for trauma should be approached transabdominally so that vascular control can be obtained before Gerota's fascia is opened. The kidney is reached by incising the retroperitoneum from the level of the ligament of Treitz to the caecum. The small bowel mesentery is placed on the abdomen in the right upper quadrant in a Lahey bag. The ligament of Treitz is incised and the retroperitoneum entered thus exposing the vessels as depicted. A large haematoma is often encountered, making identification of the retroperitoneal structures exceedingly difficult. Usually, by careful dissection immediately beneath the ligament of Treitz, the left renal vein can be identified.

Once this structure is identified, the aorta is easily approached, and the right renal artery is identified between the vena cava and aorta. The left renal artery may be a bit more difficult to identify, but again is often found immediately beneath the left renal vein. It should be noted that the origin of the superior mesenteric artery is within 1 cm of the origin of the renal artery. The superior mesenteric artery can often be confused with the renal artery and it is mandatory to confirm the nature and course of the vessel suspected of being the renal artery prior to severing it. The right renal vein is identified generally with a fair degree of ease as it is the first major vessel cephalad to the origin of the right gonadal vein.

Once these vessels are encircled with vascular loops, Gerota's fascia may be opened and the kidney approached. If there is obvious separation of the parenchymal tissue, that which is separated is removed, the borders of the kidney are debrided and full-thickness sutures bring the margins together.

7

Major renal parenchymal injuries which are to be explored must be approached through the abdomen so that vascular control can be obtained before Gerota's fascia is opened. Small bowel contents are swept to the right and placed in a Lahey bag. The retroperitoneum is opened immediately adjacent to the ligament of Treitz, thus exposing the vessels as depicted.

8a–d

A collecting system injury associated with a parenchymal fracture requires debridement of the parenchyma and a watertight closure of the collecting system. Non-viable renal parenchyma is excised (a) and bleeding vessels suture-ligated with fine chromic suture (b). The collecting system is closed with fine chromic suture (c). The capsule is closed (d). If the capsule is not sufficient for closure, a piece of peritoneum or fascia may be used in its place (see *Illustration 9d*). Major lacerations, if explored, are brought together with chromic sutures over buttresses of fat or Gelfoam.

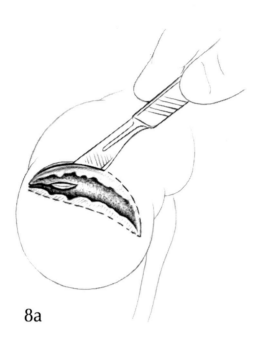

8a

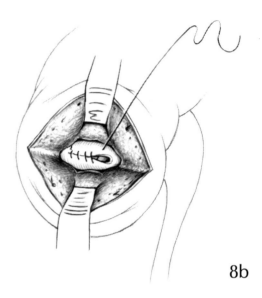

8b

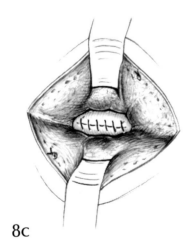

8c

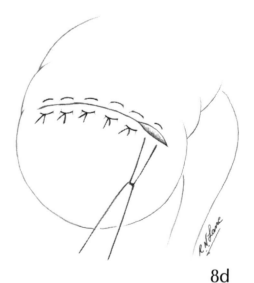

8d

9a–d

On occasion a heminephrectomy is required if the injured parenchyma is extensively fractured and localized to one pole of the kidney. The devitalized tissue is excised, preserving as much capsule as possible(a). The collecting system is closed in a watertight fashion with fine chromic suture (b). The capsule is closed (c), or if it is insufficient, a piece of peritoneum is sutured over the parenchyma (d).

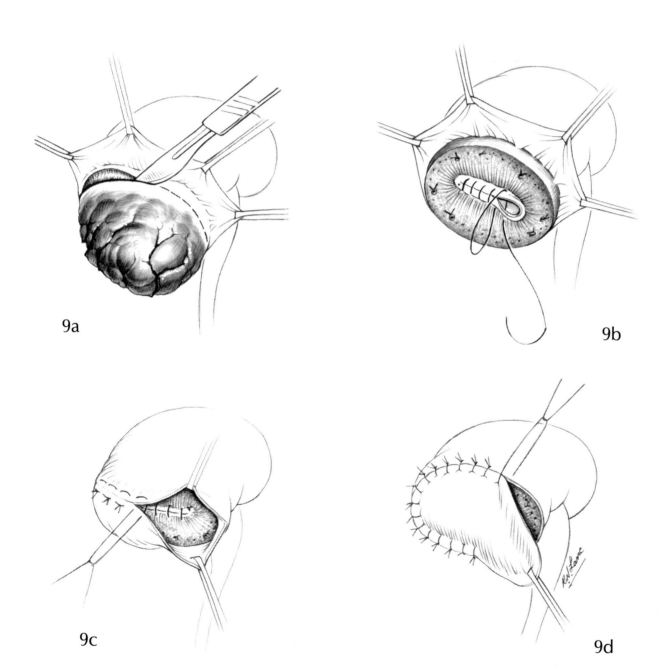

9a

9b

9c

9d

10a–d

Finally, vascular injuries are repaired with 6/0 Prolene sutures. If an intimal tear is present, the segment involved is excised and the ends primarily reanastomosed (a). Alternatively, the origin of the renal artery is ligated at the aorta (b) and the renal artery itself or a graft is sutured directly into the aorta (c). Patch grafts may be necessary in some instances in order to prevent compromise of the small vessel lumen (d). If necessary, either Gore-Tex or saphenous vein may be used as an interposed segment. The anastomosis is best made with the aid of magnification, since accuracy is absolutely mandatory for a successful outcome. Prior to occluding the renal artery, an infusion of mannitol is helpful in protecting the kidney from ischaemia and promoting diureses following restoration of renal bloodflow.

When the kidney is injured and there is a major duodenal, pancreatic or vascular injury, the kidney must be separated from these structures. If this cannot be accomplished by reapproximating Gerota's fascia and draining the area away from the above-named structures, then the kidney should either be removed or autotransplanted (see chapter on 'Renal transplantation', pp. 201–212, for the technique of autotransplantation). A nephrostomy should be performed if the kidney is left in situ in such instances, since if urine bathes wounds of the pancreas, duodenum or great vessels complications and a high mortality rate are inevitable.

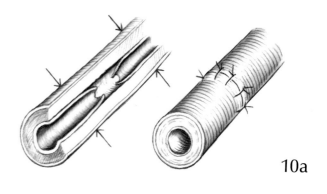

10a

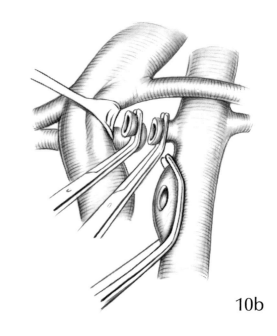

10b

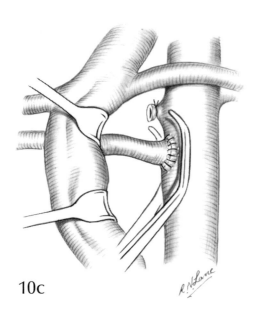

10c

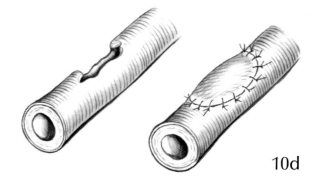

10d

Complications of renal trauma

There are numerous complications of renal trauma which may occur within the first few weeks or as late sequelae. Early complications include haemorrhage, sepsis, urinary extravasation, perinephric abscess, fistula formation, vascular suture line disruption, pancreatic fistula, duodenal fistula, and acute renal failure.

Late complications include hypertension, generally as a result of a compromised vessel or constriction of the kidney (Page kidney), hydronephrosis, chronic renal failure, calculus disease, arteriovenous fistulae, haematocele and non-functioning kidney.

Renal injury in children

Children's kidneys are much more vulnerable to injury than adults' because the retroperitoneal area is not as well protected by fat as it is in adults'. Most children with renal injuries, save for those of the pedicle and complete fracture of the kidney with separation of parts, should be observed initially. They may be explored after being stabilized between the second and the fifth post-injury day if there is urinoma formation, continued haemorrhage, or the extent of the original injury was underestimated. Immediate exploration, of course, should be performed in patients with expanding flank masses or pedicle injury, or in whom major segments of parenchyma are disrupted and disassociated from the remaining kidney with continued bleeding.

Further reading

Bergquvist, D., Hedelin, H., Lindblad, B. Blunt renal trauma, Scandinavian Journal of Urology and Nephrology 1980; 14: 177–180

Cass, A. S. Immediate radiological evaluation and early surgical management of genitourinary injuries from external trauma. Journal of Urology 1979; 122: 772–774

Emanuel, B., Weiss, H., Gollin, P. Renal trauma in children. Journal of Trauma 1977; 17: 275–278

McAninch, J. W., Carroll, P. R. Renal trauma: Kidney preservation through improved vascular control – a refined approach. Journal of Trauma 1982; 22: 285–290

McDougal, W. S., Persky, L. Traumatic injuries of the genitourinary system. Baltimore: Williams and Wilkins, 1981

Wein, A. J., Murphy, J. J., Mulholland, S. G., Chait, A. W., Arger, P. H. A conservative approach to the management of blunt renal trauma. Journal of Urology 1977; 117: 425–427

Williams, J. E. Renal trauma; the place of arteriography. British Journal of Radiology 1976; 49: 743–744

Illustrations by Harriet Phillips

Surgical correction of congenital ureteropelvic junction obstruction

Terry W. Hensle MD
Director, Pediatric Urology, and Associate Professor of Urology,
College of Physicians and Surgeons, New York, USA

Howard R. Goldstein MD
Pediatric Urologist and Clinical Assistant Professor of Surgery,
UMDNJ-Rutgers Medical School at Camden,
Cooper Hospital-University Medical Center, New Jersey, USA

Kevin A. Burbige MD
Associate Director, Pediatric Urology and Assistant Professor of Urology,
College of Physicians and Surgeons, New York, USA

Introduction

Obstruction at the ureteropelvic junction is most frequently diagnosed in childhood, but can be seen in patients of all ages. Presenting symptoms may vary widely with abdominal mass being common in the newborn, whereas older children usually present with abdominal pain, urinary tract infection or haematuria. Ureteropelvic junction obstruction occurs twice as often in males, and in most reports, the left kidney is more frequently involved than the right. The incidence of bilaterality varies in different series but is considered generally to be about 20–25 per cent[1-7]. Interestingly, bilateral cases have been reported more commonly in the infant population[2,6].

Pathogenesis of ureteropelvic junction obstruction

Obstruction at the ureteropelvic junction can be related to either extrinsic or intrinsic lesions of the collecting system. Regardless of the aetiology the end result is a poorly propelled urinary bolus across the ureteropelvic junction which results in hydronephrosis. The obstruction may lead to varying degrees of renal parenchymal destruction, and in its most severe form, seen with proximal ureteral atresia, the result will be the development of a multicystic kidney. The association of ureteropelvic junction obstruction in the contralateral kidney of those infants with unilateral multicystic kidney would suggest that the aetiology is often a bilateral ureteral bud defect[3,7].

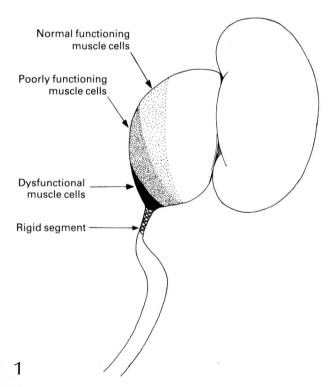

Normal functioning muscle cells

Poorly functioning muscle cells

Dysfunctional muscle cells

Rigid segment

1

In most instances a congenital intrinsic lesion is responsible for ureteropelvic junction obstruction. The histopathology of the obstruction has been shown to be very similar to that of primary obstructive megaureter. There is an abundance of intracellular ground substance and collagen present within the ureter as well as smooth muscle cell dysplasia most strikingly seen at the point of maximal obstruction and decreasing in severity proximal to the obstruction. This has all been convincingly demonstrated in electron microscopic and histochemical studies by Hanna et al.[8,9] and Gosling and Dixon[10].

Other conditions such as aberrant lower pole vessels, ureteral bands, kinks, high insertion of the ureteral ostium on the renal pelvis, intraluminal polyps and ureteral valves[11] have been proposed as an aetiology for some ureteropelvic junction obstructions. The controversy as to whether polar vessels are primarily responsible for ureteropelvic junction or whether the redundant hydro-nephrotic renal pelvis merely drapes over the vessel is long standing[8, 11]. Most investigators today agree that the primary lesion is intrinsic and that the ballooning of the renal pelvis over polar vessels is usually secondary to the intrinsic lesion[12].

Ureteropelvic junction obstruction may also be encountered in association with vesicoureteral reflux[13]. Whether the upper ureteral obstruction is a concomitant anomaly or a direct result of the reflux is often difficult to determine. When significant ureteropelvic junction obstruction is found in the presence of low grades of reflux, the obstruction is usually an independent lesion. When ureteropelvic junction obstruction is associated with massive degrees of reflux, however, it is usually caused by tortuosity and kinking of the upper ureter from the reflux[13]. In either case the degree of obstruction should be quantified before antireflux surgery is performed. In most instances, if the obstruction at the ureteropelvic junction is mild, it will subside once the reflux has been corrected. If, however, significant obstruction coexists with significant reflux, it should be corrected before undertaking antireflux surgery since the resultant oedema at the ureterovesical junction may further compromise renal drainage.

Presentation and diagnosis

In infancy, ureteropelvic junction obstruction presents most commonly as an abdominal mass. In older children and adults, the presenting symptoms are most often abdominal or flank pain, urinary tract infection or haematuria. Gross haematuria can occur in the adolescent with ureteropelvic junction obstruction after minor flank or abdominal trauma[1-7]. Children with vague abdominal symptoms mimicking gastrointestinal disorders have frequently been recognized to have symptoms caused by ureteropelvic junction obstruction alone[2]. Many of the symptoms of ureteropelvic junction obstruction may be intermittent and only occur during rapid diuresis. In suspected cases of intermittent obstruction; a diuretic excretory urogram or radionuclide scan may not only reproduce the symptoms but also simultaneously confirm the obstruction radiographically[12, 13].

Several authors have advocated abdominal ultrasound or radionuclide scans as initial diagnostic procedures. While these modalities are helpful the cornerstone of diagnosis remains the excretory urogram. Obstruction may cause marked delay in the excretion of contrast medium and unless late films are obtained, the renal pelvis may not be visualized. High dose intravenous drip infusion urography and nephrotomography will improve the diagnostic yield. However, confirmation of the diagnosis is often needed. In these instances we prefer the Tc99 DTPA diuretic renogram as popularized by Koff et al.[14-16] which provides an objective assessment of renal parenchymal function as well as quantitation of the degree of obstruction. Percutaneous antegrade pyelography and pressure flow studies also can be helpful[17-19] in delineating clearly the ureteropelvic anatomy and assessing the degree of obstruction. In very sick infants or where the ultimate function of an obstructed kidney is in question, a percutaneous nephrostomy may easily be left in the renal pelvis at the time of antegrade studies to facilitate assessment of renal function after decompression. This information may be helpful in deciding whether a primary nephrectomy or pyeloplasty is indicated.

Voiding cystourethrography should be carried out in all patients with ureteropelvic junction obstruction to rule out the presence of concurrent vesicoureteral reflux, although the routine use of retrograde pyelography as a diagnostic tool other than as a confirmatory study just prior to pyeloplasty is not indicated. Retrograde pyelography in the presence of obstructed renal pelvis may precipitate urosepsis and should be done only immediately prior to surgery.

Surgical correction of ureteropelvic junction obstruction

Historically, the surgical correction of ureteropelvic junction obstruction has been approached in many ways. In 1937 Foley[20] reported his technique of Y-V plasty, and this remains a useful operation for situations in which there is a high insertion of the ureter on the renal pelvis. Davis[21] first described intubated ureterostomy in 1943, and in 1949 Anderson and Hynes[22] introduced the dismembered pyeloplasty which remains popular today. In the 1950s a variety of pyeloplasties using renal pelvic flaps were introduced. Scardino and Prince[23] advocated a vertical flap technique, while Culp and DeWeerd[24] suggested the use of a spiral flap. Both these techniques are extremely useful in long, proximal ureteral strictures where dismembered pyeloplasty cannot be accomplished without tension.

The dismembered pyeloplasty

The dismembered pyeloplasty remains the most versatile of the ureteropelvic reconstructive procedures. It allows removal of the primary pathology and creation of a dependent funnel-shaped pelvis which, after surgical tapering, can initiate a strong enough peristaltic wave to carry a urinary bolus across the reconstructed uretero-pelvic junction. Hanley[25] has described a normal funnel-shaped renal pelvis and a box-like abnormal renal pelvis which is more likely to develop ureteropelvic junction obstruction during diuresis. His data would indicate that the creation of a dependently draining funnel-shaped renal pelvis is likely to result in a favourable outcome after plastic repair.

Surgical technique of the dismembered pyeloplasty

Adherence to rigid principles in surgical technique offers the best chance of obtaining favourable results in ureteropelvic junction reconstruction, no matter what technique is used. We attempt to use the operation that best fits the patient's anatomical defect. However, the Anderson-Hynes dismembered pyeloplasty, because of its simplicity, has become our preferred procedure as it has at most centres around the world.

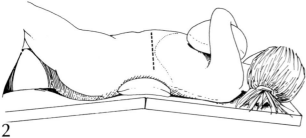

2

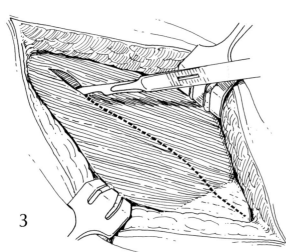

3

2

The patient is placed in a supine position with a sandbag under the flank. The table is flexed modestly to facilitate the anterior approach to the renal pelvis. An incision is made from the tip of the 12th rib and carried medially in a transverse fashion to a point two fingerbreadths lateral to the rectus abdominis muscle and two fingerbreadths above the umbilicus. This incision allows the surgeon direct access to the renal hilum and ureteropelvic junction. The tip of the 12th rib may be resected if additional exposure is needed, but we have not found this to be necessary in most paediatric patients.

3

The external and internal oblique muscles are incised in the direction of the skin incision. Laterally the latissimus dorsi is incised just enough to provide sufficient relaxation of the posterior aspect of the wound. The transversus abdominis is split in the direction of its fibres and the lumbodorsal fascia is sharply incised. The peritoneum is bluntly displaced medially and Gerota's fascia incised. At this point, the Denis Browne self-retaining ring retractor is placed in the wound for maximal exposure.

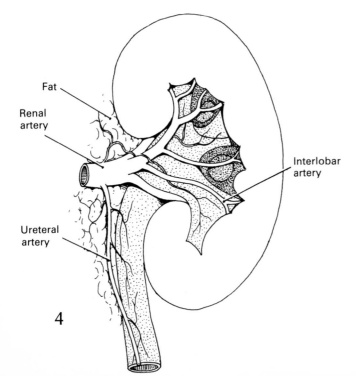

4

4

Great care must be taken to minimize trauma to the upper ureter. The blood supply of this region is best maintained by minimal dissection of the upper ureter and reconstruction of the ureter and pelvis *in situ*[26].

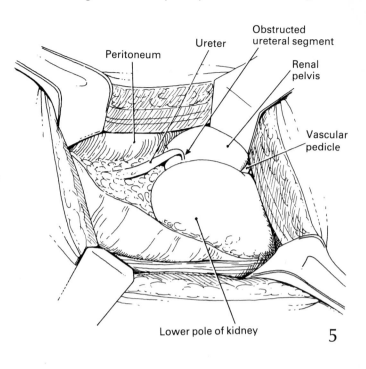

Peritoneum   Ureter   Obstructed ureteral segment   Renal pelvis   Vascular pedicle

Lower pole of kidney   5

5

Once the area of obstruction is exposed, attention is directed to designing the repair.

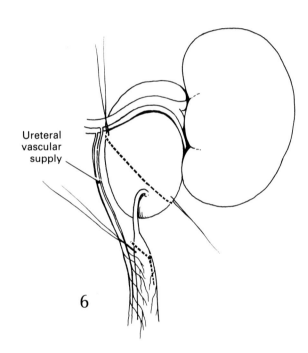

Ureteral vascular supply

6

6

Stay sutures are placed in the superior medial and inferior lateral renal pelvis as well as in the adventitial layer of the upper ureter. Methylene blue is useful for marking out the line of resection once the pelvis is decompressed.

7

The upper ureter is transected obliquely and spatulated laterally for about 1 cm, leaving the medial blood supply undisturbed. The reanastomosis of the ureter and resected renal pelvis is accomplished using interrupted 5/0 or 6/0 absorbable sutures with knots tied outside the lumen.

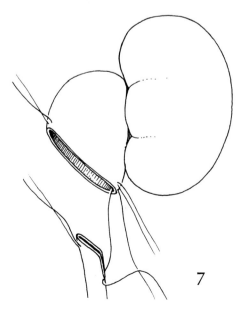

7

8

Once several sutures have been secured, a lower pole nephrostomy or pyelostomy is placed in the kidney by simply pushing a right-angled clamp through a thin area in the lower pole of the kidney or pelvis and grasping an 8 Fr Silastic paediatric feeding tube to bring the tip into the renal pelvis. This feeding tube is fixed to the renal capsule or pelvis with 4/0 chromic catgut and brought out to the skin at the lateral edge of the wound. Creating extra drainage holes in the end of the feeding tube facilitates urinary drainage postoperatively. A small feeding tube or red rubber catheter of appropriate size may be used as a temporary stent to facilitate the anastomosis.

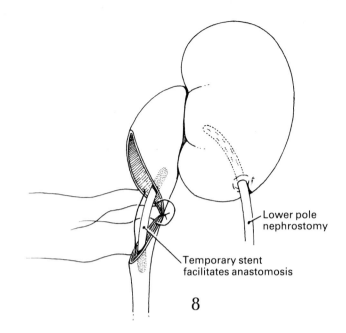

Lower pole nephrostomy

Temporary stent facilitates anastomosis

8

9

The stent must be removed before the anastomosis is completed and the tapered renal pelvis is closed. At this point, gentle irrigation of the nephrostomy tube will ensure patency of the anastomosis and display any leaks, which can then be closed with additional sutures. The repair is drained postoperatively with a soft Penrose drain which is placed dependently and brought out through the posterior aspect of the incision. Wound closure is accomplished in layers using continuous absorbable suture. The nephrostomy tube and drain are fixed to the skin using silk sutures.

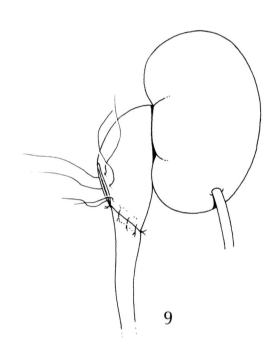

9

Whether stenting a ureteropelvic anastomosis is beneficial or not remains controversial. Recent evidence from several authors suggests that there are fewer long-term problems in dismembered pyeloplasty done without stenting catheters passing through the anastomosis[26, 27]. However, a strong case for using proximal urinary diversion after pyeloplasty can be made from data provided by Caine and Hermann[35] who have demonstrated in cineradiographic studies that normal ureteral peristalsis does not return for about 3 weeks after anastomosis.

The nephrostomy tube is left to dependent drainage for 3–4 days postoperatively and then clamped intermittently and residuals measured. In most instances the patient is discharged on the 5th postoperative day with the tube clamped. At 10 days a nephrostogram is performed with fluoroscopy. If the renal pelvis drains well, the nephrostomy or pyeloplasty tube is removed. If contrast medium is retained in the renal pelvis, the patient may be sent home again with the tube in place and re-examined in a similar manner after several weeks. The nephrostomy tract can on rare occasions be used for endoscoping the anastomosis if persistent obstruction is present.

Other pyeloplasty techniques

Each of the major types of non-dismembering pyeloplasty techniques has specific advantages and applications which will allow maximal surgical results when these operations are applied for particular pathological anatomy. The Foley Y-V plasty[20] is, for example, particularly helpful in reconstructing the high insertion type of ureteropelvic junction obstruction.

The surgical technique in all the non-dismembering operations is the same as the Anderson-Hynes procedure described above until the point where the ureteropelvic junction is approached.

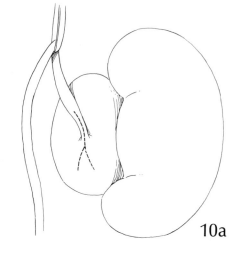

10a

10a, b & c

In the Foley Y-V plasty a widely based V-flap is designed from the inferolateral aspect of the renal pelvis and carefully outlined with a tissue marker or methylene blue. The ureter, which is best left *in situ*, is spatulated laterally and the apex of the V-flap is brought down and anastomosed to the lowest point of spatulation.

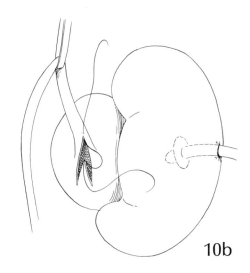

10b

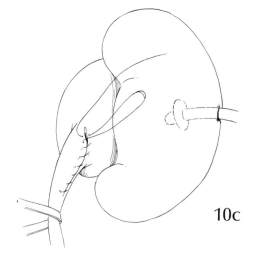

10c

11a, b & c

A very similar procedure has been described which is particularly helpful with a high insertion ureteropelvic junction obstruction and in a horseshoe kidney with an anteriorly placed renal pelvis.

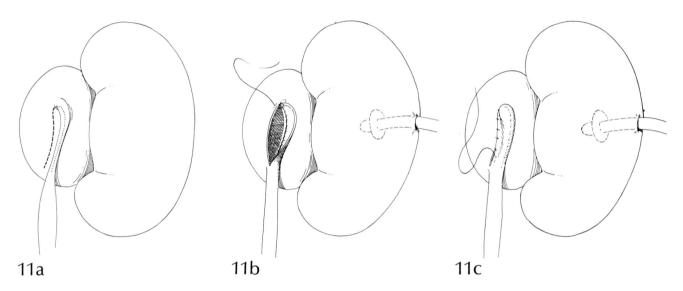

11a   11b   11c

The various flap procedures are similar in principle to the Foley Y-V plasty in that a wide-based flap of redundant pelvis is rotated inferiorly and anastomosed beyond a spatulated narrowed ureteropelvic junction. The two most popular flap procedures have been the Culp-DeWeerd spiral flap[24] and the Scardino-Prince procedure.

12a, b & c

The Culp-DeWeerd operation involves creation of a long flap of pelvis which when rotated laterally and inferiorly will oppose the spatulated narrowed segment or proximal ureter. The spatulation is generally performed on the anteromedial aspect of the ureter and should extend just beyond the narrowed segment. This procedure as well as the Scardino-Prince flap procedure[23] have particular application to long proximal ureteral strictures.

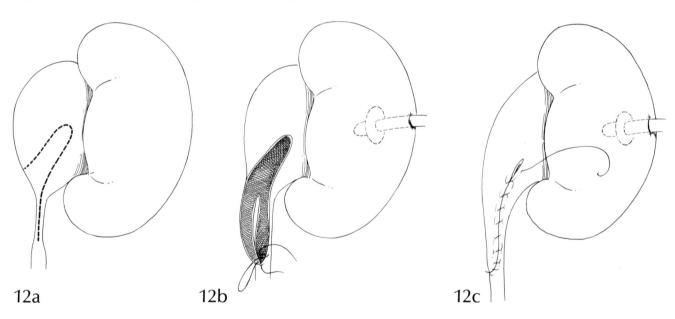

12a   12b   12c

13a, b & c

The Scardino-Prince operation differs from the Culp procedure only in that a vertical flap of redundant pelvis is rotated inferiorly and anastomosed to the spatulated proximal ureteral stricture.

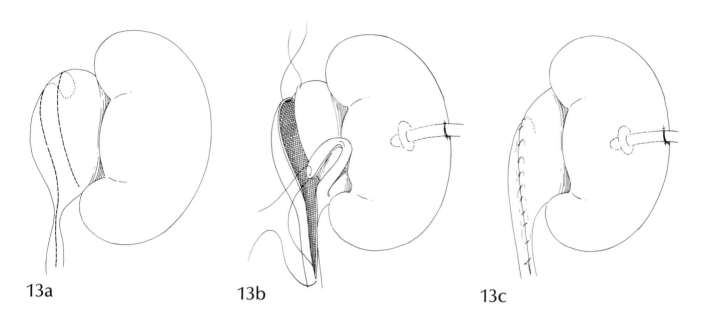

13a   13b   13c

Nephrectomy

Nephrectomy is rarely necessary as a form of primary therapy in the paediatric population with ureteropelvic junction obstruction. In the 1960s Uson et al.[27] reported a 36 per cent primary nephrectomy rate in a series of 136 kidneys, and Kelalis[28] had a nephrectomy rate of 24 per cent. In the late 1970s reports of fewer primary nephrectomies appeared. In Great Britain Williams[4] and Johnston[6] reported a 4.8 per cent and 10 per cent primary nephrectomy rate respectively while in the United States Hendren reported a primary nephrectomy rate for ureteropelvic junction obstruction of only 5 per cent[1,29]. This improvement is consistent with improved surgical technique.

Postoperative follow-up

Following successful surgical correction of ureteropelvic junction obstruction, all patients are maintained on antibiotic suppression for a period of 3 months. Excretory urography is performed at 3 months, 1 year and 5 years postoperatively in order to follow renal growth and assess the patency of the pyeloureteral anastomosis.

References

1. Hendren, W. H., Radhakrishnan, J., Middleton, A. W., Jr. Pediatric pyeloplasty. Journal of Pediatric Surgery 1980; 15: 133–144

2. Zincke, H., Kelalis, P. P., Culp, O. S. Ureteropelvic obstruction in children. Surgery, Gynecology and Obstetrics 1974; 139: 873–878

3. Robson, W. J., Rudy, S. M., Johnston, J. H. Pelvic ureteric obstruction in infancy. Journal of Pediatric Surgery 1976; 11: 57–61

4. Williams, D. I., Kenawi, M. M. The prognosis of pelviureteric obstruction in childhood: a review of 190 cases. European Urology 1976; 2: 57–63

5. Smith, P., Roberts, M., Whitaker, R. H., Garousche, A. R. Primary pelvic hydronephrosis in children: a retrospective study. British Journal of Urology 1976; 48: 549–554

6. Johnston, J. H., Evans, J. P., Glassberg, K. I., Shapiro, S. R. Pelvic hydronephrosis in children: a review of 219 personal cases. Journal of Urology 1977; 117: 97–101

7. Williams, D. I., Karlaftis, C. M. Hydronephrosis due to pelvi-ureteric obstruction in the newborn. British Journal of Urology 1966; 38: 138–144

8. Hanna, M. K. Some observations on congenital ureteropelvic junction obstruction. Urology 1978; 12: 151–159

9. Hanna, M. K., Jeffs, R. D., Sturgess, J. M., Baskin, M. Ureteral structure and ultrastructure. Part II: Congenital ureteropelvic junctions obstruction and primary obstructive megaureter. Journal of Urology 1976; 116: 725–730

10. Gosling, J. A., Dixon, J. S. Functional obstruction of the ureter and renal pelvis: a histological and electron microscopic study. British Journal of Urology 1978; 50: 145–152

11. Kelalis, P. P. Ureteropelvic junction. In: Kelalis, P. P., King, L. R., eds. Clinical pediatric urology, Vol. 1. Philadelphia: W. B. Saunders Co., 1976: 239–257

12. Johnston, J. H. The pathogenesis of hydronephrosis in children. British Journal of Urology 1969; 41: 724–734

13. Lebowitz, R. L., Johan, B. G. The coexistence of ureteropelvic junction obstruction and reflux. American Journal of Radiology 1982; 140: 231–238

14. Koff, S. A., Thrall, J. H., Keyes, J. W., Jr. Diuretic radionuclide urography: a non-invasive method for evaluating nephroureteral dilation. Journal of Urology 1979; 122: 451–454

15. Koff, S. A., Thrall, J. H., Keyes, J. W., Assessment of hydroureteronephrosis in children using diuretic radionuclide urography. Journal of Urology 1980; 123: 531–534

16. O'Reilly, P. H., Testa, H. J., Lawson, R. S., Farrar, D. J., Edwards, E. C. Diuresis renography in equivocal urinary tract obstruction. British Journal of Urology 1978; 50: 76–80

17. Whitaker, R. H. Investigating wide ureters with ureteral pressure flow studies. Journal of Urology 1976; 116: 81–82

18. Whitaker, R. H. The Whitaker test. Urologic Clinics of North America 1979; 6: 529–539

19. Whitfield, H. N., Britton, K. E., Fry, I. K., et al. The obstructed kidney – correlation between renal function and urodynamic assessment. British Journal of Urology 1977; 49: 615–619

20. Foley, F. E. B. A new plastic operation for stricture at the ureteropelvic junction: report of 20 operations. Journal of Urology 1937; 38: 643–672

21. Davis, D. M. Intubated ureterotomy: a new operation for ureteral and ureteropelvic stricture. Surgery, Gynecology and Obstetrics 1943; 76: 513–523

22. Anderson, J. C., Hynes, W. Retrocaval ureter: a case diagnosed preoperatively and treated successfully by plastic operation. British Journal of Urology 1949; 21: 209–214

23. Scardino, P. L., Prince, C. L. Vertical trap ureteropelvioplasty. Southern Medical Journal 1953; 46: 325–331

24. Culp, O. S., DeWeerd, J. H. A pelvic flap operation for certain types of ureteropelvic obstruction: observations after 2 years' experience. Journal of Urology 1954; 71: 523–529

25. Hanley, H. G. The pelvi-ureteric junction: a cinepyelographic study. British Journal of Urology 1959; 31: 377–384

26. Caine, M., Hermann, G. The return of peristalsis in the anastomosed ureter. British Journal of Urology 1970; 42: 164–170

27. Uson, A. C., Cox, L. A., Lattimer, J. K. Hydronephrosis in infants and children II. Surgical management and results. Journal of the American Medical Association 1968; 205: 327–332

28. Kelalis, P. P., Culp, O. S., Stickler, G. B., Burke, E. C. Ureteropelvic obstruction in children: experience with 109 cases. Journal of Urology 1971; 106: 418–422

29. Crooks, K. K., Hendren, W. H., Pfister, R. C. Giant hydronephrosis in children. Journal of Pediatric Surgery 1979; 14: 844–850

Illustrations by James Suchy

Renal transplantation

Andrew C. Novick MD
Chief, Renal Transplant Service, Department of Urology,
Cleveland Clinic Foundation, Cleveland, Ohio, USA

Introduction

During the last 15 years renal transplantation has become a safe and effective method to treat patients with end-stage renal failure. Transplantation is now being done successfully in many high-risk patients and the pool of potential transplant recipients continues to increase. In 1980, approximately 40 000 patients with end-stage renal disease were treated with either dialysis or transplantation in the United States.

Renal transplant patients are particularly susceptible to poor healing and infection because of the complications of uraemia and the altered host response induced by immunosuppressive therapy. These considerations demand meticulous attention to detail in performing transplantation surgery with careful handling of tissues and strict adherence to basic operative principles of asepsis and haemostasis. Equally important in minimizing the morbidity associated with renal transplantation are anticipation of and prompt treatment of surgical complications, when these occur.

Selection and preparation of recipients

In recent years the criteria for acceptance into most transplant programmes have expanded to encompass many high-risk patients with end-stage renal failure[1]. These include conditions such as age less than 10 or greater than 45 years, an abnormal lower urinary tract, prior cured malignancy, coronary artery disease, persistent hepatitis B antigenaemia, tuberculosis or systemic diseases, such as diabetes mellitus, systemic lupus erythematosus, cystinosis, polyarteritis, scleroderma or Wagener's granulomatosis. Renal transplantation currently is contraindicated only in the management of chronic renal failure owing to oxalosis, or in patients with active infection, uncontrolled or recently treated malignancy, or such severe extrarenal disease as to render prohibitive the risk of anaesthesia for a major operation.

In most cases renal transplantation is not performed until chronic dialysis has been initiated, and patients maintained on chronic peritoneal dialysis are now acceptable candidates as well. Transplantation for chronic renal failure is recommended before dialysis in patients with diabetic nephropathy to obviate progression of extrarenal manifestations of this disease, such as retinopathy or neuropathy. In patients who present before dialysis with an HLA identical living-related donor, transplantation often is scheduled for the time when the patient would otherwise require initiation of chronic dialysis.

Before transplantation all candidates undergo a residual urine determination and a voiding cystourethrogram, while a cystometrogram is also obtained in diabetic patients. No other urological studies are done routinely unless the history suggests an abnormality of the upper or lower urinary tracts. In patients whose bladder cannot be used for transplantation, because of severe neurogenic disease or refractory postinflammatory contracture, transplantation is done into a prefashioned intestinal conduit.

All transplant candidates with diabetes, symptoms of coronary artery disease or age greater than 40 years undergo coronary arteriography in our programme[2]. A coronary artery bypass operation is performed prior to transplantation in patients with significant occlusive disease. This approach has reduced significantly the cardiac risk associated with transplantation surgery, particularly in older or diabetic patients.

In patients with documented remote or active peptic ulcer disease, an acid-reducing gastric procedure is done before transplantation to lessen the potential for postoperative steroid-induced gastrointestinal haemorrhage. Recently selective vagotomy has become the operation of choice and these patients are also treated with cimetidine during the initial transplant hospitalization. Pretransplant splenectomy is done in patients with evidence of hypersplenism, particularly those with leukopenia.

The indications for pretransplant bilateral nephrectomy must be balanced with the advantages derived from retained native kidneys in patients on dialysis. Definite indications for preliminary nephrectomy are pyelonephritis, structural abnormalities of the urinary tract, reninmediated hypertension, and polycystic kidneys which have led to urinary infection or significant haematuria. Less common indications are renal malignancy, immunologically active renal disease, severe proteinuria, or the unusual syndrome of cachexia, hypertension and ascites experienced by some chronic dialysis patients. When preliminary nephrectomy is indicated, bilateral posterior surgical incisions are employed because of a reduced operative morbidity observed with this approach[3].

Numerous studies have demonstrated improved allograft survival rates in patients receiving blood transfusions before cadaver transplantation[4]. This beneficial effect occurs with a single transfusion and appears to be dose-related with the best graft survival in those patients receiving more than 20 transfusions. The mechanism of this effect remains unclear but may include recipient or donor selection or nonspecific immunological effects of blood transfusion. Unresolved issues in this regard include the optimum timing of transfusion, the best type of blood product, the amount of blood to be given with transfusion, the value of random versus donor-specific transfusions and the benefit of intraoperative transfusions. The poor results seen in nontransfused patients argue convincingly against transplantation in these patients.

Renal preservation

Immediate flushing of the donor kidney with a cold electrolyte solution is routinely used in both living-related and cadaver transplantation. Living-related donor kidneys are flushed with a cold extracellular electrolyte solution and transplantation into the recipient is then performed immediately with a short preservation time. Cadaver donor kidneys are flushed with an intracellular electrolyte solution and preservation is accomplished either by simple cold storage or by hypothermic pulsatile perfusion.

In simple cold storage, the flushed kidney is placed in a plastic container and immersed in another container packed with crushed ice. The principal disadvantage of this method is that the period of preservation is limited to about 24 hours, particularly if there has been any significant warm renal ischaemic time. Hypothermic pulsatile perfusion is generally preferable when the anticipated period of preservation exceeds 24 hours: this has been successfully used to preserve kidneys for up to 72 hours. A variety of perfusates may be employed for perfusion preservation, including cryoprecipitated plasma, plasma protein fraction and modifed albumin solution. An additional advantage of pulsatile perfusion is in allowing viability testing to be performed after donor nephrectomy and prior to transplantation.

Basic renal transplant operation

In selecting the iliac fossa for implantation of the allograft, one should consider both the anteroposterior relationships of the renal vessels and the anticipated method of arterial anastomosis. When end-to-end arterial anastomosis to the hypogastric artery seems likely, as in performing single artery transplantation in younger patients, it is customary to place the right kidney in the left iliac fossa and vice versa. When end-to-side arterial anastomosis to the external or common iliac artery is expected, as in older patients or when employing a Carrel aortic patch with multiple donor arteries, the right kidney will lie more comfortably in the right iliac fossa and the left kidney in the left iliac fossa. It should be stressed that these are only relative considerations and, with careful attention to positioning the graft and renal vessels, each kidney may be inserted into the right or left iliac fossa with either method of arterial anastomosis. In general, the author prefers to employ the right iliac fossa, regardless of the side from which the donor kidney was harvested, because the right iliac vein has a more horizontal course than the left and is more accessible for the venous anastomosis. This may assume clinical significance when transplanting a kidney with an unusually short renal vein.

In patients with a history of lower extremity thrombophlebitis, silent thrombosis of the iliac veins may have occurred and transplantation should be performed preferentially into the opposite iliac fossa. If ipsilateral transplantation is being considered, preoperative venography should be done to verify iliac venous patency. In patients with a prior failed renal transplant, the second graft is always placed in the unoperated contralateral iliac fossa.

When the recipient is anaesthetized, an 18 Fr Silastic Foley catheter is inserted in the bladder. A urine specimen is sent for culture or, if the patient is anuric, the bladder is irrigated with saline and this fluid is cultured. The bladder is filled by gravity with 100–200 ml of 1 per cent neomycin sulphate solution, and the catheter is clamped and connected to a closed drainage system. Shaving of the operative site is done in the operating room and the skin is prepared with an iodine solution for 10 minutes. Prior to commencing the operation, a single intravenous bolus of broad-spectrum antibiotics is given. This consists of ampicillin 2 g, Nafcillin 2 g and tobramycin 2 mg/kg. In patients allergic to penicillin, clindamycin 400 mg is substituted for ampicillin and nafcillin[5].

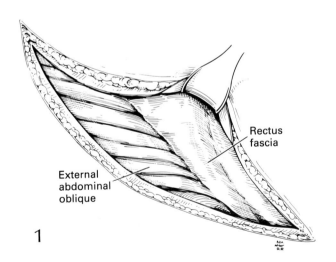

Rectus
fascia

External
abdominal
oblique

1

1

A lower quadrant transverse semilunar skin incision is made extending from the midline to just above the anterior superior iliac spine. Throughout the operation, care is taken to achieve absolute haemostasis and to minimize blood loss. The external oblique, internal oblique and transversus abdominis muscles are divided in line with the incision. The inferior epigastric vessels are identified lateral to the rectus muscle and are secured and divided. The rectus muscle is either retracted medially or, if exposure of the bladder is not adequate, this muscle is divided at its tendinous insertion into the symphysis pubis. In the female the round ligament is ligated and divided. The spermatic cord in the male is mobilized and retracted medially to obviate postoperative hydrocele formation which commonly occurs following high cord ligation.

2

Extraperitoneal exposure of the iliac fossa is obtained by reflecting the peritoneum superiorly to the common iliac artery and medially to the bladder. A self-retaining ring retractor is inserted to maintain exposure of the operative field. The lateral blade of the retractor is doubly padded to avoid injury to the lateral femoral cutaneous nerve[6]. The superior retractor blade is positioned to avoid compression of the common iliac artery, which may interfere with allograft perfusion following revascularization.

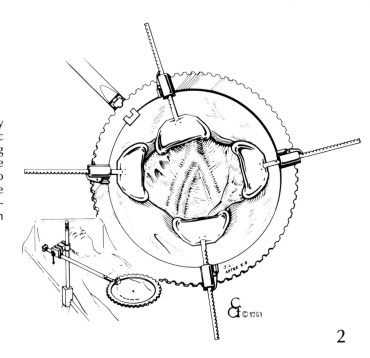

2

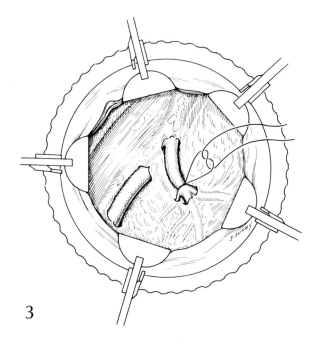

3

3

The external iliac vein is mobilized from the internal iliac origin to the femoral junction. To avoid postoperative lymphatic complications, all overlying lymphatic tissue is ligated and divided[7]. If the donor kidney has a short renal vein, the internal iliac vein is divided to allow elevation of the external iliac vein and thereby facilitate the venous anastomosis. End-to-end anastomosis of the renal artery to the hypogastric (internal iliac) artery is preferred, and the latter vessel is mobilized from its origin to the major anterior and posterior branches. Again, all overlying lymphatic vessels are ligated and divided. In such cases, it is unnecessary to mobilize the common and external iliac arteries.

4

Vascular clamps are placed proximally and distally on the external iliac vein. A venotomy is performed by excising a narrow longitudinal elipse from the anterolateral aspect of the vein. The hypogastric artery is temporarily occluded proximally, its major branches are ligated distally and the artery is divided proximal to the ligatures. If mild atherosclerosis of the hypogastric artery is present, endarterectomy is performed to render this vessel suitable for anastomosis to the renal artery. Heparin solution is instilled into the lumen of the hypogastric artery and external iliac vein. The kidney is brought into the operative field and the artery and vein are examined. Any residual tissue surrounding the origin of these vessels is removed and, if the renal vein appears short, it is mobilized from the renal sinus to obtain greater length. The kidney is lowered into the incision and end-to-side anastomosis of the renal vein to the external iliac vein is performed with a continuous 5/0 silk suture. End-to-end anastomosis of the renal artery to the hypogastric artery is performed with interrupted 6/0 silk, after aligning these vessels carefully to avoid angulation or kinking. After the arterial anastomosis is completed, all vascular clamps are removed and circulation to the kidney is restored.

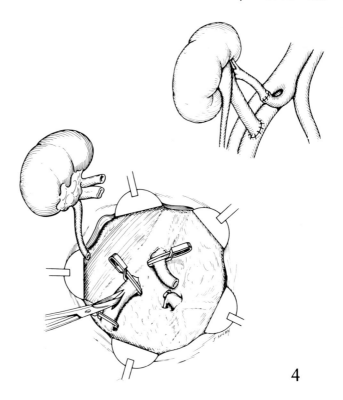

4

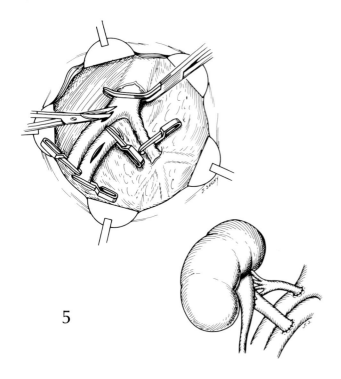

5

5

The indications for end-to-side arterial anastomosis to the common or external iliac artery are: extensive atherosclerosis of the hypogastric artery, significant discrepancy in size between the renal and hypogastric arteries, or multiple donor renal arteries encompassed by a Carrel aortic patch. In such cases, the external iliac artery and a contiguous segment of the common iliac artery are mobilized, while the hypogastric artery is left undisturbed. Vascular clamps are placed across the common iliac, hypogastric and external iliac arteries, and an arteriotomy is performed in the recipient vessel. In general, our preference is to perform end-to-side arterial anastomosis to the common iliac artery because of its larger calibre. This may not be possible when there is either insufficient renal arterial length or significant atherosclerosis of the common iliac artery. In such cases, the artery is anastomosed to the external iliac artery which lies in closer proximity to the renal hilus and is less often diseased. An interrupted suture technique with 6/0 silk is employed unless anastomosis of a Carrel aortic patch is performed, in which case a continuous suture of 5/0 silk is used.

6, 7 & 8

After completion of the vascular anastomoses, urinary tract reconstruction is achieved by ureteroneocystostomy. This method is preferred over ureteroureterostomy or ureteropyelostomy because of a lower incidence of postoperative urinary fistulae[8]. The bladder is opened through an anterior cystotomy and a stab incision is made in the posterolateral bladder wall just above and lateral to the ipsilateral ureteral orifice. This opening should be in a relatively fixed portion of the bladder, although not necessarily on the trigone, to prevent kinking of the ureter with bladder filling. The donor ureter is brought through a stab incision, and a wide 2–3 cm long submucosal tunnel is fashioned, directed toward the bladder neck. The ureter is brought through the tunnel taking care to avoid torsion on its longitudinal axis. Since the allograft ureter receives its blood supply exclusively from renal artery branches, the shortest length of ureter should be used that will reach the bladder without tension. With these considerations in mind the ureter is spatulated and anastomosed to the bladder with interrupted 5/0 chromic sutures. The sutures fixing the distal aspect of the ureter to the bladder are inserted deeply into the muscularis while the remaining sutures are placed only through the bladder mucosa. The mucosa overlying the stab incision is closed with a continuous 5/0 chromic suture.

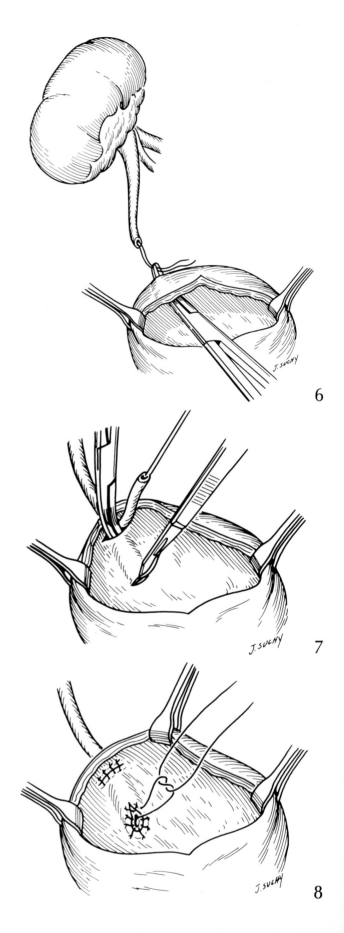

6

7

8

9

The cystotomy incision is closed in three layers to ensure a watertight repair. The first layer is of continuous 4/0 chromic for the mucosa, the second of continuous 4/0 chromic for the muscularis, and the third of interrupted 3/0 chromic for the adventitia, fat and muscularis. The second and third layers should slightly overlap the immediate underlying layer at each end of the cystotomy closure to avoid extravasation at these two points.

After all anastomoses have been completed and adequate haemostasis has been achieved, the wound is irrigated with 2000 ml of normal saline. This is an important local measure both in debriding the wound of small nonviable pieces of tissue and in minimizing the influence of inadvertent intraoperative contamination. The wound is irrigated with an additional 500 ml of 1 per cent neomycin solution. The transplant incision is always closed without drainage in two separate musculofascial layers. The subcutaneous layer and the skin are also closed separately. A pressure dressing is then used to cover the wound.

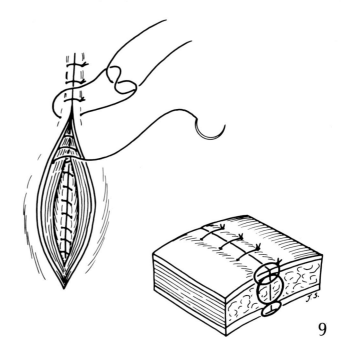

9

SPECIAL SURGICAL PROBLEMS

Multiple renal arteries

Multiple renal arteries occur unilaterally and bilaterally in 23 per cent and 10 per cent of the population respectively. When donor kidneys with multiple arteries are transplanted, failure to recognize and preserve an accessory renal artery may eventuate in ureteral necrosis, graft rupture, segmental renal infarction, postoperative hypotension or calyceal fistula formation. A variety of techniques are available for performing multiple artery renal transplantation[9]:

10

Carrel aortic patch

Anastomosis of a Carrel aortic patch encompassing all renal arteries to the recipient common or external iliac artery is the preferred method for arterial anastomosis of cadaver kidneys with multiple arteries. This requires that cadaver donor nephrectomy be performed *en bloc* with the aorta and vena cava. Use of such an aortic patch is not possible when kidneys are harvested separately, when polar vessels are injured inadvertently during removal, when there is significant atherosclerosis of the perirenal aorta and when the renal arteries are widely separated on the aorta. Likewise, in living-related transplantation, a cuff of aorta should never be taken because of the increased risk to the donor.

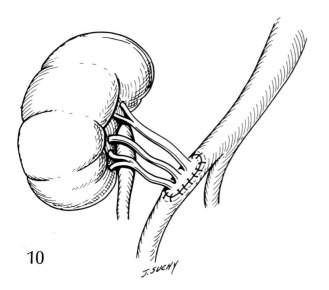

10

J. SUCHY

11

Conjoined arterial anastomosis

When two adjacent renal arteries of comparable size are present, the method preferred by the author is extracorporeal side-to-side anastomosis of the two vessels to create a common ostium. This is done just before implantation, with the kidney cooled in ice saline solution. Continuous 6/0 or 7/0 vascular sutures are employed for the repair, with optical magnification provided by 3.5× ophthalmological loupes. Revascularization in the recipient involves only a single arterial anastomosis, preferably end-to-end to the hypogastric artery, with no increase in the warm renal ischaemic time. This method is technically simple and, haemodynamically, yields less resistance to flow than separate vascular anastomoses because of the greater cross-sectional area of the coapted vessels.

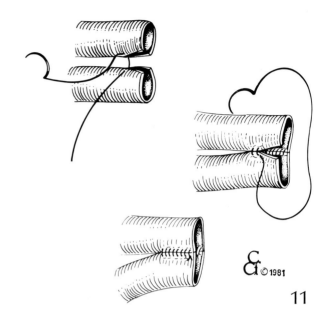

11

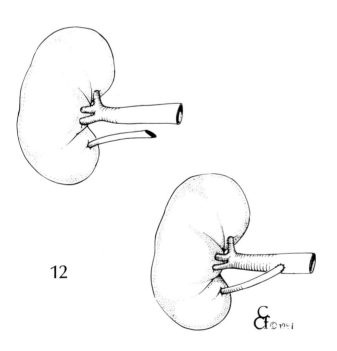

12

12

Reimplantation of polar artery into main renal artery

This is the author's method of choice to transplant kidneys supplied by two renal arteries of disparate calibre. With the kidney cooled in ice saline solution, extracorporeal microvascular end-to-side anastomosis is performed of the smaller artery to the larger one. A short linear arteriotomy is made in the side of the main renal artery, without removing any of the vessel wall to obviate narrowing of the arterial lumen. After the polar vessel is spatulated, end-to-side anastomosis to the main renal artery is done with interrupted 7/0 vascular sutures, using microvascular instruments and 3.5× ophthalmological loupes for magnification. A small catheter or probe may be placed through the suture line during its construction to prevent accidental entrapment of the back wall. For vessels less than 1.5 mm in diameter, 9/0 vascular suture material is used, and the repair is performed under the operating microscope. The completed anastomosis is tested for patency and integrity by gentle perfusion of the main renal artery. The transplant operation is done as with a single renal artery. The advantages of this method are: (1) it is technically simple; (2) it involves anastomosis of vessels which are similar in thickness; (3) only one arterial anastomosis is required in the recipient; and (4) warm renal ischaemic time is not prolonged. This technique is also readily applicable to reconstruction of kidneys supplied by more than two renal arteries of varying calibre.

13

Extracorporeal repair with autogenous branched vascular graft

Another method for transplanting kidneys with multiple renal arteries involves fashioning these into a single artery before implantation with a branched graft of autogenous hypogastric artery. If atherosclerosis is present in the hypogastric artery, this can be removed after its procurement using the eversion endarterectomy technique. Donor arterial repair is done extracorporeally under surface hypothermia with end-to-end anastomosis of the graft branches to the distal renal arteries. The kidney is transplanted as with a single renal artery, with no added warm ischaemic time. This technique is particularly useful for transplanting kidneys with more than two renal arteries or when insufficient arterial length is present to permit use of the previous two methods described. Should extensive calcification of the hypogastric artery render it unsuitable as a reconstructive graft, a branched saphenous vein graft can be used in the same fashion.

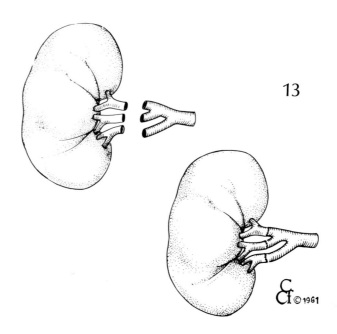

13

14a–d

Other techniques

Additional techniques for performing multiple artery transplantation are: (a) separate arterial anastomoses to the hypogastric and external iliac arteries; (b) separate arterial anastomoses to the external and/or common iliac arteries; (c) arterial anastomoses to the branches of the hypogastric artery; and (d) polar artery anastomosis to the inferior epigastric artery. These techniques all require performance of multiple arterial anastomoses *in situ* which results in a prolonged warm renal ischaemic time. Therefore, when a Carrel aortic patch is not available, the author prefers to perform extracorporeal arterial reconstruction employing one of the three methods described above. These latter techniques have proved to be readily applicable, either individually or in combination, to most anatomical variants presented by kidneys with multiple arteries.

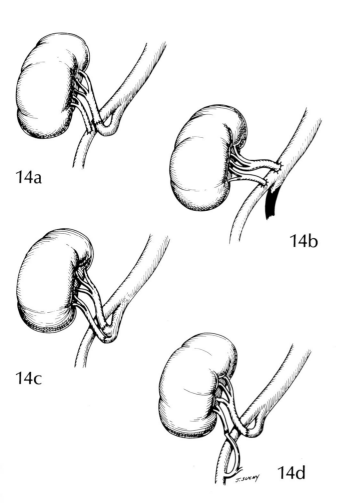

14a

14b

14c

14d

Multiple renal veins

Multiple renal veins are less common than multiple arteries and more frequently involve the right kidney. Small renal veins can simply be ligated without risk. When double renal veins of approximately equal size are present, both must be preserved to avoid increased intrarenal venous pressure after revascularization. The optimum method involves implanting these together with a cuff of vena cava obtained at the time of nephrectomy. When this is not available, extracorporeal venous reconstruction is performed as decribed for multiple arteries, generally with a conjoined anastomosis of the two veins.

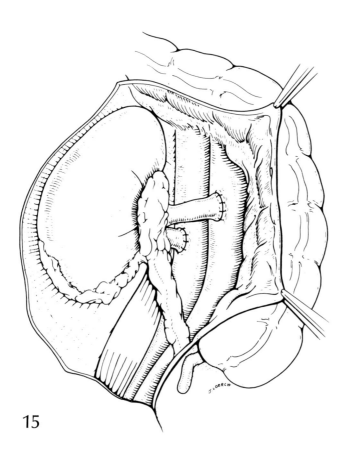

15

Transplantation in children

15

There are special surgical considerations when renal transplantation is performed in paediatric patients. In children weighing less than 20 kg, the iliac fossa is too small to accommodate a kidney from an adult donor. In this event, a midline transperitoneal incision is made, and the caecum and ascending colon are reflected medially to expose the aorta, the vena cava and common iliac vessels. The graft is placed retrocaecally with end-to-side anastomosis of the renal vein either to the vena cava or to the right common iliac vein[10]. The renal artery is anastomosed end-to-side either to the aorta or to the right common iliac artery. Immediately following revascularization of the allograft, 300 ml of blood or albumin are administered as an intravenous bolus to replenish the suddenly depleted intravascular volume and to ensure adequate renal perfusion. The ureter generally reaches the bladder easily, remaining retroperitoneal throughout its course, and a ureteroneocystostomy is performed. Very small children, weighing less than 8 kg, will require transplantation with a paediatric cadaver graft.

Transplantation with urinary diversion

When the bladder is unsuitable, because of either severe neurogenical disease or marked post-inflammatory contracture, renal transplantation is performed in conjunction with supravesical urinary diversion. In such cases, an ileal or colon conduit with a lower quadrant stoma is fashioned; 6 weeks later, transplantation is performed. The preferred technique is to place the allograft retrocaecally, as in paediatric transplantation, with anastomosis of the renal vessels either to the aorta and vena cava or to the common iliac vessels. This allows gravity-dependent urinary drainage and a more direct ureteroenteric anastomosis than when transplantation is performed into the iliac fossa.

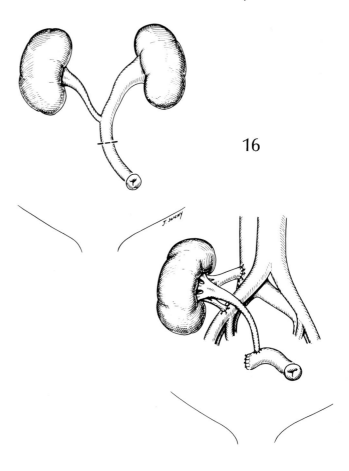

16

In some patients with end-stage renal disease where diversion with cutaneous ureterostomy has been performed, a well functioning stoma is already present. In such cases, the stoma and a short contiguous segment of distal ureter can be preserved at the time of bilateral nephrectomy. Transplantation is performed with anastomosis of the allograft ureter to the retained native ureter just below the abdominal wall, thus obviating the need for an intestinal segment. Utilizing this method, satisfactory urinary drainge is achieved through the normal peristaltic ability of the allograft ureter, and the retained dilated ureter functions solely as a short conduit and stoma.

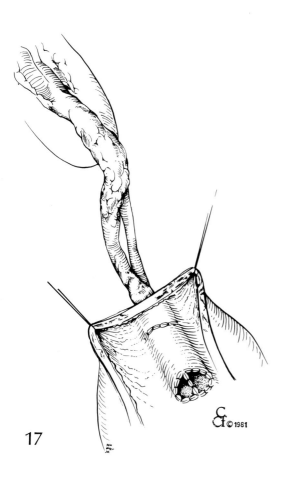

17

Double ureter

The incidence of ureteral duplication is 0.6 per cent and donor kidneys with this anomaly can be transplanted successfully. The two ureters are left in their common adventitial sheath and are brought through the posterior bladder wall and submucosal tunnel together, exactly as decribed for a single ureter. Both ureteral ends are spatulated. The medial ends are sutured together and the lateral and distal aspects are anastomosed to the bladder as with a single ureter.

Postoperative care

In early postoperative period, fluid and electrolyte balance is maintained by monitoring central venous pressure, blood pressure, pulse rate, urinary output and body weight. When oligoanuria is present, despite normovolaemia, mannitol 12.5 g and furosemide (frusemide) 40 mg are given intravenously. This amount of furosemide may be doubled to a maximum dose of 160 mg. Some cadaver allograft recipients will remain oliguric following these measures due to vasomotor nephropathy. This diagnosis can be established only after excluding hyperacute rejection or technical problems by examining the incision for drainage, ensuring a patent urethral catheter and obtaining a cystogram and renal scan. By contrast, living related allograft recipients often experience a profound postoperative osmotic diuresis which requires vigorous fluid and electrolyte replacement.

Within the first 24 hours postoperatively a technetium renal scan is done routinely to verify patency of the transplant renal artery. If there is absent or questionable uptake of isotope by the allograft, renal arteriography should be performed to evaluate the possibility of arterial thrombosis or hyperacute rejection[11]. The initial surgical dressing is removed 48 hours postoperatively and is changed daily thereafter using strict sterile technique. Systemic antibiotic therapy is administered only to patients with a documented infection. A urethral catheter is left indwelling for 7 days in all patients, and the sutures from the transplant wound are removed 14 days postoperatively.

In evaluating patients with impaired allograft function following renal transplantation, it is necessary to distinguish between immunological, ischaemic and technical problems. Serial isotope renography with ^{131}I orthoiodohippurate provides an excellent, noninvasive functional assessment and can differentiate vasomotor nephropathy reliably from acute rejection[12]. Nevertheless, the clinical stigmata of acute rejection may be identical to postoperative complications such as ureteral obstruction, urinary fistula or perinephric fluid collections which are not readily diagnosed by isotope renography. In our programme CAT scanning following intravenous injection of 50 ml of 60 per cent sodium and meglumine diatrizoate has proved an accurate, noninvasive complementary method of evaluating such patients by demonstrating in detail the cross-sectional anatomy of the graft in relation to surrounding pelvic structures[13]. Ultrasonography has also been described as an effective method for diagnosing pelvic fluid collections. These noninvasive techniques have reduced significantly the indications for open renal biopsy or transplant angiography; the latter studies are now largely reserved for patients with acute rejection unresponsive to high-dose steroid therapy in order to determine whether further attempts to salvage the graft are warranted.

Acknowledgement

Illustrations 3–8 and 13–15 are reproduced from Novick[14].

References

1. Novick, A. C., Braun, W. E., Magnusson, M., Stowe, N. Current status of renal transplantation at the Cleveland Clinic. Journal of Urology 1979; 122: 433–437

2. Braun, W. E., Phillips, D., Vidt, D. G., et al. Coronary arteriography and coronary artery disease in 99 diabetic and nondiabetic patients on chronic hemodialysis or renal transplantation programs. Transplantation Proceedings 1981; 13: 128–135

3. Novick, A. C., Ortenberg, J., Braun, W. E. Reduced morbidity with posterior surgical approach for pretransplant bilateral nephrectomy. Surgery, Gynecology and Obstetrics 1980; 151: 773–776

4. Opelz, G., Terasaki, P. Dominant effect of transfusions on kidney graft survival. Transplantation 1980; 29: 153–158

5. Novick, A. C. The value of intraoperative antibiotics in preventing renal transplant wound infections. Journal of Urology 1981; 125: 151–152

6. Vaziri, N. D., Barnes, J., Mirahmadi, K., Ehrlich, R., Rosen, S. M. Compression neuropathy secondary to renal transplantation. Urology 1976; 7: 145–147

7. Braun, W. E., Banowsky, L. H., Straffon, R. A. et al. Lymphoceles associated with renal transplantation. American Journal of Medicine 1974; 57: 714–729

8. Salvatierra, O., Jr, Olcott, C., Amend, W. J., Cochrum, K. C., Feduska, N. J. Urological complications of renal transplantation can be prevented or controlled. Journal of Urology 1977; 117: 421–424

9. Novick, A. C., Magnusson, M., Braun, W. E. Multiple-artery renal transplantation: emphasis on extracorporeal methods of donor arterial reconstruction. Journal of Urology 1979; 122: 731–735

10. Starzl, T. E., Marchioro, T. L., Morgan, W. W., Waddell, W. R. A technique for use of adult renal homografts in children. Surgery, Gynecology and Obstetrics 1964; 119: 106–108

11. Hamway, S., Novick, A. C., Braun W. E., et al. Impaired renal allograft function: a comparative study with angiography and histopathology. Journal of Urology 1979; 122: 292–297

12. Salvatierra, O., Powell, M. R., Price, D. C., Kountz, S. L., Belzer, F. O. The advantages of I[131]-orthoiodohippurate scintiphotography in the management of patients after renal transplantation. Annals of Surgery 1974; 180: 336–342

13. Novick, A. C., Irish, C., Steinmuller, D., Buonocore, E., Cohen, C. The role of computerized tomography in renal transplant patients. Journal of Urology 1981; 125: 15–18

14. Novick, A. C. Surgery of renal transplantation and complications. In: Novick, A. C., Stratton, R. A. eds. Vascular problems in urologic surgery. Philadelphia, London: W. B. Saunders, 1982: 233–260

Illustrations by Francis E. Steckel

Donor nephrectomy

John A. Libertino MD
Director of Transplantation, Department of Urology;
Vice Chairman, Division of Surgery, Lahey Clinic Medical Center, Burlington, Massachusetts, USA

Introduction

Donor nephrectomy for transplantation can be from either a living, related or cadaver donor. Whatever the source of the organ, nephrectomy must be carried out with the same gentle, meticulous technique. The surgeon who performs donor nephrectomy must provide the transplant surgeon with a kidney which has proper lengths of artery, vein and ureter. The blood supply to the ureter must also be preserved. The harvesting surgeon should be aware of and provide the transplant surgeon with a Carrel patch of the aorta when polar arteries are present and a cuff of vena cava with the right renal vein.

Living, related donor nephrectomy can be carried out through an anterior transperitoneal or supracostal 11th rib approach. Cadaver donor nephrectomy is performed through an anterior transperitoneal approach that allows for bilateral nephrectomy and *in situ* cooling.

The operations

LIVING DONOR NEPHRECTOMY

The living, related donor is given 1500 ml of dextrose saline solution intravenously the night before operation and intraoperatively receives mannitol 50 g or frusemide (Lasix) 40 mg to induce a diuresis.

1

For a transabdominal left donor nephrectomy, an incision is made from the tip of the left 11th rib to the lateral border of the right rectus muscle.

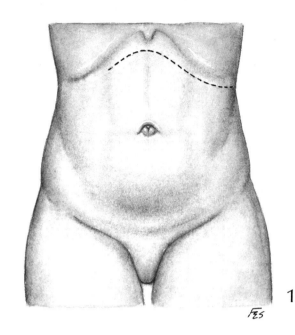

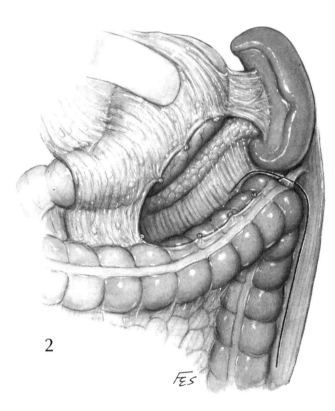

2

The splenic flexure of the colon is mobilized from the mid-transverse colon to the mid-descending colon. Care is taken to preserve the integrity of the spleen and pancreas.

3

After the splenic flexure has been reflected, the left renal vein is identified and mobilized. The left renal artery lies at the upper border of the left renal vein.

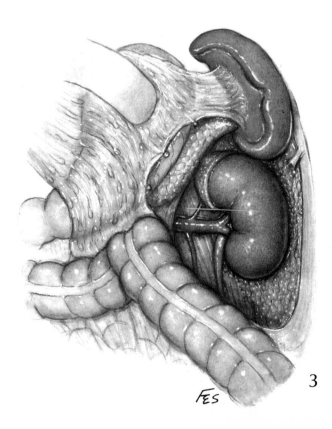

4

When a right donor nehrectomy is carried out, access to the right renal pedicle is obtained by mobilizing the hepatic flexure of the colon and the duodenum.

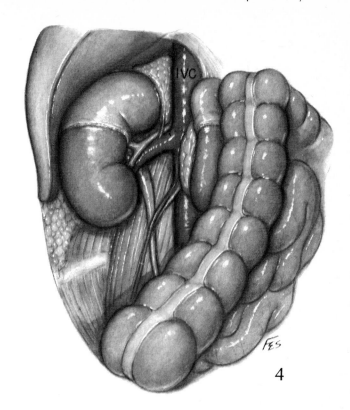

4

5

The origin of the retrocaval right renal artery is best found at its aortic origin. The renal artery is taken at its origin to provide the transplant surgeon with sufficient vascular length.

5

6

Another approach for donor nephrectomy is the 11th supracostal incision. This is an extraperitoneal extrapleural incision, the one favoured at the Lahey Clinic for living donor nephrectomy.

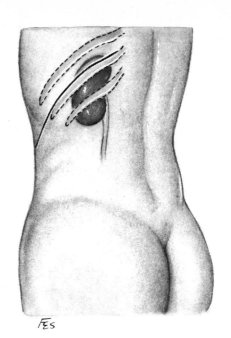

6

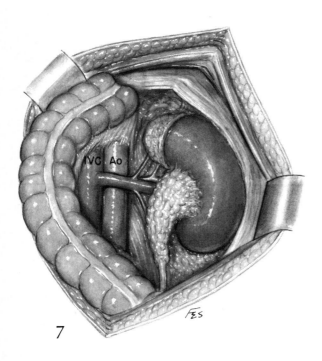

7

7

The colon is reflected anteriorly through the left flank and the left renal pedicle is identified.

8

The left adrenal and gonadal veins are divided. The renal vein can now be mobilized safely to expose the left renal artery.

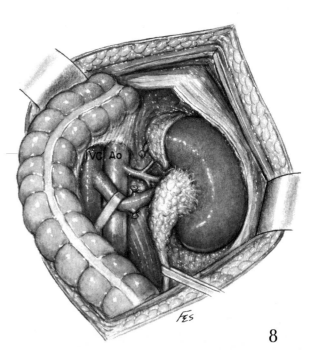

8

9

The artery and vein are ligated and divided at their origins. The ureter is divided where it crosses the iliac vessels. The donor's renal artery and vein are doubly ligated with 0 silk sutures.

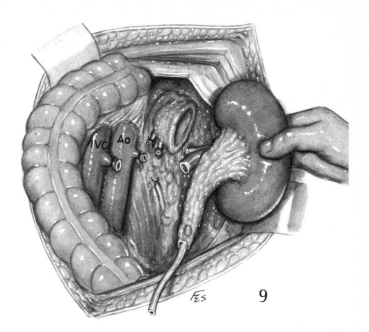

9

10

The kidney is placed in iced, slush saline solution. An angiocath (polyethylene sheath only) is inserted into the renal artery. A mixture of 1 litre of lactated Ringer's solution with 50 mg of heparin is used to flush the kidney until the effluent from the renal vein is clear. The kidney is now ready for transplantation.

10

CADAVER DONOR NEPHRECTOMY

Cadaver donor nephrectomy is carried out in the operating room under sterile conditions. When the criteria for cerebral death have been met, kidneys may be removed from a cadaver with an intact circulation. The donor may be supported with intravenous fluids, heparin, mannitol, frusemide, and dopamine, depending on the status of the urinary output and blood pressure. Vasoconstrictor agents for support of blood pressure are to be avoided.

11

The kidneys are removed by a transverse upper abdominal incision, a long midline incision, or a combination of both incisions depending on the body habitus of the cadaver.

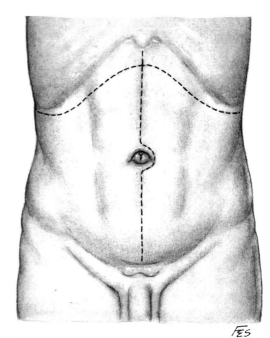

11

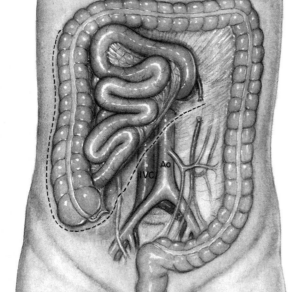

12

12

Incision of the posterior parietal peritoneum is used to mobilize the intestines so that they may be placed in a Lahey bag and put onto the cadaver's chest. The inferior mesenteric vein is divided to enhance exposure.

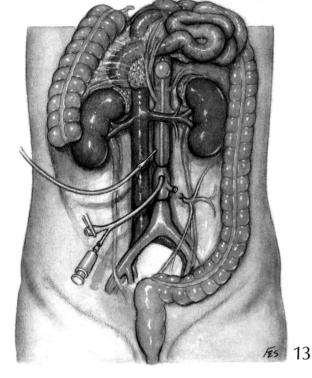

13

13

The distal aorta is ligated. A Foley catheter is inserted proximally into the aorta and the balloon inflated above the renal arteries. The kidneys are then perfused, cooled and preserved *in situ* with Collin's or Sack's solution dripped into the aorta as shown.

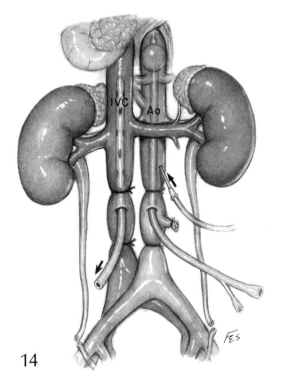

14

14

The distal vena cava is ligated and a large abdominal suction tube is placed proximally to evacuate the venous blood and ensure perfusion of the kidneys.

15

The aorta is transected above and below the renal arteries. It is then divided longitudinally so that a large cuff of aorta accompanies the renal artery or arteries. In this way multiple renal vessels are taken with an aortic patch. The left renal vein is divided at the vena cava and the ureter at the level of the iliac artery.

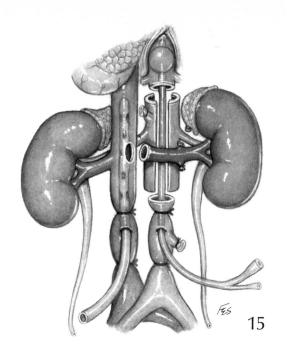

15

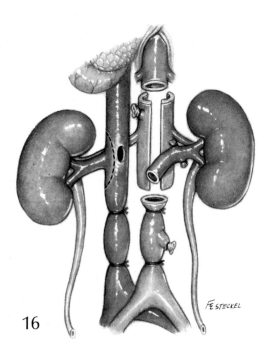

16

16

The right renal vein is taken with a Carrel patch of vena cava.

17

The kidneys, with their appropriate patches of aorta and vena cava, are now removed and preserved in anticipation of transplantation.

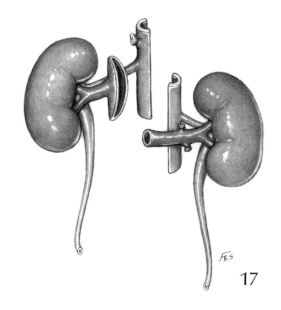

17

Further reading

Ackermann, J. R., Snell, M. E. Cadaveric renal transplantation: a technique for donor kidney removal. British Journal of Urology 1968; 40: 515–521

Collins, G. M., Halasz, N. A. Current aspects of renal preservation. Urology 1977; 10: Suppl.: 22–32

Freed, S. Z., Veit, F. J., Tellis, V., Whittaker, J., Gliedman, M. L. Improved cadaver nephrectomy for kidney transplantation. Surgery, Gynecology and Obstetrics 1973; 137: 101–103

Uehling, D. T., Maledk, G. H., Wear, J. B. Complications of donor nephrectomy. Journal of Urology 1974; 111: 745–746

Illustrations by Robert N. Lane from originals by Richard G. Notley

Surgical anatomy and exposure of the ureter

Richard G. Notley MS, FRCS
Senior Consultant Urological Surgeon, Royal Surrey County Hospital, Guildford, Surrey, UK

Surgical anatomy

In the adult the ureter is a thick-walled tube about 24–30 cm in length which can be seen arising within the renal sinus as a funnel-shaped dilatation termed the renal pelvis. Into this open the calyces and the renal pyramids. The renal pelvis funnels down into the narrow ureter which runs caudally on the posterior abdominal wall, plastered to the muscles of the back by the parietal peritoneum. It runs along the surface of the psoas major muscle, across psoas minor if that muscle is present, in the line of the tips of the lumbar transverse processes and crossing the genitofemoral nerve to dip into the pelvic cavity in the region of the bifurcation of the common iliac vessels. During its downward course on psoas the ureter is crossed obliquely by the testicular or ovarian vessels.

On the right side the renal pelvis and upper ureter are usually covered by the second part of the duodenum, and, as it runs caudally, the ureter lies immediately lateral to the inferior vena cava where it is crossed by the right colic and ileocolic vessels. Just before it crosses the pelvic brim the right ureter passes behind the lower part of the small bowel mesentery. On the left the ureter is crossed by the left colic vessels and the pelvic mesocolon.

Having crossed the pelvic brim at the bifurcation of the common iliac vessels over the sacroiliac joint, the ureter continues its extraperitoneal course downwards as far as the spine of the ischium. The internal iliac artery and its branches, together with the obturator nerve, lie on its lateral side. Having reached the ischial spine, the ureter runs forwards and medially to reach the base of the bladder. As it turns forward it is crossed by the vas deferens in the male and the uterine artery in the female.

Throughout its length from the kidney to the bladder the ureter is closely applied to the parietal peritoneum lining the posterior abdominal wall and pelvis so that when the peritoneum is stripped up the ureter is elevated with it. This has the advantage of making surgical access to the ureter relatively simple, but this also means that the ureter is vulnerable to accidental ligature or clamping during the repair of the pelvic peritoneum after surgery. The lowermost part of the ureter may also be damaged during hysterectomy by inaccurate clamping of the nearby uterine artery. This part of the ureter is the most awkward to expose surgically, requiring division of the superior vesical pedicle and the obliterated umbilical artery (and sometimes the inferior vesical pedicle) to demonstrate its union with the base of the bladder.

The blood supply to the ureter is derived from several sources, but, unlike the gut, it receives no regular segmental blood supply. The renal pelvis and the upper ureter are supplied by branches of the renal artery or arteries. The lower ureter receives branches from the inferior and superior vesical arteries, and, in between these extremes, numerous variable vessels reach the ureter from the gonadal arteries and often, too, from the common iliac arteries. All these vessels make longitudinal anastomoses with each other in the adventitia of the ureter. The veins of the ureter drain into the renal, gonadal and internal iliac veins. The lymphatic vessels run back alongside the arteries, from the abdominal portion into the para-aortic lymph nodes and from the pelvic portion into the nodes alongside the internal iliac arteries on the pelvic side wall.

Exposure of the abdominal ureter

Surgical exposure of the ureter is most commonly required for the relief of ureteric obstruction by calculus. It may also be necessary for the relief of extrinsic obstruction, for the repair of injury or for removal of the ureter in combination with the kidney (for transitional cell carcinoma of the ureter or renal pelvis). The surgeon may also wish to expose the ureter in order to affect temporary or permanent diversion of the urine from the bladder.

Lying as it does in intimate relationship to the posterior parietal peritoneum, the ureter may be exposed either by the transperitoneal or extraperitoneal routes. If the object is to open the ureter, the problems of peritoneal contamination and urine drainage make the transperitoneal route less safe than the extraperitoneal, unless the intention is to join the ureter to the bowel intraperitoneally. Bilateral extrinsic obstruction of the ureters due to retroperitoneal fibrosis may be dealt with transperitoneally, but by far the most usual route of exposure is extraperitoneal.

The extraperitoneal approach to the ureter may be carried out either by the lumbar or the abdominal route, each having its own advantages. In general, in dealing with obstructive lesions and injuries, preliminary radiological investigation will permit accurate localization of the site to be exposed. When such accurate localization of the lesion can be achieved the abdominal extraperitoneal route affords good exposure of the required region and has the advantage for the patient of a smaller, anterior skin-crease incision. The exact site of the incision can be matched to the part of the ureter to be exposed, from renal hilum to pelvic brim (see *Illustration 6*). When the lesion is ill defined, or there is a risk that the obstructing calculus may dislocate upwards or downwards, wider exposure of the ureter may be required and the lumbar extraperitoneal approach is then indicated.

The anterior approach to the kidney and the upper ureter has much to commend it in the operation of nephroureterectomy. This approach to the kidney can be combined with the necessary lower abdominal incision without delay and without altering the position of the patient on the table, as will be necessary if the kidney is exposed by the lumbar route.

Position of patient

When the abdominal approach is used the patient is placed in a supine position on the operating table. A small sandbag placed behind the lower ribs on the affected side tilts the trunk sufficiently to facilitate the extraperitoneal approach to the ureter.

Positioning for a lumbar approach is more complex. The patient is placed on his side with the break point of the table level with the waistline. The lower thigh and knee should be flexed and the uppermost leg extended over them to stretch the lateral abdominal muscles, thus increasing exposure when the latter are divided. The table should then be 'broken' to its full extent to create as much lateral flexion of the spine as is feasible for that particular patient. In this way the loin to be operated upon is opened out as the incision proceeds. The patient should be stabilized in this position of full lateral flexion with the upper arm carried forward and secured to an angled arm-rest placed in front of the chest at the level of the shoulder. The pelvis is most conveniently fixed by a length of 3-inch non-stretch adhesive strapping passed across the hips at the level of the greater trochanter and fixed to the operating table on each side. An alternative to 'breaking' the table is to use inflatable pneumatic cushions beneath the loin to achieve the required lateral flexion. Whatever approach is used it is advisable for the surgeon to arrange the position of the patient to his own satisfaction before operating on the kidney or ureter.

THE ANTERIOR APPROACH

1

With the patient supine and a small sandbag beneath the lower ribs on the side of the ureter to be exposed, the incision is planned. Study of the radiographs demonstrating the lesion enables an incision to be made which brings the surgeon accurately to the required part of the ureter. To reach the upper third of the ureter and the pelviureteric segment the incision should commence between the tips of the 10th and 11th ribs, crossing the costal margin laterally by 1 cm or so. The incision runs medially and slightly downwards in the line of the ribs to about midway across the rectus sheath, a total length of 12–15 cm being all that is necessary.

1

2

After the skin and subcutaneous tissues have been incised, the external oblique muscle fibres are demonstrated laterally, while more medially these fibres give way to aponeurosis which runs medially to form the rectus sheath, exposed at the medial end of the incision. The external oblique muscle fibres and its aponeurosis are divided in the line of the skin incision, the incision being carried on to the rectus sheath to expose the vertical fibres of the rectus muscle.

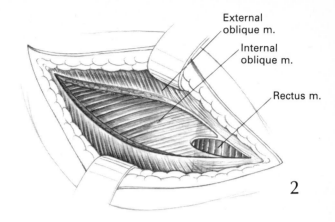

External oblique m.

Internal oblique m.

Rectus m.

2

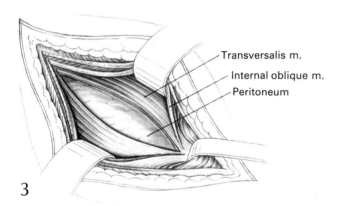

Transversalis m.

Internal oblique m.

Peritoneum

3

3

The exposed fibres of the internal oblique, running at right angles to those of the external oblique, are now incised to expose the horizontal fibres of the transversalis muscle. This incision is carried medially into the posterior rectus sheath for 1 cm or so, the rectus muscle being retracted medially to permit this. The transversalis muscle is split carefully along its fibres in the depths of the muscle incision to expose the underlying anterior parietal peritoneum.

4

The peritoneum is separated carefully from the anterior abdominal wall muscles. The more medial the incision the more adherent and delicate is the peritoneum and the more care is necessary to separate it from the overlying muscles without breaking its continuity. Gentle blunt dissection with the fingers is usually the most effective method of achieving separation of the intact peritoneum. Once the peritoneum is separated from the muscles for 2–3 cm along both edges of the incision the separation is carried laterally around the flank, down into the gutter lateral to the psoas muscle. The floor of this gutter is the quadratus lumborum muscle. The dissecting fingers must now climb anteriorly, up the steep side of psoas, before continuing the medial lifting of what is now the posterior parietal peritoneum until the great vessels are reached in the midline.

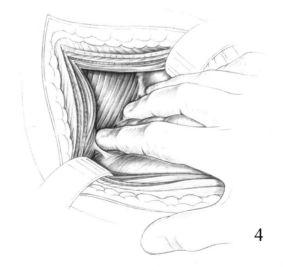

4

5

A suitable self-retaining retractor is inserted to separate the upper and lower edges of the incision. The peritoneum is retracted medially by an assistant using a wide-bladed, blunt retractor. The ureter is now identified, often lifted off the psoas with the peritoneum to which the ureter tends to adhere. The lower pole of the kidney is exposed and the union of pelvis and ureter can be visualized with a little blunt dissection medial to the kidney. Care must be taken to identify and preserve any lower polar vessels to the kidney during such dissection.

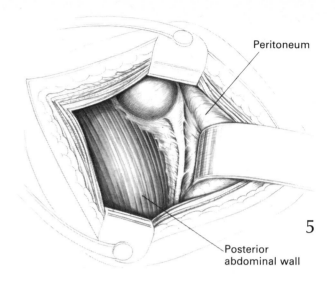

Peritoneum

Posterior abdominal wall

5

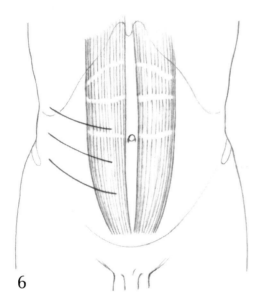

6

6

Access to the lower regions of the abdominal ureter may be obtained by siting the incision lower on the anterior abdominal wall. The precise level may be ascertained by accurate radiological localization of the lesion, but it is important to bear in mind that the lesion always seems to be located more cranially than may appear from the radiographs.

7

A precisely similar method of approach as described above will achieve access to the ureter at the pelvic brim, through the lowermost incision shown (*see Illustration 6*).

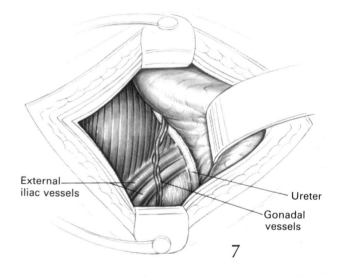

External iliac vessels

Ureter

Gonadal vessels

7

THE LUMBAR APPROACH

When localization of the lesion in the ureter is less precise, the lumbar approach to the abdominal ureter has advantages. The disadvantage to the patient of a long incision affecting his back and loin muscles is offset by the surgeon's ability to expose and explore the ureter from the renal hilum to the pelvic brim through a single incision. This approach has particular advantage if it is thought that the risk of upward dislocation of a calculus is high as the whole of the renal pelvis and kidney are accessible through a single incision.

8

With the patient in the lateral position an oblique incision is made in the loin. This incision may be the classical incision excising the anterior end of the 12th rib (see chapter on 'Surgical exposure of the kidney', pp. 21–32) or it may be made as an intercostal incision between the 11th and 12th ribs. This incision necessitates careful localization of these ribs so that the knife passes accurately between them. After incision of the skin the anterior fibres of latissimus dorsi and the posterior part of the external and then the internal oblique muscles are divided in the same line. The aponeurotic fibres of transversalis may be pierced just above the tip of the 12th rib to enter the perinephric space and thus achieve early localization of the region to be explored. The fibres of transversalis then separate easily in the line of the incision in front of the surgeon's finger. The peritoneum pushes easily away.

The intercostal neurovascular bundles will remain unseen in the layers of this incision if it is kept at the correct oblique angle, but it is wise to keep a sharp lookout for them as it is very easy to be a few degrees off course. By keeping fairly close to the upper edge of the 12th rib, damage to the 11th intercostal bundle can be avoided. As the incision in between the ribs is extended backwards it is necessary to watch out for the lower extent of the pleura which must be identified and preserved. This part of the incision can be deepened conveniently with

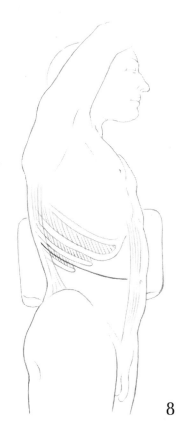

8

scissors so that the pleura can be preserved, if necessary dividing some slips of diaphragm which come down to the 12th rib. If the pleura is inadvertently opened it is best left until the wound is being sutured at the end of the operation to effect proper closure. Under such circumstances it is usually not necessary to do more than ensure that the lung is fully inflated before closing the pleura with a continuous catgut suture. Underwater seal drainage to the pleural cavity is not usually necessary.

9

To complete the exposure the incision should be carried posteriorly into the paravertebral muscle mass until the articulation of the 12th rib can be freed from the transverse process. The 12th rib can be swung down and the incision held wide open with a suitable self-retaining retractor. Blunt dissection then enables the posterior peritoneum to be lifted forward to expose the ureter from renal hilum to pelvic brim after opening the perinephric space. The kidney and upper ureter may also be exposed from behind by way of the lumbotomy incision. The exposure of this region through a vertical posterior lumbotomy incision is slightly more difficult. However, it permits a smoother and shorter postoperative course with minimal morbidity. The approach has great advantages where exposure of the kidney is concerned, but for the upper ureter it has little or no advantage over the anterior approach outlined above.

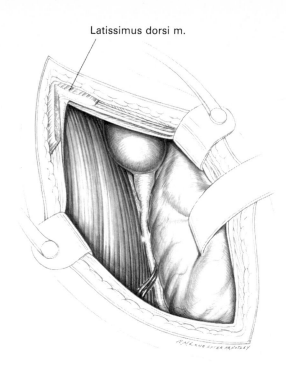

Latissimus dorsi m.

9

Wound closure

Both the anterior and lumbar approach incisions to the ureter require accurate, layer-by-layer closure of the separated muscles. It is a matter of personal choice whether absorbable or non-absorbable sutures are used or whether the sutures are continuous or interrupted as long as the stitches do not strangulate the closed muscles. Drainage of the ureter after incision of its wall is essential; a tube drain placed adjacent to the site is brought out below the main incision and connected to a drainage bag.

This drain may be removed as soon as it ceases to drain significant amounts and in all cases should be removed by the 4th or 5th day after operation. The temptation to leave it in position any longer should be resisted even if large amounts of urine are still draining. A drain of this kind offers the line of least resistance for the escape of urine and may perpetuate a urinary fistula which would close spontaneously within a day or two after removal of the drain as long as no distal ureteric obstruction remains.

Exposure of the lower ureter and ureterolithotomy

R. E. Williams   MD, ChM, FRCS(Ed), FRCS
Consultant Urologist, The General Infirmary and
St James's University Hospital, Leeds, UK

Principles

Ureterolithotomy is probably the commonest indication for exposure of the lower ureter. Other indications include nephroureterectomy; the repair of injuries, usually following pelvic surgery; urinary diversion by ileal conduit, ureterosigmoidostomy or cutaneous ureterostomy; the relief of ureteric obstruction from extrinsic causes such as retroperitoneal fibrosis or tumour.

Methods of approach

The ureter runs retroperitoneally throughout its course, has a close relationship to the posterior parietal peritoneum and is usually approached extraperitoneally. While it can be approached by the transperitoneal route, this may lead to extravasation of urine into the peritoneal cavity with the risk of infection, and this approach is used only when ureterointestinal anastomosis is intended or when fibrosis or disease has obliterated the extraperitoneal plane. Extraperitoneal exposure may also be difficult when there is severe spinal deformity.

Preliminary investigation with intravenous urography, retrograde ureterography or micturating cystography will have provided the diagnosis, an indication of the site of the ureter to be exposed and the functional activity of both kidneys.

Position of patient

The patient is placed on the operating table in the supine position and dissection deep in the pelvis is made easier if the head end of the table is tilted downwards and if the bladder is empty.

Anaesthesia

The operation is usually done under a general anaesthetic using an endotracheal tube and a suitable muscle relaxant drug.

Exposure of the lower ureter

1

The incisions

The ureter follows the curve of the cavity of the pelvis from the brim downwards and is deeply placed in the pelvis as it approaches the bladder. A modified *Gibson oblique incision* (A) may be used; this begins near the anterosuperior iliac spine and curves inwards and medially to a point above the symphysis pubis. If disease is suspected in the bladder also, a lateral extension of the *Pfannenstiel transverse suprapubic incision* (B) will give satisfactory exposure of bladder and lower ureter. The most popular incisions are by an extraperitoneal approach through a *midline incision* (C), extending from the umbilicus to the symphysis pubis, or through a *paramedian incision* (D), especially if transperitoneal exposure is intended for urinary diversion.

In female patients a catheter is passed to ensure an empty bladder, and in male patients the external genitalia are prepared and draped as well as the lower abdominal wall so that a urethral catheter can be passed at any time during the operation. If preliminary cystoscopy has been done, one should make sure the bladder is empty at the end of that procedure.

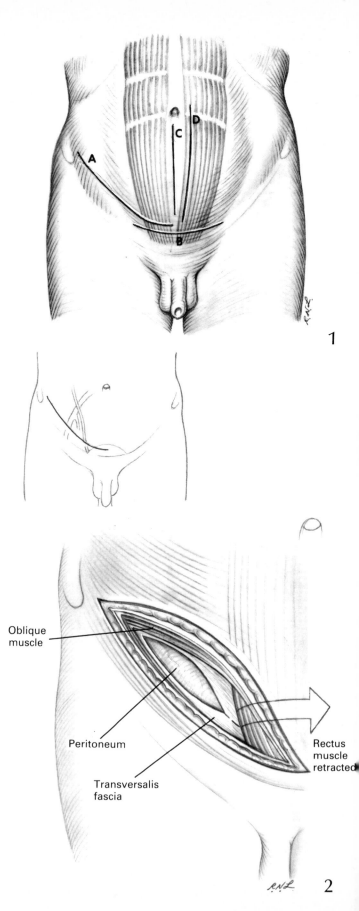

1

2

Modified Gibson incision

This hockey stick incision runs parallel to the inguinal fold and 2.5 cm above it. It starts 2.5 cm medial to the anterosuperior iliac spine and curves inwards and medially to a point one finger's breadth above the symphysis pubis; it may be extended to the opposite side. The skin, superficial fascia and external oblique aponeurosis are divided in this line, as are the external oblique muscle fibres. Medially, the rectus fascia can be divided to the midline and the belly of the rectus muscle retracted medially without being incised. The external and internal oblique muscle fibres may be split bluntly with the scalpel handle or divided with the scalpel blade. The transversalis fascia should be divided carefully by lifting it with forceps, making a nick in it and then separating off the underlying peritoneum by blunt dissection. This is continued until the peritoneum can be retracted medially to expose the ureter in the retroperitoneum where it may remain adherent to the posterior surface of the peritoneum. It may be necessary to divide the deep epigastric vessels and also sometimes the uterine artery overlying the ureter in the female. The ureter is identified high in the incision, encircled by loops and traced downwards.

Oblique muscle

Peritoneum

Transversalis fascia

Rectus muscle retracted

2

The Pfannenstiel approach

This incision may be satisfactory if there is no need to expose the ureter at a higher level than the true pelvis, if there are other lesions affecting the bladder which have to be dealt with simultaneously or if a bilateral approach to the lower ureters is indicated. It heals well with a minimum of scarring but identification of the ureter in the depth of the pelvis may prove to be rather more difficult than when this structure has been identified previously at a higher level as in the other incisions. A slightly curved transverse suprapubic incision is carried through skin, subcutaneous fascia and rectus sheath, after which the rectus bellies may be spread laterally.

3

Midline extraperitoneal approach

The midline incision gives excellent exposure of the lowest part of the ureter and with the extraperitoneal approach an incisional hernia is rare. Most surgeons prefer to stand on the side of the patient opposite to that of the ureter involved so that the assistant surgeon can retract the lower abdominal muscles. The skin, subcutaneous tissues and anterior rectus sheath are divided in the line of the incision and then the lateral surface of the bladder can be swept off the side wall of the pelvis from the pubic ramus upwards until the iliac vessels are exposed. The first objective should be to identify the ureter as it crosses the iliac vessels at the pelvic brim where the peritoneum arches across the front of vessels and ureter. When a deep-bladed retractor is used to lift this peritoneal arch the ureter will be displaced medially, and will be found lying in a thin layer of connective tissue adherent to the peritoneum. Once the ureter is identified, a sling should be passed under it and then, if ureterolithotomy is intended, round it a second time to occlude its lumen.

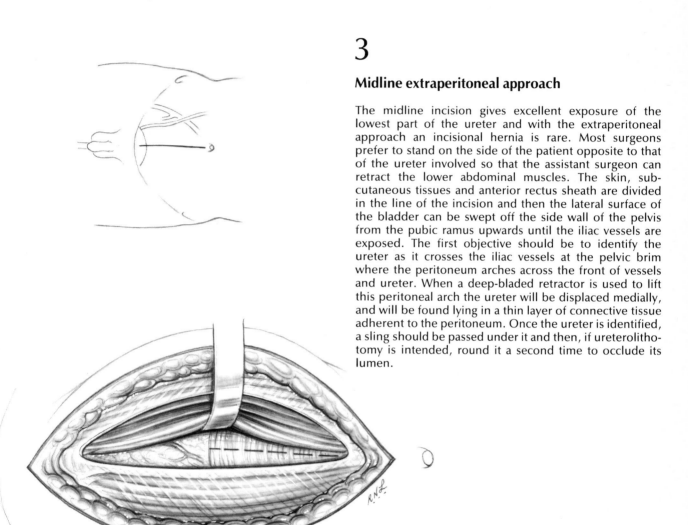

3

Paramedian extraperitoneal approach

In the paramedian approach the rectus sheath is incised longitudinally, the muscle is retracted laterally and the posterior rectus sheath is divided in the upper third of the wound to expose the peritoneum throughout the length of the incision. The peritoneum may be separated from the parietal pelvic wall for the extraperitoneal approach or opened for the transperitoneal approach.

Ureterolithotomy

Preoperative

Indications

A round or oval ureteric stone less than 5 mm wide which has a smooth surface is likely to pass spontaneously. A stone larger than 5 mm wide which has a spiculated surface and has not descended in the ureter after 1 week's observation is less likely to pass. Other factors that would indicate surgical removal of the stone are urinary infection and evidence of persistent ureteric obstruction as shown by ureteric dilatation on X-ray or by impaired renal function. Recurrent attacks of severe colic without progression of the stone are also an indication for operative relief. Sometimes a stone may lie symptomless in the ureter for many months and there may be gradual onset of renal damage. In the author's opinion, a stone that has not moved after 1 year should be removed, even though it is not producing symptoms.

Preoperative procedure

Usually an intravenous urogram will have been performed to establish the diagnosis. If the patient is in pain a dense nephrogram will develop with delayed excretion of contrast medium on the affected side and the appearance of a dilated collecting system. Follow-up films may be required at 12 hour intervals before function is sufficient to outline the ureter down to the site of the stone. A stone in the lower ureter may be obscured by the dye in the bladder unless a satisfactory postmicturition film is obtained. If the patient is not in pain, the ureter will fill quickly with dye. When more than one suspicious opacity is present, an oblique film will demonstrate which opacity is within the ureter. It is essential that a plain X-ray of the renal tract be taken on the way to the operating theatre to confirm the position of the stone before surgical exposure is begun.

If urinary infection is present preoperative antibiotics should be given but it is unlikely that the infection will be cleared completely until the obstructing stone is removed.

Preliminary cystoscopy and ureteric catheterization should not be done unless there is some doubt about the diagnosis of a ureteric stone. If a ureteric catheter is passed up to or beyond the suspicious opacity, X-rays with anteroposterior and oblique views will confirm whether or not it is in the ureter. The ureteric catheter may be left in place to help identify the ureter at operation. Care must be taken to ensure that the stone is not pushed into a dilated upper ureter. If no opaque stone can be seen on plain X-ray, retrograde ureterography may demonstrate the presence of a uric acid stone, a ureteric tumour or a sloughed renal papilla. The bladder should be emptied before removing the cystoscope.

Initial stages

When ureterolithotomy has been decided upon, the ureter should be exposed by any of the methods described previously. The author's preference is for a lower abdominal midline incision.

The operation

4a & b

Identification of stone

Often a large stone can be palpated easily and this may help in the identification of the ureter. More often it will be too small to feel or will be surrounded by periureteric fibrosis, and in all cases it is better to identify the ureter at the pelvic brim and dissect downwards from there. The ureter is secured with a controlling tape passed round it twice and then is followed under the arcades of blood vessels crossing from the internal iliac vessels to the bladder.

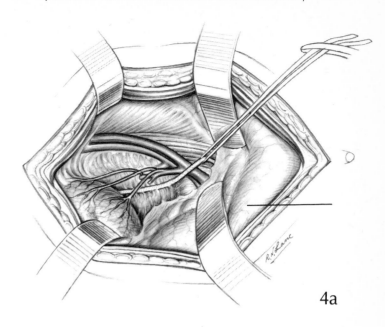

4a

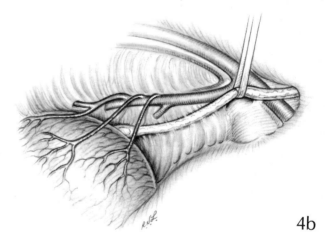

4b

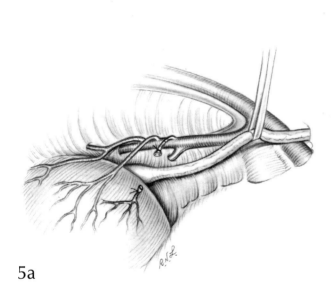

5a

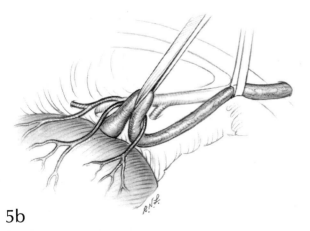

5b

5a & b

Sometimes it is advantageous to divide these arcades (a) while on other occasions the ureter can be pulled out through an opening in the arcades and another tape placed round it there (b). Care should be taken to avoid injuring the ureteric vessels which run parallel to the ureter. The dissection is continued downwards until the stone can be felt through the wall of the ureter. If the stone is very low in position it may be necessary to dissect the intramural portion of the ureter. The final arcade of vessels covering the stone may be ligated and divided if this makes exposure of the terminal ureter easier. At this stage another sling may be passed round the ureter below the stone.

6

Incision

A longitudinal incision can then be made into the ureteric wall on to the stone and the stone can be removed. The ureter must never be opened unless it is certain the stone is present there.

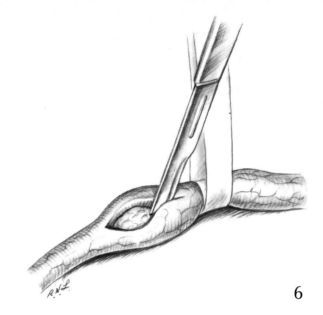

6

7, 8 & 9

Removal of stone

The stone may be removed by using gentle leverage with a blunt dissector and then grasping it with a pair of stone forceps. It is important to make sure that removal is complete and that no fragments have been left behind. If the proximal tape is loosened a flow of urine will appear and some of this can be sent for bacteriological culture.

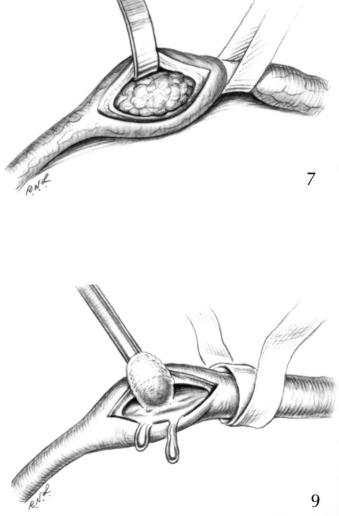

7

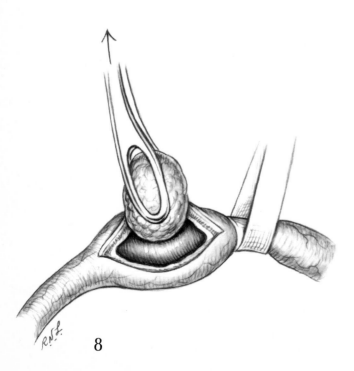

8

9

10

Patency of distal ureter

Once the stone is removed it is essential to ensure that the ureter below that level is not obstructed by a further calculus which might lead to a urinary fistula. A large catheter, preferably of the Braasch bulb type, should be passed down into the bladder.

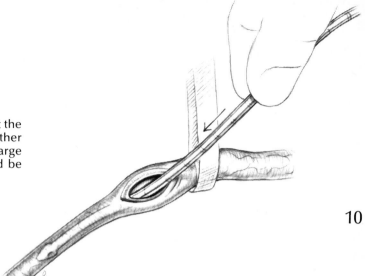

10

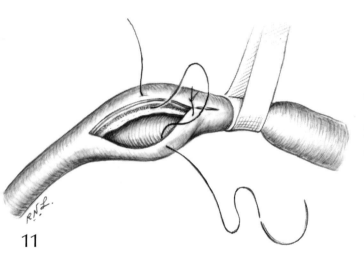

11

11

Closure of incision in ureter

A few interrupted sutures of plain catgut may be placed in the ureteric wall to include the fibrous and muscular coats only. There is no evidence that these sutures help ureteric healing and many surgeons believe that suturing of this incision may be omitted.

Drainage and closure of the wound

A drain is passed through a separate stab incision down to the opening in the ureter. The main wound may now be closed in layers. The drain should be shortened on the third or fourth postoperative day and removed on about the fifth or sixth day depending on the volume of leaking urine.

The removed stone should be sent for analysis.

SPECIAL PROBLEMS

No stone can be found

In these circumstances either the ureter has not yet been dissected far enough down into the pelvis, the stone may have slipped down into the bladder or the suspected opacity may never have been a stone at all! The ureter should be followed into its intramural portion and palpated carefully. If necessary, an X-ray is taken of the patient's abdomen on the operating table to see if the opacity is still present. If the position is still the same, the bladder is opened and a metal probe passed up the ureter until it can be felt to grate on the stone; if necessary further X-rays are taken with oblique and anteroposterior views. If all these attempts fail, the bladder and the wound are closed. The ureter must never be opened unless the stone can be identified with certainty.

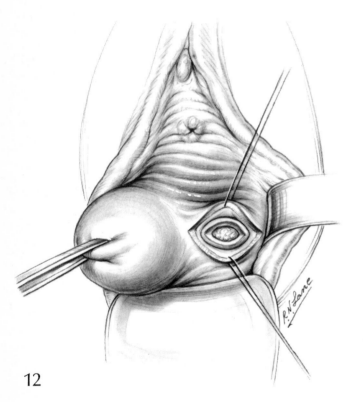

12

Repeat ureterolithotomy

When a previous ureterolithotomy has been done and now a new stone has formed and lodged at the same site in the ureter, further surgery there may prove difficult. Often, dense adhesions around the ureter will prevent extraperitoneal dissection and it may be necessary to open the peritoneal cavity, mobilize the caecum on the right or the sigmoid colon on the left and remove the stone intraperitoneally. In these circumstances urinary leakage may be lessened if a stent is left in the ureter, if the peritoneum is closed over the ureter and if an extraperitoneal drain can be left down to the site of the incision.

Persistent urinary leakage

If urine continues to leak from the drainage site after the 12th postoperative day, an X-ray of the abdomen should be taken to make certain that no further calculi are present and then a ureteric catheter should be passed at cystoscopy under anaesthesia. This ureteric catheter may be kept in place by attaching it to a Foley catheter in the bladder and left for several days until the leakage stops.

12

VAGINAL URETEROLITHOTOMY

This method has limited usefulness but may be used when an easily palpable stone can be felt in the vaginal fornix. With a vaginal speculum holding back the posterior wall, the cervix is grasped with forceps and pulled downwards and towards the contralateral side. An incision is made through the vaginal wall at the lateral margin of the cervix and extended outwards. The vaginal mucosa is dissected to expose the ureter and care must be taken to avoid the uterine vessels. Babcock clamps placed on either side of the stone may prevent it from being dislodged. A longitudinal ureteric incision allows the stone to be removed and the distal ureter to be probed. The ureteric wall should be carefully sutured and the vaginal mucosa closed over it except where a small soft rubber drain has been placed (see chapter on 'Vaginal ureterolithotomy', pp. 240–242).

Illustrations by Robert N. Lane from originals by Richard G. Notley

Transurethral and transvesical ureterolithotomy

Richard G. Notley, MS, FRCS
Senior Consultant Urological Surgeon, Royal Surrey County Hospital, Guildford, Surrey, UK

Introduction

A calculus lodged in the intramural ureter presents particular problems in removal. While small calculi may be extracted endoscopically using a Dormia extractor (*see* chapter on 'Extraction of ureteric calculi', pp. 751–754), larger calculi may be inaccessible since they can prevent the passage of the stone basket up the ureter. In such circumstances transvesical ureterolithotomy becomes necessary. The obstructing calculus is localized radiographically at the lowermost end of the ureter. Before proceeding to surgery it is wise to cystoscope the patient as even the most obdurate calculus occasionally falls into the bladder during the patient's journey from bed to operating table.

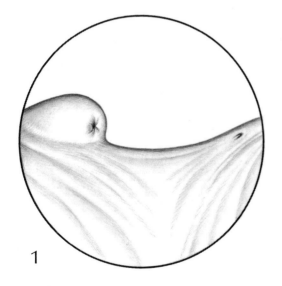

1

1

When a stone is impacted in the intramural ureter the cystoscopic appearances are usually unmistakable. The ureteric orifice on the side in question is usually oedematous and the intramural ureter bulges. In contrast the other ureteric orifice is normal in appearance. A stone in this position may be removed transvesically, but the experienced endoscopic surgeon will prefer to use the transurethral route.

The operations

TRANSURETHRAL URETEROLITHOTOMY

2

The cystoscope is removed from the bladder and replaced by the resectoscope

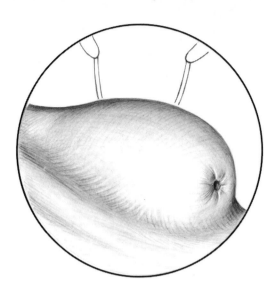

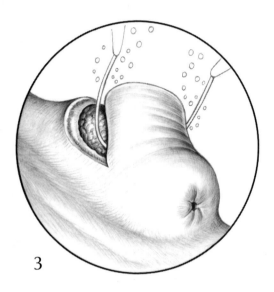

3

The loop of the resectoscope is used to decapitate the bulging intramural ureter.

4

This will reveal the stone lying within the intramural ureter.

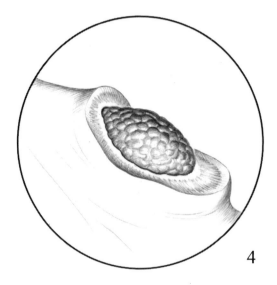

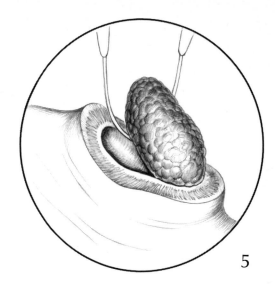

5

The stone is dislodged with the resectoscope loop and is extracted from the bladder. Haemostasis is obtained.

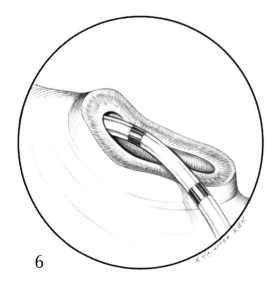

6

A suitably sized ureteric catheter is passed up the ureter to the renal pelvis (checking its precise siting radiographically). This catheter is left *in situ* for 48 hours, strapped to an 18 Fr Foley catheter left draining the bladder.

OPEN TRANSVESICAL URETEROLITHOTOMY

Transurethral ureterolithotomy relieves a patient of an obstructing ureteric calculus painlessly and reduces the length of stay in hospital. However, for the surgeon unfamiliar with the resectoscope it is safer to proceed to open transvesical ureterolithotomy.

7

Once the radiographic diagnosis has been confirmed by cystoscopy a Pfannensteil incision is made with the patient supine and tilted 5–10° head down to facilitate access to the pelvis.

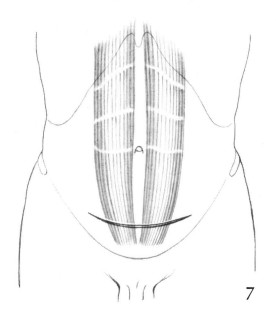

8

The flap of anterior rectus sheath is raised to exposed the two rectus muscles. The recti are separated from the anterior sheath above and below the incision.

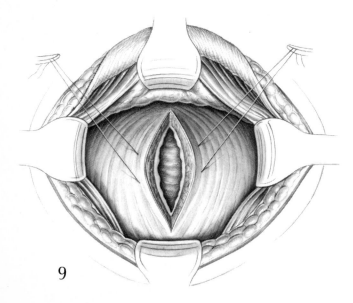

9

The recti are then separated from each other and the retropubic space is developed by blunt dissection. The peritoneum is pushed upwards to expose the bladder. The incision is held open with a suitable self-retaining retractor and the bladder opened vertically between two stay sutures.

10

The self-retaining retractor is repositioned with its blades inside the bladder. The bulging intramural ureter with its contained stone is visualized. An incision is then made over the stone in the line of the ureter and the stone is removed. It is unnecessary to suture the open intramural ureter. It is sensible to pass a probe up the ureter to ensure that there is no obstruction higher up, but it is not usually necessary to drain the ureter.

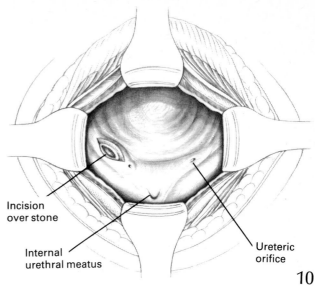

Incision
over stone

Internal
urethral meatus

Ureteric
orifice

10

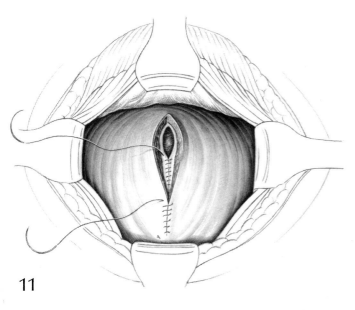

11

11

The bladder should be drained with a self-retaining catheter passed *per urethram*. The self-retaining retractor is repositioned outside the bladder to permit closure in two layers with continuous catgut.

12

A tube drain is inserted through a separate small incision to drain the retropubic space. The recti are approximated with a few loose sutures and the rectus sheath closed with a continuous suture of absorbable or non-absorbable material according to the surgeon's personal preference. The drain should be removed on the 4th or 5th postoperative day and the catheter in 8–10 days.

Note: A suitable self-retaining retractor is the Millin retractor used in combination with a Joll thyroid retractor to hold the upper and lower flaps of rectus sheath apart. The Denis Browne ring retractor modified by Turner-Warwick is also a convenient self-retaining retractor for retropubic and intravesical surgery.

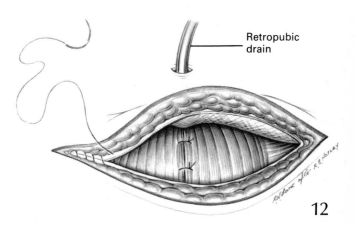

Retropubic
drain

12

Further reading

McLean, P A., McDermott, T. E., Walsh, A. Transurethral ureterolithotomy. British Journal of Urology 1980; 52: 439–442

Illustrations by Daniel S. Beisel

Vaginal ureterolithotomy

Thomas J. Rohner, Jr MD
Professor of Surgery (Urology), Chief, Division of Urology, Pennsylvania State University College of Medicine and The Milton S. Hershey Medical Center, Hershey, Pennsylvania, USA

Introduction

The vaginal approach to ureterolithotomy was described in 1890 by Kelly, with Emmett receiving credit for performing the first procedure in 1884. This approach gained a certain degree of popularity and several small series of successfully managed patients appeared during the first half of this century[1-3]. In recent years it has been little used and current urological textbooks do not recommend this procedure[4].

However, vaginal incision to carry out ureterolithotomy can be considered for removal of a palpable distal ureteral calculus which is located just outside the bladder in a multiparous patient. The main advantage of this approach is that it avoids an abdominal incision and postoperative discomfort is minimal. Major disadvantages include the close apposition of ureteral and vaginal incisions with the possibility of persistent ureterovaginal fistula and lack of access to the proximal ureter should the stone move upwards during the procedure.

Preoperative

Indications

The indications for vaginal ureterolithotomy are the same as for ureterolithotomy using other surgical techniques for ureteral exposure, and include sepsis, significant upper tract obstruction or intractable pain. In addition, the patient being considered for the vaginal approach should be multiparous to permit satisfactory vaginal exposure. The stone should be palpable on vaginal examination but not visualized by cystoscopic examination. If the stone is within the intramural or intravesical portion of the ureter, then an endoscopic or open intravesical procedure is used to remove it.

1

The stone should therefore be located 2–4 cm from the ureteral orifice in the lower ureter outside the bladder.

Preoperative preparation

The patient should have the vagina prepared with iodine-povidone solution the evening before surgery and receive a broad-spectrum antibiotic 2 hours before the operation is due to begin.

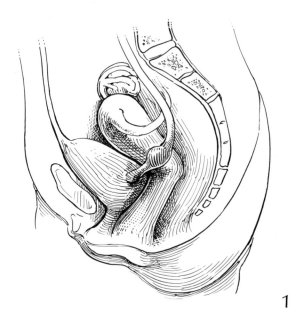

1

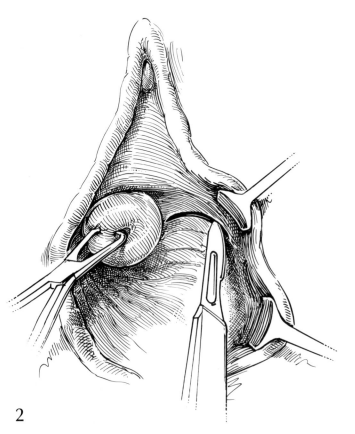

2

The operation

The patient is placed in the exaggerated lithotomy position with the knees and thighs well padded. The vagina and introital areas are scrubbed and draped appropriately. A plain film of the abdomen should be made, confirming the unchanged location of the stone and cystoscopy done to be certain the stone has not moved into the bladder. A cystoscope should be available for use throughout the course of the operation.

2

Exposure of the vagina is improved by sewing the labia laterally with interrupted 2/0 silk sutures and using a weighted vaginal speculum posteriorly. If the stone is still palpable, the cervix is grasped with a tenaculum and downward and lateral traction is exerted to the side opposite the stone. A 2–3 cm transverse incision is made in the vagina slightly anterior and lateral to the cervix or directly over the palpable stone.

In this position the ureter will be found running in an anterior–posterior direction. The index finger should be used to open the vaginal incision further, with dissection done laterally to avoid the bladder base. The uterine artery will be above and medial to the ureter. Continued lateral and posterior blunt dissection with the index finger will permit mobilization of the ureter above the stone.

3

The ureter should be grasped with a Babcock clamp above the stone and a knife used to incise the ureter over the stone.

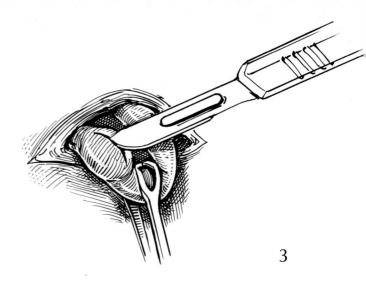

3

4

After stone removal, a catheter should be passed distally into the bladder and proximally, to be certain no obstruction remains.

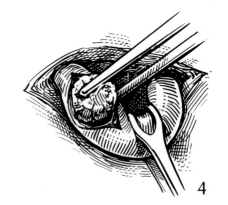

4

5

A few interrupted 5/0 chromic sutures can be used to close the ureteral adventitia loosely.

A small Penrose drain should be used to drain the area and led out through the vaginal incision. The vaginal incision should either be left open or approximated loosely.

If, after the ureter has been mobilized, the stone is not present, cystoscopy should be done to see if it has passed into the bladder. If the stone has moved a short distance proximally as determined by a plain film of the abdomen, one can consider introducing a stone basket through the ureterotomy and attempting to retrieve the stone.

After successful removal of the stone, cystoscopy can be done and a ureteral catheter passed up the ureter to provide a stenting catheter and perhaps decrease the chance of fistula. Although a persistent ureterovaginal fistula has been reported as a complication of this procedure, the chance of this occurring is apparently small.

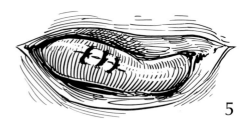

5

References

1. Bergman, R. T. Vaginal ureterolithotomy. Journal of Urology 1941; 45: 176–185

2. Shaw, E. C. Vaginal ureterolithotomy. Journal of Urology 1936; 35: 289–299

3. Garvey, F.K., Gomberg, D. Vaginal ureterolithotomy. Journal of Urology 1946; 56: 49–56

4. Persky, L., Hoch, W. H., Kursh, E. D. Transvaginal approach to the ureter. In: Campbell's Urology, Vol. 3., 4th ed. Philadelphia: W. B. Saunders, 1979: 2197–2198

Retroperitoneal fibrosis

J. Dermot O'Flynn   MCh, FRCS, FRCSI
Consultant Urological Surgeon, Meath Hospital, Dublin;
Lecturer in Urology, Trinity College, Dublin, Ireland

Introduction

Retroperitoneal fibrosis may be primary (idiopathic RPF) or secondary to, or associated with, inflammatory bowel disease, vascular disease, radiotherapy, trauma and malignant disease.

In all forms one or both ureters become engulfed by the fibrotic process. Progressive ureteric narrowing and medial (and sometimes forward) displacement of the ureter occur and the resulting upper tract obstruction causes ureterectasis, pyelocalyectasis and ultimately uraemia.

Strong indications for the diagnosis of idiopathic RPF are a history of severe chronic abdominal pain or backache, a persistently raised ESR and the fact that both the obstructed ureters are usually easily catheterized. Hypertension is frequently present and thromboembolism may also occur. In addition there is a definite association with prolonged methysergide intake.

The condition may be self-limiting, and, in the early stages, at least, steroid therapy will cause regression. Some cases may be treated satisfactorily by corticosteroids combined with temporary ureteral catheterization, pyelostomy or nephrostomy and surgical operation may not be necessary. Stopping methysergide therapy has also resulted in regression in some cases.

The preoperative differential diagnosis between idiopathic and other forms of RPF may be impossible and even at operation may be sometimes very difficult. Intravenous, retrograde and antegrade pyelography, tomography and ultrasound study will usually give an accurate picture of the level and extent of the lesion and this will help to exclude malignant and other conditions of which ureteral obstruction is a complication. Before operating it is vital to establish as accurately as possible the extent of the lesion as this will greatly influence the surgical approach.

Preoperative

Most (60 per cent) of patients present with some degree of uraemia and a small number (13 per cent) may be anuric. This is best treated by percutaneous nephrostomy or pyelostomy, done with X-ray control. This should be considered a preliminary procedure in all patients, whether uraemic or not. Diversion of this type relieves the upper urinary tract obstruction and provides a means of antegrade pyelography. In addition, the ureteral dilatation diminishes and the ureter returns to near-normal calibre, becomes less friable and is easier to manipulate. Ureteral catheterization will also decompress the upper urinary tract, but it is not as useful as percutaneous nephrostomy for diagnostic purposes and is less reliable for prolonged drainage.

In idiopathic RPF the ureter is compressed but not infiltrated by the fibrosis. The peritoneum is usually not adherent and will peel off fairly easily and the ureter is released without much difficulty.

In secondary RPF the fibrosis may be dense and infiltrate the ureteral wall so extensively that it may be impossible to mobilize part or all of the ureter, making ureteral replacement or diversion necessary. If the diagnostic study indicates this may be necessary, the patient should be prepared accordingly.

Ureterolysis alone is not sufficient to prevent reinvolvement of the ureter. The ureter must be freed widely from the fibrosis, fixed in a new position well away from the area of fibrosis and prevented from becoming involved once more in the fibrotic process. This may be done by interposing the peritoneum between the fibrotic mass and the ureter or by wrapping the ureter in omentum. Opinions differ as to which of these two methods is the better because both have been known to fail. Where the condition is relatively localized, intraperitonealization of the ureter may be effective, but, in extensive disease, omental wrapping is mandatory.

Where vascular complications are evident or predominate preoperatively a vascular surgeon's opinion and help may be necessary. In some cases the ureteral surgery may be a small part of an extensive vascular procedure.

Preoperative preparation

As the projected operation may be long and difficult it is important that the patient should be as fit as possible. Many patients with RPF are very ill, usually due to upper urinary tract obstruction and uraemia, and the first step should be the establishment of percutaneous ('stab') nephrostomy and active treatment of the uraemic state. If the preoperative investigation indicates that the disease is very extensive and that the dissection may involve bowel trauma or the possibility of diversion to bowel, then appropriate bowel sterilization should be carried out preoperatively. Because of the danger of haemorrhage from large vessels involved in the fibrosis, adequate blood replacement should be available.

Anaesthesia

General anaesthesia is satisfactory and controlled hypotension may be helpful. Spinal anaesthesia may be used for low and localized lesions.

Choice of approach

Depending on the preoperative findings, either an intraperitoneal or extraperitoneal approach may be used. The intraperitoneal approach is most commonly used and is indicated for bilateral ureteral obstruction and especially those cases where the obstruction extends deep into the pelvis. It may have some limitations if the obstruction extends high up in the ureter or involves the renal pelvis. The extraperitoneal approach is useful in unilateral cases and where the length of the ureter involved is short.

Careful consideration should be given to the type of approach and the choice will be determined by the investigational findings and whether or not a simple intraperitoneal transposition or an omentoplasty is envisaged. If omentoplasty is proposed the intraperitoneal approach must be used if the omentum is to be mobilized satisfactorily.

The operation

INTRAPERITONEAL APPROACH

1

With the patient in a moderate head-down supine position a vertical paramedian or midline incision is made, extending from the symphysis pubis to (or nearly to) the xiphisternum. The peritoneum is opened and the intestines packed away.

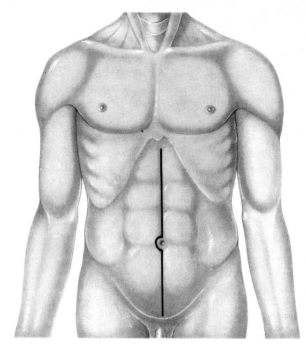

1

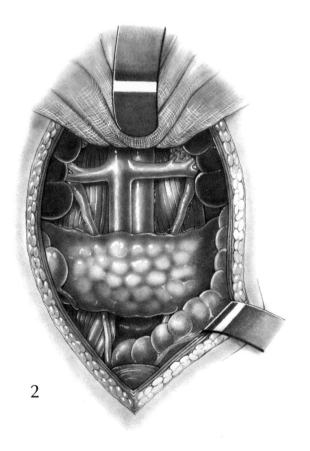

2

2

Inspection and palpation will now reveal the fibrotic pink-white, tumour-like mass behind the peritoneum and usually extending from the fourth lumbar vertebrae to the top of the sacrum and laterally across the posterior abdomen. Usually it has ill defined edges which fade away on either side lateral to the iliac vessels and over the psoas muscle and it extends upwards and downwards lateral to the iliac vessels for a variable distance. (This is the most common finding, but great variation may occur in the extent of the lesion. Its exact extent should have been well defined by the preoperative workup, but it may be found to be more extensive than the preoperative study indicated.)

3

In a thin person the ureters may be seen entering the mass, or emerging below it, although no ureter may be visible or palpable. It should, therefore, be sought through a vertical incision in the posterior peritoneum several cm above the level of the mass well lateral to and above the common iliac artery. If the ureter is palpable or visible below the mass the dissection may be started here. Sometimes there is no lead to the site of the ureter and a careful and tedious dissection may be necessary during which it may be impossible to distinguish between the ureter and large blood vessels. Any doubtful tubular structure encountered should be aspirated with a fine hypodermic needle and syringe before being mobilized. The ureter is mobilized by blunt dissection, taped and freed as far as the mass.

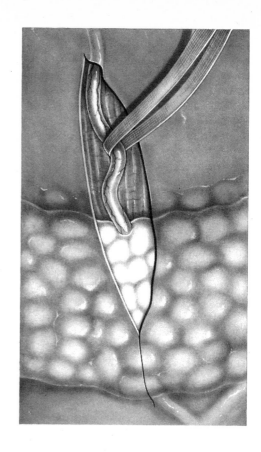

3

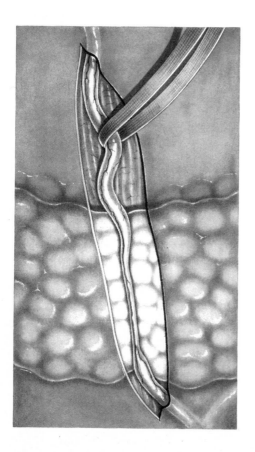

4

4

The incision is now extended over the mass and if possible its lower level is defined and the peritoneum reflected. The peritoneum is usually not involved and its dissection from the mass presents no special problem. The area of retroperitoneal fibrosis can now be shown as a pinkish white rubbery mass with a dilated ureter entering it at the upper border and, on occasion, the normal ureter emerging from the lower part of the mass.

5a, b & c

At this stage formal mobilization of the large bowel may be necessary, especially on the left side. This is achieved by extending the posterior peritoneal incision vertically along the paracolic gutter.

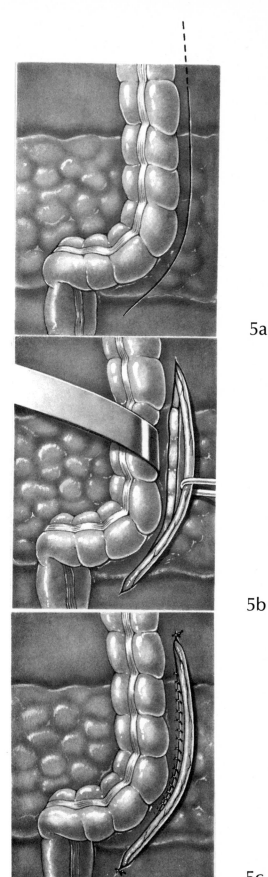

5a

5b

5c

6

The caecum is more easily mobilized on the right side.

If the ureter is to be intraperitonealized, it is important that this incision should be sited well laterally in order to provide an adequate leaf of peritoneum on the outer side of the colon so that the peritoneum can be sutured behind the ureter. If, on the other hand, omentoplasty is proposed, then a wide peritoneal leaf on the bowel is not important. In extensive disease it may be necessary to mobilize the colon right up to the level of the renal pelvis. On the right side the caecum and ascending colon will be mobilized and care should be taken at the upper end of the incision that the duodenum is not injured.

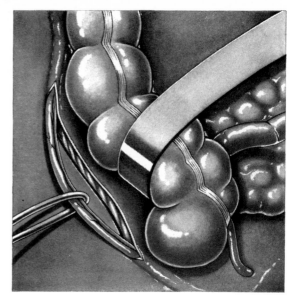

6

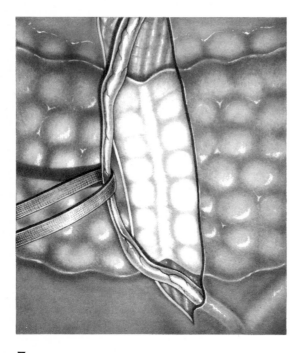

7

7

Biopsy for frozen section is now taken (note that the absence of the malignant cells in the biopsy does not necessarily exclude malignancy as a cause of the RPF) and the mass is now incised vertically approximately in the line of the ureter. In favourable cases ureterolysis is now a simple procedure as the ureter peels easily from the surrounding tissue where it is seen to lie in a trough. It is released by blunt dissection, care being taken not to incise or puncture the ureter or dissect into its wall.

In some cases the ureter may be infiltrated and completely stuck within the mass. Sharp dissection with scissors and knife may be the only means of liberating it and here there is a high risk of ureteric damage.

Because of the denseness of the fibrosis and the loss of anatomical landmarks, the dissection may now be exceedingly difficult and any of the large vessels or their branches or the gonadal vessels may be damaged. The ureter should be extensively mobilized well beyond the apparent limit of the fibrosis and this may take a considerable time to achieve satisfactorily.

8

Intraperitoneal transposition of the ureter

The lateral leaf of the incised posterior peritoneum is now pulled medially under the ureter and the peritoneal incision closed with interrupted or continuous 3/0 catgut sutures. The ureter is displaced laterally and fixed with interrupted sutures on its lateral side which pick up the adventitial part of the ureteral wall and the peritoneum and retroperitoneal fat as far laterally as is possible without kinking the ureter. Interrupted nylon or chromic catgut sutures are suitable for this. The procedure is repeated on the opposite side.

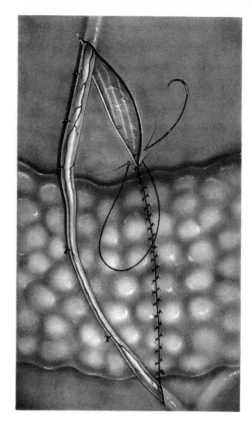

8

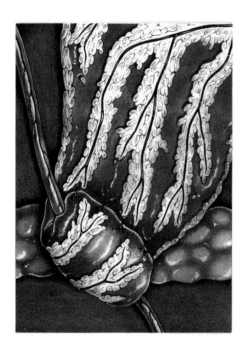

9

Omentoplasty

9

In most cases wrapping the ureter in omentum will prevent it from again becoming involved in the RPF. If only a short segment of ureter is involved, the adjacent omentum may be pulled around the ureter and sutured to itself, thus insulating the ureter from the RPF mass.

10

When the ureteral involvement is extensive, the avascular edge of omentum is first detached from the colon and the short gastroepiploic vessels are then divided along the greater curve of the stomach, care being taken that the main blood supply to the omentum at either end of the stomach is not compromised. The vessels should be individually tied and divided between ligatures.

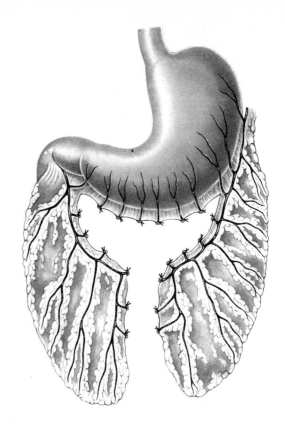

10

11

The omentum is then split vertically to produce two aprons which can be pulled downwards and laterally and wrapped around the ureters. The apron of omentum should be passed laterally behind the ureter and sewn to itself with fairly thick catgut, enclosing the ureter very loosely.

The peritoneum and abdomen are closed in the usual way. Wound drainage is usually necessary, especially if oozing or urinary leakage has been a problem.

11

Operative difficulties

The technique described is suitable for uncomplicated ideopathic retroperitoneal fibrosis. Operative difficulties arise because the fibrotic mass is more extensive than anticipated or the ureter is either partially or totally invaded by the fibrotic process.

The ureter is perforated during mobilization

12

This is best dealt with by passing a suitable catheter (12–14 Fr) distally through the perforation and completing the dissection.

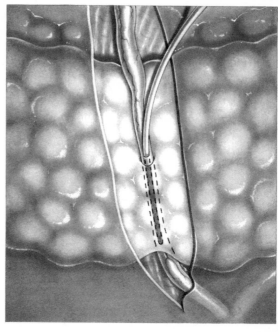

12

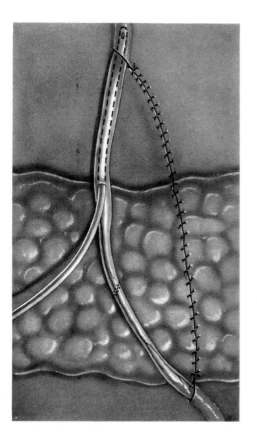

13

13

After ureterolysis the defect may be repaired with fine chromic catgut if the nephrostomy is satisfactory. If a preoperative nephrostomy has not been accomplished, ureterostomy should be performed above the level of the repair.

A segment of ureter cannot be mobilized

Short segment loss

14

If a segment of ureter cannot be mobilized, the ureter should be divided obliquely above and below the level of the segment and the two ends spatulated. If necessary an end-to-end anastomosis should be performed obliquely over a ureterostomy tube or, if this is not convenient, over a polyurethane splint passed into the bladder and recovered later with cystoscopic biopsy forceps. If a polyurethane splint is used it should have several holes cut in it above the below the level of the repair.

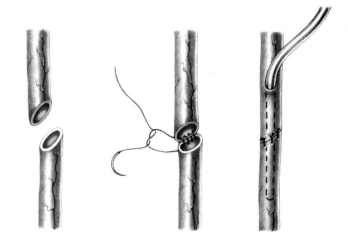

14

Long segment loss

Where a long segment of ureter cannot be mobilized, one of the following procedures may be necessary.

15

Reimplantation of the ureter into the bladder The bladder is mobilized, the superior vesical pedicle divided and the ureter implanted laterally into the dome of the bladder using chromic catgut sutures. This may be a direct anastomosis but if sufficient ureter is available a tunnel technique may be used.

Division of the superior vesical pedicle greatly facilitates bladder mobilization and when this has been done quite a large segment of bladder can be pulled upwards to bridge the ureteral gap. This should always be fixed to the psoas muscle ('psoas hitch') with chromic catgut or unabsorbable sutures. In most cases of reimplantation this will make construction of a Boari flap unnecessary (*see* chapter on 'Surgery of genitourinary tuberculosis', pp. 158–163).

When this is not possible, replacement of a segment of ureter with ileum, relocation of the kidney, or urinary diversion by either ureterocolic anastomosis or ileal loop may have to be considered (*see* chapter on 'Ileal conduit diversion', pp. 273–281).

15

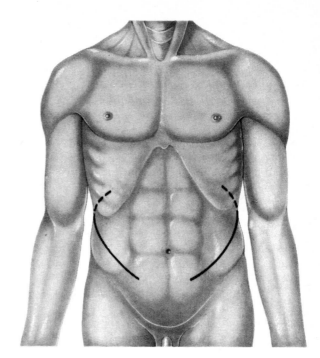

16

EXTRAPERITONEAL APPROACH

16

This may be done through a muscle-cutting incision (Rutherford Morison), which may need to be extended upwards. Extension of this incision may give adequate exposure of the whole ureter and renal pelvis.

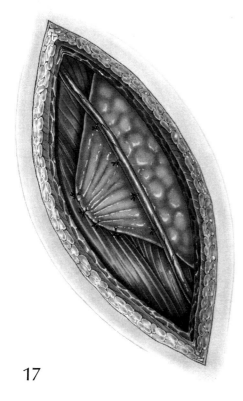

17

17

After the peritoneum has been peeled off intact, the ureter is exposed and mobilized as indicated and displaced medially. Without being opened, the double layer of peritoneum is then pulled behind the ureter and fixed to the posterior muscles and the ureter is then lateralized and fixed to the peritoneum with 3/0 chromic catgut. Mobilization of the peritoneum may not be satisfactory in some cases and, if this manoeuvre is not possible, the peritoneum should be opened and the ureter intraperitonealized as described. If for any reason satisfactory insulation of the ureter from the fibrotic mass is not achieved, the adjacent omentum should be wrapped around the ureter as described. Whichever procedure is adopted the peritoneum should be closed carefully either by suturing it to itself or to the omentum.

Postoperative care

For simple ureterolysis no special postoperative care is necessary. Where an extensive operation has been necessary the standard postoperative care for large intra-abdominal procedures should be initiated. Both ileus and thrombophlebitis are special hazards. The nephrostomy tubes may be removed in 7–10 days provided the intravenous urogram or nephrostogram shows satisfactory renal drainage and no ureteral leakage.

Where the RPF has been shown to be of malignant origin the appropriate radiotherapeutic or oncological treatment should be instituted.

All cases of idiopathic retroperitoneal fibrosis should be followed up radiographically for an indefinite period, as there is a risk of recurrence either due to surgical failure or to extension of the disease process. This applies especially to patients with an initial apparent unilateral lesion.

Corticosteroids have been shown to be effective in preventing recurrence. After wound-healing is complete, these should be given for a period of 3–6 months or until the ESR has returned to normal.

Further reading

Abercrombie, G. F., Vinnicombe, J. Retroperitoneal fibrosis. Practical problems in management. British Journal of Urology 1980; 52: 443–445

Lepor, H., Walsh, P. C. Idiopathic retroperitoneal fibrosis. Journal of Urology 1979; 122: 1–6

Mitchinson, M. J., Whithycombe, J. F. R., Jones, R. A. The response of ideopathic retroperitoneal fibrosis to corticosteroids. British Journal of Urology 1971; 43: 444–449

Saxton, H. M., Kilpatrick, F. R., Kinder, C. H., Lessof, M. H., McHardy-Young, S., Wardle, D. F. H. Retroperitoneal fibrosis. Quarterly Journal of Medicine 1969; 38: 159–181

Wagenknecht, L. V., Hardy, J. C. Value of various treatments for retroperitoneal fibrosis. European Urology 1981; 7: 193–200

Illustrations by Harriet Phillips

Surgery of dilated ureters and ureteral tailoring (megaureter repair)

Terry W. Hensle MD
Director, Pediatric Urology and Associate Professor of Urology,
College of Physicians and Surgeons, New York, USA

Howard R. Goldstein MD
Pediatric Urologist and Clinical Assistant Professor of Surgery,
UMDNJ-Rutgers Medical School at Camden,
Cooper Hospital-University Medical Center, New Jersey, USA

Kevin A. Burbige MD
Associate Director, Pediatric Urology and Assistant Professor of Urology,
College of Physicians and Surgeons, New York, USA

Introduction

In general the term megaureter simply describes ureters of larger than normal calibre. The increased calibre is usually a result of ureteral decompensation due to a pathological anatomical situation at a more distal level in the lower genitourinary tract. Fusiform dilation of the mid and distal ureter with a normal appearing renal pelvis was first described in 1923 by Caulk[1] in a patient with a normal trigone and ureter orifices. He coined the term 'mega-loureter' (megaureter) to describe this constellation and also noted that the lower ureters could either be free from obstruction or have a 'small ureteral valve'.

From the time of Caulk's first description of megaureter, the literature has been at best confusing with regard to the aetiology, definition, classification, diagnosis and management of these dilated ureters. Until recently, the pathogenesis of megaureter has been largely speculative. However, electronmicroscopic and histochemical techniques have revealed many of the pathological mechanisms responsible for megaureter[4-9].

Ureteral embryology

The ureter arises as a diverticulum of the Wolffian duct (ureteral bud) at approximately the 5th week of embryological development. Aberrations in its formation will frequently result in a number of abnormalities of the ureterovesical junction. Vesicoureteral reflux, orthotopic ureterocele, complete ureteral duplication with or without ectopic ureterocele, ureteral ectopy and primary obstructive megaureter are all conditions associated with large dilated ureters and can all be traced to ureteral bud abnormalities.

Many attempts have been made to describe the anatomical pathology of megaureters through a variety of names, including megaloureter, aperistaltic megaloureter, primary megaureter, simple megaureter, primary obstructive megaureter, achalasia of the ureter, atonic distal ureteral segment, functional stenosis of the ureter, adynamic distal ureteral segment, aperistaltic distal ureteral segment, non-occlusive dilation of the ureter and congenital ureteral stricture[10]. Many authors have proposed different classification schemes for dilated ureters based on either aetiology, pathological findings or radiographic appearance[11,12].

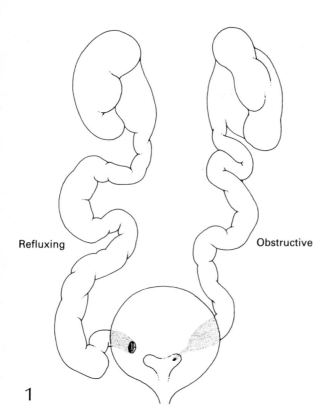

Refluxing   Obstructive

1

1

We feel, however, that a simplified approach which divides megaureter into either obstructive or refluxing is most appropriate. Essentially this system is a slightly modified version of Hendren's classification and is set out below.

Obstructive
Primary   – congenital
Secondary – iatrogenic
Associated   with ureterocele

Refluxing
Primary   – associated with high grade reflux
Secondary – to vesical or urethral pathology or neurogenic bladder
Associated   with duplication of ureter
Associated   with Prune-belly syndrome

In addition, we feel the term primary obstructive megaureter should be reserved to describe the syndrome of fusiform distal ureteral dilatation associated with a lesser degree of involvement of the renal pelvis and calyces. Primary obstructed megaureters all have a distal dysfunctional segment which accounts for the radiographic and gross anatomical features noted[10-16]. The material presented in this chapter regarding the diagnosis and management of megaureter will largely relate specifically to primary obstructive megaureter: however, the general principles are applicable to all types of megaureters.

Aetiology of megaureter

In 1923 Caulk[1] speculated that the pathogenesis of these dilated ureters represented a congenital defect in the ureteral wall which was comparable to Hirschsprung's disease of the sigmoid colon. Since that time, various authors have proposed a myriad of aetiologies[12–25]. However, it was not until 1969 that reports of abnormal histological findings in these distal ureters began to appear, along with attempts at establishing a cause and effect relationship[8].

Recent electronmicroscopic studies of abnormal ureteropelvic and ureterovesical junction tissue have demonstrated that effective ureteral peristalsis may be impeded by increased amounts of collagen present in the interstitial spaces. This evidence establishes a strong case for a similar pathogenesis in both congenital ureteropelvic junction obstruction and primary megaureter[26, 27].

Hanna et al.[4–7] in 1976 expanded this concept in a series of histological and clinicopathological studies which demonstrated that in both ureteropelvic junction obstruction and primary obstructive megaureter, disturbed plexuses from intracellular collagen resulted in a poorly distensible ureteral segment. This concept seems to account for the fact that in their series a small catheter or probe could be passed retrograde through the area of functional obstruction but antegrade propulsion of a bolus of urine could not be effectively accomplished.

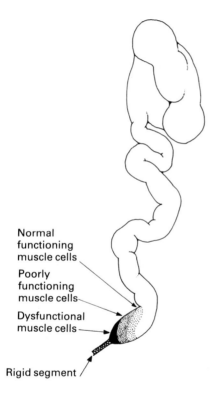

Normal functioning muscle cells

Poorly functioning muscle cells

Dysfunctional muscle cells

Rigid segment

2

These same authors demonstrated that the smooth muscle cells of the ureter proximal to the functionally obstructed area became progressively more compromised as one neared the obstruction.

Further evidence confirming the aetiological similarity of primary megaureter and congenital ureteropelvic junction obstruction was contributed in 1978 by Gosling and Dixon[9], who undertook an exquisite study utilizing light microscopy, histochemical methods and electronmicroscopy. They found that there was a marked reduction in pseudocholinesterase activity in the smooth muscle cells proximal to and at the point of maximal collagen deposition in the cellular interstitium. This was indeed a major step forward in understanding the pathogenesis of megaureters.

2

Diagnosis of megaureter

3

The diagnosis of primary obstructive megaureter is most frequently made by excretory urography.

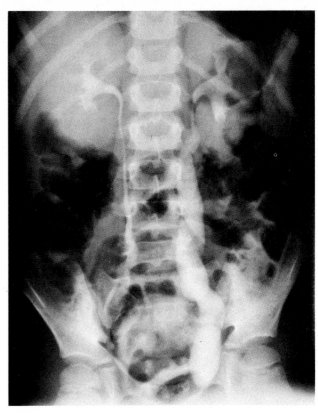

3

Primary obstructive megaureter as demonstrated by IVP. Note protection of renal pelvis and upper collecting systems

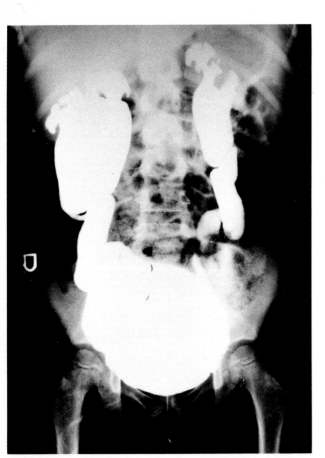

4

Refluxing megaureter demonstrated on voiding cystourethrogram. Note loss of normal upper collecting system architecture

4

Refluxing megaureter is best demonstrated by voiding cystourethrography, performed usually as part of an evaluation for urinary tract infection or haematuria[25-31].

In primary obstructive megaureter adjunctive radiographic examinations can be useful in defining the secondary effect of obstruction on renal function as well as the anatomy of the obstruction itself. Percutaneous antegrade pyelography with pressure-flow studies, as described by Whitaker[31,32,43], can supply some of this crucial information. However, the development of the diuretic radionuclide renogram has added a simple non-invasive method not only of measuring renal function: it also quantifies the degree of obstruction present. Radionuclide scanning also provides a simple means of monitoring the physiological status of the kidney and ureter after reconstructive surgery[34,35].

Surgical repair of the megaureter

Surgical intervention in the management of primary obstructive megaureter is at times controversial. Although there exists a subgroup of patients who may not experience upper tract deterioration with conservative treatment, there is no definitive way of selecting this group from all patients with primary obstructive megaureter. Therefore, if one opts for non-operative therapy, careful long-term radiographic follow-up is mandatory to prevent renal functional impairment. Certainly, those patients who have evidence of renal compromise when first seen, or who present with urinary infection, are unquestionably candidates for reconstructive surgery. In cases of refluxing megaureter, surgical intervention is generally indicated in order to create an effective antirefluxing mechanism, which is of paramount importance in the preservation of renal function as well as the eradication of chronic infection in these grossly dilated ureters[11, 15, 44-47].

The surgical approach to megaureter has changed over the years. Caulk in 1923[1] and Hurst and Gaymer-Jones in 1931[17] advocated ureteral meatotomy alone and reported favourable results, although the long-term data are not available. Vermooten in 1939[20] performed ureteral dilatation as a primary treatment, while Carver in 1948[39] advocated presacral neurectomy in managing megaureter. The first suggestion that a reconstructive operation might be beneficial in the management of megaureter was made by Crabtree in 1935[40] and later by Wayman in 1949[41]. Nesbit and Withycombe[42] in 1954 reported poor results with the operative treatment of megaureters and felt that therapeutic efforts should be directed at the antibacterial control of infection and less towards the correction of the ureteral dilatation.

During the 1950s a variety of surgical manoeuvres were tried which all sought to enhance peristaltic coaptation of the ureteral walls during urine transport. Included in these procedures was psoas muscle transplantation[44] and various ureteral wrapping procedures using small bowel[45, 46, 47], as well as total ureteral replacement with ileum.[23] The majority of these procedures produced poor results, most likely because they did not deal with the true obstructive nature of the distal ureteral segment.

Bischoff and others[10, 16, 29, 30, 48-52] have stressed that early repair of megaureter is essential in order to maintain renal function. It is Bischoff, however, who should be credited with the first resection and tapering of ureters, while Johnston[53] in 1966 and Creevy in 1967[25] later emphasized the technical points which they felt were crucial in reconstructive surgery on these dilated ureters.

The long-term goals of ureteral remodelling are: good urinary drainage, eradication of urinary infection, effective ureteral peristalsis and an antirefluxing ureterovesical anastomosis[29, 30, 36, 37]. It has been shown by many investigators[29, 30, 36, 37] that, in order for effective propulsion of a urinary bolus to occur without retrograde regurgitation, an ideal ureteral diameter must be created which will allow proper coaptation of the ureteral walls during peristalsis. These principles form the basis for our present approach to primary megaureter, which was established in the late 1960s by Hendren[10, 16, 29, 50]. His results with distal ureteral resection, ureteral tailoring and reimplantation have set the standard for modern megaureter surgery.

As far as timing is concerned, temporary urinary diversion has been advocated by some authors for early stabilization of the infant with megaureter. We have felt, however[38], that definitive surgical reconstruction at the time of presentation was the correct approach, and, with advances in both paediatric anaesthesia and neonatal intensive care, we have achieved favourable long-term clinical results using this approach.

Differing opinions also exist among those who have proposed one-stage remodelling of the entire dilated ureter[36] and those who advocate a staged reconstruction. Surgery to the lower ureteral segment is performed allowing clinical follow-up and physiological testing to determine if upper ureteral reconstruction is needed to improve drainage[10, 38]. It has been our experience that total ureteral reconstruction is rarely necessary, but it may be useful for the massively dilated, tortuous ureter often seen in the child with Prune-belly syndrome.

The operation

Surgical technique

Meticulous surgical technique, careful handling of tissue and attention to fine detail are the cornerstones for obtaining favourable long-term results in primary megaureter repair. Our approach to the correction of primary obstructive megaureter involves these principles and the technique is described below.

5

The patient is placed in a frog-leg position, the bladder filled to the point of being palpable through the anterior abdominal wall. A Pfannenstiel suprapubic incision is made. In cases where there has been prior surgery on the lower ureter, and where additional procedures might be employed (i.e. transureteroureterostomy), a lower mid-line transperitoneal approach is probably best.

In routine cases, the incision is carried through skin, subcutaneous tissue and Scarpa's fascia down to the rectus fascia.

Skin flaps are then elevated superiorly to an area just below the umbilicus and inferiorly to the symphysis pubis, using sweeping motion with a No. 15 scalpel blade. Haemostatic control of perforating vessels is obtained and a Denis Browne self-retaining ring retractor is placed in the wound, exposing the linea alba in the infraumbilical area. The rectus fascia is incised in the midline and the bladder mobilized laterally and inferiorly to the bladder neck. The lateral blades of the Denis Browne ring retractor are then placed in the wound at 3 and 9 o'clock, and a midline cystotomy is made down to the bladder neck, taking great care not to injure the circular fibres in the area of the bladder neck. A lip of bladder is left at the dome in order to accommodate a hand-held retractor.

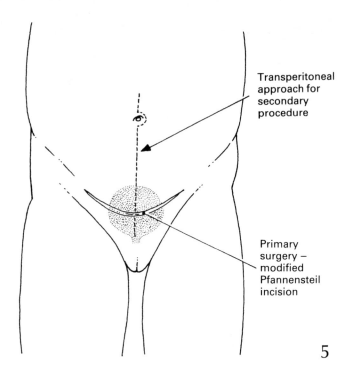

Transperitoneal approach for secondary procedure

Primary surgery – modified Pfannensteil incision

5

6

Lateral bladder retraction is accomplished by placing traction sutures at the 2, 4, 8 and 10 o'clock positions of the cystotomy and draping them over the ring retractor. The orifice of the megaureter is intubated with a 5 Fr Silastic infant feeding tube, which is fixed to the ureter at the 12 o'clock position with a 5/0 silk.

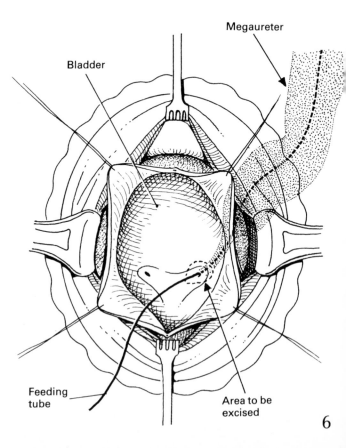

Megaureter

Bladder

Feeding tube

Area to be excised

6

7

The bladder mucosa is then incised in a tear-drop fashion around the orifice, and intravesical mobilization of the ureter is accomplished using fine scissors and taking great care to assure haemostasis of vessels in the muscular wall of the bladder. Care must be taken at this point so as not to skeletonize and devascularize the ureter.

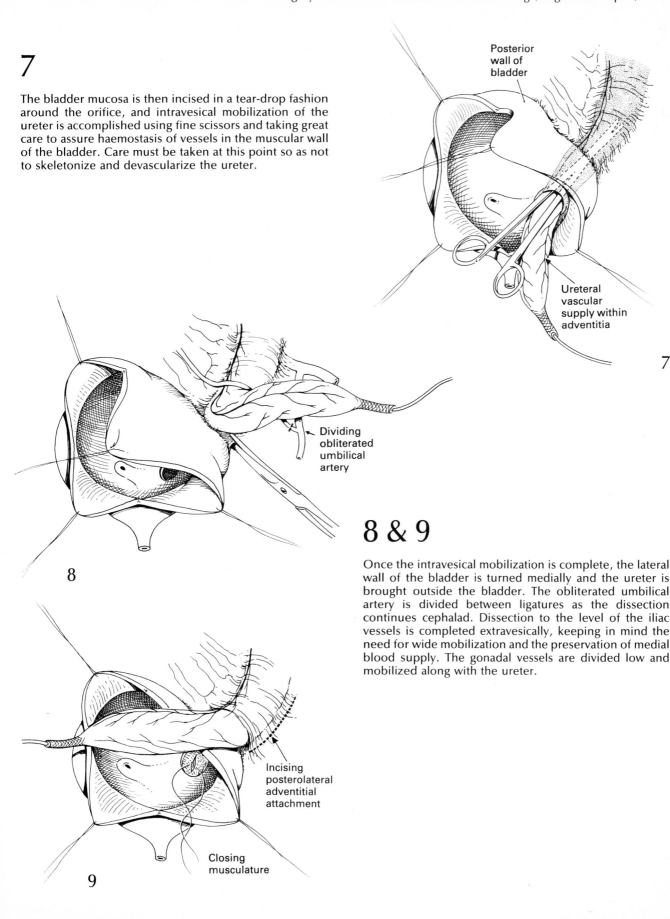

Posterior wall of bladder

Ureteral vascular supply within adventitia

7

Dividing obliterated umbilical artery

8

8 & 9

Once the intravesical mobilization is complete, the lateral wall of the bladder is turned medially and the ureter is brought outside the bladder. The obliterated umbilical artery is divided between ligatures as the dissection continues cephalad. Dissection to the level of the iliac vessels is completed extravesically, keeping in mind the need for wide mobilization and the preservation of medial blood supply. The gonadal vessels are divided low and mobilized along with the ureter.

Incising posterolateral adventitial attachment

Closing musculature

9

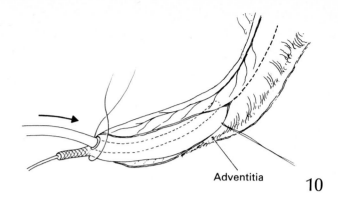

Adventitia

10

10, 11 & 12

Once the ureter has been mobilized a 12 Fr or 14 Fr catheter is placed in the lumen of the megaureter through a small incision just proximal to the stenotic segment. Ureteral remodelling is accomplished over this stenting catheter. Once the catheter is in place, the adventitial covering of the ureter is incised sharply on its lateral aspect and peeled off much like two leaves of a book in order that it may be used as a covering after the tapering has been accomplished. Specifically designed Hendren megaureter clamps are then placed along the course of the catheter to the approximate level of the iliac vessels and the lateral tissue is excised. In some instances we distend the megaureter with saline and then use methylene blue to outline a wedge of ureter for resection.

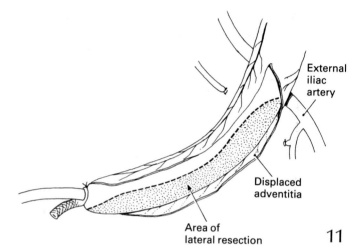

External
iliac
artery

Displaced
adventitia

Area of
lateral resection

11

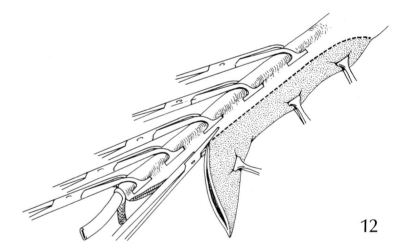

12

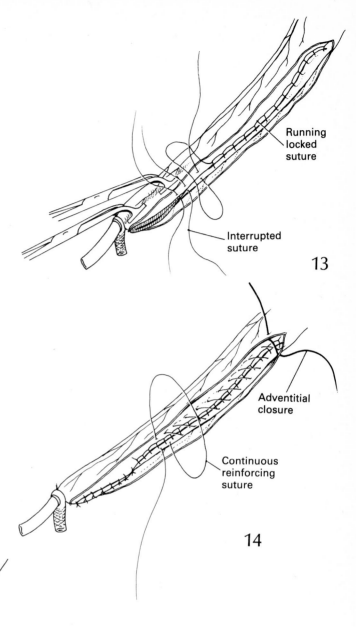

Running locked suture

Interrupted suture

13

Adventitial closure

Continuous reinforcing suture

14

13 & 14

Reapproximation of the ureteral wall is begun proximally over the catheter. We try to obtain a watertight multi-layered closure of well-vascularized tissue, using a continuous 5/0 absorbable suture for the first layer followed by a loose reinforcing continuous layer of 6/0 absorbable suture for the adventitia. The distal portion of the ureter is closed with interrupted sutures in order that the resection of any redundant distal ureter does not interfere with the running suture lines.

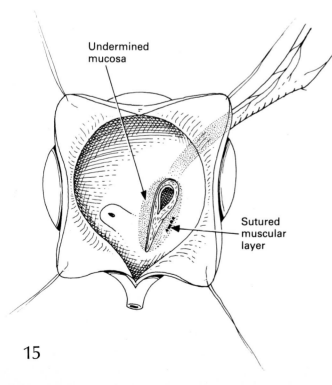

Undermined mucosa

Sutured muscular layer

15

15

Once tapering has been completed, attention is turned to reimplantation of the tailored distal ureter into the bladder. This is accomplished in a modified Politano-Leadbetter technique[58]. We feel that an optimal sub-mucosal tunnel to ureteral diameter ratio of 5:1 is important in ensuring an antirefluxing anastomosis. Care must be taken in closing the original muscle hiatus before going ahead with reimplantation in order to prevent an iatrogenic bladder diverticulum and poor muscular backing for the new submucosal tunnel. By adequate mobilization of the urothelium adjacent to the old hiatus, the detrusor muscle can be securely closed using interrupted 3/0 or 4/0 absorbable sutures. The mobilized urolothelium can then be used in the creation of a submucosal tunnel or simply closing it if it is too far lateral to be incorporated into the ureteroneocystostomy.

16

The new hiatus in the posterior wall of the bladder is created by using cutting cautery from the outside of the bladder over an appropriately placed gauze dissector from the inside. Great care must be taken in choosing the new hiatus for the tapered ureter in order to provide not only a sufficiently long submucosal tunnel, but also a medially placed hiatus which prevents post-operative kinking and obstruction of the ureter with bladder filling. Once the hiatus has been created, a small incision is made with electrocautery at the 6 o'clock position in the detrusor muscle in a further effort to prevent any angulation as the ureter enters the bladder. A submucosal tunnel of appropriate length and width is then created sharply with fine scissors.

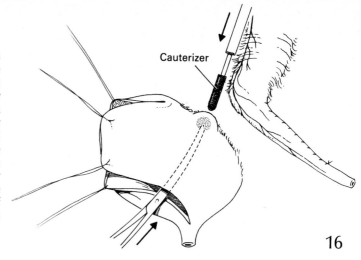

16

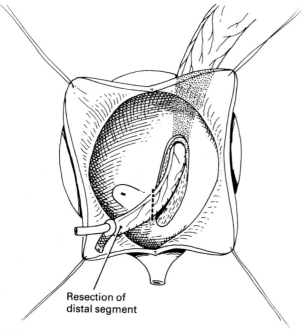

Resection of
distal segment

17

17

The ureter is brought through this tunnel and any redundant distal ureter is resected.

18

Fixation of the ureter begins at 6 o'clock with a deep suture of 4/0 absorbable suture including muscle and urothelium. The remainder of the ureterovesical approximation is mucosa to mucosa and done with 5/0 absorbable suture at 3, 9 and 12 o'clock. Additional mucosal sutures may be included if needed. The urothelium is then reapproximated over the reimplanted ureter using running 5/0 absorbable suture. The tapered ureter is stented using a 5 or 8 Fr Silastic infant feeding tube which is brought out through a stab cystostomy in the contralateral bladder wall and lateral to the skin incision. This stent also serves to divert urine away from the tapered segment, therefore additional side holes are cut in the end of the feeding tube to ensure adequate drainage.

The bladder is drained via a straight catheter of appropriate size which also has additional drainage holes cut in the end. This urethral catheter is fixed to the prepuce or the labia majora using non-absorbable suture material. We do not use balloon retention catheters as they have a narrower relative internal diameter, as well as making postoperative bladder spasms worse by irritative action of the balloon on the bladder base.

The bladder is then closed in two layers of absorbable suture material and the area is drained with a latex drain. We close all wounds with absorbable suture material of appropriate strength and use a subcutaneous drain under our mobilized skin flaps for 3 days postoperatively.

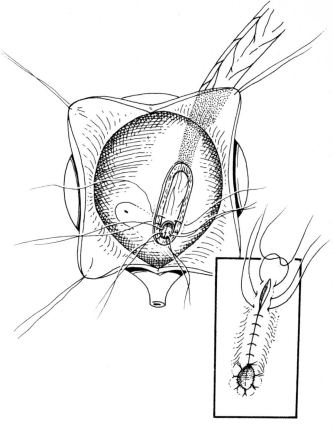

18

Postoperative care

Prophylactic broad-spectrum antibiotics and anticholinergics are used routinely in the postoperative period. Stenting-drainage tubes are left in place for 10–12 days, at which time a stent contrast study is done under fluoroscopic control to ensure intact suture lines before removing the stent. Once the stenting catheter has been removed, the bladder catheter is left in place for an additional 24 hours and then removed. Patients are kept on low-dose suppressant antibiotics for a minimum of 3 months following surgery.

Radiographic and bacteriological follow-up is done postoperatively at 3 months, 1 year, 3 years and 5 years. An excretory urogram is done at each of these intervals in order to assess renal parenchymal growth. Voiding cystourethrography is done at 3 months and 1 year to ensure the adequacy of our antirefluxing ureterovesical anastomosis.

Complications of megaureter surgery

Complications of ureteral tapering and reimplantation may be encountered early and late. Early complications consist of extravasation, which can easily be treated by simply leaving the stenting catheter in for a longer period of time, and early ureteral obstruction secondary to oedema, which can be dealt with in a similar fashion.

Late complications are most commonly persistent reflux and obstruction. Most reflux encountered after megaureter repair is secondary to inadequate tapering or ureteroneocystostomy, while most obstruction is due to devascularization of the lower end of the ureter. Management of these complications is reviewed elsewhere[13].

References

1. Caulk, J. R. Megaloureter – the importance of the ureterovesical valve. Journal of Urology 1923; 9: 315–330

2. Saintu, O. Note sur un cas de retention d'urine chez le foetus avec permeabilités due canal de l'urethre. Journal de Medicine de Paris 1896; 8: 332–333

3. Fortescue-Brickdale, J. M. A note on congenital dilatation of the ureters with hydronephrosis. Bristol Medico-Chirurgical Journal 1905; 23: 231–233

4. Hanna, M. K., Jeffs, R. D., Sturgess, J. M., Barkin, M. Ureteral structure and ultrastructure. Part I. The normal human ureter. Journal of Urology 1976; 116: 718–724

5. Hanna, M. K., Jeffs, R. D., Sturgess, J. M., Barkin, M.Ureteral structure and ultrastructure. Part II. Congenital ureteropelvic junction obstruction and primary obstructive megaureter. Journal of Urology 1976; 116: 725–773

6. Hanna, M. K., Jeffs, R. D., Sturgess, J. M., Barkin, M. Ureteral structure and ultrastructure. Part III. The congenitally dilated ureter (megaureter). Journal of Urology 1977; 117: 24–27

7. Hanna, M. K., Jeffs, R. D., Sturgess, J. M., Barkin, M. Ureteral structure and ultrastructure. Part IV. The dilated ureter, clinopathological correlation. Part IV. Journal of Urology 1977; 117: 28–32

8. McKinnon, K. J., Foote, J. W., Wigglesworth, F. W., Biennerhassett, J. B. The pathology of the adynamic distal ureteral segment. Transactions of the American Association of Genito-Urinary Surgeons 1969; 61: 63–67

9. Gosling, J. A., Dixon, J. S. Functional obstruction of the ureter and renal pelvis. A histological and electron microscopic study. British Journal of Urology 1978; 50: 145–152

10. Pfister, R. C., Hendren, W. H. Primary megaureter in children and adults. Urology 1978; 12: 160–176

11. Cussen, L. J. The morphology of congenital dilatation of the ureter; intrinsic ureteral lesions. The Australian and New Zealand Journal of Surgery 1971; 41: 185–194

12. King, L. R. Megaloureter: definition, diagnosis and management. Journal of Urology 1980; 123: 222–223

13. Hendren, W. H. Complications of ureteral reimplantation and megaureter repair. In: Smith, R. B., Skinner, D. C., eds. Complications of urologic surgery: prevention and management. Philadelphia: Saunders, 1976: 151–208

14. Hendren, W. H. Complications of megaureter repair in children. Journal of Urology 1975; 113: 238–254

15. Hanna, M. K., Jeffs, R. D. Primary obstructive megaureter in children. Urology 1975; 6: 419–427

16. Hendren, W. H. Operative repair of megaureter in children. Journal of Urology 1969; 101: 491–507

17. Hurst, A. F., Gaymer-Jones, J. A case of megaloureter due to achalasia of the ureterovesical sphincter. British Journal of Urology 1931; 3: 43–52

18. Kretschmer, H. L., Hibbs, W. G. A study of the vesical end of the ureter in hydronephrosis. Surgery, Gynecology and Obstetrics 1933; 57: 170–186

19. Hutch, J. A., Tanagho, E. A. Etiology of non-occlusive ureteral dilatation. Journal of Urology 1965; 93: 177–184

20. Vermooten, V. A new etiology for certain types of dilated ureters in children. Journal of Urology 1939; 41: 455–463

21. Gloor, H. U. Veber die Ursachen der Megaloureter bildung. Schweizerische Medizinische Wochenschrift 1939; 69: 1080–1084

22. Swenson, O., MacMahon, H. E., Jaques, W. E., Campbell, J. S. A new concept of etiology of megaloureters. New England Journal of Medicine 1952; 246: 41–46

23. Swenson, O., Fisher, J. H., Cendron, J. Megaloureter: investigation as to the cause and report on the results of newer forms of treatment. Surgery 1956; 40: 223–233

24. Grana, L., Kidd, J., Idriss, F., Swenson, O. Effect of chronic urinary tract infection on ureteral peristalsis. Journal of Urology 1965; 94: 652–657

25. Creevy, C. D. The atonic distal ureteral segment (ureteral achalasia). Journal of Urology 1967; 97: 457–463

26. Tanagho, E. A. Intrauterine fetal ureteral obstruction. Journal of Urology 1973; 109: 196–203

27. Notley, R. G. Electron microscopy of the upper ureter and the pelvi-ureteric junction. British Journal of Urology 1968; 40: 37–52

28. Notley, R. G. Electron microscopy of the primary obstructive megaureter. British Journal of Urology 1972; 44: 229–234

29. Hendren, W. H. III: Restoration of function in the severely decompensated ureter. In: Johnston, J. H., Scholtmeijer, R. J., eds. Problems in paediatric urololgy. Amsterdam: Excerpta Medica, 1972: 1–56

30. Williams, D. I., Hulme-Moir, I. Primary obstructive megaureter. British Journal of Urology 1970; 42: 140–149

31. Whitaker, R. H. Investigating wide ureters with ureteral pressure flow studies. Journal of Urology 1976; 116: 81–82

32. Whitaker, R. H. The Whitaker test. Urologic Clinics of North America 1979; 6: 529–539

33. Jaffe, R. B., Middleton, A. W., Jr. Whitaker test: differentiation of obstructive from nonobstructive uropathy. American Journal of Roentgenology 1980; 134: 9–15

34. Koff, S. A., Thrall, J. H., Keyes, J. W., Jr. Diuretic radionuclide urography: a noninvasive method for evaluating nephroureteral dilation. Journal of Urology 1979; 122: 451–454

35. Koff, S. A., Thrall, J. H., Keyes, J. W., Jr. Assessment of hydroureteronephrosis in children using diuretic radionuclide urography. Journal of Urology 1980; 123: 531–534

36. Hanna, M. K. New surgical method for one-stage total remodeling of massively dilated and tortuous ureter. Urology 1979; 14: 453–464

37. Tanagho, E. A. Ureteral tailoring. Journal of Urology 1971; 106: 194–197

38. Hendren, W. H. A new approach to infants with severe obstructive uropathy: early complete reconstruction. Journal of Pediatric Surgery 1970; 5: 184–199

39. Carver, J. H. Megaloureter: report of 2 cases. British Journal of Surgery 1948; 36: 168–172

40. Crabtree, E. G. Plastic operation for the short stricture at the uretero-pelvic juncture. Transactions of the American Association of Genito-Urinary Surgeons 1937; 30: 311–322

41. Wayman, T. B. Surgical treatment of megaloureter and presentation of artificial ureter. Journal of Urology 1949; 61: 883–903

42. Nesbit, R. M., Withycombe, J. F. The problems of primary megaureter. Journal of Urology 1954; 72: 162–171

43. Stephens, F. D. Treatment of megaureters by multiple micturition. The Australian and New Zealand Journal of Surgery 1957; 27: 130–134

44. Carlson, H. E. The intrapsoas transplant of megaloureter. Journal of Urology 1954; 72; 172–177

45. Hirschorn, R. C. The ileal sleeve. II. Surgical technique in clinical application. Journal of Urology 1964; 92: 120–126

46. Wrenn, E. L., Jr. Proposed operation for megaloureter Surgery 1963; 54: 950–952

47. Grana, L., Swenson, O. A new surgical procedure for the treatment of aperistaltic megaloureter. American Journal of Surgery 1965; 109: 532–535

48. Bischoff, P. Operative treatment of megaureter. Journal of Urology 1961; 85: 268–274

49. Bjordal, R. I., Stake, G., Knutrud, O. Surgical treatment of megaureter in the first few months of life. Annales Chirurgiae et Gynaecologiae 1980; 69: 10–14

50. Hendren, W. H. Functional restoration of decompensated ureters in children. The American Journal of Surgery 1970; 119: 477–482

51. Kalicinski, Z. H., Kansy, J., Kotarbinska, B., Joszt, W. Surgery of megaureters – modification of Hendren's operation. Journal of Pediatric Surgery 1977; 12: 183–188

52. Mayor, G., Genton, N., Torrado, A., Guignard, J-P. Renal function in obstructive nephropathy; long-term effect of reconstructive surgery. Pediatrics 1975, 56; 740–747

53. Johnston, J. H. Reconstructive surgery of megaureter in childhood. British Journal of Urology 1967; 39: 17–21

54. Hanna, M. K., Wyatt, J.K. Primary obstructive megaureter in adults. Journal of Urology 1975; 113: 328–334

55. Hodgson, N. B., Thompson, L. W. Technique of reductive ureteroplasty in the management of megaureter. Journal of Urology 1975; 113: 118–120

56. Derrick, F. C., Jr. Management of the large, tortuous, adynamic ureter with reflux, Journal of Urology 1972; 108: 153–155

57. Bishop, M. C., Askew, A. R., Smith, J. C. Reimplantation of the wide ureter. British Journal of Urology 1978; 50: 383–386

58. Politano, V. A., Leadbetter, W. F. An operative technique for the correction of vesicoureteral reflux. Journal of Urology 1958; 79: 932–941

59. Hendren, W. H. Megaureter. In: Harrison, J. H., Gittes, R. F., Perlmutter, A. D., Stamey, T. A., Walsh, P. C., eds. Campbell's Urology, Vol. 2, 4th ed. Philadelphia: W. B. Saunders, 1979: 1697–1742

Illustrations by C. Willem and M. Lemaire

Ureteric duplication

Emile de Backer MD
Conference Chairman, Catholic University of Louvain;
Chief of Urology Service, The Institute of Saint Elizabeth, Brussels, Belgium

Introduction

Duplications of the ureter not infrequently complicate other pathological conditions of the urinary tract or may themselves be responsible for the presenting symptoms. In its most minor form ureteric duplication consists of a bifurcation of the ureter at some point between the renal pelvis and the ureterovesical junction. A complete duplication occurs when both ureters enter the bladder, often quite close together, though with the upper pole of the kidney draining through the lower and medial orifice in the bladder. Complete duplication may be accompanied by an ectopic opening where the upper pole ureter enters the urinary tract at the bladder neck or in the urethra, or communicates with the genital tract, the vagina or vulva in the female, the ejaculatory duct or seminal vesicle in the male.

Incomplete duplication

This is generally a radiological discovery in cases with no specific pathology and no relevant symptoms. Surgical treatment may, however, be required in certain circumstances where there is reflux or peristaltic incoordination.

1a–c

When the junction is very near the bladder the ureterovesical implantation can be affected, predisposing to reflux. If so, it is easy to reimplant both ureters in their sheath after resecting the bifurcation.

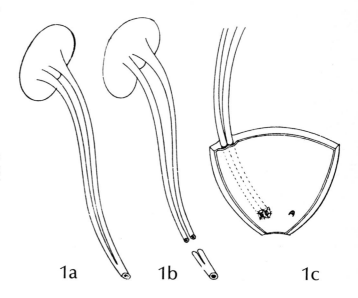

1a   1b   1c

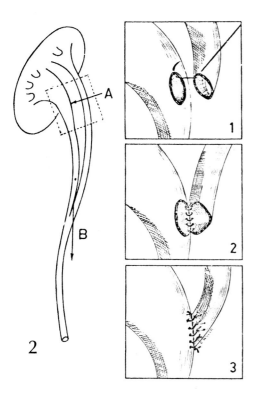

2

When the junction is situated in the midureter, ureteroureteric reflux can occur, producing a moderate or temporary dilatation of one or both branches. This is due to an incoordination of the peristaltic contraction of the ureters, either with or without retroperistalsis. Clinically this can give rise to urinary infection or pain, but before attributing symptoms to this malformation, one has to be sure that there is no other cause, which is sometimes difficult. It has to be proved by cineradiology that the ureteroureteric reflux does exist. Only then, and only if conservative treatment fails, is surgery indicated. The bifid ureter should be converted into a bifid pelvis: the upper ureter is anastomosed to the lower renal pelvis (A) and the rest of its length is excised (B), flush down to the bifurcation.

Blind bifid ureter or ureteric diverticulum is very rare: the accessory ureteric bud does not come into contact with the metanephric cells. This anomaly can give rise to urinary infections and sometimes has to be removed.

Complete duplication

The pathology of duplex ureters depends upon the situation of the ureteric opening. It should be borne in mind that the ureter draining the upper pole of the kidney always opens lower in the urogenital tract than its twin draining the lower pole.

3

Orthotopic openings

When both ureters open into the bladder the lower ureteric orifice (upper renal element) lies closer to the bladder neck on the interureteric bar and implantation is usually normal. This means that its antireflux mechanism is normal. However, the upper ureteric orifice (lower renal element) opens above the trigone and is not sufficiently surrounded by muscles, so that reflux may easily occur, producing lower pole pyelonephritic scarring.

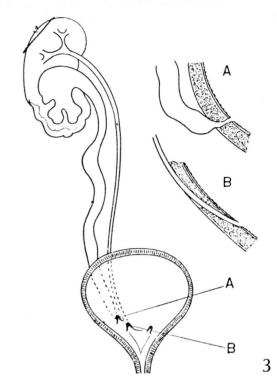

3

When the pyelonephritis has destroyed the lower pole, heminephrectomy and ureterectomy should be performed. These operations have been described in the chapters on partial nephrectomy and heminephrectomy, and nephrectomy, though in duplications the operation is very often facilitated by the fact that not only is there nearly always a separate vascularization of each pole, but that the scarred tissue is very well defined. On the other hand if the infection has gone on for a long time, dissection of the lower end of the ureter can be extremely difficult. One has to be careful not to sever or damage the good ureter and, if this is inevitable, it requires a reimplantation of this ureter.

In cases where it is still possible to conserve the lower pole, ureteric reimplantation or antireflux plasties have to be done on both ureters, leaving them together in their common sheath. This procedure is much easier and much safer than trying to reimplant the affected ureter only, after a difficult dissection. When the condition is diagnosed in an acute state, with high temperatures resisting antibiotics, it can be necessary to do a temporary pyelostomy or nephrostomy. This intermediate step amounts to a 'rescue operation' which makes the second intervention much easier and safer.

If the lower end of the ureter is too damaged to be reimplanted, one might envisage anastomosing the lower pelvis to the good ureter. This, however, should not be done because of the risk of damaging the good ureter while having little chance of keeping a poor lower pole. Partial nephroureterectomy is a much better solution.

Reflux can affect both ureters, even when the lower ureteric orifice lies in a normal position. The anomaly of the ureterovesical junction is then just the same as when reflux occurs in a single ureter.

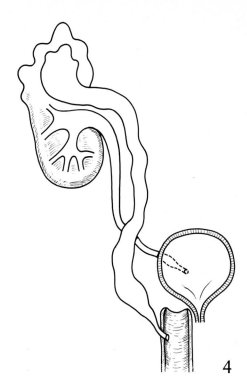

Ectopic ureters

4

In the more severe anomalies one or both ureters can open lower than the trigone. Most frequently the ureter draining the lower pole of the kidney opens at the normal site, while the other draining the upper pole opens into the bladder neck or urethra, or even into the genital tract.

4

For several reasons this condition is often overlooked since the typical dribbling incontinence is rarely severe and the symptoms are apt to be those of a sore vulva or a little discharge in the male. This is due to the fact that the upper pole involved is often very small and contains only immature nephrons; likewise the abnormal orifice is narrow so that hydroureter and hydronephrosis occur. If infection then supervenes, the pyelonephretic upper pole will produce little urine. Moreover, the X-ray features, although characteristic may be so slight as to pass unrecognized. For these reasons the diagnosis is often made late in childhood or even in adult life when the affected upper pole has been destroyed and the corresponding ureter is grossly dilated and flaccid. The only solution will then be heminephrectomy and ureterectomy. In male patients it may be necessary to remove the seminal vesicles if they too are infected.

If the diagnosis is made during an acute stage of infection, when the ureter has become a pouch full of pus, it is wiser not to embark directly on heminephrectomy but to drain the ureter. Through a short lumbar incision at the tip of the 11th or 12th rib, it is easy to locate extraperitoneally the bulging ureter full of pus and drain it by means of two catheters, one going up and one going down the ureter. Ten to 12 days is the optimum time which should be allowed to elapse between this drainage and the definitive operation. By then the general health of the patient will be much better and the dissection from healthy tissues much safer and easier, especially on the right side where it can be difficult to separate the ureter from the vena cava and the second part of the duodenum.

Given early diagnosis of the condition, there is the chance of discovering an upper pole still functioning as well as a relatively unimpaired ureter. Dissection of the lower end of this ureter and reimplantation is not then a great problem.

Ectopic ureterocele

5

A special mention has to be made of this anomaly, which occurs chiefly in the female and can be bilateral. When the ureter from the upper pole opens into the bladder neck, either just above or beneath, the last centimetre of its wall can be reduced to a mucosal coat. This factor, associated with the usual pinpoint opening of the ureter, gives rise in such cases to a sort of cyst at the lower end of the ureter, blowing up in the bladder. The opening of the lower pole ureter lies on this 'cyst'.

The upper pole ureter and corresponding renal cavities are uniformly dilated with the usual consequences. Occasionally in big ureteroceles the lower pole and its ureter are also dilated.

The ureterocele can prolapse in the urethra and sometimes appears at the urethral meatus in girls, causing dribbling incontinence, dysuria or, occasionally, retention. In this way the opposite urinary tract can also be affected.

Treatment always necessitates the uncapping of the ureterocele, accompanied by conservative or radical surgery of the upper pole and sometimes of the lower pole. The decision concerning the upper pole depends, of course, on its relative value as well as that of the lower pole and sometimes of the other kidney.

6a–d

Uncapping the ureterocele is best done transvesically through a low abdominal incision. Transurethral section of the ureterocele often gives reflux and may only be tried in small ureteroceles. The entire wall of the 'cyst' is excised, great care being taken not to sever the other ureteric orifices (a). The muscular edges of the bladder are then sutured (b) by a few separate stitches after the lower end of the upper pole ureter has been separated from inside or outside the bladder. The mucosal flap of the lower pole ureteric orifice is then fixed downwards and the remaining mucosal edges are sutured (c, d).

When the ureterocele opens in the urethra itself, the incision can be rather difficult. However, it can be done by lifting the posterior wall of the bladder upwards and dissecting the posterior part of the bladder neck and urethra from the vagina.

Where the upper urinary tract is concerned, total nephroureterectomy is indicated if the entire kidney has been destroyed. If only the upper pole has been destroyed, heminephroureterectomy is advisable, using a similar lower abdominal incision to free the lower end of the ureter as that used for the uncapping.

If the upper pole, although impaired, is still functioning, it should be kept, especially when the lower pole and the other kidney are affected. Ureteropelvic anastomosis and excision of the remaining upper pole ureter are then required.

In cases where the function of both kidneys is impaired the life-saving step of a temporary ureterostomy will be required.

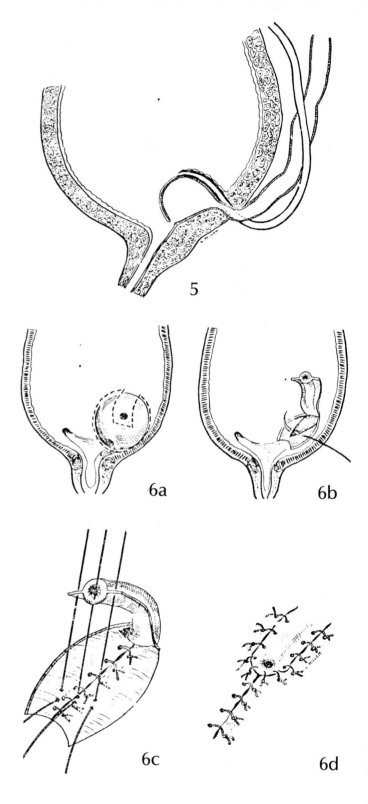

5

6a

6b

6c

6d

Acknowledgement

The author would like to thank Mrs Duroux for her help with the preparation of the chapter.

Illustrations by Ladislao Tinao

Ileal conduit diversion

José A. Martínez-Piñeiro MD
Associate Professor in Urology,
La Paz Hospital, Faculty of Medicine, Universidad Autónoma, Madrid, Spain

Introduction

The technique of cutaneous ureteroileostomy or ileal conduit diversion was first proposed by Nissen in 1929 and used by Seiffert in 1935 before falling into oblivion until 1950, when Bricker rediscovered and launched this method of urinary diversion to its present popularity. The short-term results reported thereafter were very satisfactory and the general feeling was that an almost ideal procedure of urinary diversion had been attained, since it was free of the feared complications of the cutaneous ureterostomy and ureterosigmoidostomy and the operative mortality was moderate (1.2–8 per cent). That this was a premature conclusion was demonstrated by the study of long-surviving patients, such as children with congenital malformations of the excretory tract or congenital neurogenic bladder dysfunctions. Indeed, long-term follow-up showed that although ileal conduit diversion prevented deterioration in 60–70 per cent of the renal units and was free of the typical complications of other forms of diversion, it created delayed problems which were not easily solved.

On the whole, morbidity rates vary between 58–98 per cent. Intestinal obstruction, stomal dysfunction, pyelonephritis, calculi, ureteroileal stenosis and/or reflux and electrolytic disturbances are the most common sources of trouble[1–8]. Time revealed that many of the complications were due to:

1. inadequate patient selection – mainly children with severely dilated and atonic ureters and/or patients with poor renal function.
2. faulty surgical technique, including errors such as ileal loop segments that were too long, failure to peritonealize the ureteroileal anastomosis, use of irradiated bowel for anastomosis and defective stoma construction.

Improved understanding of the factors which increased the vulnerability of these patients to infection and stone formation[9], in particular the role of reflux, ureterointestinal stenosis and back-flow[10–16], led to revision of the indications, to surgical refinements[13, 16–21], to better collecting appliances, and consequently to a significant improvement in the early and late complication rates.

Preoperative

Indications

Supravesical urinary diversion is indicated mainly in the following circumstances:

1. Irreversible bladder and/or urethral dysfunction causing urinary incontinence not manageable by reconstructive surgery, intermittent catheterization, electronic devices or external appliances.
2. Severe impairment of the upper urinary tract due to congenital malformations or acquired diseases, especially after failure of operative reconstruction.
3. Malignant lesions of the pelvic organs and/or urogenital sinus, requiring radical excisions.

The diversion may be temporary or permanent. Generally speaking, benign lesions should be treated by a temporary diversion, because diversion-mediated renoureteral improvement is to be expected, which in turn may bring about the possibility of a secondary reconstruction[22-25]. In particular, all children with lesions other than a neurogenic bladder should be considered as candidates for secondary urinary tract reconstruction. Therefore, simple temporary diversion procedures such as the cutaneous loop or sling ureterostomy, or the cutaneous Y-transureteroureterostomy, should be preferred to an ileal or colonic conduit. This does not mean that urinary tract reconstruction would not be feasible after conduit diversion – in fact, it facilitates reconstruction in some instances[26] – but it is evident that the simpler primary procedures are less aggressive and offer easier reconstructive prospects. Many urologists consider the cutaneous Y-ureteroureterostomy as the best method both for temporary and definitive diversion in children and adults, whenever at least one of the ureters is wide, long and has good peristalsis.

In malignant lesions where the ureters are normal and the pelvis has been irradiated, the ileal or colonic conduit is currently the most commonly recommended technique for permanent urinary diversion. There are, of course, cases in which other forms of diversion are preferable – for instance, patients with a very short life expectancy operated on palliatively, or high-risk patients who would not tolerate a long and stressful operation[27].

With these considerations in mind, the general indications for an ileal or colonic conduit diversion are the following:

1. Benign diseases
   (a) Congenital
   As primary treatment or as a secondary procedure after failure of reconstructive attempts or other diverting techniques.

   Bladder exstrophy.
   Urethral agenesis.
   Imperforate anus with recto-urethral fistula.
   Primary or secondary megaloureter.
   Prune-belly syndrome.
   Neurogenic bladder dysfunction due to spinal dysraphism and/or sacral agenesis.

   (b) Acquired

   Neurogenic bladder dysfunction due to trauma, inflammation, degenerative disease or neoplana. Contracted bladder associated with irreparable urethral stenosis.
   Trauma to the lower urinary tract: irreparable rupture of the urethra; obstetrical lesions of the bladder and/or urethra.

2. Malignant diseases
   As a means of diverting urine after radical excisions or as a palliative procedure:
   (a) Malignant tumours

   Bladder cancer.
   Prostatic sarcomas.
   Tumours of the urogenital sinus.
   Uterine cancer.
   Rectal and/or sigmoid cancer.
   Sacrococcygeal teratomas.

   (b) Complications of irradiation to the pelvis

   Contracted bladder.
   Vesicovaginal fistula.
   Vesicorectal fistula.
   Frozen pelvis.

Contraindications

Gross debilitation is a relative contraindication, whereas impaired renal function with a creatinine clearance rate below 20 ml/min is practically the only absolute contraindication for any type of transintestinal urinary diversion. The high surgical risk involved and the deterioration of renal function secondary to urine reabsorption and electrolytic disturbances must be weighed against the potential benefits of diversion.

Choice between ileal or colonic conduit

Great interest in the use of the defunctioned pelvic colon as a conduit arose after Mogg's report in 1965[19] but long-term follow-up has revealed conflicting results[28-32]. For some, the rate of complications appears significantly less than that seen previously in patients with ileal loop diversion, whereas for others the incidence of stomal stenosis, ureterocolic stenosis, ureterocolic reflux and upper tract deterioration shows no advantage for the use of colon.

The theoretical major advantage of the colonic conduit lies in the possibility of performing effective antireflux ureterocolonic anastomosis, but recent reports suggest that reflux and back-flow can also effectively be prevented in ileal conduits by nippled ureteroileal anastomosis[33] and/or intussusception of the ileum[13, 14, 16].

Another distinct advantage of the colonic conduit is the possibility of using non-irradiated segments of the large intestine (i.e. transverse colon[28, 34]). Problems are not to be expected in cases treated with adjuvant preoperative radiotherapy, either 4000–4500 rad in 4 weeks or 1500–2000 rad in 2–4 days, but when radical treatments (up to 6500 rad) have failed, salvage surgery and urinary diversion yield a significantly higher complication rate of anastomotic dehiscence, stenosis, infection and wound disruption. A transverse colonic conduit seems to be a good choice in these instances, despite the optimistic results with the use of ileal conduits in irradiated patients reported by certain groups[35, 36].

Among the disadvantages of the colonic conduit, technical difficulties are often encountered in obese patients, who usually have very short mesenteriums.

I recommend sigmoid conduit diversion in benign conditions, especially in children – where in general there are no technical problems and in whom the possibility of reconstruction should always be kept in mind. The transverse colon conduit is recommended in salvage surgery after failure of pelvic radiotherapy, and the ileal conduit in other patients if cutaneous Y-transuretero-ureterostomy is contraindicated. The small bowel must be used if a left colostomy has already been used for faecal diversion.

Preoperative preparation

Early morbidity may be decreased by preoperative preparation which must include: stomal site selection and skin preconditioning; bowel cleansing; and improvement of the patient's general condition.

One week before operation in malignant cases and 2 or 3 weeks in benign cases, a site in the abdomen is selected for the stoma. The stomal position will depend on factors such as obesity, existing scars, type of work or sport (a right-sided golf player should wear the collecting appliance on the left side, for instance), lower-extremity bracings, the level at which the upper urinary tract will be diverted and the intestinal segment to be used (colon left, ileum right usually). An appliance is cemented on the selected place and filled with a small amount of water or saline to see if it fits correctly and if there is any skin sensitivity to the cement or to the components of the appliance; every 2 or 3 days it should be removed and reapplied in the presence of the family, who become acquainted with its use. During this period, any correction can easily be made, the skin hardens and the patient adapts himself psychologically to diversion.

Bowel preparation begins 5–7 days before the operation with a low-residue diet and mild laxatives. Erythromycin plus paromomycin are administered the day before. Colonic lavage or whole-gut irrigation are mandatory when the large bowel is to be used as a conduit[37]. Anaemia, hypoproteinemia and electrolytic imbalance should be corrected.

Technique

Many problems related to the performance and sequelae of intestinal conduit diversion can be prevented by paying attention to the following basic rules:

1. Avoid irradiated tissues for anastomoses.
2. Avoid excess length and tortuous course of the conduit to prevent residual urine, urinary infection and reabsorption. Adequate lengths are 10–15 cm in children and 20–25 cm in adults.
3. Avoid using large and atonic ureters which could perpetuate urinary stasis. It is preferable to perform a pyeloileal cutaneous diversion in these cases.
4. Avoid kinks, torsion or devascularization of the ureter which has to be transposed under the mesenteric arcade.
5. Avoid anastomosis where there are doubts about the blood supply.
6. Retroperitonealize the ureterointestinal anastomosis and leave a drain in the vicinity.
7. Carefully suture the mesenteric defects, the space between the lower border of the mesentery of the loop and the posterior peritoneum to avoid intestinal obstruction.
8. Always perform an appendicectomy.
9. Do not try to reperitonealize the pelvic floor if a simultaneous radical procedure has been performed. A tight peritoneal suture will give way in the following days, increasing the risk of internal herniation.
10. Suture the abdominal wall meticulously with non-absorbable materials. Monofilament sutures are best for irradiated patients.
11. Fix the loop to the abdominal wall with two layers of suture to avoid parastomal hernias.
12. Form a protruding nipple. This has distinct advantages over a flush stoma as far as comfort and prevention of backflow from the collecting device is concerned.

Usual types of uretero- and pyelo-intestinal anastomosis

1a & b

End-to-end

(a) The Wallace technique where the ureters are anastomosed to one another and to the end of the ileal segment.
(b) End-to-end anastomosis between the ileum and a single ureter or between the ileum and the renal pelvis.

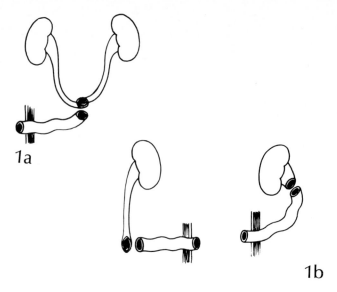

1a

1b

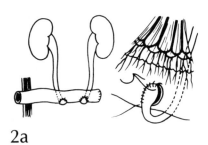

2a

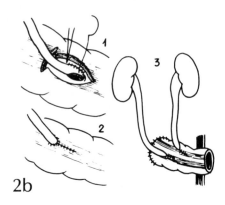

2b

2a & b

End-to-side

(a) Anastomosis between the ureter and the ileum on the end-to-side principle with direct mucosa-to-mucosa suture.
(b) Non-refluxing (tunnelled) ureterocolic anastomosis.

3

Combined

Variants on the use of pyelointestinal anastomosis.

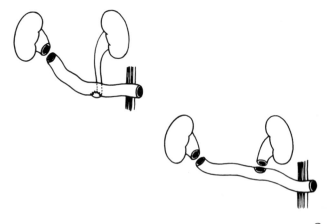

3

The operation

4

The ureters are isolated at the pelvic brim, preserving the adventitial blood supply, and transected. A stay suture is attached to each ureter and the distal stump is ligated. Loose-fitting Levene gastric tubes 4–12 Fr are inserted high into the ureteric lumen.

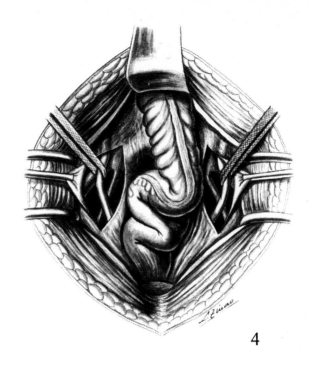

4

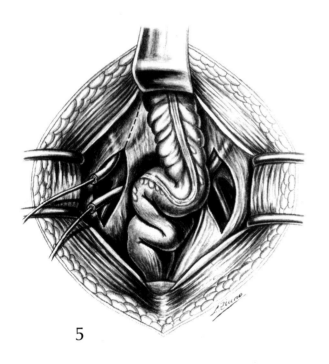

5

5

A broad tunnel is created under the mesocolon and posterior peritoneum by means of blunt dissection, and the left ureter is transposed to the right side, avoiding kinks or torsions. Either the right-sided posterior peritoneal incision, used for the right ureteric dissection, is prolonged upwards and medially to enable both ureters to be drawn out laterally; or a separate central peritoneal incision is made for this purpose.

6

An ileal loop of adequate length is selected, avoiding use of the last 20 cm of the small intestine. The length will depend on the patient's age and somatic characteristics, and can be calculated by measuring the distance between the posterior peritoneum and the skin plus three finger widths.

The mesenteric vascular pedicle is prepared with the help of transillumination, preserving at least two primary vascular arcades, supplied by two large arteries. The distal mesenteric incision should be longer than the proximal, to enable exteriorization of the distal end of the loop through the abdominal wall.

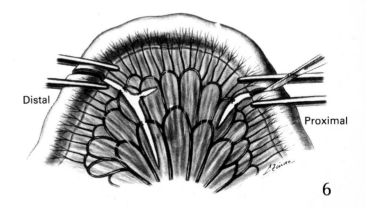

Distal

Proximal

6

7

The ileum is sectioned obliquely between clamps. Verify that the isolated intestinal loop is not longer than required, and straighten its distal end by incising the mesentery parallel to the loop, proximal to the secondary vascular arcade. The length of this incision should be equal to the thickness of the abdominal wall in order to allow for the creation of a protruding stoma without undue traction on the mesentery.

   The conduit is displaced to an inframesenteric position, and intestinal continuity is restored with a single layer of interrupted 2/0 silk seromuscular stitches. The mesenteric defect is repaired afterwards, stitching both peritoneal leaves; care has to be taken to avoid injury to the vascular pedicle of the conduit when reaching the root of the mesenteric incision.

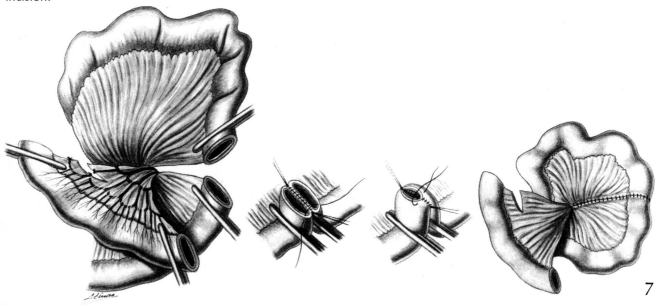

7

8

The ureters are trimmed and spatulated to a length similar to the diameter of the ileal conduit; then, both ureters are stitched one to each other with a continuous 4/0 Dexon or chromic catgut suture, to form an elliptical common stoma (Wallace II). The splinting tubes are now fixed to the ureters with a 6/0 absorbable stitch.

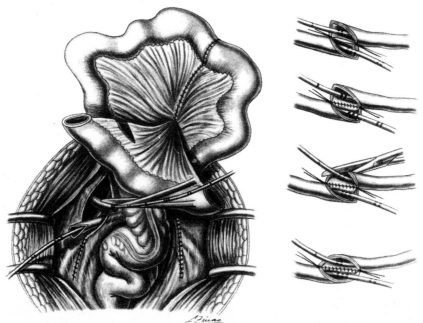

8

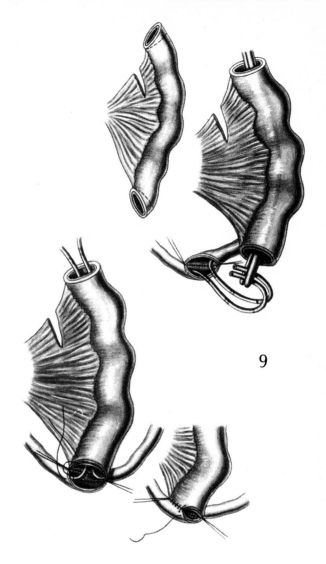

9

The ends of the ileal conduit are now cut back, discarding any excess of tissue on the antimesenteric border and the protruding mucosa is trimmed away. A clamp is passed through the conduit and the ureteric splinting tubes are withdrawn through the loop. The proximal end of the conduit is brought close to the ureteric stoma and two stay sutures are inserted. The ureteroileal anastomosis is then performed with a continuous running 3/0 or 4/0 Dexon or chromic catgut suture, picking up all the ureteric layers and the intestinal seromuscular layer. Some reinforcing stitches are inserted afterwards.

9

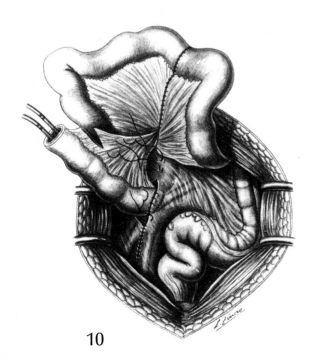

10

10

The edges of the posterior peritoneal incision are stitched to the conduit 1 cm distal to the ureteroileal anastomosis, in order to extraperitonealize this suture line; a suction drain is left in the vicinity. The proximal border of the mesenteric pedicle of the conduit is sutured to the posterior peritoneum, to avoid internal herniation.

11

A cylinder of abdominal wall is excised at the selected stomal site. If the skin has been preconditioned, the central defect of the collecting appliance leaves an excellent outline for this excision. About eight Dexon or chromic catgut 3/0 stitches are now inserted, picking up the edge of the peritoneum and of the posterior transversus fascia or posterior rectus sheath depending on the position of the stoma. The ends of these sutures are clipped and left long.

The conduit is brought out through the opening, so that 4 or 5 cm protrude above the skin level without tension. It is then sewn to the peritoneum and posterior transversus fascia using the previously inserted sutures. With a second layer of stiches, the conduit is fixed to the muscle and superficial aponeurotic sheath. No attempt should be made to suture the mesentery to the abdominal wall as this would endanger the stomal blood supply.

The redundant ileum is everted for about 2 cm and its free edge is sutured to the seromuscular layer, flush with the skin level. There is no need to sew the resulting bud to the skin unless a collecting device is to be cemented immediately. The ureteral splinting tubes are anchored to the stoma with a pair of stiches.

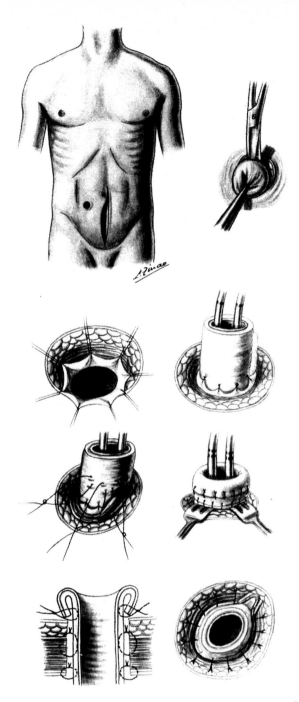

11

Postoperative management

Postoperative intestinal decompression by tube gastrostomy or by nasogastric tube is maintained until the reappearance of intestinal peristalsis, around the 3rd to 5th day. Management includes fluid and electrolyte replacement, protein-sparing therapy, antibiotics (*Editor's comment:* antibiotics are not often used in the UK or USA) and early ambulation. The ureteric splints are removed around the 10th day if there are no anastomotic leaks.

The collecting appliance may be cemented and left in place immediately after the operation (in which case the ureteric splints are cut almost flush with the stomal bud) or when the wound is completely healed, in which case the conduit is drained by a large-bore Foley catheter during the immediate postoperative period. The most appropriate collecting appliances are the expendable ones with a no-return valve. At first these should be permanently connected to a Uribag, but after the stoma has healed they are used only during sleep to prevent backflow of urine.

References

1. Engel, R. M. Complications of bilateral uretero-ileo cutaneous urinary diversion. A review of 208 cases. Journal of Urology 1969; 101: 508–512

2. Schwarz, G. R., Jeffs, R. D. Ileal conduit urinary diversion in children: computer analysis of followup from 2 to 16 years. Journal of Urology 1975; 114: 285–288

3. Stevens, P. S., Eckstein, H. B. Ileal conduit diversion in children. British Journal of Urology 1977; 49: 379–383

4. Bystrom, J. Early and later complications of ileal conduit urinary diversion. Scandinavian Journal of Urology and Nephrology 1978; 12: 233–237

5. Pitts, W. R. Jr., Muecke, E. C. A 20-year experience with ileal conduits: the fate of the kidneys. Journal of Urology 1979; 122: 154–157

6. Dunn, M., Roberts, J. B. M., Smith, P. J. B., Slade, N. The long-term results of ileal conduit urinary diversion in children. British Journal of Urology 1979; 51: 458–461

7. Bergman, B. Studies on patients with ileal conduit diversion with special regard to renal infection. Scandinavian Journal of Urology and Nephrology 1978; Suppl. 47: 1–32

8. Mayo, M. E., Chapman, W. H. Stomal obstruction of ileal conduits in children: a urodynamic study. Journal of Urology 1979; 121: 68–70

9. Dretler, S. P. Pathogenesis of urinary tract calculi occurring after ileal conduit diversion: I. Clinical study. II. Conduit study. III. Prevention. The Journal of Urology 1973; 109: 204–209

10. Strohmenger, P. Le conduit intestinal. Le rôle de l'infection de l'anse isolée et du reflux intestino-rénal. Acta Urologica Belgica 1975; 43: 424–428

11. Richie, J. P., Skinner, D. G. Urinary diversion: the physiological rationale for non-refluxing colonic conduits. British Journal of Urology 1975; 47: 269–275

12. Woodside, J. R., Borden, T. A., Damron, J. R., Kiker, J. D. Isotope loopography, a new test: comparison with standard loopography and its relationship to renal function in patients with ileal conduit urinary diversion. Journal of Urology 1978; 119: 31–34

13. Bergman, B., Nilson, A. E. V. Intussusception of the ileal loop: an operative method for preventing urinary backflow in ileal conduits. The Journal of Urology 1974; 112: 735–738

14. Leisinger, H. J., Schauwecker, H., Sauberli, H. Dynamics of the continent ileal bladder. An experimental study in dogs. Investigative Urology 1977; 15: 49–54

15. Middleton, A. W. Jr., Hendren, W. H. Ileal conduits in children at the Massachusetts General Hospital from 1955 to 1970. Journal of Urology 1976; 115: 591–595

16. Reiner, W. G., Jeffs, R. D. Ileal intussusception as an antireflux mechanism in urinary diversion for myelomeningocele. Journal of Urology 1979; 121: 212–216

17. Wallace, D. M. Ureteric diversion using a conduit: a simplified technique. British Journal of Urology 1966; 38: 522–527

18. Clark, P. B. End-to-end ureteroileal anastomoses for ileal conduits. British Journal of Urology 1979; 51: 105–109

19. Mogg, R. A. The treatment of neurogenic urinary incontinence using the colonic conduit. British Journal of Urology 1965; 37: 681–686

20. Mahoney, E. M., Harrison, J. H. Successful prevention of ileal conduit stomal stenosis: experience during a 12-year period. Journal of Urology 1980; 123: 475–477

21. Bryniak, S. R., Bruce, A. W., Awad, S. A. Skin flap technique in formation of urinary conduit stoa. Urology 1980; 15: 275–277

22. Monfort, G. Harnwegrekonstruktion nach Ileum-und-Colon-Conduit beim Kind. Aktuelle Urologie 1975; 6: 147–156

23. Firlit, C. F., Sommer, J. T., Kaplan, W. E. Pediatric urinary undiversion. Journal of Urology 1980; 123: 748–753

24. Bauer, S. B., Colodny, A. H., Hallet, M., Khoshbin, S., Retik, A. B. Urinary undiversion in myelodissplasia: Criteria for selection and predictive value of urodynamic evaluation. The Journal of Urology 1980; 124: 89–93

25. Martínez-Piñeiro, J. A. Derivaciones urinarias. Hospital General 1980; 20: 227–232

26. Skinner, D. G., Gottesman, J. E., Richie, J. P. The Isolated sigmoid segment: its value in temporary urinary diversion and reconstruction. Journal of Urology 1975; 113: 614–618

27. Martínez-Piñeiro, J. A., Arocena, F., Hernandez Armero, A. La derivación de orina en los tumores vesicales. Archivos Españoles de Urología 1975; 28: 109–140

28. Morales, P., Golimbu, M. Colonic urinary diversion: 10 years of experience. Journal of Urology 1975; 113: 302–307

29. Altwein, J. E., Jonas, U., Hohenfellner, R. Longterm follow-up of children with colon conduit urinary diversion and ureterosigmoidostomy. Journal of Urology 1977; 118: 832–836

30. Althauser, A. F., Hagen Cook, K., Hendren, W. H. Non refluxing colon conduit: experience with 70 cases. The Journal of Urology 1978; 120: 35–39

31. Elder, D. D., Moisey, C. U., Rees, R. W. M. A long-term follow-up of the colonic conduit operation in children. British Journal of Urology 1979; 51: 462–465

32. Dagen, J. E., Sanford, E. J., Rohner, T. J. Jr. Complications of the non-refluxing colon conduit. Journal of Urology 1980; 123: 585–587

33. Patil, U., Glassberg, K. I., Waterhouse, K. Ileal conduit surgery with a nippled ureteroileal anastomosis. Urology 1976; 7: 594–597

34. Schmidt, J. D., Hawtrey, C. E., Buchsbaum, H. J. Transverse colon conduit: a preferred method of urinary diversion for radiation treated pelvic malignancies. Journal of Urology 1975; 113: 308–313

35. Malgieri, J. J., Persky, L. Ileal loop in the treatment of radiation-treated pelvic malignancies: a comparative review. Journal of Urology 1978; 120: 32–34

36. Mansson, W., Colleen, S., Stigsson, L. Four methods of uretero-intestinal anastomosis in urinary conduit diversion. A comparative study of early and late complications and the influence of radiotherapy. Scandinavian Journal of Urology and Nephrology 1979; 13: 191–199

37. Ackermann, D., Weirich, W., Riedmiller, H., Hutschenreiter, G. Sinnvolle Kolonvorbereitung in der Urologie. Aktuelle Urologie 1981; 12: 74–76

Colonic conduits

Alan B. Retik MD
Chief, Division of Urology, Children's Hospital Medical Center, Boston, Massachusetts;
Professor of Surgery (Urology), Harvard Medical School, Boston, Massachusetts, USA

Introduction

The increasing number of late complications following ileal conduit diversion has prompted the use of the colon as a urinary conduit. The occurrence of pyelonephritis following diversion with an ileal conduit has been attributed to reflux with infection. Richie et al.[1] have also shown in animal experiments the increased incidence of histological pyelonephritis with freely refluxing ileal conduits when compared with non-refluxing colon conduits. In addition, stomal stenosis appears to be seen less frequently with the colon than with the small bowel. The methods of diversion to be described below are being employed in children with increasing frequency as methods of permanent or, in some instances, temporary urinary diversion. The initial results with these procedures have been excellent. The incidence of reflux, ureteral obstruction and stomal stenosis has been low with relatively short-term follow-up.

The operations

SIGMOID CONDUIT

The indications for sigmoid conduit diversion are similar to those for the ileal conduit, i.e. children with neurogenic bladder dysfunction with repeated attacks of pyelonephritis or severe incontinence unresponsive to conventional therapy and some tumours of the lower urinary tract.

Stomal considerations are analogous to those for most intestinal stomas with the exception that the stoma may be located on either side of the abdomen. In children with ileal conduits being converted to sigmoid conduits, we prefer to use the previously located stomal site. The mobility of the sigmoid colon in children readily allows this.

1

The abdomen is opened through a paramedian incision and the ureters isolated and divided as they cross the pelvic brim. The lateral attachments of the sigmoid colon are incised and a 15 cm segment chosen, with due care, to ensure a broad blood supply. The isolated segment may be placed lateral or medial to the bowel anastomosis, which is done in standard fashion. The conduit is rotated 180° to make it isoperistaltic and the proximal end closed with a Parker-Kerr stitch of chromic catgut and interrupted fine silk Lembert sutures.

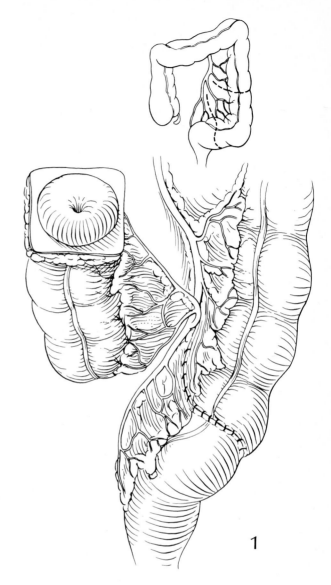

1

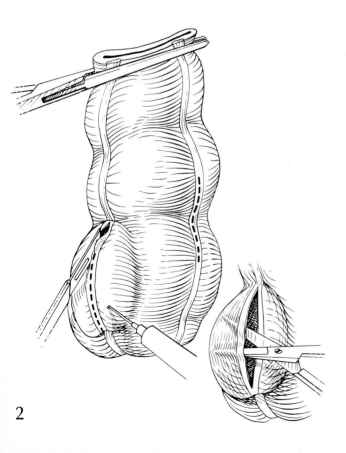

2

2

The ureteral anastomoses, done by a submucosal tunnel technique, should provide a tunnel length of 4–5 cm. The tunnels are staggered along the tenia, which are infiltrated with dilute adrenaline (epinephrine) solution to minimize bleeding and help establish the correct plane. Each tenia is incised and the seromuscular wall reflected from the submucosa. Most of the undermining is done laterally to avoid devitalizing the medial portion between the two ureteral tunnels. It is important to provide a tunnel adequate in width as well as length.

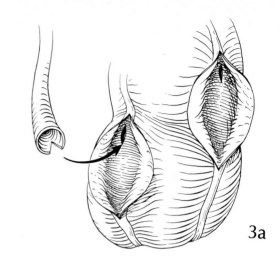

3a

3a, b & c

The mucosa is incised at the distal portion of the tunnel and the ureter is spatulated slightly and anastomosed to the mucosa with interrupted 5/0 chromic catgut.

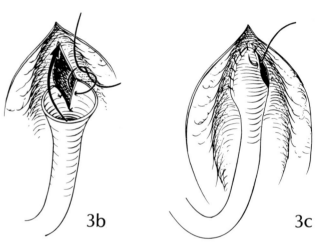

3b   3c

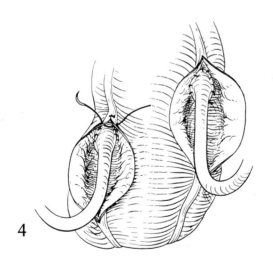

4

4

The seromuscular layer is then closed over the ureter with interrupted 4/0 silk.

5

It is important to be able to insert a right-angled clamp easily into the entrance of the tunnel to ensure that the ureter is not constricted.

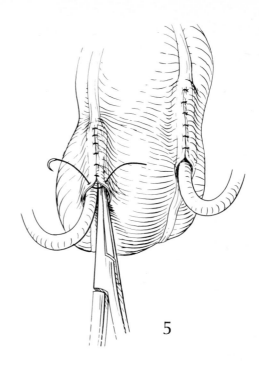

5

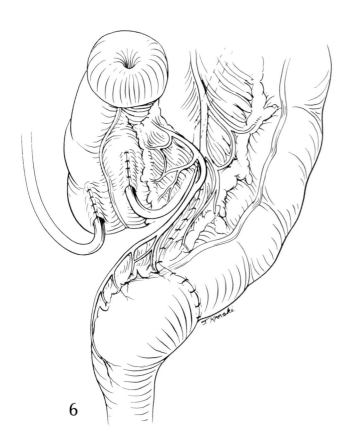

6

6

The completed sigmoid conduit has been reported to have encouraging results. Althausen et al.[2] experienced no cases of stomal stenosis, a 10 per cent incidence of ureterocolic stenosis and 14 per cent incidence of low-pressure reflux in 40 children with sigmoid conduits followed-up from 1 to 8 years. Others[3,4] have also reported satisfactory results.

However, it is imperative to reserve enthusiasm for any of the non-refluxing colon conduits until further long-term results become available.

THE ILEOCAECAL CONDUIT

The ileocaecal segment has been used for many years, primarily for bladder augmentation. The use of this segment of bowel as a urinary conduit did not receive much attention. In 1975 Zinman and Libertino[5] reported its use in this regard and emphasized the effectiveness of the ileocaecal valve as an anti-refluxing mechanism.

The ileocaecal segment has certain anatomical advantages as a conduit over other colonic segments. The ileocolic vessels supplying it are constant and are easily mobilized, with a long mesentery providing an excellent blood supply to the bowel. These vessels can be isolated accurately in obese children with thick mesenteric attachments by palpation of the ileocolic and right colic arteries. Ileocaecal segments can be added to a pre-existing ileal segment if the uretero-ileal anastomoses are functioning well and are probably the procedure of choice for absent, short or dilated ureters. They have minimal

stomal problems, can be readily taken down if necessary, and may lower the incidence of tumour development following internal diversion.

In our series of more than 50 children who have had ileocaecal segments performed, approximately 80 per cent had failed ileal conduits. The majority of these were patients with myelodysplasia. We have also employed this method of diversion in the few children with neurogenic bladder dysfunction which cannot be successfully managed by intermittent catheterization, pharmacological means, bladder neck surgery or implantation of an artificial sphincter. It has also been used in children with malignant bladder or prostatic tumours and as a temporary method of urinary diversion as part of a series of operations to reconstruct complex anomalies such as exstrophy of the bladder or cloaca, severe female epispadias with maldevelopment of the bladder, and bilateral single ectopic ureters.

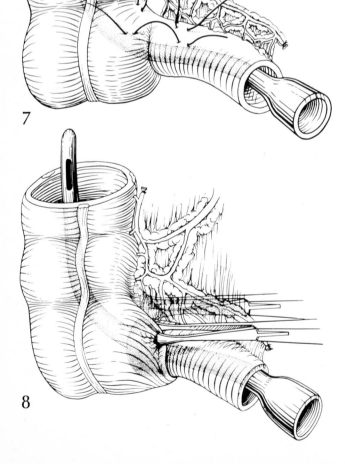

7

7

Through a midline incision the caecum, right colon and hepatic flexure are mobilized. The right ureter is isolated below the pelvic brim. The constant ileocolic vessels are identified and the ileum divided approximately 10 cm proximal to the ileocaecal valve. The ascending colon is divided proximal to the right colic artery and the mesentery incised appropriately. A 28 Fr catheter is introduced into the ileum, through the ileocaecal valve, to emerge through the colonic end; the antireflux mechanism is obtained by plicating the caecum around the terminal ileum in a collar-like fashion. The use of a catheter avoids too much narrowing of the distal ileum during this process. The ileum is intussuscepted into the caecum for 2–3 cm with several seromuscular sutures of 3/0 Tevdek.

8

The anterior and posterior walls of the caecum are then wrapped like a collar around the terminal 4 cm of ileum in a 270° encircling fashion with interrupted seromuscular Tevdek incorporating ileum and caecum on either side of the mesentery.

After this is completed, the large red rubber catheter is removed and the anti-reflux mechanism tested by inflating the ascending colon and measuring pressures. The valve mechanism should be continent to at least 50 cmH$_2$O. It is also advisable to make absolutely certain that the plication has not caused obstruction by allowing fluid to pass in antegrade fashion from the ileum to the colon. The left ureter is then isolated lateral to the sigmoid colon and brought under the sigmoid mesentery through the peritoneal opening on the right side.

9–13

The author prefers a conjoint ureteroureterostomy which is constructed by incising the ureters medially for 3 cm, suturing their walls with interrupted 5/0 chromic catgut, and anastomosing the resultant single opening to the open proximal ileum.

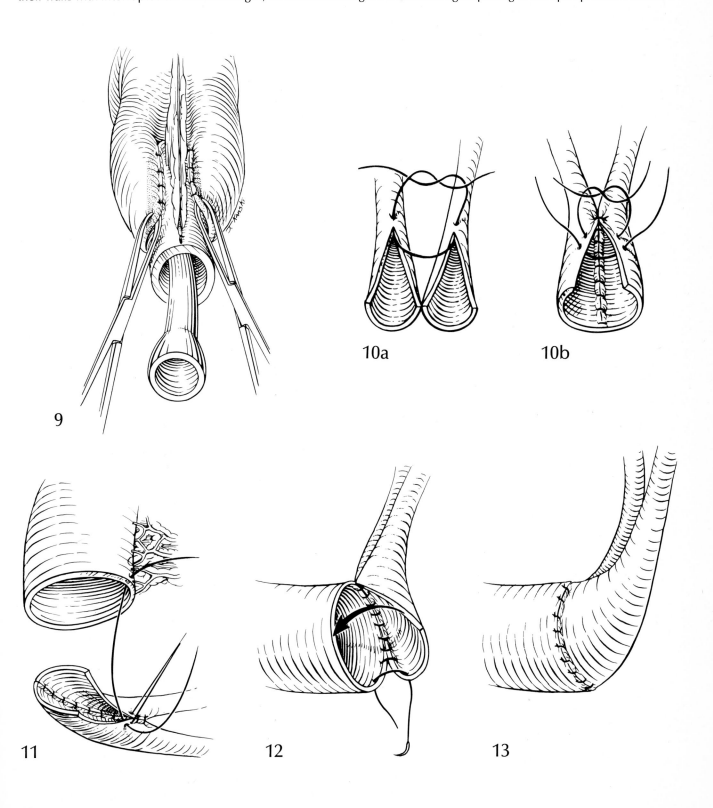

9

10a   10b

11   12   13

14

The results of the completed ileocaecal conduit diversion have been excellent. Zinman[5] has reported almost uniform success with the anti-reflux mechanism which he outlined. The incidence of obstruction has been minimal. Long-term results of the ileocaecal conduit in children are lacking, although the short-term results are encouraging. The incidence of obstruction is negligible and the incidence of low-pressure reflux minimal.

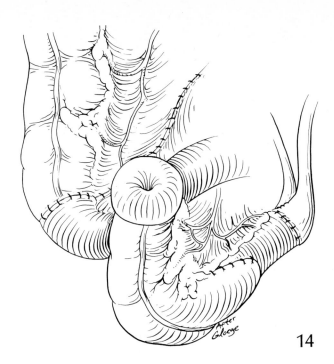

14

References

1. Richie, J. P., Skinner, D. G., Waisman, J. The effect of reflux on the development of pyelonephritis in urinary diversion: an experimental study. Journal of Surgical Research 1974; 16: 256–261

2. Althausen, A. F., Hagen-Cook, K., Hendren, W. H. Non-refluxing colon conduit; experience with seventycases. Journal of Urology 1978; 120: 35–39

3. Altwein, J. E., Jonas, U., Hohenfellner, R. Long-term follow-up of children with colon conduit urinary diversion and ureterosigmoidostomy. Journal of Urology 1977; 118: 832–836

4. Morales, P., Golimbu, M. Colonic urinary diversion: ten years of experience. Journal of Urology 1975; 113: 302–307

5. Zinman, L., Libertino, J. A. The ileo-cecal conduit for temporary and permanent urinary diversion. Journal of Urology 1975; 113: 317–323

Ureterosigmoidostomy

Hermann Dettmar MD
Director of the Urological Clinic, University of Düsseldorf, West Germany

Preoperative

Indications and contraindications

As a method of diversion ureterosigmoidostomy has the great advantage of avoiding any abdominal stoma or appliance for the collection of urine, and is, therefore, widely acceptable to patients. It requires an intact anal sphincter, however, and involves a greater risk of ascending urinary infection than does a skin diversion. It is widely employed in the treatment of some non-malignant disorders of the lower urinary tract where reconstructive surgery is impossible or has failed: for instance, in severely contracted bladder resulting from inflammation or irradiation; in incurable vesicovaginal fistula; following traumatic destruction of the urethra; and in exstrophy of the bladder. For diversion following total cystourethrectomy for bladder tumours it has many advantages, though some urologists prefer to avoid it when surgery is combined with radiotherapy. It is not suitable for the treatment of severe bladder symptoms which often accompany the terminal stages of pelvic malignancies as anal control is unlikely to be adequate, and for the same reason it should not be employed in any neurological disorder.

Preoperative preparation

It is important that the colon should be empty at the time of operation. Oral purgatives should be avoided, and oral antibiotics such as neomycin are unnecessary, but cleansing enemas should be given for 3 days prior to surgery, and the patient should be placed on a low-residue diet.

The operation

1

The abdomen is opened by a lower abdominal midline or suprapubic transverse incision. The peritoneal cavity is opened and the small bowel packed off into the upper abdomen. The ureter is then identified most easily at the point where it crosses the iliac vessels. The peritoneum over it is incised. The ureter is mobilized and dissected free towards the bladder, and is cut and tied at its lower end. It is convenient to start by isolating the right ureter; then the left can be freed in the same way, lateral to the sigmoid colon, which it is sometimes necessary to mobilize first.

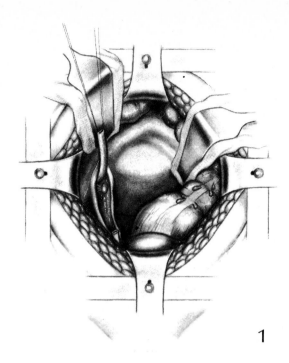

1

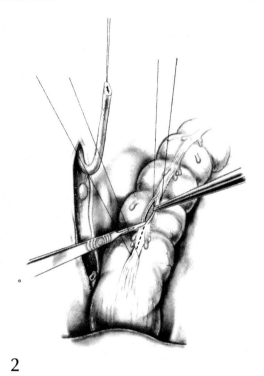

2

2

Stay sutures are placed in the proximal cut end of the ureter and preparations are made at a corresponding level in the bowel; the upper part of the rectum or rectosigmoid is appropriate. Two silk sutures are placed in the taenia and the seromuscular layer is then incised longitudinally.

3

The seromuscular layer on each side is held up by a stay suture and dissected laterally to expose the mucosa. At the distal end of the space so formed a transverse incision is made in the mucosa where the ureter is to be reimplanted.

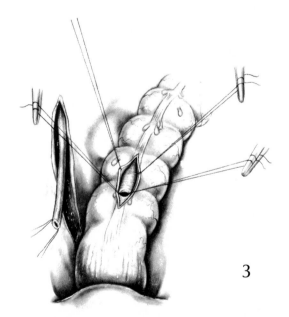

3

4

The ureter is now laid in the prepared bed and anastomosed in the mucosal opening with a series of 4/0 chromic catgut sutures.

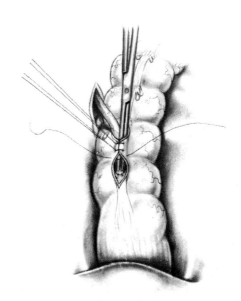

4

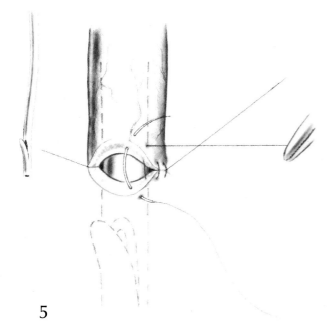

5

5

This anastomosis is more easily accomplished if the ureter is splinted. It is, however, important to use a splint which cannot slip upwards into the ureter. A short catheter with an expanding end may be used or a little flap at the side of the splint (as illustrated) may be raised as a barb.

6

The seromuscular layers of the colon are now closed over the ureter using interrupted or continuous silk sutures. The suture line should be started distally and in order to prevent a tight closure around the ureter a slightly opened sinus forceps should be put in the submucosal channel while the sutures are placed.

6

7

The medial border of the posterior peritoneal incision through which the ureter was brought is now fixed to the pelvic colon lateral to the anastomosis by a series of interrupted stitches.

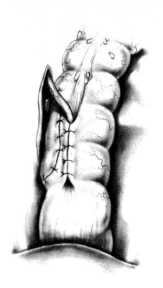

7

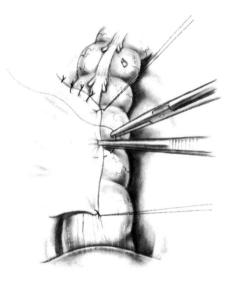

8

8

The lateral margin of the peritoneal incision is now fixed medial to the taenia, thus covering and extraperitonealizing the anastomosis.

9

The procedure is repeated on the left side at a slightly higher level in the sigmoid colon, leaving the bowel without tension in an S-shaped form. This is important to avoid any kinking or tension at the site of implantation.

At the end of the operation the rectal sphincter is dilated and a rectal tube inserted for 4–5 days. A forced postoperative diuresis is important and should be induced by intravenous administration of fluid. Any severe degree of ileus is very unusual and a bowel action should be induced after a day or two. The splints will be passed out with the first faecal movement.

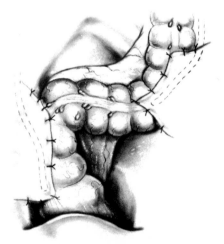

9

Postoperative care

Careful supervision is required to ensure early recognition of any dysfunction of the new implantation either by obstruction or reflux. Biochemical investigations should include estimation of serum electrolytes and urea. Not infrequently it will be necessary to administer bicarbonate on a regular basis to control acidosis. Intravenous urography should be performed as a routine between 3 and 6 months after operation and then at intervals. Early obstruction of the ureter may indicate the need for a further operative procedure. Later onset of fevers due to pyelonephritis with increasing upper tract dilatation may demand revision to a different form of diversion.

Illustrations by C. Willem and Patrick M. Elliott

Cutaneous ureterostomy

Emile de Backer MD
Conference Chairman, Catholic University of Louvain,
Chief of Urology Service, The Institute of Saint Elizabeth, Brussels, Belgium

Introduction

When cutaneous diversion is necessary, a simple cutaneous ureterostomy is generally preferable to an ileal or colonic conduit ureterostomy if one or both ureters are tortuous and dilated. In these circumstances the technique is simpler and the operative shock much less than with the intestinal conduit. Local complications are less frequent and there is no metabolic disturbance.

When, however, the upper urinary tract is not dilated, stoma problems often occur. In the case of single kidney or when the intestinal conduit must be avoided (for instance after irradiation or because of high risk), ureterostomy is indicated.

Preoperative

Positioning of the cutaneous stoma is critical. Theoretically the best site is on a line between the anterior superior iliac spine and the umbilicus as far from the spine as is necessary, according to the age of the patient, to allow the appliance to fit. It is, however, necessary to adapt the stoma to the circumstances, especially in the case of obese or wheelchair patients. A few days before the operation the appliance should be placed at the best point and its position checked after a few hours of normal activity.

The operations

SINGLE CUTANEOUS URETEROSTOMY

1

An oblique iliac incision makes it easy to find the lower third of the ureter extraperitoneally at the point where it crosses the iliac vessels. After section close to the bladder and ligature of the lower stump, the lower third of the ureter is freed, great care being taken not to mobilize it too high and to handle it with care to preserve the small blood vessels. Close dissection and stripping of the ureter is to be avoided. Mobilization should be carried out to the point where the ureter can be brought without tension to the abdominal wall at the appropriate site.

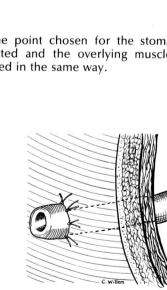

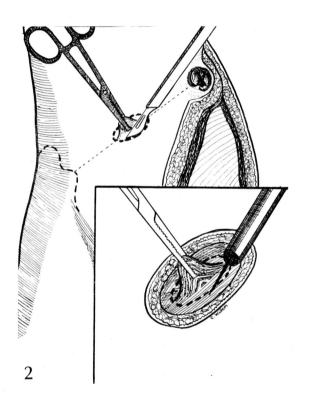

2

At the point chosen for the stoma a patch of skin is resected and the overlying muscles and aponeuroses excised in the same way.

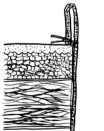

3

The ureter is brought out through this opening and a nipple formed by everting it and stitching it to the skin. This nipple must be at least 1 or 2 cm high in order to form a satisfactory stoma for appliances. The formation of the nipple is, however, only possible when the ureter is dilated. If simple eversion leaves the circumference rather tight, it may be incised on one side and a flap of skin brought up.

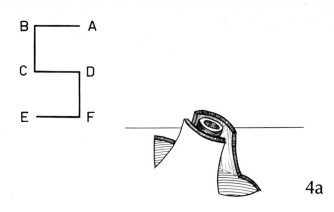

4a & b

Where the ureter is not sufficiently dilated to form a good nipple, a projecting stoma may be formed from skin flaps as shown by the S technique. The skin incision is made at the usual site and the underlying muscle and aponeurosis excised as before. The end of the ureter is then split for a distance of 0.5 cm and stitched to the skin edges.

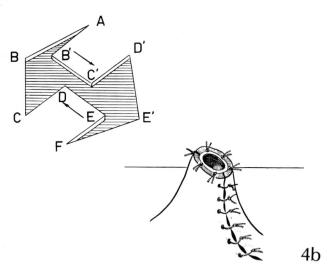

4a

4b

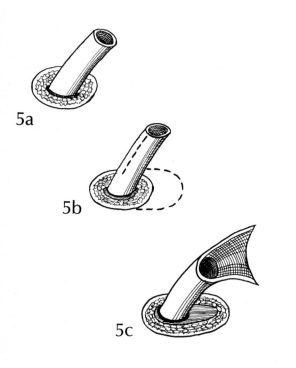

5a

5b

5c

5a–d

If the ureter is too short to fashion a nipple, it may be better to use an ileal conduit, but in an emergency the end of the ureter may be spatulated and sutured to the skin after excision of a corresponding area of epidermis.

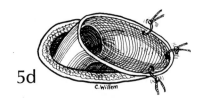

5d

C. Willem

DOUBLE CUTANEOUS URETEROSTOMY

Cutaneous ureterostomy with two separate stomas – one on each side – must be avoided, since it is cumbersome to the patient.

Cutaneous transureteroureterostomy is the best solution when one or both ureters are dilated. The less dilated ureter is brought across the midline retroperitoneally and anastomosed to the other, and this in turn is anastomosed to the skin. The dissection can also be made intraperitoneally (see chapter on transureteroureterostomy, pp. 00–00). This technique can be extended to less dilated or nearly normal ureters: using microsurgical techniques, end-to-side anastomosis of the ureters is made with 5/0 or 6/0 sutures.

6

A lower paramedian incision is made. The right lateral extraperitoneal space is exposed by blunt dissection and the right ureter isolated. This is cut across at the vesical as for single cutaneous ureterostomy.

A similar manoeuvre is performed on the left side and then by blunt finger dissection a retroperitoneal tunnel is made above the inferior mesenteric artery at the level of the fourth or fifth lumbar vertebra. The left ureter is brought through this tunnel to be anastomosed to the right ureter end-to-side. A longitudinal incision is made in the right ureter appropriate to the width of the left one. The anastomosis should be at least 1 cm in length. Interrupted sutures of 4/0 or 5/0 atraumatic catgut are suitable. Catheters may be left in the ureters, but this is not usually necessary.

The cutaneous stoma is as already described.

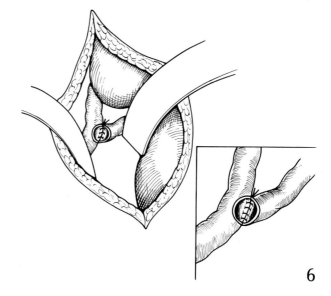

6

DOUBLE-BARRELLED URETEROSTOMY

7a & b

After extraperitoneal dissection, the opening of both ureters can be placed either in the midline (*a*) or in the lateral position at the ordinary site of cutaneous diversion (*b*).

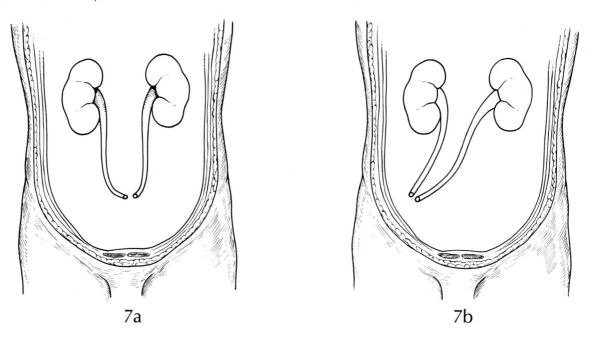

7a   7b

8a, b & c

The ureterocutaneous anastomosis is made as shown in the accompanying illustrations. This technique allows the formation of the nipple even where the ureters are small.

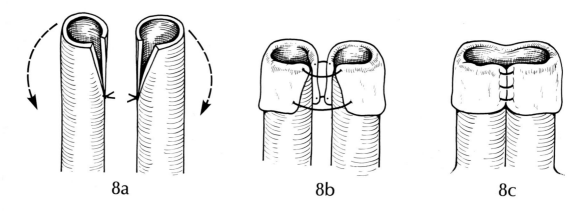

8a   8b   8c

TEMPORARY CUTANEOUS URETEROSTOMY

In infants with extremely dilated ureters, especially where renal function is impaired, it may be desirable to make a temporary cutaneous ureterostomy. The simplest form is the loop ureterostomy.

9

A short lumbar incision is made at the tip of the 12th rib.

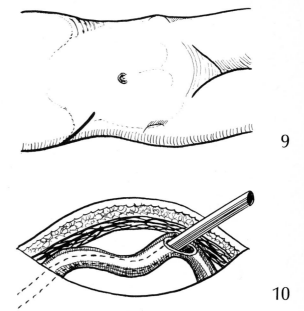

10

The ureter is found extraperitoneally and a portion of it mobilized sufficiently to bring it to the surface. Only very dilated and tortuous ureters are suitable for this procedure.

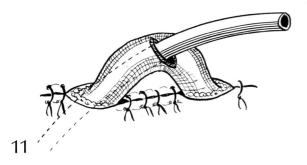

11

The musculoaponeurotic layers are closed beneath the loop, leaving a free passage for the ureteric arch.

12

A longitudinal incision 1–2 cm long is made in the ureter and its edges sutured to the skin. Alternatively the skin may be closed behind the loop.

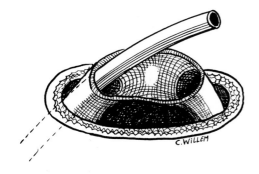

Illustrations by Jean Perry

Ureteroneocystotomy: reimplantation of the ureter

S. Joseph Cohen FRCS, MRCP
Consultant Paediatric Surgeon and Urologist, Booth Hall Children's Hospital Manchester;
Royal Manchester Children's Hospital, Saint Mary's Hospital, Manchester;
Lecturer in Paediatric Surgery, University of Manchester, UK

Introduction

The vesicoureteric junction has a very effective valve mechanism which allows free flow of urine from the ureter into the bladder but prevents reflux in the opposite direction even during a forceful act of micturition. The mechanism may fail where there is incompetence allowing vesicoureteric reflux or stenosis causing ureteric obstruction.

Preoperative

Indications for surgery

Reimplantation may be required whenever there is a disorder at the vesicoureteric junction.

Reflux

This is the most common condition necessitating reimplantation. The degree of reflux covers a spectrum varying from the mildest Grade I, where there is only a whisp of reflux into the lower ureter, to the most severe Grade 5, where there is gross reflux into a very dilated and tortuous ureter with pelvicalyceal hydronephrosis[1]. The renal parenchyma may show varying degrees of pyelonephritic scarring[2].

Primary reflux In this condition patients with urinary symptoms have reflux in the absence of bladder or urethral obstruction and without a neurogenic bladder. These cases are first treated with long-term antibiotics but, if the reflux persists and is severe, reimplantation is advisable. However, gross scarring and/or hypertension may be a contraindication to surgery.

Secondary reflux This is seen in association with obstructive lesions of the urethra, such as urethral valves, or in association with neurogenic bladders as in myelomeningocele. The obstruction must first be adequately treated, and a period of months or even years must be allowed for the bladder to return to normal. Only then, and if the reflux persists, should reimplantation be undertaken. It was previously the practice to resort to urinary diversion in the neurogenic bladder, but, with intermittent catheterization, reimplantation has become a more favoured adjunct to treatment.

Ureterovesical obstruction In children the condition of stenosed or obstructed megaureter is due to a neuromuscular incoordination at that site. It necessitates excision of the affected segment and ureteric reimplantation. A ureterocele in children is more commonly associated with complete duplication of the ureters, and reimplantation is often a necessary part of treatment.

Operative procedures on the bladder neck and urethra In cases of ectopia vesicae or epispadias where the trigonal area is used for the construction of the neourethra, it is advantageous to reimplant the ureters in a higher position in the bladder. These ureters are often incompetent and refluxing, and deserve reimplantation in their own right.

Operative technique

Many methods have been devised for reimplantation of ureters. They can be divided broadly into two groups: those where the primary approach is mainly intravesical, such as the Hutch[3], Politano-Leadbetter[4], Glenn-Anderson[5], Paquin[6] and Cohen[7] techniques; and those where the approach is purely extravesical – best exemplified by the Liche-Gregoir[8] technique.

The operations

1

The incision

A low skin crease incision of the Pfannensteil type is used. This heals with very little disfigurement and does not deter girls from wearing bikinis in later years.

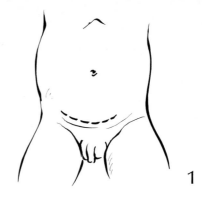

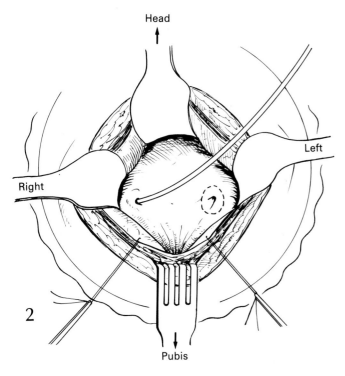

Exposure

2

The bladder is exposed after separating the recti and is then opened vertically between two stay sutures. A retractor of the Denis Browne type is inserted. The ureteric orifices are first inspected for number, position, shape and competence, and their tunnels are measured for length. A fine infant feeding tube, either 3½ or 5 Fr is inserted into the ureter, as shown, on the patient's right. A stay suture is placed around the meatus and loosely tied over the feeding tube. The ureteric meatus is then circumcised by an incision around the ureter as indicated by the dotted line on the patient's left.

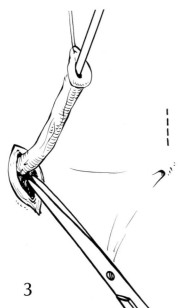

3

The ureter is now carefully dissected from its attachment to the muscles of the bladder and trigonal area, great care being taken not to damage the blood supply which runs along the surface of the ureter. The dissection is facilitated by gentle traction on the suture. All bleeding vessels are carefully diathermied, avoiding those running on or supplying the ureter itself. Care must be taken at this stage not to damage the peritoneum, which is closely applied to the ureter. It can be gently teased away from the back of the ureter using a pledget or by careful blunt dissection. Eventually the ureter is completely freed from all its attachments and a sufficient length of well vascularized ureter obtained for an adequate reimplantation.

This is the essential basis for all intravesical ureteric reimplantations and it must be carried out meticulously.

THE COHEN OR TRANSTRIGONAL METHOD OF REIMPLANTATION

4

The dissection described above may have enlarged the hiatus to such a degree that it could allow diverticulum formation. It should therefore be narrowed by the insertion of two or three Dexon sutures as shown, making sure that the ureter can still move freely in and out of the hiatus.

The new tunnel is commenced by incising the mucosa at a point above and slightly lateral to the opposite ureteric orifice, as indicated by the dotted line in *Illustration 3*. The next manoeuvre is facilitated by mild traction, using a pair of fine Allis forceps applied to the lateral aspect of this incision. The new submucosal tunnel is made by gently opening and closing a blunt pair of scissors and advancing them in a gradual curve towards the hiatus or origin of the ureter for reimplantation. The tunnel should be large enough to allow the ureter to fit comfortably and long enough to prevent reflux.

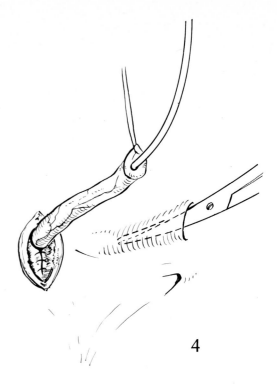

4

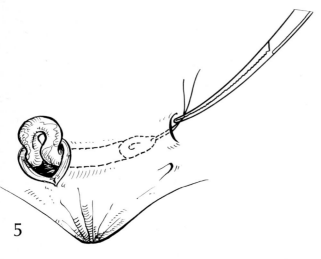

5

5

The ureter is now gently threaded through its new tunnel by traction on the ureteric stay suture until its fits comfortably in its new position.

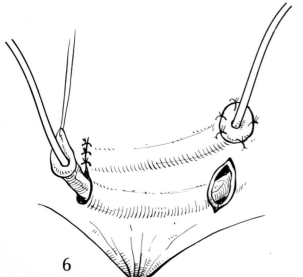

6

6

The cuff of the ureteric meatus is anchored in its new position by a lateral 3/0 Dexon suture through the full thickness of muscle of both the ureter and the bladder. This prevents retraction. The mucosa is then sutured to the bladder mucosa with 3 or 4 fine Dexon sutures (4/0 or 5/0). The mucosa of the original meatal entrance is closed with fine Dexon sutures. This is shown here in the upper ureter. The reimplanted ureter becomes a gently curved extension of the ureteric entrance into the bladder.

BILATERAL REIMPLANTATION

The second ureter is freed in exactly the same way as in *Illustrations 2, 3* and *4*. Its tunnel is then formed from its entrance, through the trigone to the orifice of the opposite side, in a gentle curve parallel to the upper tunnel. This is shown in the lower tunnel in *Illustration 6* and is fixed in position in the same manner. The mucosal cuff should be preserved if possible, but one should not hesitate to resect the terminal portion of ureter where it has been traumatized or its vascularity compromised. It is of course obligatory to resect the affected segment in cases of stenosed megaureter and ureterocele.

Bladder closure

This is carried out in the routine manner using a continuous Dexon suture to the mucosa and interrupted Dexon sutures for the bladder musculature. Ureteric stents (3½ or 5 Fr feeding tubes) are left in the reimplanted ureter and a suprapubic Malecot catheter left in the bladder. The retropubic space is drained by a suction drain and the skin closed in layers with a subcuticular Dexon suture.

POLITANO-LEADBETTER TECHNIQUE

The dissection of the ureter is carried out as in *Illustrations 2* and *3*.

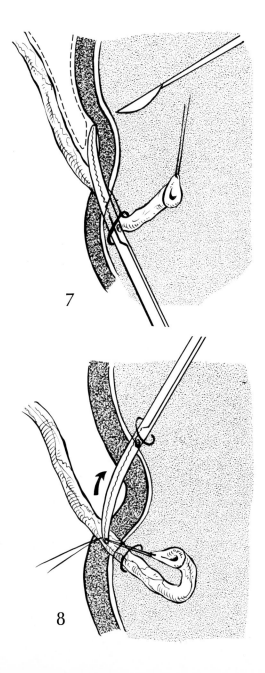

7

Further dissection is now carried out through the hiatus and the peritoneum is freed from the back of the bladder by blunt dissection. This plane is enlarged upwards towards the dome of the bladder, care being taken not to open the peritoneum (shown by the dotted lines in the illustration) or to damage any of the intraperitoneal structures. If any difficulties are encountered at this stage it is safer to proceed with an added extravesical dissection of the ureter. A pair of forceps is now inserted through the hiatus into this plane and the tip pressed into the bladder wall as shown. An incision is made at this point creating the new hiatus of entrance of the ureter.

8

A second pair of forceps is grasped by the first and is led into the lower orifice in the bladder. The ureteric stay suture is then gently drawn up into the bladder bringing the ureter into its new entrance.

9

The new tunnel is fashioned by blunt scissor dissection between the old hiatus and the new. Once this has been adequately prepared, the stay suture on the ureter is grasped and gently threaded through the new tunnel.

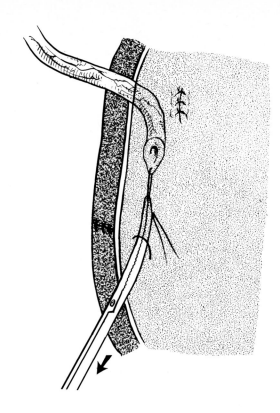

9

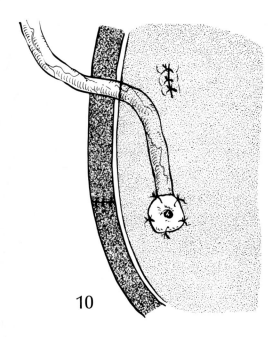

10

10

The old meatus is then resutured back to its old site. If there has been any damage to the end of the ureter, or if there is any relative stenosis, the end should be excised and a better ureteric termination formed.

11

This schematic drawing indicates the difference between the two techniques. The stippled ureter indicates the method of Politano-Leadbetter and shows its new hiatus of entrance and new tunnel down to the original meatus; the danger area indicated by the arrow is where the peritoneum and its structures can be damaged or where an S-bend can be formed if care is not taken.

In the cross-trigonal method one can see clearly why these problems do not arise, and how the new ureteral tunnel is a gentle prolongation of the curve of the ureter.

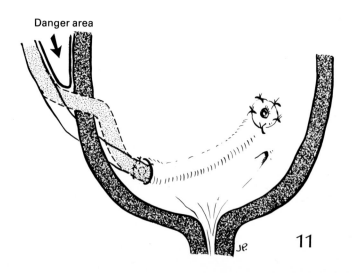

Danger area

11

EXTRAVESICAL TECHNIQUE

12

The Liche-Gregoir technique exposes the bladder in the normal way and then rotates it to the opposite side and slightly forward. The ureter is exposed by dividing the obliterated umbilical artery and the few vessels which cross the ureter at this point. Once the ureter has been exposed, the incision is made as indicated by the dotted line. Note that this is on the back wall of the bladder.

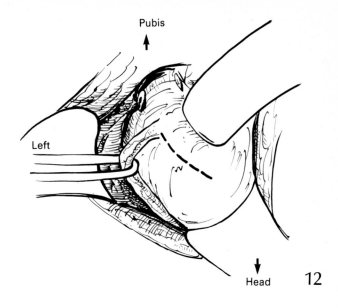

13

The incision is carried down to the bladder mucosa taking care not to injure the mucosa, and freeing the muscle sufficiently to allow mucosa and muscle to be sutured over the ureter. An important point is that the dissection must be carried out well down to the junctional area between the ureter and the bladder musculature; a shelf must not be left here.

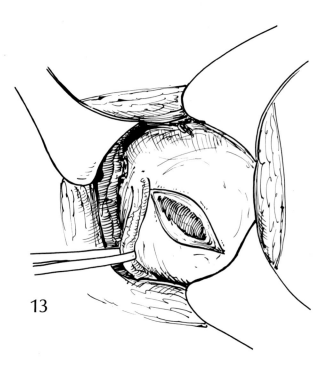

14a & b

Once this is carried out, resuturing commences. Interrupted Dexon sutures are inserted, beginning at the proximal end of the tunnel as indicated and making sure the ureter is not constricted by the sutures. A two-layer closure is recommended and care must be taken to ensure that the ureter is not strangulated anywhere along its reimplanted length. The bladder is then allowed to fall back into its position and the ureter assumes its natural course but with a larger submucosal segment.

The problem with this technique is that it can only be used in moderately dilated ureters.

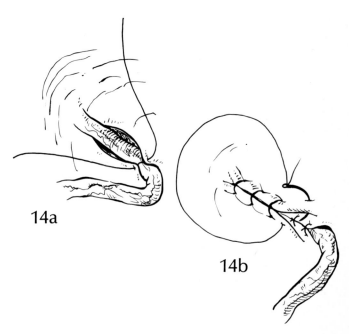

REIMPLANTATION OF THE GROSSLY DILATED URETER

15

If the ureter is dilated to such a degree that it does not allow for an adequate reimplantation, then tailoring or remodelling should be carried out[9]. The ureter may be fully mobilized intravesically, but this is achieved more easily by added extravesical dissection. The kinks and bends must be straightened out and great care taken not to damage the blood supply. This often allows many centimetres of ureter to be mobilized so one can safely excise a centimetre or two from the end and still have sufficient length for reimplantation.

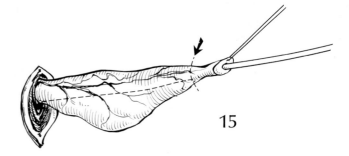

16

An 8 Fr feeding tube is now threaded up the ureter and special clamps applied, preserving the blood supply to the ureter which is remodelled. The excess ureter is then trimmed away as indicated.

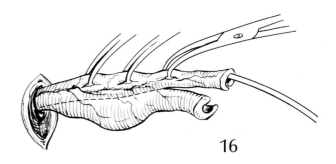

17

Resuturing of the ureter is then commenced from above downwards. A continuous Dexon suture commences at the proximal end of the remodelled ureter. It is preferable to use an inverting suture of the Connell type, and to strengthen it with several interrupted Dexon sutures.

The newly remodelled ureter is now ready for reimplantation and can be reimplanted as in *Illustrations 4, 5 and 6*.

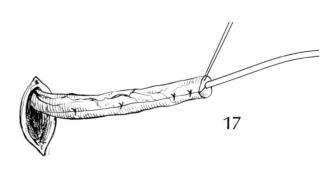

Conclusions

Reimplantation of the ureters is a recognized technique for correction of abnormalities at the ureterovesical junction. The results of surgery are improving, and the complication rate in ureters with only moderate dilatation and without any bladder abnormality should be in the region of 1–4 per cent. In the grossly dilated ureter and in cases where the bladder is trabeculated as a result of obstruction or a neurogenic effect, the complication rate is higher. Nevertheless this should not deter the surgeon from carrying out this operation.

References

1. Dwoskin, J. Y., Perlmutter, A. D. Vesicoureteral reflux in children: A computerised review. Journal of Urology 1973; 109: 888–890

2. Smellie, J., Edwards, D., Hunter, N., Normand, I. C. S., Prescod, N. Vesicoureteric reflux and renal scarring. Kidney International 1975; 8: Suppl. 4: 565–572

3. Hutch, J. A. Ureteric advancement operation: anatomy, technique and early results. Journal of Urology 1963; 89: 180–184

4. Politano, V. A., Leadbetter, W. F. An operative technique for the correction of vesicoureteral reflux. Journal of Urology 1958; 79: 932–941

5. Glenn, J. F., Anderson, E. E. Distal tunnel ureteral reimplantation. Journal of Urology 1967; 97: 623–626

6. Paquin, A. J. Jr. Ureterovesical anastomosis: the description and evaluation of a technique. Journal of Urology 1959; 82: 573–583

7. Cohen, S. J. Ureterozystomeostomie: eine neue antireflux technik. Aktuelle Urologie 1975; 6: 1–8

8. Gregoir, W., Van Regemorter, G. Le reflux vésico-urétéral congénital. Urologia Internationalis 1964; 18: 12–136

9. Hendren, W. H. III. Operative repair of megaureter in children. Journal of Urology 1969; 101: 491–507

Illustrations by Babara Rankin

Ureteral injuries

W. Scott McDougal MD
Professor and Chairman, Department of Urology
Vanderbilt University Medical Center, Nashville, Tennessee, USA

Introduction

Ureteral injuries are rare, constituting less than 0.1 per cent of all surgical admissions. They are classified according to whether they are due to violent trauma (penetrating or blunt) or to operative misadventure. Over 90 per cent of non-operatively injured ureters have as their cause penetrating trauma. About 17 per cent of patients presenting with genitourinary trauma due to penetrating injuries will have a ureteral injury. Moreover, about 2 per cent of all patients who present to hospital with a penetrating injury will have a ureteral injury. Blunt trauma resulting in injury to the ureter usually occurs as a result of a hyperextension injury, or as a consequence of displaced spicules of bone penetrating the ureter. Almost all penetrating injuries and most blunt injuries have associated lesions. Damage to the small bowel and colon is the most common concomitant injury.

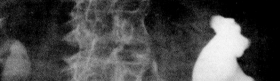

1

Iatrogenic injuries are often associated with significant morbidity, as only 20–30 per cent are recognized at the time of injury. The procedure most commonly associated with ureteral injury is a hysterectomy. Urological manipulation, rectosigmoid colon resection and aortoiliac surgery account for the majority of the remainder.

Often the diagnosis is not suspected, as associated injuries or a recent operative procedure generally draw attention away from the ureter. Renal colic, particularly in the postoperative period, may suggest the diagnosis. Haematuria, which occurs in 80 per cent of cases due to blunt or penetrating trauma, and in only 10 per cent of cases due to iatrogenic or operative injury, may also suggest the diagnosis. Other clinical findings include ileus and, rarely, hyperchloraemic metabolic acidosis. The diagnosis is made by intravenous pyelography, which demonstrates the lesion approximately 90 per cent of the time. Ultrasonography, when the injury results in hydronephrosis, may also be helpful. Retrograde pyelography is fully diagnostic. A helpful technique intraoperatively, if a ureteral injury is suspected, is to inject indigo carmine or methylene blue plus mannitol intravenously. This will establish a diuresis and the dye may then become apparent within the wound. In selected circumstances an open cystotomy and retrograde cannulation from the bladder may be required to make the diagnosis

Iatrogenic ureteral injury. Notice that the retrograde catheter lies outside the confines of the ureter

Treatment

The general principles involved in treating ureteral injuries include: adequate debridement with removal of all non-viable tissue; adequate mobilization of the ureter with a tension-free anastomosis; and a watertight anastomosis which is excluded and drained away from other injured structures. When a concomitant duodenal, pancreatic or major vessel injury occurs, proximal urinary diversion and stents are required.

URETERAL LIGATION AND DELIGATION

Ureters which have been ligated during an operative procedure may be deligated if recognized immediately. Care must be taken to assure that the ligature has not caused necrosis of the ureter, for this will inevitably result in a fistula. Ureters which have been ligated with absorbable sutures should not be left with the hope that the absorbable suture will dissolve and the obstruction will be relieved. In fact, the suture resorption is generally not rapid enough to prevent major loss of renal function.

In selected circumstances, ureteral ligation has been advocated when the ureteral injury is extensive, the contralateral side is normal and the patient is a poor risk. This procedure, which often results in fistula formation and may lead to sepsis, is generally not recommended.

URETEROURETEROSTOMY

This procedure is generally indicated for injuries which involve the middle and upper third of the ureter. The injuries should not be extensive and both ends of the ureter must be easily brought together after debridement. Mobilization of the kidney and inferior nephropexy will provide additional length if required.

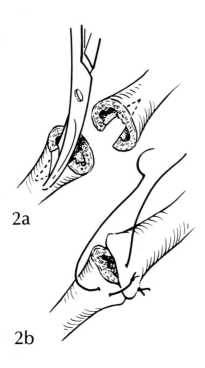

2a

2b

2a & b

Following debridement, both ends of the ureter are spatulated (a) and sutured with interrupted 4/0 or 5/0 chromic catgut (b). The anastomosis should be tension-free and watertight.

Many advocate the use of a stent, suggesting that this structure will prevent periureteral extravasation of urine and thus lessen scar tissue formation. If the stent is to be used, it should not be occlusive. Others suggest that, as the use of a stent may irritate the anastomosis and increase scar formation, it should be used only under extenuating circumstances. A stent and proximal diversion are mandatory, however, if there is an associated duodenal, pancreatric or great vessel injury.

TUBE URETEROSTOMY

A tube ureterostomy is performed as a temporizing procedure when there are severe associated injuries which preclude prolonged ureteral surgery.

3

A Foley catheter is threaded up the proximal ureter to the renal pelvis and the balloon inflated. The distal margin of the ureter is tied about the catheter. The catheter is then brought out through a separate stab wound and the retroperineal area drained. The distal ureter should be sought if time permits and tagged with a non-reabsorbable suture to facilitate reconstructive surgery.

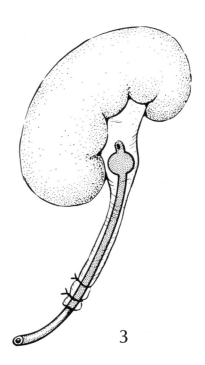

3

URETERONEOCYSTOSTOMY

For lower ureteral injuries in which the ureter may be mobilized sufficiently, a ureteroneocystostomy is the procedure of choice. The technique for this procedure is described in the chapter on 'Ureteroneocystomy: reimplantation of the ureter', pp. 300–306.

Boari-Ockerblad flap

When lower ureteral injuries are extensive and a primary ureteroneocystostomy cannot be performed, or when a psoas hitch does not allow enough length for a tension-free anastomosis to be made, a Boari-Ockerblad flap may be used to bridge the gap. This procedure is illustrated in the chapter on 'Surgery of genitourinary tuberculosis', pp. 156–161. Technical points to remember when constructing this flap are that contralateral mobilization of the bladder is essential; a psoas hitch should be performed on the ipsilateral side; and the base of the flap should be wide. The ureter may be sutured either into the tube flap end-to-end or into a non-refluxing submucosal tunnel. Long-term complications include strictures of the flap with obstruction of the renal segment.

TRANSURETEROURETEROSTOMY

This procedure is rarely indicated in the immediate post-traumatic period for repairing the injured ureter since it requires extensive retroperitoneal mobilization and considerable operative time. It is clearly contraindicated in patients who have a prior history of retroperitoneal fibrosis, tuberculosis, transitional cell carcinoma of the ureter and pelvis, or obstruction of the recipient ureter. If the procedure is to be performed, the recipient ureter must not be mobilized and the crossover should be made above the inferior mesenteric artery to prevent tension. The technique for this procedure is illustrated on pp. 315–318.

Autotransplantation and ileal substitution procedures may be used to bridge large gaps of ureteral loss. Autotransplantation is performed as described in the chapter on 'Renal transplantation' pp. 199–210, and ileal substitution as described in the chapter on 'Ileal ureteral replacement', pp. 310–314.

Further reading

Carlton, C. E., Scott, R., Guthrie, A. G. The initial management of ureteral injuries: a report of 78 cases. Journal of Urology 1971; 105: 335–340

McDougal, W. S., Persky, L. Traumatic injuries of the genitourinary system. Baltimore: Williams & Wilkins, 1981

Zinman, L. M., Libertino, J. A., Roth, R. A. Management of operative ureteral injury. Urology 1978; 12: 290–303

Illustrations by Frank E. Steckel

Ileal ureteral replacement

John A. Libertino MD
Director of Transplantation, Department of Urology;
Vice Chairman, Division of Surgery, Lahey Clinic Medical Center, Burlington, Massachusetts, USA

Joseph B. Dowd MD
Chairman, Department of Urology, Lahey Clinic Medical Center, Burlington, Massachusetts, USA

Introduction

Ileal replacement of the ureter is indicated when a segment of ureter is lost or destroyed or when patients who have recurrent stones require a 'stone shoot' to facilitate the passage of renal calculi. The procedure is a complex one, not to be undertaken lightly.

General indications for ileal ureteral replacement are loss or destruction of a long segment of ureter resulting from trauma, radiation damage, extensive scarring, radical surgery, or as a 'bailout' procedure for previously failed ureteropelvic junction reconstruction or ureteroneocystotomy beyond salvage by ordinary reconstructive measures. The bladder must be physiologically normal. Contraindications include incontinence, vesical neck obstruction, neurogenic vesical dysfunction and malignant disease in a patient who has a limited expected survival.

Preoperative

Preoperative preparation includes oral antibiotics, low-residue diet, laxatives and enemas. In patients who have had many reconstructive ureteral operations and when identification of a scarred ureter may be difficult, passage of a 6 or 7 Fr ureteral catheter preoperatively will make identification of the ureter simpler at operation. If retrograde catheterization is not possible, percutaneous antegrade nephrostomy and advancement of a catheter may be helpful. For patients in whom prior reconstructive procedures have failed and who present with an obstructed renal segment and urosepsis, percutaneous nephrostomy is helpful in managing the septic component; it also helps to restore the metabolic status sufficiently to allow ileal replacement of the ureter.

The operation

1

A midline incision is preferred, extending from the xiphoid process to the pubis.

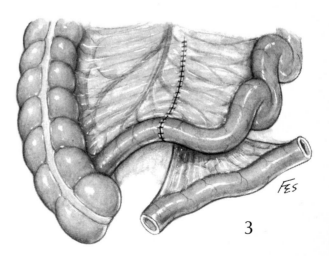

2

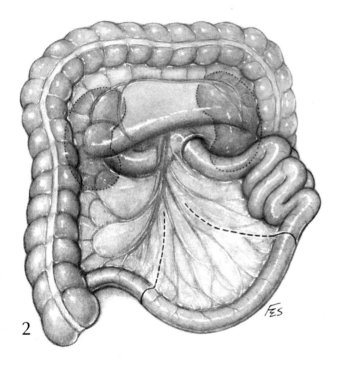

A mobile segment of ileum, 25–35 cm in length, is selected. The length chosen should be slightly greater than the measured distance from the renal pelvis to the bladder. Because it is impossible to straighten the ileum completely in its course and because of the length of the mesentery, the ileal segment selected should be longer than is anatomically required. It is always easier to trim a generous segment from the ileum than to stretch an inadequate bowel segment and have suture lines under tension.

3

The continuity of the ileum is restored with a standard two-layer bowel anastomosis. The bowel anastomosis is accomplished anterior to the isolated ileal segment. The openings in the mesentery are closed to avoid internal herniation. The technique for isolating the segment of ileum is identical with that used to create an ileal conduit.

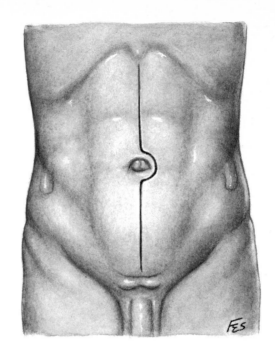

4

The isolated loop of bowel is irrigated with warm saline solution to wash out mucus and faecal material before it is placed in its retroperitoneal position.

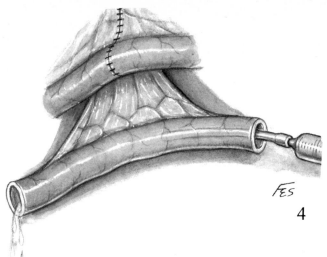

5

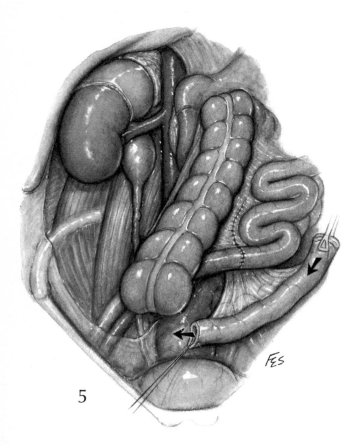

The colon is mobilized by sharp dissection, incising the peritoneum along the white line of Toldt. Mobilization of the colon allows placement of the ileal ureter in its retroperitoneal position and also enables good access to the renal pelvis. It is important to maintain the isoperistaltic nature of the ileal segment. On the right side, the caecum and ascending colon must be mobilized medially to enable this manoeuvre to take place. On the left side, the descending and sigmoid colon are mobilized, and a window is created in the mesentery of the descending colon so that the ileal segment can approach the bladder with ease without kinking over the rectosigmoid colon in the pelvis.

6

The ileoureteral segment is now visualized in its retroperitoneal position. The diseased ureter is ligated or removed as required by the clinical situation. At this point, care must be exercised to prevent injury to the vasculature of the isolated ileal segment by the rotation which is necessary to preserve its isoperistaltic direction.

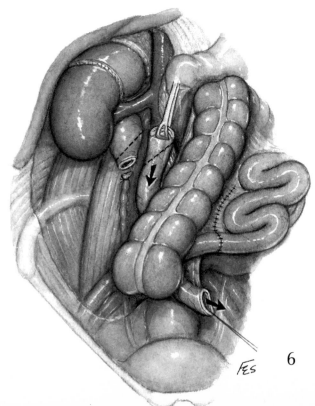

7

The ureter and pelvis are spatulated in a 45° angle so the opening in the pelvis and the isolated ileal segment are exactly the same length. The anastomosis between the renal pelvis and the ileum is carried out using interrupted 2/0 chromic sutures. Before completion of the anastomosis a nephrostomy tube and ureteral stent are placed in the kidney. The stent is made to lie through the ureteropelvic anastomosis.

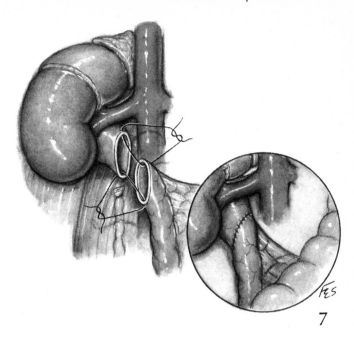

8

When both ureters are to be replaced, a long segment of ileum is isolated so that it may pass from one renal pelvis to the other and then descend to the bladder. This technique is preferable to using two loops of ileum in a Y formation.

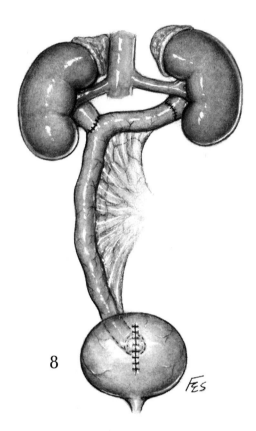

9

Anastomosis of the distal end of the ileum to the bladder is accomplished through the posterior wall of the bladder. A large, full-thickness button of the bladder wall is excised posteriorly to create a new orifice of the correct circumference to accommodate the ileum. The bladder is opened anteriorly to facilitate the anastomosis. A clamp is passed from within the bladder outwards through the posterior window.

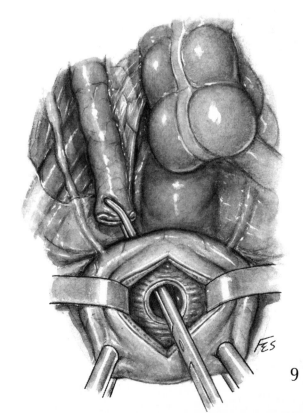

10

The ileal segment is brought into the bladder and straightened as much as possible in its course from the kidney towards the bladder. The excess length of ileum protruding into the bladder is excised. The opened end of the ileum is anastomosed to the bladder. The seromuscular layer of the ileum is anastomosed to the seromuscular layer of the bladder with interrupted 2/0 chromic sutures. A second anastomosis between the mucosa of the ureter and the mucosa of the bladder is carried out with 4/0 interrupted sutures. Several seromuscular sutures are placed between the ileum and the serosa of the bladder on its posterior surface to reduce tension on the suture line.

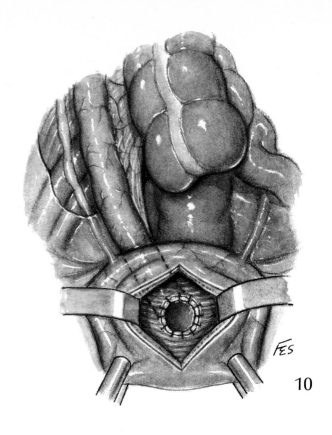

10

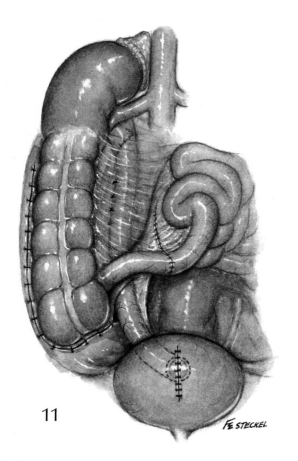

11

11

The ileoureteral substitute, seen here with retroperitonealization of the right colon, is completed with the closure of the anterior wall of the bladder.

References

1. Moore, E. V., Weber, R., Woodward, E. R., Moore, J. G., Goodwin, W. E. Isolated ileal loops for ureteral repair. Surgery, Gynecology and Obstetrics 1956; 102: 87–97

2. Goodwin, W. E., Cockett, A. T. K. Surgical treatment of multiple, recurrent branched, renal (staghorn) calculi by pyelonephroileal-vesical anastmosis. Journal of Urology 1961; 85: 214–222

3. Skinner, D. G., Goodwin, W. E. Indications for the use of intestinal segments in the management of nephrocalcinosis. Journal of Urology 1975; 113: 436–442

4. Boxer, R. J., Fritzsche, P., Skinner, D. G. et al. Replacement of the ureter by small intestine – clinical application and results of ileal ureter in 89 patients. Journal of Urology 1979; 121: 728–731

Illustrations by Sylvia Barker

Transureteroureterostomy

J. C. Smith MS, FRCS
Consultant Urological Surgeon, The Churchill Hospital, Oxford, UK

1a, b & c

The principle

Transureteroureterostomy is defined as an operation which joins one ureter to its fellow across the midline. The operation includes the joining of ureters in a urinary diversion, the Y-anastomosis when both kidneys are present and the use of the opposite ureter to drain a solitary kidney.

Indications

The chief indication is in ureteric injuries, whether accidental in the course of abdominal or pelvic surgery or deliberate in the excision of extensive neoplasms. Other indications, such as failure of a ureteric reimplantation, long stricture of the ureter or in the treatment of vesicoureteric reflux, occur less commonly.

Contraindications

Gross infection or disease in one kidney with a normal contralateral kidney makes the operation unwise. The operation is seldom indicated in transitional cell neoplasms of the urinary tract.

In injuries to the lower ureter, reimplantation of the ureter utilizing the Boari flap or psoas hitch is preferable if technically possible.

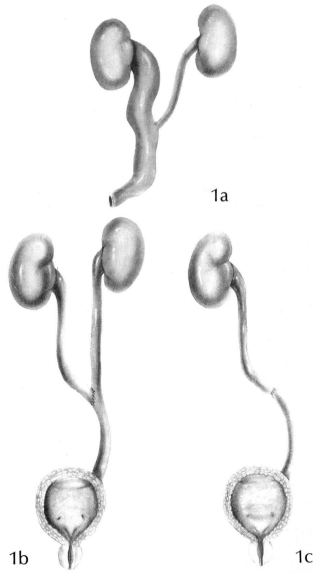

1a

1b

1c

The operation

2

The incision

Any incision that gives adequate access to the damaged and contralateral ureter can be utilized. The author prefers a transverse incision unless a previous operation causing the injury has been performed via a vertical incision, in which case the previous incision may be reopened. If a Pfannenstiel incision has been used, then a new incision (either transverse, oblique or vertical) is necessary to obtain access to the ureter above the pelvic brim.

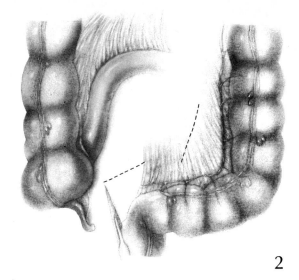

2

3

Following mobilization of the small intestine (which may be adherent to the pelvis following previous surgery), the intestine is turned upwards including the caecum to show the right ureter. If this is injured it is mobilized and divided at the point of injury. Mobilization of the ureters should include periureteric tissue to preserve blood supply. The incision in the posterior peritoneum is continued across the brim of the pelvis and the left ureter located by incision of the pelvic mesocolon. If this proves difficult, then the pelvic colon may be mobilized medially and the ureter located retroperitoneally. It is then mobilized and brought towards the midline through the mesocolon.

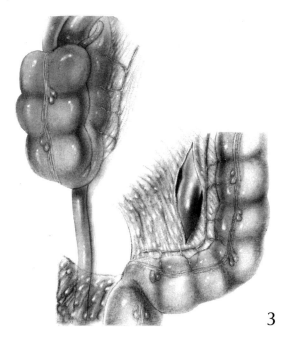

3

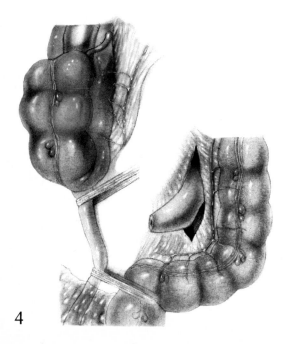

4

4

The normal ureter should be pulled gently towards the midline with two tapes and the injured ureter, which has previously been divided, brought across the midline to lie in approximation without tension.

5–8

The normal ureter is incised for 1–1.5 cm and the end of the divided ureter reimplanted into it using 4/0 chromic catgut either interrupted or continuous sutures. It is helpful to cannulate the upper and lower ends of the anastomosis with a soft tube during the suturing, completing the anastomosis in the middle of the anterior layer.

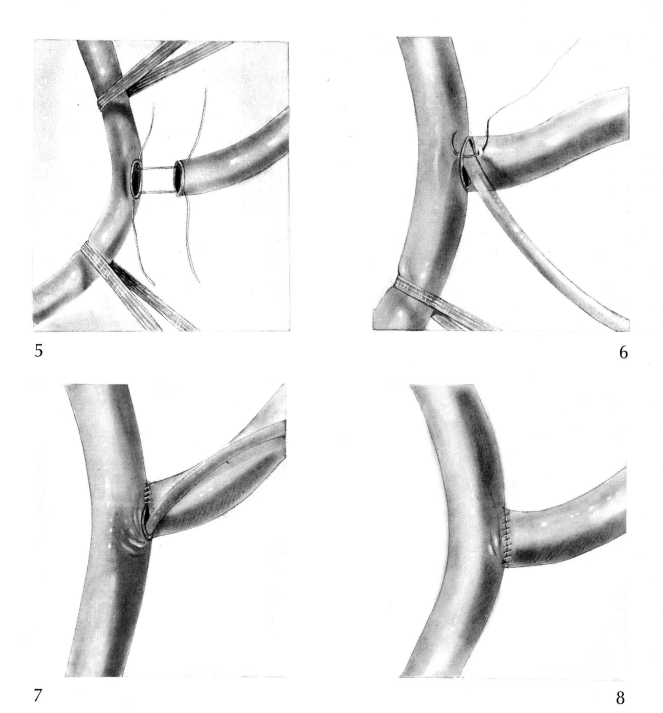

5

6

7

8

Postoperative care

The author does not employ stents but other surgeons use this method. In draining a solitary kidney with the opposite ureter, a diverting nephrostomy or ureterostomy may be employed, particularly if the lower ureter has been non-functioning for some time. A vacuum drain down to the site of the anastomosis should be left for 5 days or until drainage ceases, whichever is the longer. A urethral catheter may be employed to keep the bladder empty but this is not essential.

In the absence of other indications, follow-up excretory urography should be deferred for 6 months to allow the temporary postoperative hydronephrosis time to resolve.

Further reading

Smith, I. B., Smith, J. C. Transureteroureterostomy: British experience. British Journal of Urology 1975; 47: 519–523

Udall, D. A., Hodges, C. V., Pearse, H. M., Burns, A. B. Transureteroureterostomy – a neglected procedure. Journal of Urology 1973; 109: 817–820

Drainage of the bladder

John P. Blandy   MA, DM, MCh, FRCS
Professor of Urology, The London Hospital Medical College;
Consultant Urologist, St Peter's Hospital, London, UK

Preoperative

Thanks to the modern non-irritating latex plastic and silicone rubber catheters, and to the general application of those principles of catheter care that prevent infection, an indwelling catheter may be used in nearly every case where it is necessary to drain the bladder for a prolonged period of time. With the advent of intermittent self-catheterization, many patients formerly condemned to a lifetime of diversion or indwelling catheter drainage are now able to look after themselves with minimal long-term morbidity and a new freedom from apparatus and the risk of infection.

Today suprapubic drainage is needed relatively infrequently. The indications fall into two main categories: when it is impossible to pass even a narrow Gibbon-type catheter or where any kind of catheterization is likely to make things worse (e.g. in certain selected cases or urethral trauma); or as a form of prolonged drainage, in order to protect the bladder while it is healing after an operation for stone or reimplantation of the ureter, or to protect a particularly difficult and delicate operation on the urethra. In the latter category come also those patients with widespread sepsis and extravasation in the perineum due to some injury or lesion of the urethra, where diversion of the urine is essential as part of the strategy of clearing up the septic process.

As a permanent method of urinary diversion of choice, suprapubic cystostomy has almost been eclipsed. On the one hand it has been replaced by intermittent self-catheterization, and on the other, by the use of the ileal conduit. Nevertheless, one must recognize that in a few, selected, very special patients, a suprapubic cystostomy may be the lesser of several evils. Just occasionally the chairbound paraplegic, unable to cope with the stoma of an ileal conduit, is well served by being given a permanent suprapubic catheter.

The operations

TEMPORARY SUPRAPUBIC DRAINAGE

A number of suprapubic catheter kits are now available. Essentially they consist of a stiff trochar inside a plastic catheter, which may or may not be provided with a Foley-type balloon to keep it from slipping out of the bladder. When working in difficult circumstances, a little ingenuity will enable the surgeon to do almost the same procedure using locally available material. There are two important steps: to make sure that the bladder is really full; and to find out how far down it is situated from the level of the skin. In most cases the patients for whom such a diversion will be used are ill, and one must insert the catheter under local anaesthesia.

First, the bladder must be distended fully. If the patient is already in retention of urine, there is no difficulty. If not, a catheter must be passed deliberately to distend the bladder with enough sterile saline to make it easily palpable above the pubis.

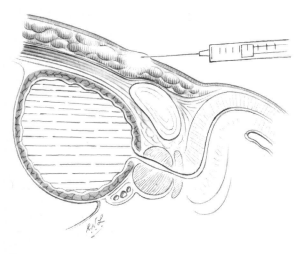

1

1

The skin is shaved and prepared in the usual way.

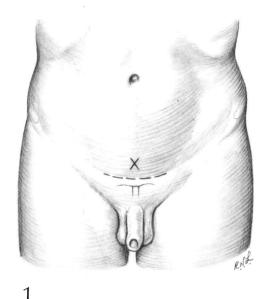

2

2

A syringe with 1 per cent lignocaine is used to raise a bleb in the skin 2 cm above the pubis (one fingerbreadth).

3

A bigger and longer needle, aimed at the anus – i.e. slightly downwards rather than in a vertical direction – is used to infiltrate and aspirate as the needle is advanced to the bladder. When urine is aspirated – which is usually very obvious – a forceps is placed on the needle to show how far down from the surface of the skin the bladder is situated. This is a very useful dodge, since patients vary so much in the depth of their suprapubic fat.

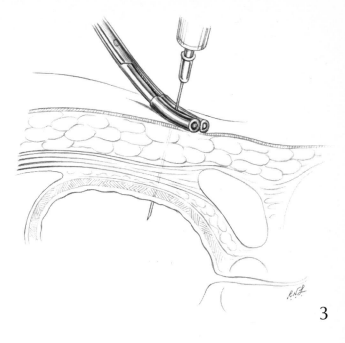

3

4

Now the trochar and cannula are used to measure off the distance from the skin to the bladder which has just been discovered with the needle used for the local anaesthetic.

5

The trochar and cannula are firmly held and aimed once more in the direction of the anus, making sure that they cannot penetrate more than 2 cm farther than the measured distance from skin to bladder. An adequate nick is made through the skin weal so that the trochar and cannula slide easily through the skin. The trochar is thrust firmly down into the bladder. The trochar is withdrawn and the cannula is passed right down and onwards into the bladder.

In the Supracath type of cannula, which has no balloon, there are two tabs to be sutured to the skin either side of the small incision to hold the cannula in position. In other types the surgeon has to inflate the Foley balloon with the appropriate volume of sterile water. In either case, it is a wise precaution to complete the manoeuvre by stitching the tube to the skin. It is also wise to make sure that a bit of the tube is stuck to the skin with adhesive tape to prevent accidental dislodgement.

The advantages of these forms of suprapubic drainage lie in their simplicity, speed and safety. The fact that there is no catheter lying in the urethra to cause pressure necrosis or paraurethral gland infection is of particular advantage in children and paraplegics. The disadvantages are few but important. The plastic tube easily kinks where it emerges from the skin, or is blocked by pus or a blood-clot.

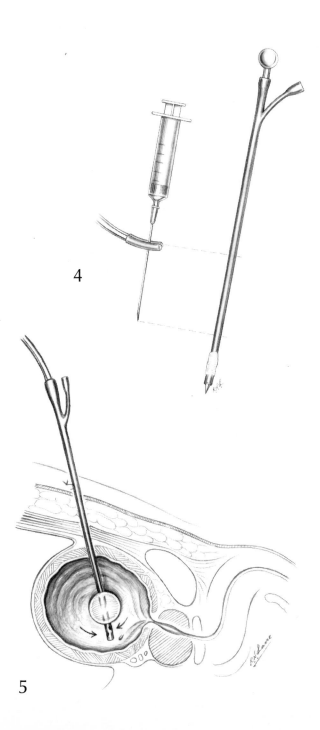

4

5

SUPRAPUBIC CYSTOSTOMY

A suprapubic cystostomy is often a difficult operation because of previous incisions and operative scars in the suprapubic region. It is an operation which should always be taken very seriously and not delegated to the least experienced member of the team. The chief danger is that one may fail to recognize a tethered loop of small intestine, stuck to the front of the bladder after previous infection or surgery, and make a small bowel fistula. The greater the experience of the urologist, the more wary he or she becomes of this operation.

Incision

6

A common error is to make the suprapubic incision too near the symphysis. It should be at least as high as the halfway point between umbilicus and symphysis, and in a chairbound patient even higher. Just as care is taken to site the opening of an ileal conduit to suit the contours of the patient's abdominal wall, especially in paraplegics, so care should be taken to ensure that the opening of the suprapubic cystotomy is accessible to the patient, and not hidden, kinked or covered by an apron of abdominal fat. Equally, the track of the suprapubic tube must not come too close to the cartilage of the symphysis pubis, or there is the risk of osteitis pubis and necrosis of the symphyseal cartilage.

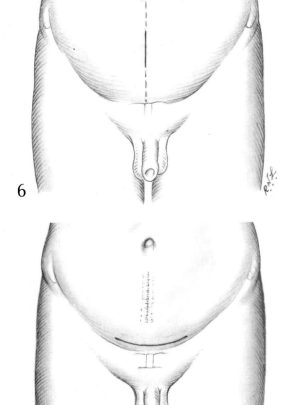

6

7a

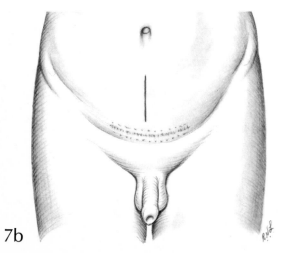

7b

7a & b

The surgeon must decide whether to make a midline or a Pfannenstiel incision. If there is a choice (i.e. if there are no previous scars), then a neat and unobtrusive incision is the Pfannenstiel (a). Otherwise, a vertical incision is used, its highest point coming at least halfway between umbilicus and symphysis (b).

A Pfannenstiel incision is made in the usual way. A vertical incision should be carried down in the midline through skin and subcutaneous fat, opening the linea alba in the midline and retracting the fascia laterally to expose the recti. These are separated and held in a self-retaining retractor.

8

The peritoneum is identified and wiped off the front of the bladder, which is already filled. This is by no means easy when the patient has been operated on before. The bladder is identified by its characteristic coarse crisscross muscle fibres, but if there is any uncertainty, its contents can be aspirated with a fine needle and syringe. It is vital at this stage to make quite certain that there is no risk of injuring the bowel.

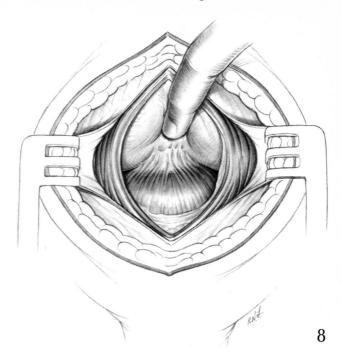

8

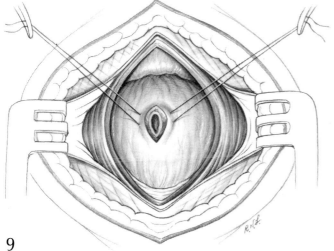

9

9

Once the bladder is identified, a pair of stay sutures are put in and it can be lifted up. The bladder is opened with a diathermy needle and the urine inside aspirated with a sucker.

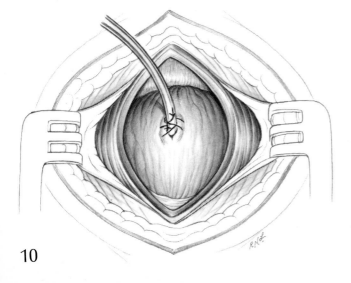

10

10

The catheter of choice can now be inserted. For most purposes a 20 Fr latex or silicone rubber catheter is ideal, either a Malecot or a Foley type. In either case, the catheter is secured to the skin with a strong suture for the first week.

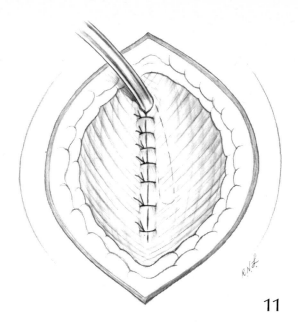

11

11 & 12

Closure

The wound is closed with interrupted chromic catgut sutures, never using any non-absorbable material. Closure is made over the catheter in such a way that the tube runs in a long oblique tunnel from bladder to the highest point of the midline incision, at least halfway from symphysis to umbilicus. If a Pfannenstiel incision has been used, the tunnel is made under the superior skin-and-muscle flap.

In hospital, the catheter is led to a sterile collecting bag, preferably containing a suitable antiseptic such as chlorhexidine or hydrogen peroxide. On going home, the patient may wear a portable bag of suitable design.

The suprapubic catheter should be changed roughly every 4 weeks where modern silicone rubber Foley-type catheters are used. The rate at which the catheter becomes encrusted and blocked with phosphatic debris varies from one patient to another.

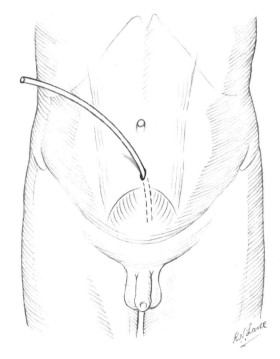

12

VESICOSTOMY

There is seldom a good indication for making a vesicostomy as a means of permanent urinary diversion. In selected patients, however, it may have a role[1,2], and the operation is one to be remembered for the exceptional case where it is indicated.

13

The bladder is exposed through the Pfannenstiel incision in the skin crease above the symphysis and a U-shaped flap of bladder formed between stay sutures. A U-shaped flap of skin is similarly outlined, taking care that this is given a broad base.

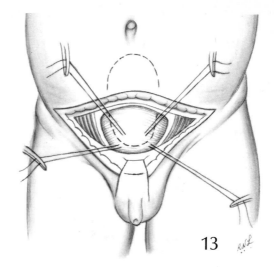

13

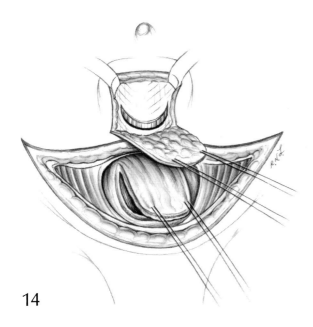

14

14

After elevating the full-thickness skin flap, a U-shaped incision is made in the rectus aponeurosis. The bladder flap is sewn to this in order to take tension off the subsequent suture line.

15 & 16

Then the skin flap is folded down under the fascia and sewn to the bladder, while the bladder flap is brought up and sewn to the skin, catgut being used throughout.

The advantage of this operation is that no indwelling catheter is required. The disadvantage is that patients are often not continent. For this reason Naudé's 'continent' tubed vesicostomy[3] offers certain advantages.

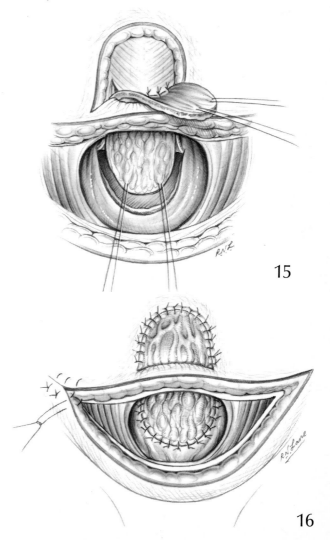

15

16

Naudés operation

17–20

In Naudé's operation the base of the bladder tube is sited inferiorly and the Boari-type bladder flap formed into a tube by sewing it around an inert splint of silicone rubber.

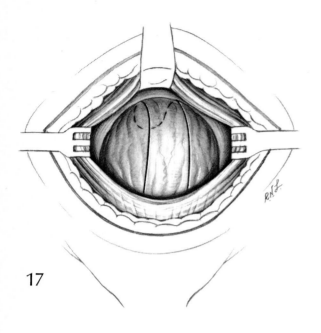

17

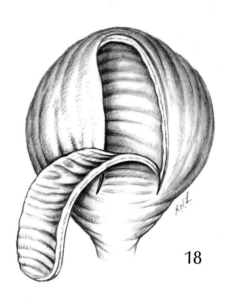

18

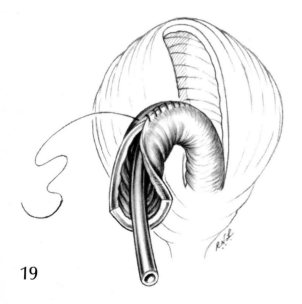

19

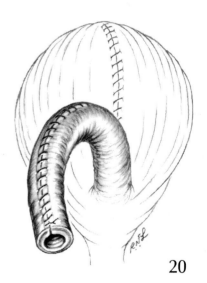

20

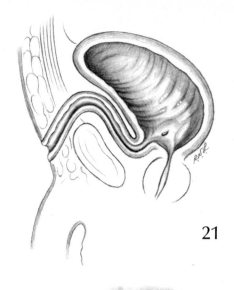

21

21 & 22

The tube is then brought above the symphysis and out through the skin near the base of the penis in males, or in females just within the vulva. In either sex the opening is inconspicious.

These patients are continent, but have no way of emptying the bladder voluntarily. Instead, they must use a catheter, but this is easily done in the privacy of the bathroom, and the diversion has the supreme advantage that it is invisible. It may, however, be necessary to perform a separate procedure to close off the urethra and bladder neck in some patients for whom this type of diversion is contemplated.

References

1. Lapides, J., Ajemian, E. P., Lichtwardt, J. R. Cutaneous vesicostomy. Journal of Urology 1960; 84; 609–614

2. Lapides, J. The abdominal neourethra. Journal of Urology 1966; 95: 350–355

3. Naudé, J. H. The hidden vesicostomy. British Journal of Urology 1982; 54: 686–688

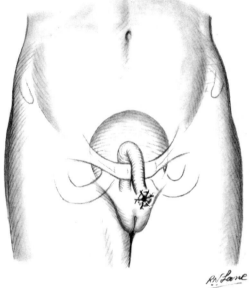

22

Illustrations by Robert N. Lane

Vesical lithotomy and diverticulectomy

John P. Blandy   MA, DM, MCh, FRCS
Professor of Urology, The London Hospital Medical College;
Consultant Urologist, St. Peter's Hospital, London, UK

Exposure of the bladder

1

For nearly all purposes the best approach to the urinary bladder is provided by Pfannenstiel's incision, though the very wide exposure required in a total cystectomy or evisceration may require a long midline or paramedian incision. If there has been a previous operation, one may just as well make use of the old scar.

The incision is placed in the skin crease just cephalad to the symphysis pubis. A common error is to site this incision too far cephalad: the convexity of the incision should be only 1.5 cm above the symphysis.

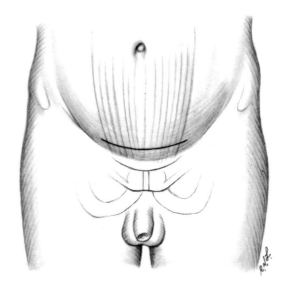

1

2

The incision is carried down through the fat, taking care to secure a constant superficial vein at each corner of the wound. Following the same line as the skin incision, the rectus aponeurosis is incised and its upper leaf elevated to display the recti and pyramidalis muscle, when present.

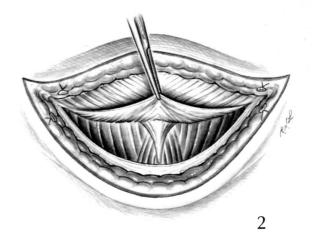

2

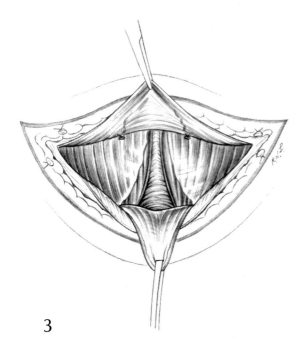

3

3

The upper leaf of rectus aponeurosis is dissected cranially, making sure that a constant artery entering its deep surface from the rectus muscle is coagulated before it is divided to avoid troublesome bleeding. Having elevated the upper leaf of aponeurosis, the pyramidalis is separated, and with it the lower leaf of rectus aponeurosis dissected off the inferior insertion of the rectus muscle bellies. A triangular defect is thus exposed, which may be entered with the finger, or occasionally with the touch of the knife.

The peritonal reflection is now swept upwards off the front of the bladder with a finger protected by a gauze swab. A Millin's self-retaining retractor or similar device is inserted to retract the muscle bellies of the rectus.

What follows at this stage must depend upon what has to be done to the bladder.

REMOVAL OF A BLADDER STONE

Although there are few calculi in adults which cannot be removed by means of the lithotrite, occasions arise when it is more convenient to remove them by cystotomy: want of experience or a suitable instrument, presence of multiple diverticula, or an intractable stricture of the urethra may make suprapubic lithotomy safer than an attempt at litholapaxy.

4

Two stay sutures are placed in the bladder, which has been displayed by means of the Pfannenstiel incision. The bladder is incised, preferably using the diathermy needle to avoid needless loss of blood. The urine is aspirated with the sucker.

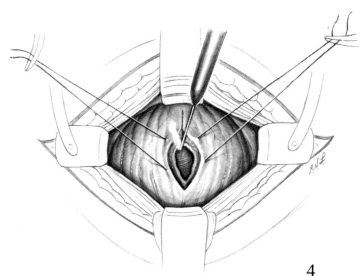

4

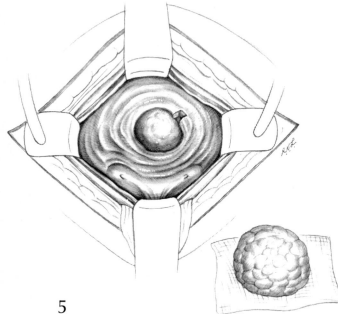

5

5

The Millin's retractor is now readjusted so as to reveal the calculus, which is lifted out. A biopsy should be taken of any suspicious area of adjacent vesical mucosa in view of the occasional complication of squamous carcinoma.

6

A self-retaining Foley catheter of appropriate size (e.g. 18–20 Fr) is left in the bladder, which is closed in one or two layers of continuous 3/0 chromic catgut.

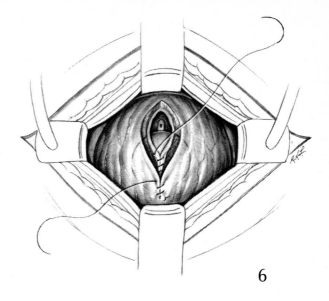

6

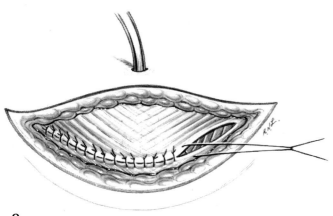

7

7 & 8

A tube drain (about 20 Fr) is led out through the upper skin flap from the suture line in the wall of the bladder and secured with a stitch. The muscle bellies of the rectus are approximated with one or two loosely tied catgut sutures, one of them catching up the apex of pyramidalis when it is present. The aponeurosis of the rectus is now closed with continuous or interrupted 3/0 catgut and the skin with interrupted silk or nylon.

In most cases where the bladder has been thus opened and closed, it is advisable to leave the urethral catheter in the bladder for 8 days, but the suprapubic wound drain may be taken out after 48 hours. The skin sutures are removed on the ninth or tenth day.

8

DIVERTICULECTOMY

There are few diverticula in which there is not an associated bladder outflow obstruction. In most instances this is caused by stenosis of the neck of the bladder, usually with some degree of hypertrophy of the prostate, and so it is usually futile to remove a diverticulum unless the obstruction at the bladder neck is dealt with as well.

Nowadays it is, in general, far more satisfactory to resect the obstructing bladder neck tissue transurethrally before opening the bladder to deal with the diverticulum, since a far more precise and controlled operation can be per-formed endoscopically than can be accomplished across the open bladder.

In the following description it has been assumed either that the bladder neck is normal, or that it has been dealt with already.

It is easier to perform the diverticulectomy if the bladder is filled with urine or saline before making the incision, which will be the Pfannenstiel approach unless there is a good reason to make a midline or paramedian incision.

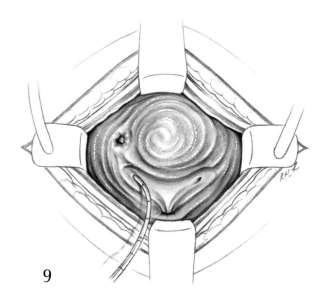

9

9

Once exposed the bladder is opened between two stay sutures and its contents aspirated as described above. One should take care not to bruise the trigone with the sucker, or else it may be difficult (particularly in a bladder which is already somewhat inflamed) to identify the orifices of the ureters. The next step is to catheterize the ureter or ureters on the side of the diverticulum or diverticula. Occasionally a ureter may be tightly bound to the wall of a diverticulum, and it is a considerable help to be able to feel a catheter in its lumen and know where the ureter is situated at any given moment in the subsequent dissection.

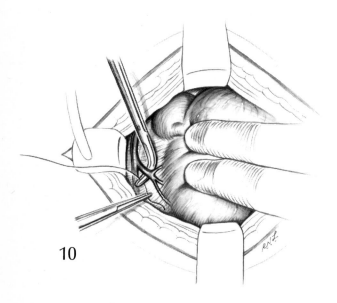

10

10

The second step is to mobilize the side of the bladder on which the diverticulum is situated. This is done by ligating the superior vesical pedicle, which is usually very easily found by following down the so-called obliterated umbilical artery. Once doubly ligated, the superior vesical leash is divided, and this simple manoeuvre liberates the bladder and allows the diverticulum to be rotated into the wound.

11

If the fundus of the diverticulum is easily identified, it should be seized with an Allis forceps. When its wall is thickened, inflamed and fibrotic, a more useful manoeuvre is to put a finger into its orifice via the opening which has been made into the bladder, and so identify it at its neck. The fibromuscular tissues which tether the neck of the diverticulum to the main part of the wall of the bladder are now dissected away, until the neck of the diverticulum has been opened, and the lumen of the bladder, or the operator's finger, can be seen. At this stage it is helpful to insert a 3/0 catgut suture, the start of the running stitch which will be used to close off the orifice of the diverticulum bit by bit as it is defined.

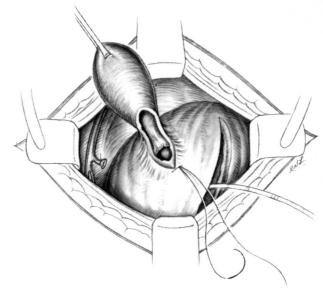

11

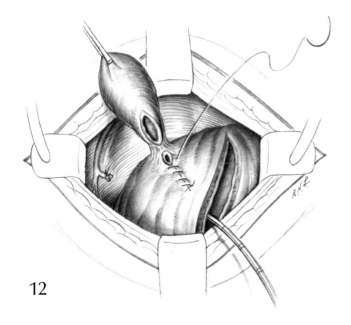

12

12

Eventually, in most cases, the diverticulum is left attached to the bladder only by a shred or two of fibrous tissue and muscle strands. The hole in the bladder wall is closed off with the running suture and the diverticulum detached and removed. Commonly, in a thickened and inflamed diverticulum of long standing, one must dissect it down, back and behind the bladder in order to remove it completely, and there are from time to time very difficult cases where it is surgical folly to continue with a difficult dissection and risk making an accidental hole in the anterior wall of the rectum. In such a case it is perfectly safe to leave the remnant of the fundus of the diverticulum *in situ*, and lead a drain out from that region. What is left of the diverticulum will be removed in the course of time by organization and the drain seldom discharges for more than a few days.

13 &14

Many diverticula are seen which are shallow and easily pulled inside out. So long as the ureter has been protected by means of a catheter this is a perfectly safe procedure, but it does not apply to any but small examples. The everted diverticulum is cut off and its base secured with a transfixion suture.

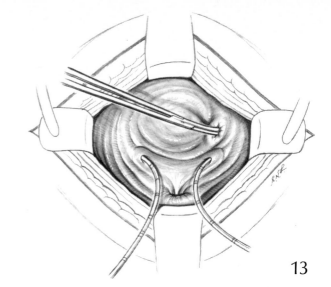

13

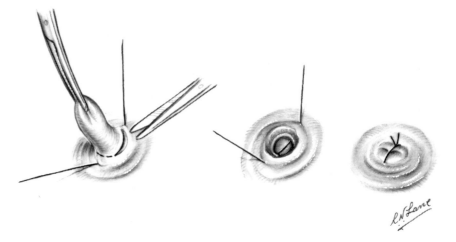

14

Cystoplasty

W. Gregoir MD
Chief of the Department of Urology, University of Brussels, Belgium

F. d'Udekem MD
Department of Urology, University of Brussels, Belgium

There are two types of cystoplasty, depending on whether the purpose is to enlarge or replace the bladder or, on the contrary, to reduce its size where it is congenitally enlarged or secondarily distended.

ENLARGEMENT OR SUBSTITUTION INTESTINOCYSTOPLASTY

Indications for enlargement

Enlargement of the bladder is indicated in all permanently contracted bladders severe enough to disrupt the patient's social life. The common pathological conditions are: tuberculosis; bilharziasis; interstitial cystitis (Hunner's ulcer) after failure of distension treatment and steroid therapy; rare cases of hypertonic neuropathic bladder; and late contraction following irradiation or chemical cystitis. In these conditions enlargement is indicated not only because of subjective symptoms, frequency and dysuria, which may become intolerable, but also because of upper tract damage. Any dilatation of the renal excretory system, either because of an obstruction or of reflux, is an imperative indication for enlargement: reimplantation of the obstructed ureter into the intestinal graft is an indispensable concomitant.

Indications for substitution

Disseminated papillomatosis or very superficial malignant metaplasia are the only justifiable indications for total replacement cystoplasty. Infiltrating malignant tumours requiring preoperative irradiation and radical cystectomy with lymphadenectomy are unsuitable and urinary diversion should be preferred. Even with appropriate indications, total replacement requires an intact external sphincter, absence of obstructive disease of the ureter, absence of pelvic irradiation and absence of neoplastic change in the urethra.

In the case of a superficial neoplastic lesion, radical cystectomy is performed, with removal of the prostate and the seminal vesicles, leaving as the basis for reconstruction the membranous urethra and in this event the risk of incontinence is considerable. In the case of totally benign papillomatosis, the bladder neck may be preserved and then only a simple subtotal cystectomy, without removal of the seminal vesicles should be performed. The risk of serious sphincteric disorder is then much smaller and, in some favourable cases, erection and ejaculation may be preserved.

Choosing the intestinal segment

A distinction should be made between enlargement and substitution cystoplasty. In the first case, any intestinal segment can be used. In the second, the choice must be determined by the physiological aspect of the intestinal graft. In vesical enlargement, the sphincteric mechanisms are not interfered with and the physiological properties of the graft should not be a cause for concern. The ileum, sigmoid and caecum are perfectly suitable reservoirs and hence their choice depends more on local conditions, mobility and mesenteric length. In substitution, on the contrary, the ileum, which is a transit organ, is less appropriate than the colon. When an isolated ileal loop is gradually filled, it shows an unceasing peristaltic activity, the amplitude of which increases as it becomes more distended. By contrast the physiological response of the colon is much more comparable to that of the vesical detrusor; it can easily be distended and can, without any reaction, almost reach its maximum capacity; it then reacts with a strong expelling contraction.

A preliminary radiological study of the intestine is indispensable to exclude diverticulosis or other abnormality.

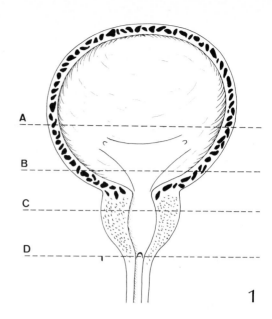

1

1

Intestinoplasty techniques

The difference between enlargement and substitution cystoplasty lies essentially in the level at which one performs the anastomosis between the intestinal segment and the urinary tract. Enlargement takes place after partial cystectomy, usually a hemicystectomy (A). Substitution is subtotal when the bladder neck is preserved but total when it is removed. Following resection, anastomosis between the graft and the urethra is performed either at the bladder neck (B), at the prostatic apex (C) or even in the membranous urethra (D).

It is mandatory in certain cases to remove completely the vesical lesion, especially when cystoplasty is performed in cases of interstitial cystitis, since if a lesion is left in the lower part of the bladder, as after hemicystectomy, pain and frequency will persist in spite of the enlargement.

Good vascularization is vital for the survival of an isolated intestinal graft. Its preparation involves precise examination of the mesentery by transillumination and the intestinal arteries are cut and tied with a view to preserving the maximum arterial supply to the graft. The technique for performing the graft is the same in principle whether enlargement or substitution is performed, but in the second case, the graft has to be lowered much further to the pelvic floor. An ileal segment can be lowered by a short transverse incision along the mesentery, but this involves some afferent arteries and is only safe provided their deficiency is compensated by more distal arcades. In order to lower the sigmoid colon, it is sometimes necessary to free the descending colon by incising the left paracolic groove and by freeing the splenic angle.

The length of the intestinal graft is varied according to the degree of enlargement to be obtained. The average for an ileal graft is 25 cm. The anastomosis between the intestine and the urinary tract should be in two layers: one joining the bladder adventitia or prostatic apex to the intestinal adventitia and the other an internal layer. Sutures are usually interrupted and must be of absorbable material.

Implantation of the ureter into the isolated graft can be carried out in different ways. The simplest is by bevelling the distal end of the ureter and passing it through an oblique tunnel in the intestinal wall, securing the end by a transfixing U-formed stitch. Alternatively an end-to-side elliptical anastomosis in one layer with interrupted sutures may be performed, or, where the ureter is grossly dilated, an end-to-end implantation into the proximal end of the graft which is closed in a racket-shaped suture line. It is not essential to drain reimplanted ureters by ureteric catheters, but it is a safe practice as it prevents urine leaks through the sutures during the first days after the operation. Moreover, it allows easier monitoring of individual kidney function.

Preoperative

The patient is placed on a low-residue diet for 3 or 4 days before the operation and undergoes systematic intestinal disinfection: 3 g sulfaguanidine per day will suffice. Antibiotics which disturb the intestinal flora should be rejected. When the use of colon is considered, the patient should undergo extensive washouts during the 2 days preceding the operation.

The operations

ELARGEMENT ILEOCYSTOPLASTY

2

The abdominal incision is subumbilical and median. The peritoneum on the vesical dome is incised transversely and pushed back off both sides of the bladder. The detrusor cap is cut off (in a case of upper hemicystectomy). It may be necessary because of vesical lesions to perform a more extensive resection and an intestinal graft should never be implanted into a simple incision on the vesical dome, because this is followed by rapid constriction of the anastomosis.

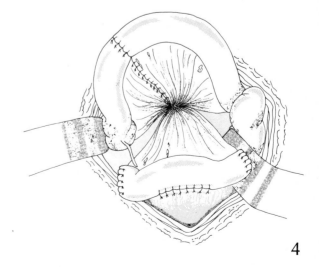

2

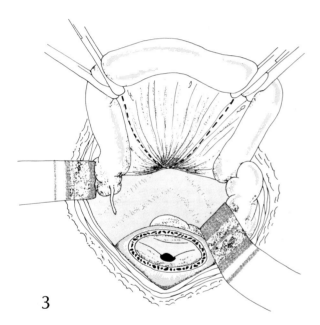

3

3

The ileal graft is usually taken from the last or last but one loop. The mesenteric vessels are individually ligated and great care is taken to preserve the vascularization of the graft. Intestinal continuity is re-established by an end-to-end ileoileal anastomosis with interrupted sutures, using one layer of 3/0 silk. The mesenteric defect under this anastomosis is carefully closed on both aspects to avoid internal hernia formation.

4

When only a portion of the detrusor cap has been removed, the anastomosis is carried out in two layers after opening the intestine on its antimesenteric edge. One layer is peritoneal and involves the vesical peritoneum on one hand and the intestinal serosa on the other. The second layer is total. Wound drainage is not required, but a catheter should be left in the bladder.

4

When a larger vesical resection is performed, the posterior peritoneum should be sutured first to the posterior side of the mesentery. The graft should then be anastomosed in two layers and finally the front part of the peritoneum should be sutured to the front of the mesentery. The anastomosis alone can be extraperitonealized, leaving both extremities of the graft free in the abdominal cavity. Complete extraperitonealization involves the risk that the graft will be constricted by subperitoneal sclerosis. In this case, the rigid and flattened loop loses its function and the benefit of the operation vanishes.

The bladder neck deserves very careful investigation. The slightest sclerosis requires resection of the posterior lip, as even a minor obstruction here inevitably causes retention in a bladder the wall of which consists of intestine.

5–8

Technical variants

The intestinovesical anastomosis may be carried out in a form of a U or a J (*Illustrations 5* and *6*). The bladder may also be enlarged by the intestinal patch or open flap technique (*Illustrations 7* and *8*). From the functional point of view, however, there does not seem to be any salient advantage to these methods. The J form is mainly indicated in cases which it is necessary to replace a ureter at the same time as enlarging the bladder.

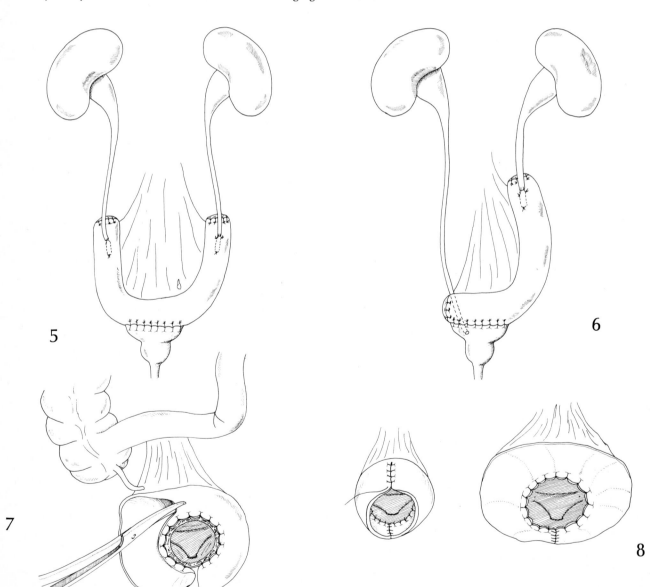

5

6

7

8

SUBSTITUTION SIGMOIDOCYSTOPLASTY

The classical Gil-Vernet method for total substitution of the bladder by a sigmoid graft is performed as follows.

9

The abdomen is opened through a paramedian incision and the dome of the bladder freed from the pelvic peritoneum so that an extraperitoneal cystectomy can be performed. When the bladder neck can be preserved the bladder is incised just above the vesicoprostatic groove. An incision is carried round laterally and posteriorly, leaving only the bladder neck after removing its mucosa. Next the posterior aspect of the bladder is dissected backwards, passing the cleavage plane between the bladder and the seminal vesicles, which are left in place. The peritoneum is incised transversely to allow for the passage of the sigmoid loop.

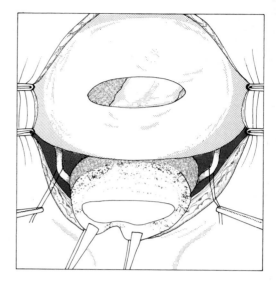

9

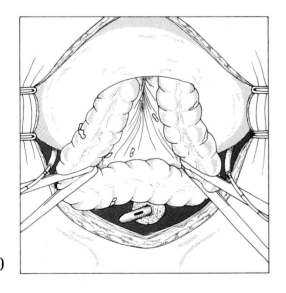

10

10

Once the cystectomy has been completed, the sigmoid is lowered through the peritoneal opening. The graft, 15 cm or more in length, is isolated in the position that allows easiest mobilization. Colonic continuity is re-established by end-to-end anastomosis and the isolated graft is completely extraperitonealized by suturing the anterior and posterior peritoneum to the mesosigmoid.

11

Both ends of the graft are closed, but an opening is made in the middle to facilitate reimplantation of the ureters into the posterior aspect. Indwelling ureteric catheters are placed in position and taken out through the urethra.

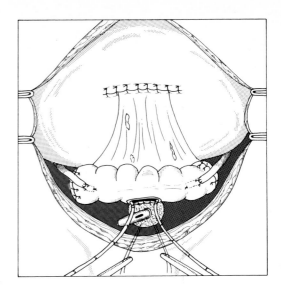

11

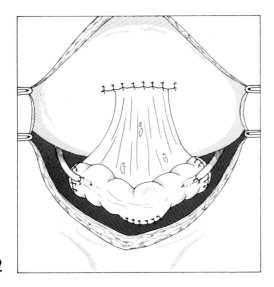

12

12

The anastomosis between the graft and the prostatic apex or the urethra is performed using two layers of interrupted sutures with 2/0 chromic catgut. A urethral catheter is placed alongside the ureteric catheters and drainage of the pelvic cavity is ensured by two lateral drains.

CAECOCYSTOPLASTY

The isolated caecum may be used to enlarge or replace the bladder. The ileum is sectioned a little above the ileocaecal valve, an appendicectomy is performed and the caecum is isolated from the ascending colon at a level corresponding to the desired capacity. Intestinal continuity is re-established by ileocolic or ileotransverse anastomosis.

13 & 14

A 180° rotation allows the caecum to be anastomosed to the dome of the bladder. The ureter is implanted into the terminal ileum. If necessary the ileum may be used to replace the entire right ureter up to the renal pelvis or to replace both ureters up to the lumbar level. The caecocystoplasty is, therefore, particularly useful when vesical enlargement must be combined with a ureteric substitution. The ileocaecal valve has the added advantage of preventing or reducing or reducing reflux into the ureters.

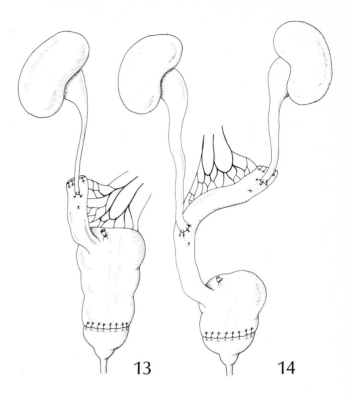

13   14

Postoperative care

Anal dilatation at the end of the operation facilitates emptying of the rectosigmoid. Gastric intubation is maintained for 3–4 days until satisfactory resumption of peristalsis. Extensive antibiotic coverage is initiated for 24 hours before operation and carried on afterwards. The ureteric catheters are maintained in place for 5–8 days if possible, but if they become obstructed they are removed. The urethral catheter is removed on the 12th day. Until that time it may require irrigation because it is frequently obstructed by mucous plugs. These sometimes require irrigation with saturated bicarbonate solution. Regular estimations of serum electrolytes must be performed during the first 5–6 postoperative days and note must be taken of the possible loss of proteins in the intestinal secretion which can cause a fall in plasma protein levels. This can be remedied by infusing 1 litre of human plasma or its equivalent in albumin.

REDUCTION CYSTOPLASTY

The purpose of reduction cystoplasty is to decrease the size of an excessively distended bladder while preserving the whole detrusor, with the aim of obtaining better evacuation. The theoretical advantage of reduction over simple partial cystectomy is complete preservation of the detrusor. The thickness of the latter will be doubled, at least over a large part of the wall. Indications are rare and limited to examples of severe and persistent disorders of evacuation following adequate removal of bladder outflow obstruction. Thus there are occasional cases of bladders of enormous capacity and persistent retention following prostatectomy, after a long period of catheterization. There are also a few examples of congenital megabladders which cannot be emptied satisfactorily either by manual pressure or by bladder neck resection and reduction cystoplasty may be justifiable.

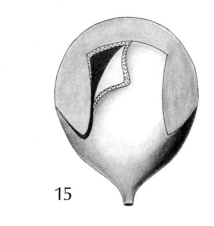

15

15 & 16

After median subumbilical incision, the dome of the bladder is completely freed from the peritoneum and the sides of the bladder are cleared. The bladder is incised following a specific 'tennis ball' pattern after locating the angles of its outline. The bladder is then widely opened and shows three flaps: one anteroinferior flap and two lateral flaps.

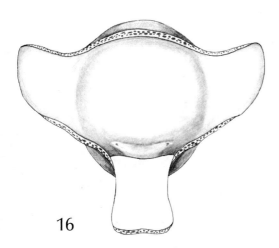

16

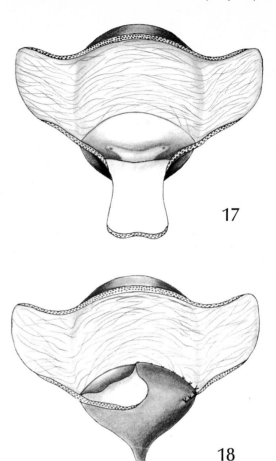

17

18

17 & 18

The whole mucosal lining of the vesical dome is then cut away from the lateral flaps and on the posterior side of the bladder up to a horizontal line passing 3 cm above the ureteric orifices. The bladder base mucosa and the anterior flap mucosa are spared. The peeling of this mucosa can sometimes be very difficult, especially in late cases involved in long-standing inflammatory disease. The operation may sometimes be facilitated by infiltrating the submucosa with a saline solution.

After removing the mucosa, the anterior flap is folded back and sutured (2/0 chromic catgut) on to the posterior side of the bladder along the line of the preserved mucosa. When this suture is completed, a new vesical cavity has been formed.

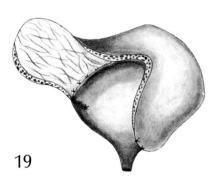

19

19 & 20

A large flap which remains from the lateral and posterior detrusor is then brought down to the front and the lateral sides of the bladder. The lateral flaps are sutured to one another in the midline and their lower edges are fastened to the bladder as close as possible to the bladder neck. Thus the newly formed bladder has a double muscle wall almost everywhere. The bladder is drained by an indwelling catheter for 12 days and a suction drain is placed between the two layers of the detrusor. Retropubic drainage is maintained for 2–3 days.

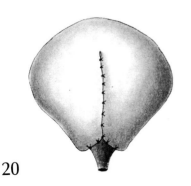

20

Further reading

Annis, D. The use of the isolated ileal segment in urology. British Journal of Urology 1956; 28: 351–362

Bourque, J. P. The indications and techniques of bowel substitution after total cystectomy: preliminary report on 25 cases. British Journal of Urology 1959; 31: 448–460

Cibert, J. Le greffon iléal en urologie d'après 105 observations personnelles. Urologia internationalis 1957; 4: 193–216

Cibert, J. L'entérocystoplastie dans le traitement de la cystite chronique tuberculeuse. Journal d'Urologie et de Néphrologic 1965; 71: 373–406

Cukier, J. Les remplacements de la vessie. In: Congrès Français d'Urologie, 6le session, Paris 1967

Gil-Vernet, J. M. Technique for construction of a functioning artificial bladder. Journal of Urology 1960; 83: 39–50

Gil-Vernet, J. M. The ileocolic segment in urologic surgery. Journal of Urology 1965; 94: 418–426

Goodwin, W. E., Winter, C. C., Turner, R. D. Replacement of the ureter by small intestine: clinical application and results of the 'ileal ureter'. Journal of Urology 1959; 81: 406–418

Heitz-Boyer, M., Hovelacque, A. Création d'une nouvelle vessie et d'un nouvel urèthre. Journal d'Urologie Médicale et Chirurgicale 1912; 1: 237–258

Küss. R., de Tourris, H., Genon, M. Une technique de colo-cystoplastie. Journal de Chirurgie 1959; 77: 423–431

Leadbetter, W. F., Clarke, B. G. Five years' experience with ureteroenterostomy by the 'combined' technique. Journal of Urology 1955; 73: 67–82

Lowsley, O. S., Johnson, T. H. A new operation for creation of an artificial bladder with voluntary control of urine and faeces. Journal of Urology 1955; 73: 83–90

Mogg, R. A. Treatment of urinary incontinence using the colonic conduit. Journal of Urology 1967; 97: 684–692

Moonen, W. A., Linssen, P. A. Geschichte der Intestinoplastiken. Urologia Internationalis 1962; 14: 173–192

Moulonguet, A. Sur la physio-pathologie de la vessie de substitution. Journal d'Urologie et de Néphrologic 1967; 73: 413–423

Murphy, J. J. Bladder substitutes. American Journal of the Medical Sciences 1956; 231: 212–217

Scheele, K. Ueber die Vergrösserungsplastik der narbigen Schrumpfblase. Beiträge zür Klinische Chirurgie 1923; 129: 414–422

Zingg, E. J. Rekonstruktion der Harnblase in Experiment und Klinik. Urologia Internationalis 1969; 24: 193–275

Illustrations by Robert N. Lane

Segmental bladder resection

John R. Richardson, Jr MD
Clinical Associate Professor of Urology,
Dartmouth-Hitchcock Medical Center, Hanover, New Hampshire, USA

Introduction

Partial resection of the bladder is most often done for invasive but localized cancer. The development and perfecting of the cystoscope in the early 20th century made it possible to diagnose these lesions and plan elective surgical removal. In 1956 Marshall published his classic monograph on segmental resection of bladder cancers, demonstrating impressive 5-year survivals in this group of patients[1]. The ideal candidate appears to be one with a single tumour mass, not amenable to transurethral resection, less than 6 cm in size, without a history of recurrent bladder cancer, and located in the mobile portion of the bladder where it is possible to get a 2–3 cm margin of resection[2,3]. Such patients are quite uncommon in our practice and this operation is infrequently performed at our institution. The aim of surgery is to remove the tumour completely, with an adequate resection margin, while preserving voiding and sexual functions. If the resection would require ureteroneocystostomy or bladder augmentation, then segmental resection is not indicated.

Preoperative

The preoperative preparation is similar to that for any major pelvic surgery. Careful medical evaluation is mandatory. Specific testing should include intravenous pyelography, cystoscopy under anaesthesia with bimanual examination of the bladder, and tests appropriate to rule out distant metastatic disease. Computed tomography of the pelvis should be considered. Bladder function and capacity should be reasonably normal. Preoperative antibiotics are used in the presence of urinary tract infection. Normally this surgery is done under general anaesthesia, although in certain circumstances a regional technique may be prefered.

The operation

The patient is placed on the table in the supine position with the head lower than the feet. An appropriate sized Foley catheter is passed through the urethra and draped into the field. A generous lower abdominal incision is utilized. We prefer the midline approach, allowing extension cephalad if necessary. The bladder is filled with 300 ml of sterile water and approached through the suprapubic incision in the usual fashion. The anterior and lateral surfaces of the bladder are bluntly exposed using finger dissection with gauze. The space of Retzius is developed and the bladder is bluntly swept from the lateral pelvic walls. A self-retaining retractor is placed within the incision and the bladder is packed away from the surrounding tissues. Knowing the cystoscopic location of the tumour, one can enter the bladder well away from the lesion.

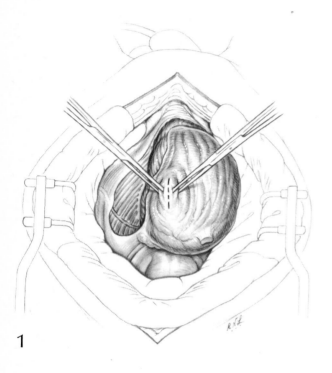

1

1

The bladder wall is grasped between two pairs of Allis forceps, drained of fluid per urethral catheter, and entered with a scalpel. This opening is elongated, with the operator's two index fingers providing traction inferiorly and superiorly. This manoeuvre provides an adequate bladder opening with minimal bleeding.

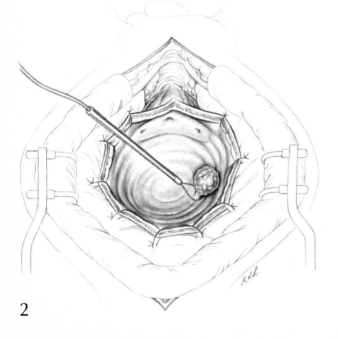

2

2

Full-thickness stay sutures of 0 silk are then placed through the bladder wall and sutured to the surrounding drapes. This is done to provide good exposure and to avoid spillage of tumour cells in the perivesical area. The decision as to operability is made at this time. One needs to be certain that the lesion is grossly confined to the bladder and that a 2 cm resection margin is possible. The lesion itself is then gently grasped and removed with large loop electroresection.

3

The portion of the bladder wall containing the tumour mass is then grasped with forceps and excised with the electrosurgical knife. This minimizes bleeding and spillage of tumour cells. After removal of the specimen, frozen section biopsies are taken of the remaining bladder wall nearest the lesion. If the biopsies are positive, further portions of the bladder wall are excised. If no tumour is found, closure is begun.

We prefer a two-layer closure with a running suture of 3/0 chromic catgut on the bladder mucosa and interrupted 0 chromic catgut sutures through the remaining bladder wall. We do not use suprapubic tubes routinely because of the danger of spreading tumour cells. A Penrose drain is left in the space of Retzius. A No. 24 Foley catheter is left indwelling in the urethra to drain the bladder. The remainder of the incision is closed in the standard fashion.

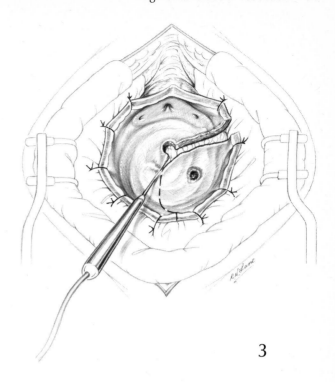

3

Postoperative care

Appropriate postoperative antibiotics are utilized until 48 hours after removal of the Foley catheter. Bladder spasms are controlled with opium and belladonna suppositories and occasionally with oral parasympatholitics. The Foley catheter is left in place for 7–10 days and removed after a cystogram has demonstrated an intact bladder. Patients are followed with intermittent cystoscopic examinations in the same fashion as those who have had a transurethral resection of their bladder tumours. In carefully selected patients, this operation seems to provide as good cancer control, stage for stage, as simple and radical cystectomy[1-4].

References

1. Marshall, V. F., Holden, J., Ma, K. T. Survival of patients with bladder carcinoma treated by simple segmental resection. Cancer 1956; 9: 568–571

2. Brannan, W., Ochsner, M. G., Fuselier, H. A., Jr., Landry, G. R. Partial cystectomy in the treatment of transitional cell carcinoma of the bladder. Journal of Urology 1978; 119: 213–215

3. Leadbetter, W. F. Bladder malignancies In: Glenn, J. F., Boyce, W. H., eds. Urologic surgery, 2nd ed. New York: Harper & Row, 1975: 323–347

4. Whitmore, W. F. The treatment of bladder tumours. Surgical Clinics of North America 1969; 49: 349–370

Illustrations by Robert N. Lane

Simple and radical cystectomy

John R. Richardson, Jr MD
Clinical Associate Professor of Urology,
Dartmouth-Hitchcock Medical School, Hanover, New Hampshire, USA

Introduction

In the first half of the 20th century, the development of satisfactory techniques of urinary diversion made the operation of cystectomy increasingly attractive to surgeons as a means of treating patients with invasive bladder cancer. The Bricker ileal conduit, described in 1950, has been the standard diversionary procedure[1]. Recently, colon conduits have enjoyed increasing use, although their superiority over the ileal operation has been disputed[2]. The addition of lymph node dissection and various doses of radiation therapy to this operation seems to increase patient survival in certain circumstances, but routine use of these modalities remains controversial[3,4,5].

1

In our hands, simple cystectomy in the male means removal of the bladder with a portion of overlying pelvic peritoneum, ureteral stumps, prostate, seminal vesicles and a portion of the membranous urethra.

2

In the female patient, the uterus, ovaries, Fallopian tubes and a portion of the vaginal vault and urethra are included in the surgical specimen.

Radical cystectomy denotes the addition of bilateral pelvic lymphadenectomy of the iliac and obturator regions to simple cystectomy. This operation is designed to remove the entire bladder, adjacent organs and the immediate lymphatic drainage areas in one surgical specimen[6]. Indications include localized invading cancers, rapidly recurring superficial cancers and endoscopically unresectable lesions[3,4]. Sexual and voiding functions are sacrificed.

Preoperative

The patient must be an acceptable medical risk for major surgery. Preoperative studies include intravenous pyelography, cystoscopy with biopsy, pelvic examination under anaesthesia and studies to rule out the presence of metastatic disease. Computed tomography of the pelvis has yet to be proved an adequate tool for staging bladder cancer[7]. In patients with normal history, physical examination, liver function tests and alkaline phosphatase levels, liver and bone scans have ordinarily not been helpful in preoperative staging[8].

Any of the standard mechanical bowel preparation routines is satisfactory. This is begun 3 days prior to surgery. We have not used routine digitalization and anticoagulation preoperatively. It is important to instruct the patient in the use of the incentive spirometer preoperatively.

Plans for location of the urinary stoma are begun a few days prior to the operation in order to familiarize the patient with the concept and appliances and to locate a satisfactory site. We try to select a flat area in the right or left lower quadrant below the belt line. The patient is asked to wear a smooth non-adherent face plate with a belt and ordinary clothes for a day – standing, sitting and lying down – in order to locate the most suitable stomal

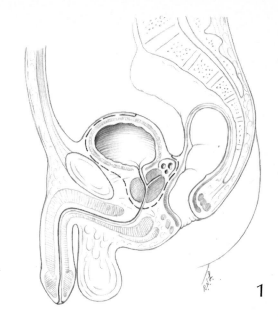

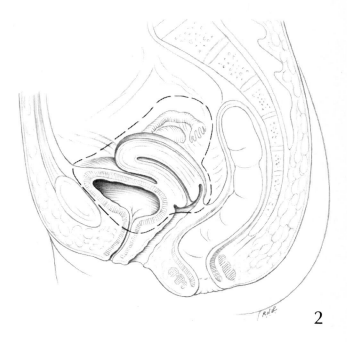

area. This is then marked with a skin pencil and inscribed with a needle in the operating room prior to skin preparation.

In cases of nutritional deficiency, hyperalimentation seems to be indicated preoperatively. Intravenous fluids are begun the night prior to surgery to avoid the hypovolaemia sometimes associated with bowel preparation.

Ordinarily the operation is performed with a single team, although a two-team approach may be useful in some situations. Concurrent urethrectomy is performed in some patients. A general anaesthetic technique is employed. Without excellent anaesthetic support and the presence of an intensive care unit, the surgeon operates at his and the patient's peril.

The operation

The patient is placed on the table in the supine head-down position, so that the intestines gravitate to the upper abdomen. The penis in the male and the vagina in the female are prepared and draped into the operative field. A 20 Fr foley catheter is inserted *per urethram* into the bladder. A midline abdominal incision is made from the upper abdomen to the pubis, skirting the umbilicus and at least 4–5 cm away from the medial aspect of the preselected stomal site. The peritoneal cavity is entered and a careful abdominal and pelvic exploration is carried out. Specific attention is paid to the iliac and obturator node-bearing areas. Frozen section specimens of any suspicious tissues are obtained, and the operation is usually terminated if there is gross evidence of metastic disease. If not, the cystectomy is begun.

A large self-retaining Balfour retractor is placed in the lower portion of the wound. Intestines are packed superiorly using three laparotomy pads and a rolled cloth towel in an inverted U-position. Next the peritoneum overlying the distal ureters is incised. On the left, one must be lateral to the sigmoid colon. The ureters are bluntly freed posteriorly, with finger dissection, from the kidney to the deep pelvis. Care is taken to preserve as much blood supply as possible. The ureters are then divided deep in the pelvis and the distal stumps are ligated with 0 chromic catgut. Sections of the proximal ureter are sent for frozen section diagnosis. If these ends are found to be healthy, they are then ligated with 4/0 chromic catgut ligatures. We believe the resulting dilatation that occurs prior to construction of the conduit facilitates the anastomosis of the ureters to the bowel; it is not associated with an increased incidence of leakage or stricture at the ureteral intestinal sites.

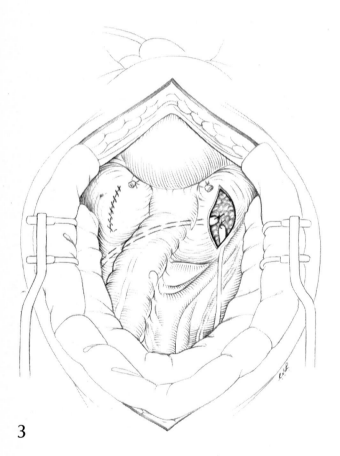

3

3

Next, using two fingers, a tunnel is made beneath the mesentery of the sigmoid colon connecting the two incisions in the posterior peritoneum. Care is taken to avoid mesenteric vessels. The left ureter is then drawn through the tunnel in a gentle arc to the peritoneal incision on the right side. One must take care to avoid excessive angulation of the left ureter which could lead to obstruction. The left peritoneal incision is closed with a running suture of 3/0 chromic catgut. The ureters remain in the right posterior peritoneal incision during the cystectomy.

4a, b & c

Using blunt dissection, the space of Retzius is developed and the bladder is separated from the lateral pelvic walls, the peritoneum being swept superiorly (*a*). The dissection is carried as far distally as the urethral catheter. The presence of the sigmoid colon makes the left side dissection somewhat more difficult. These manoeuvres are easier if the bladder has been partially filled with sterile water. At the completion of the dissection, the bladder is allowed to drain.

In the male, a generous area of pelvic peritoneum overlying the dome and posterior wall of the bladder is incised using the scalpel (*b*). The midpoint should be 2–3 cm above the peritoneal reflection in the pouch of Douglas. On both sides the vas deferens and any surrounding vessels are ligated and divided. Any remaining tissues in this area are bluntly swept towards the bladder until the lateral vesical pedicles are approached. The deep pelvic peritoneum is then sharply dissected in the midline inferiorly from the bladder for a distance of 4–5 cm (*c*). This provides a layer between the bladder wall and the rectum.

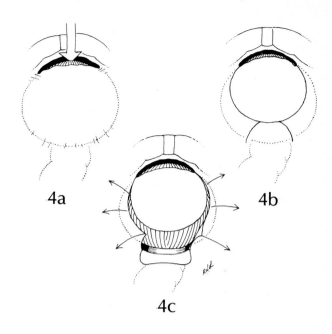

4a

4b

4c

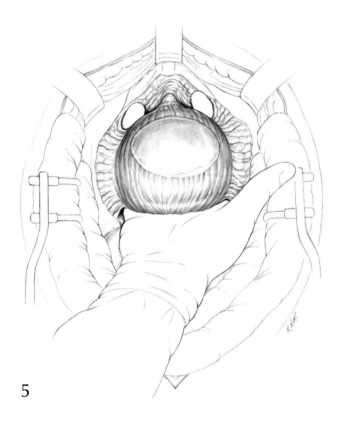

5

5

The upturned fingers and hand are worked bluntly beneath the bladder superficial to the rectum as far distally as the prostate and the urethra. With this manoeuvre two lateral wings of tissue are created containing the blood supply and lymphatic drainage of the bladder. This dissection must be done gently to avoid rectal damage, entry into the bladder and bleeding from torn veins in the area.

6

In the female, the pelvic peritoneal incisions encompass the ovaries and tubes laterally and the uterus and vaginal vault posteriorly. The bladder is freed laterally as in the male, taking care to divide and ligate the ovarian and uterine arteries and the round ligaments. Instead of creating the inferior rectovesical plane as in the male, the upper vagina and cervix are located by palpation and the vaginal vault is entered. A sponge soaked in iodine solution and inserted into the vagina preoperatively renders this manoeuvre easier and safer. The vaginal cuff is incised and whip-stitched to control bleeding. The anterior wall of the vagina is then sharply dissected from the bladder base and upper urethra containing the catheter, which can be located by palpation. When this has been done, two lateral wings of tissue containing the bladder blood supply and lymphatic drainage are created.

If pelvic lymphadenectomy is planned, it is carried out at this time. The left side is approached first as the presence of the sigmoid colon makes this dissection somewhat more difficult. The left external iliac artery is palpated on the lateral pelvic wall, and is approached with sharp dissection as far distally as the area of the inferior epigastric artery and circumflex iliac vein. Here the distal margin is marked with a silver clip. The use of these ligating clips makes the node dissection faster, easier and safer than the use of clamps and ligatures.

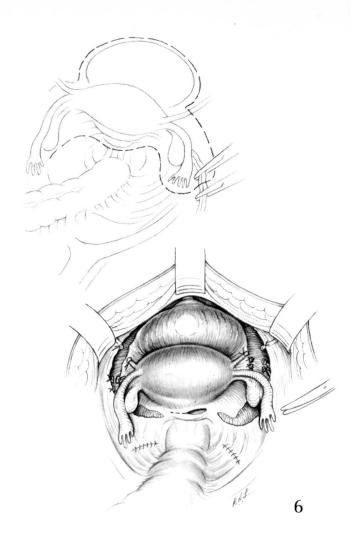

6

7

Metzenbaum scissors are then directed proximally along the wall of the artery and the overlying tissue is incised to an area just above the bifurcation of the common iliac artery. The proper plane is as close to the arterial wall as possible.

The medial and lateral tissue masses thus created are drawn inferiorly along the vessel. Vein retractors and peanut dissectors are helpful in this manoeuvre. An identical procedure is performed on the iliac vein, which lies just below the artery. Now the mass of tissue which lies below the external iliac vein is excised distally after clipping and is drawn inferomedially towards the bladder. At the bifurcation of the common iliac artery, nodal tissue is teased from the crotch. The dissection is carried down the internal iliac artery sweeping lymph-bearing tissue medially. The first two anterior branches of this artery, the superior and inferior vesical arteries, are then ligated with 2/0 silk. This deprives the bladder of its major blood supply. The tissues from the anterior portion of the internal iliac vein are likewise swept medially. Below the external iliac vein, the obturator nerve is located first by palpation and then by dissection. This is the lateral boundary of the deep node dissection. Fat- and lymph-bearing tissue is then teased from the obturator fossa with forceps and pushed medially together with the external and internal iliac specimens.

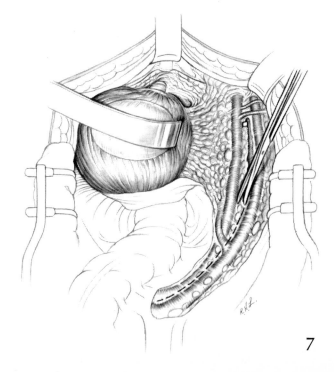

7

8

When this dissection is completed, the lateral pelvic walls and vessels should be clear of lymph-bearing tissue from just proximal to the inguinal ligament to an area just proximal to the common iliac artery bifurcation. All tissues, having been pushed medially, are removed with the bladder specimen. The same dissection is carried out on the right side.

Next the cystectomy proper is begun. If a pelvic node dissection has not been done, the internal iliac artery is exposed and the first two anterior branches are divided. Then the urethral Foley is palpated and a right-angle clamp is driven through the avascular endopelvic fascia lateral to the urethra in the female and lateral to the puboprostatic ligaments in the male. This marks the distal extent of the lateral pelvic wings of tissue on each side.

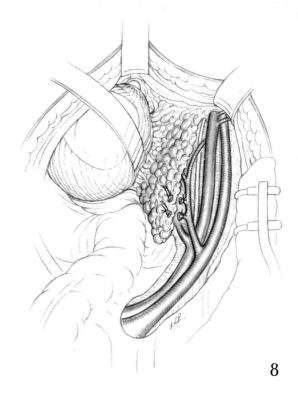

8

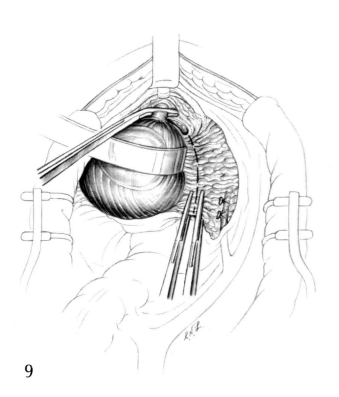

9

9

These wings are divided and suture-ligated with 0 chromic catgut between Kocher clamps. The area to be clamped is carefully palpated prior to placement of the clamps in order to avoid entering either the bladder or the rectum. When this has been accomplished, the specimen is free except for the urethra and periurethral attachments.

In the male, the puboprostatic ligaments are then sharply divided. The resultant bleeding is controlled with pressure. We have had little success in trying to suture-ligate these ligaments and the veins beneath. The urethra is then grasped with a large right-angle clamp, distal to the prostate in the male, taking care to avoid the rectum. In the female, the urethra is grasped distal to the bladder neck. The urethra is then sharply divided distal to the clamp along with the indwelling Foley catheter. This manoeuvre is not carried out if total urethrectomy is indicated.

10

The surgical specimen is removed and a 24 Fr Foley catheter with a 30 ml bag is inserted into the pelvis via the urethral remnant. The bag is inflated with 50 ml of saline and drawn down against the pelvic floor with traction, being held in place by a ring forceps applied to the catheter at the external urethral meatus. This manoeuvre successfully controls bleeding from the periurethral tissues deep in the pelvis.

The rectosigmoid is carefully inspected to make sure it is intact and a diligent search is made to locate any bleeding points in the pelvis. These are controlled with ligatures and electrocautery. Two moist laparotomy pads are then placed in the pelvis to remain there for the rest of the procedure. Appendicectomy is undertaken at this time in the standard fashion.

After the conduit has been constructed the pelvic packs are removed and a final search is made to discover any significant bleeding. Tension on the urethral Foley is removed and the periurethral area is checked to make sure there is no significant ooze. When the surgeon is satisfied, closure is begun. A nasogastric tube is placed in the stomach by the anaesthetist, the location being checked by the surgeon. Infrequently we have used gastrostomy tubes. The wound is closed with No. 2 stay sutures placed 2 cm apart through all layers of the abdominal wall, taking care not to injure the conduit or its blood supply. We place these retention sutures close together in order to provide uniform wound support and to avoid evisceration should wound infection and dehiscence occur. The peritoneal remnants, rectus fascia and subcutaneous tissues are closed in layers with absorbable sutures. A visceral retainer protects the intestines from becoming lodged between the retention sutures during the closure. The skin is closed with staples and the retention sutures are tied over two fingers of the assistant using segments of rubber catheter as bolsters. A minimal dressing is applied.

Postoperative care

Appropriate antibiotics are administered for 7–10 days. Early ambulation is essential, as is vigorous pulmonary support. The nasogastric tube is removed when the patient has passed gas or had a bowel movement. The average hospital stay is 14–18 days.

Complications have occurred in about a third of our patients. Common early problems are wound infection, prolonged ileus and ureteral intestinal leaks. Common late problems are small bowel and ureteral obstruction and stomal difficulties. The use of radiation therapy seems to increase the surgical complication rate.

In our hands, this is usually a long, difficult, tedious and bloody operation. Aggressive surgical techniques and excellent anaesthetic, medical and nursing support are essential if a good result is to be obtained. These patients require more frequent follow-up than most. About half survive for 5 years, most dying of distant metastatic

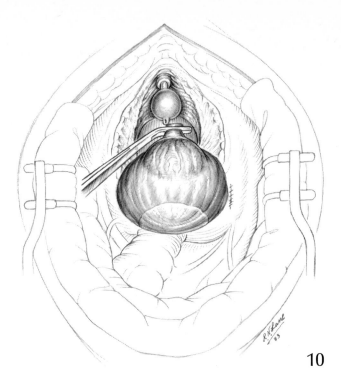

10

disease. Further increases in survival rates will probably be achieved only with the development of effective systemic anticancer therapy. Nevertheless, we feel that this surgical procedure, with or without presently available adjuvant therapy, offers most patients with aggressive and invasive bladder cancer the best chance for prolonged survival with an acceptable quality of life.

References

1. Bricker, E. M. Bladder substitution after pelvic evisceration. Surgical Clinics of North America 1950; 30: 1511–1521

2. Sullivan, J. W., Grabstald, H., Whitmore, W. F., Jr. Complications of ureteroileal conduit with radical cystectomy. Review of 336 cases. Journal of Urology 1980; 124: 797–801

3. Mathur, V. K., Krahn, H. P., Ramsey, E. W. Total cystectomy for bladder cancer. Journal of Urology 1981; 125: 784–786

4. Radwin, H. M. Invasive transitional cell carcinoma of the bladder: is there a place for preoperative radiotherapy? Urologic Clinics of North America October 1980; 7: 551–557

5. Heney, N, M., Prout, G. R., Jr. Preoperative irradiation as an adjuvant in the surgical management of patients with invasive bladder cancer. Urologic Clinics of North America 1980; 7: 543–549

6. Prout, G. R. The surgical management of bladder cancer. Urologic Clinics of North America 1976; 3: 149–175

7. Koss, J. C., Arger, P. H., Coleman, B. G., Mulhern, C. B., Pollack, H. M., Wein, A. J. CT staging of bladder carcinoma. American Journal of Roentgeneology 1981; 137. 359–362

8. Berger, G. L., Sadlowski, R. W., Sharpe, J. R., Finney, R. P. Lack of value of routine preoperative bone and liver scans in cystectomy candidates. Journal or Urology 1981; 125: 637–639

Illustrations by Kenneth Louis Clark

Cutaneous vesicostomy in children

R. Dixon Walker MD
Professor of Surgery and Pediatrics and Director of Pediatric Urology,
University of Florida College of Medicine, Gainesville, Florida, USA

Introduction

Vesicostomy can be performed as a temporary or permanent form of urinary diversion. In infants, vesicostomy is most often a temporary diversion to allow time for the child to grow and the disease process to subside until a more permanent solution can be sought. Vesicostomy, in contrast to suprapubic cystostomy, is a tubeless diversion. The importance of this to the patient is greater ease in managing bladder infections and less bladder irritation.

Although vesicostomy has been performed for many years, in the last decade Duckett[1] has popularized it as an excellent means of temporary diversion. The Blocksom, rather than the Lapides, technique is best adapted to infants and will be the one described here. The Blocksom technique creates a vesicocutaneous fistula, rather than the more permanent stoma featured in the Lapides technique.

Abnormalities involving the bladder or urethra are the primary indication for temporary cutaneous vesicostomy. Temporary decompression will allow time so that a permanent solution can be sought when the child is older and the condition possibly less complicated.

In my experience, posterior urethral valves have been the principal indication for temporary diversion in neonates. The vesicostomy is created during the neonatal period; after the child is a year old the valves are destroyed and the vesicostomy closed. Morbidity to the infant has been decreased with this method; the stricture rate has been reduced and the upper urinary tracts have often improved markedly.

The infant with myelomeningocele and areflexic neurogenic bladder is an excellent candidate for temporary cutaneous vesicostomy and, thereafter, can be so managed until intermittent self-catheterization can be taught and the vesicostomy closed.

The infant with 'prune-belly' syndrome may have a urethral obstruction that, like posterior urethral valves, will be easier to manage endoscopically when the child is older. Temporary cutaneous vesicostomy allows a delay of several years before performing a urethrotomy or similar procedure.

Repair of massive reflux in the newborn infant can be quite difficult, particularly if ureteral tapering is required. A temporary cutaneous vesicostomy permits the surgeon to wait until the patient is several years old. Frequently the ureters will become smaller, so that only simple reimplantation needs to be performed.

Preoperative

Preoperative preparation

A preoperative cystogram is essential to delineate the abnormality and assess the size of the bladder. The small contracted bladder is not suitable for vesicostomy. After a cystogram is obtained, a small 5 Fr feeding tube can be left in the bladder until the vesicostomy is performed. Before surgery, patients should be given appropriate antibacterial therapy for associated urinary tract infection. Electrolyte disturbances should be assessed and corrected. Once the decision is made to proceed with the vesicostomy, it should be performed within 24 hours of recognition of its need. The procedure does not require preoperative crossmatching of blood.

Anaesthesia

The patient is usually given preoperative medication of appropriate doses of atropine and pentobarbital. Maintenance intravenous fluids of D5-1/4 normal saline are given during the procedure and in the immediate postoperative period. During surgery the heart, temperature, blood pressure and pulse are monitored. The anaesthetic most commonly used is halothane and the patient is kept in Stage III anaesthesia, which allows mild muscle relaxation. As the procedure takes a relatively short time the patient is not usually intubated.

The operation

The patient is prepared and draped so that the lower abdomen and genitalia are exposed. A small catheter is placed in the urethra and the bladder is distended with 100–150 ml of water.

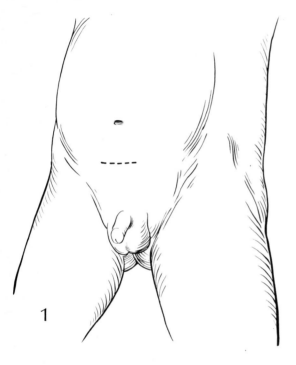

1

While the bladder is palpated, a transverse incision is made 2.5–3 cm above the symphysis pubis. The incision is approximately 2 cm long. Care should be taken not to make the incision too low. The subcutaneous tissue is dissected from the underlying rectus fascia.

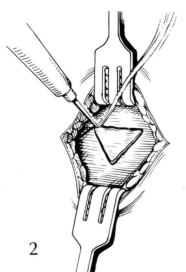

2

A triangle of anterior rectus fascia and the muscle is removed; the triangle is approximately 1 cm on each side, with its base cephalad. The prevesical space is entered caudally. The bladder is identified and the paravesical fat dissected from the bladder wall.

3

The bladder is clamped at the midline with Allis clamps, and the dome of the bladder is dissected from the paravesical fat and peritoneum. As each area of the bladder is cleaned, it is grasped with an Allis clamp to bring it clearly into view. When the urachus is reached, this indicates the most cephalad portion of the dome. The urachus is clamped, divided, and ligated with 3/0 Dexon suture.

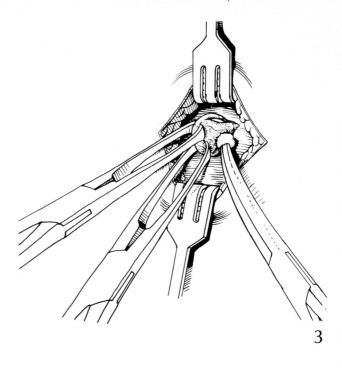

3

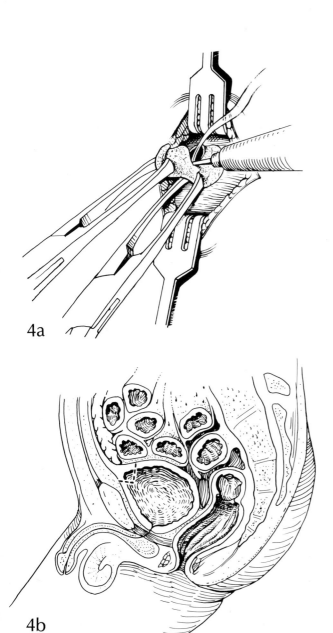

4a

4b

4a & b

The urachal segment of the bladder is then excised so that a full-thickness wedge of the bladder dome is removed with a resultant defect of approximately 1 cm in diameter. This opening should not be excessively large.

5

The bladder is elevated into the incision with Allis clamps and the bladder muscle sutured to the rectus fascia with interrupted 3/0 Dexon suture.

6

The stoma is created by approximating the urothelium and a small portion of muscle to the skin with interrupted 4/0 Dexon suture.

A dressing is applied composed of Adaptic, gauze and a nappy (diaper). No tape is needed. The urethral catheter is removed when the procedure is completed.

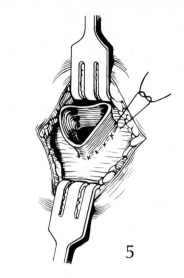

5

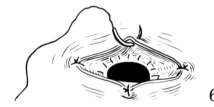

6

Postoperative care

Postoperative management is governed by the status of the kidneys. Usually these children are seen at 3–month intervals to assess the bladder and associated infection. The vesicostomy is catheterized and the urine cultured. All children are maintained on prophylactic antibacterials, usually sulphtrimethoprin combinations. Although the vesicostomy site may yield a positive culture, prophylactic treatment is not changed unless the patient becomes febrile.

The complication rate with temporary cutaneous vesicostomy is very low. Stomal stenosis may occur rarely. If it does, periodic dilatations with a catheter or plastic eye-dropper will suffice until vesicostomy closure is indicated.

Fortunately, prolapse of the bladder through the stoma is rare. This occurs more commonly after a Lapides type of vesicostomy. Adequate sedation may allow reduction of the prolapse, after which the surgeon can either close or revise the vesicostomy.

Because this approach to vesicostomy produces a temporary tubeless diversion, it must eventually be closed. In patients with posterior urethral valves this is done at the time of valve resection.

Closure is accomplished by a circumferential incision around the stoma, extended down below the fascial level. The portion of the stoma that has undergone squamous metaplasia is excised. The bladder is closed with a running 3/0 Dexon suture through the mucosa and superficial muscle, and with interrupted 3/0 Dexon sutures in the deep muscle and adventitia. The fascia is approximated with interrupted 3/0 chromic catgut sutures. The subcutaneous tissue is closed with a running 4/0 plain catgut and the skin with a 5/0 subcuticular Dexon suture. No drains are left in place and the urine is diverted for 48–72 hours with a urethral Foley catheter.

Results

Bruce and Gonzales[2] have had excellent results in 19 of 24 patients, with only 4 patients developing stomal stenosis. Allen[3] commented that prolapse did occur an appreciable number of times in his series in which a Lapides type of vesicostomy was performed. Our experience with 15 vesicostomies has been good; a prolapse developed only in the one patient who had a Lapides-type vesicostomy. Since using the Blocksom technique we have had no problems with prolapse and the occasional case of stomal stenosis is usually handled with dilatation.

References

1. Duckett, J. W. Cutaneous vesicostomy in childhood: the Blocksom technique. Urologic Clinics of North America 1974; 1: 485–495

2. Bruce, R. B., Gonzales, E. T. Cutaneous vesicostomy: a useful form of temporary diversion in children. Journal of Urology 1980; 123: 927–928

3. Allen, T. D. Vesicostomy for the temporary diversion of the urine in small children. Journal of Urology 1980; 123: 929–931

Surgery of seminal vesicles

Robert C. Flanigan MD
Assistant Professor of Surgery (Urology),
University of Kentucky Medical Center, Lexington, Kentucky, USA

Introduction

1

Surgery of the seminal vesicles is today a rare undertaking, reserved for congenital lesions (ureteral ectopia, cysts), acquired obstruction secondary to inflammatory disease of the prostate or ejaculatory ducts, and neoplastic lesions. The seminal vesicles can be approached by three general routes: anterior (transvesical, paravesical and transperitoneal); perineal; and posterior (ischiorectal, sacral and transrectal). Only the transvesical and perineal approaches will be discussed in detail.

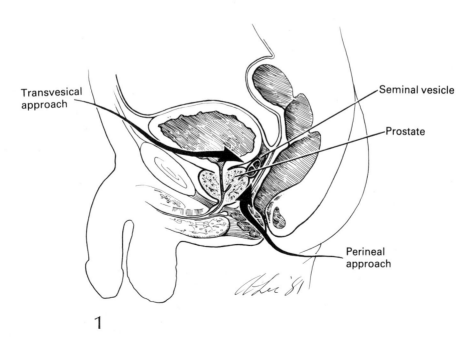

1

The operations

TRANSVESICAL APPROACH

The transvesical approach to the seminal vesicles may be useful for removal of moderately large masses of the seminal vesicles, drainage of an abscess or marsupialization of a retrovesical cyst. The bladder is exposed in the extraperitoneal space and opened in a vertical fashion adequately to expose the trigone, ureteral orifices and bladder floor.

After the upper bladder is packed with several gauze sponges, a wide malleable or Deaver retractor pulled cephalad in the bladder will often give excellent exposure. Ureteral catheterization may be helpful at this point in defining ureteral anatomy in difficult cases. Traction stitches can be placed laterally to retract the bladder walls.

2

A vertical incision through the trigone (shown) or a transverse incision 1 cm below the ureteral orifices can be used. Again, traction sutures may facilitate exposure.

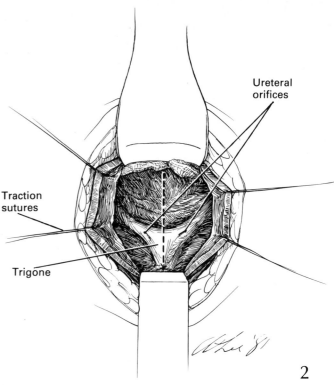

2

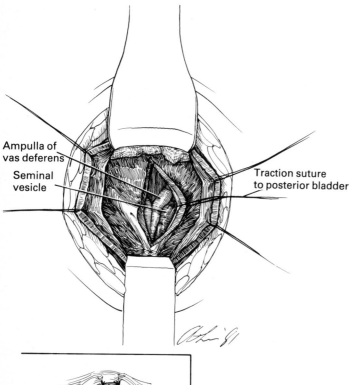

3

3

Beginning medially, the ampulla of the vas deferens is identified first and, with more lateral dissection, the seminal vesicles. Cysts of one seminal vesicle can be marsupialized using 3/0 chromic catgut to anastomose the cyst wall to the full thickness of the bladder wall (see inset). In cases where continued poor drainage of the seminal vesicle is anticipated, vesiculectomy is preferred.

PERINEAL APPROACH

The perineal approach for seminal vesicle surgery is preferred for the drainage of the unusual frank abscess and may be useful alone or in conjunction with a combined anterior approach for seminal vesiculectomy.

4

Meticulous attention to positioning of the patient in the exaggerated lithotomy position is essential. If the Young table or Palmer perineal board is not available, rolls or sandbags should be placed below the sacrum in order to thrust the perineum into a horizontal plane and allow for caudal extension of the pelvis towards the surgeon.

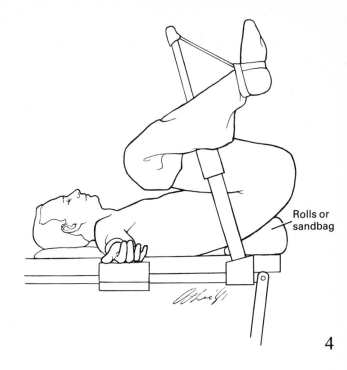

Rolls or sandbag

4

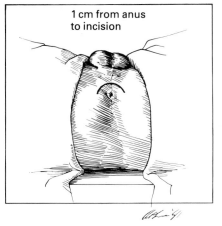

1 cm from anus to incision

5

A semicircular incision is made approximately 1 cm from the anal margin. Using the index fingers, the ischiorectal fossae are developed and the central tendon is separated from the underlying rectum and divided distal to the external anal sphincter.

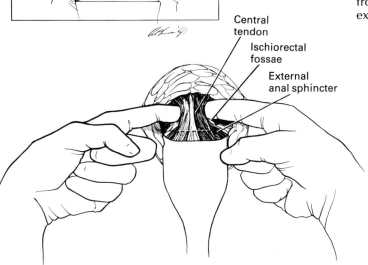

Central tendon

Ischiorectal fossae

External anal sphincter

5

6

The curved Lowsley retractor is then placed in the bladder and its jaws are separated so that cranial displacement of the retractor serves to elevate the prostate toward the surgeon.

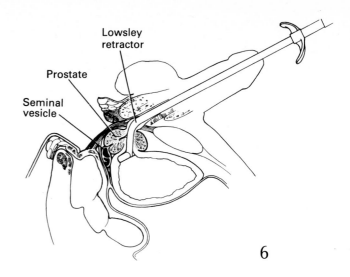

6

7

With blunt dissection, facilitated by small lateral retractors, the surgeon can develop the lateral fossae. The levator muscles are identified in the midline and swept laterally.

7

8

The rectourethralis muscle is then divided to approach Denonvilliers' fascia. It is vital at this point for the surgeon carefully to dissect the rectum away from the prostate gland to prevent rectal injury. A finger in the rectum may facilitate this step.

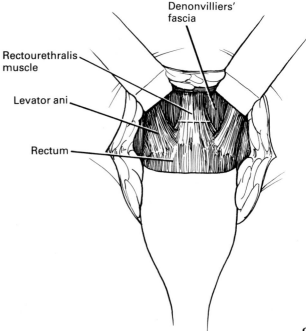

8

9

After Denonvilliers' fascia has been identified, it is incised transversely at the prostatic base.

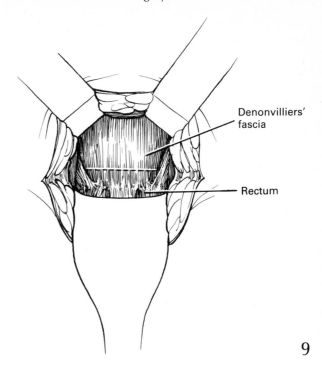

Denonvilliers' fascia

Rectum

9

10

The rectal retractor can then be used to displace Denonvilliers' fascia posteriorly, exposing the ampullae of the vas and the seminal vesicles lateral to them. Because the arterial supply to the prostate courses between layers of Denonvilliers' fascia and enters the prostate at its lateral surface, bleeding from the prostatic blood supply is usually minor.

Care must be taken during the dissection to avoid damage to the ureter as it courses posterior to the vas deferens and anterior to the seminal vesicle. Prudent use of ureteral catheterization is indicated to aid in dissection in those cases where significant inflammation or distortion of the ureter can be anticipated.

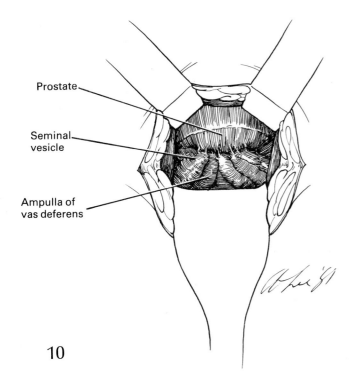

Prostate

Seminal vesicle

Ampulla of vas deferens

10

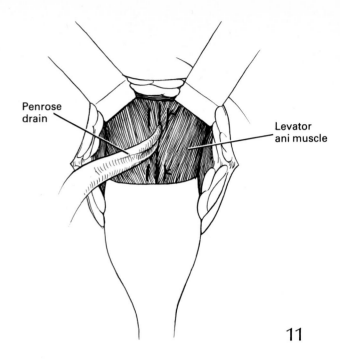

11

11 & 12

Wound closure is accomplished by approximation of the levator ani muscles in the midline and drainage is provided using a small Penrose drain brought out through the lateral margin of the incision.

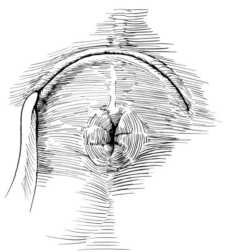

12

Further reading

de Assis, J. S. Seminal vesiculectomy. Journal of Urology 1952; 68: 747–753

Politano, V. A., Lankford, R. W., Susaeta, R. A transvesical approach to total seminal vesiculectomy. A case report. Journal of Urology 1975; 113: 385–388

Walker, W. C., Bowles, W. T. Transvesical seminal vesiculostomy in treatment of congenital obstruction of seminal vesicles. Case report. Journal of Urology 1968; 99: 324–326

Woodburne, R. T. Essentials of human anatomy. New York: Oxford University Press, 1957

Urachal disorders

Evan J. Kass, MD
Associate Professor of Urology and Child Health and Development, George Washington University School of Medicine and Health Sciences; attending Pediatric Urologist, Children's Hospital National Medical Center, Washington, DC, USA

Introduction

1

The urachus is a midline vestigial remnant which extends extraperitoneally from the apex of the bladder to the umbilicus. Normally this fistulous tract is completely obliterated at birth; however, if it remains patent, urinary drainage via the umbilicus can occur and is usually obvious immediately after birth.

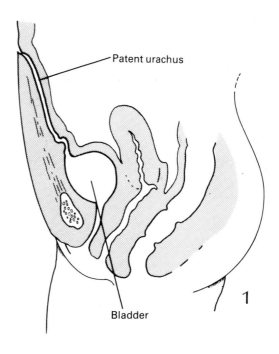

Patent urachus

Bladder

1

2

If only the most superficial portion of the urachal lumen (which is in communication with the umbilicus) remains open, then the child may present with a purulent umbilical discharge or subumbilical inflammation.

A urachal cyst can occur when both ends of the urachus become obliterated and no communication with either the bladder or the umbilicus remains. This usually manifests itself as a palpable subumbilical mass or abscess. When there is a question of urachal abnormality a voiding cystourethrogram should be performed to document the extent of the urachal remnant and to identify those few children in whom there is an associated lower urinary tract obstruction.

The management of these urachal anomalies requires a complete excision of all tissue between the bladder and umbilicus. A urachal abscess may be drained and packed initially, but complete excision should be performed following resolution of the abscess.

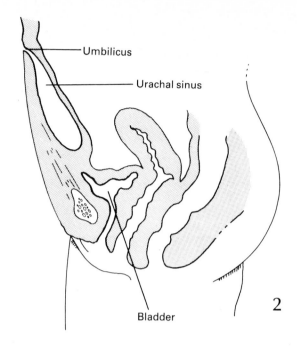

2

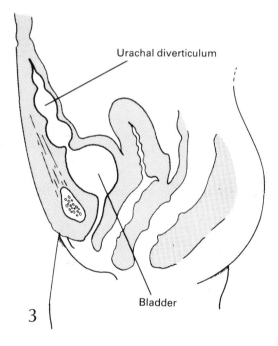

3

3

A urachal diverticulum is usually identified incidentally during a voiding cystourethrogram or cystoscopy performed for other conditions. In the abscence of any related urinary symptoms, no specific treatment is required.

Preoperative

Antibiotics are not routinely employed unless there is evidence of cellulitis, abscess or urinary infection.

Anaesthesia

General anaesthesia administered via face-mask or endotracheal tube is equally satisfactory. Intravenous fluids are administered through a small plastic cannula inserted at the time of surgery. Unless intravenous antibiotics are required postoperatively, the cannula may be removed as soon as the child is taking oral liquids.

The operation

The child is placed in the supine position and the lower trunk from the costal margins to the mid-thighs is prepared, but only the area from just above the umbilicus to the pubis is draped into the field. A catheter is placed into the bladder and fluid instilled to aid in identifying the apex of the bladder.

4

A transverse suprapubic incision in a skin fold provides excellent exposure and a satisfactory cosmetic result. The skin and subcutaneous tissues are mobilized superiorly to the level of the umbilicus and inferiorly to the pubis.

5

The rectus fascia is incised vertically in the midline and the rectus muscles are separated.

6

The bladder is identified and traced cephalad until the urachus is easily identified where it originates near the apex of the bladder.

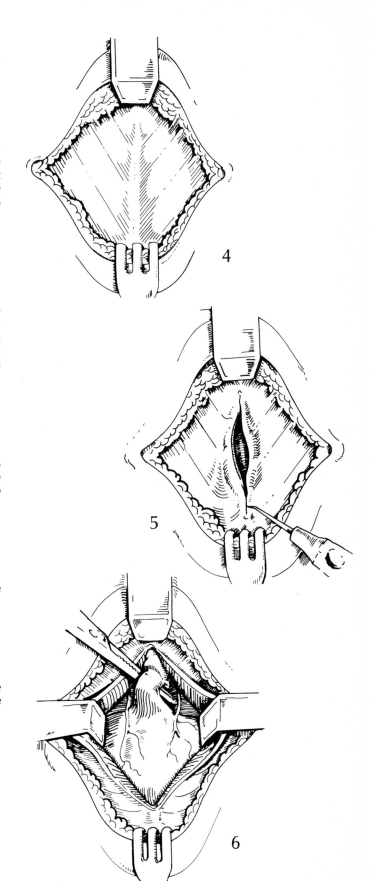

7

The urachus is then excised along with a small cuff of normal bladder.

8

The entire urachal remnant is mobilized extraperitoneally from the bladder to the posterior aspect of the umbilicus, where it is transected. The umbilicus is normally preserved unless it is grossly involved with an inflammatory process.

9

The bladder is closed in two layers with either interrupted or continuous 3/0 or 4/0 chromic sutures. A small Penrose drain is brought out below the incision separate from the original wound. A wad of gauze is placed on the umbilicus and covered with a pressure dressing in order to obliterate the dead space and provide a nice cosmetic result. The musculofascial layers are approximated with interrupted sutures of 3/0 or 4/0 chromic material and the skin is closed with a subcuticular suture of 4/0 or 5/0 nylon.

Postoperative care

A Foley catheter is not routinely employed; but if copious urinary leakage is noted via the Penrose drain, it may be necessary to leave one in place for 4 or 5 days. The Penrose drain is generally removed on the 5th postoperative day unless there is profuse urinary leakage, in which case it is left untouched until the drainage ceases. Sutures are removed on the 7th postoperative day. No postoperative X-rays are routinely performed, and postoperative urinary antibiotics are unnecessary unless there was a documented infection preoperatively.

Further reading

Bauer, S. B., Retik, A. B. Urachal anomalies and related umbilical disorders. Urologic Clinics of North America 1978; 5: 195–211

Blichert-Toft, M., Nielson, O. V. Congenital patent urachus and acquired variants. Acta Chirurgica Scandinavica 1971; 137: 807–814

Colodny, A. H., Lebowitz, R. L. Abnormalities of the bladder and prostate. In: Ravitch, M. M. et al, eds. Pediatric surgery 3rd ed., Vol. 2. Chicago: Year Book Medical Publishers, 1979: 1306–1327

Constantain, H. M., Amaral, E. L. Urachal cyst: case report. Journal of Urology 1971; 106: 429–431

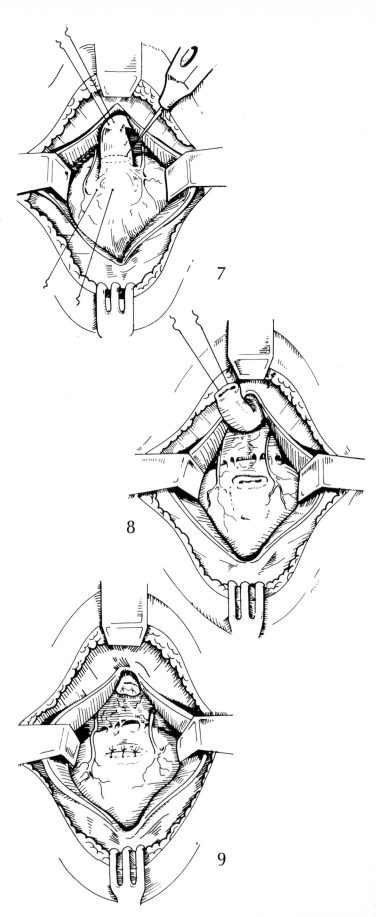

Traumatic injuries of the bladder

J. P. Mitchell   CBE, TD, MS, FRCS, FRCS(Ed)
Honorary Professor of Surgery (Urology), University of Bristol , UK

Principles of treatment

Treatment of a ruptured bladder is not a matter of extreme urgency for the first 12–24 hours after injury. Urine is normally sterile, and therefore the inevitable extravasation is unlikely to cause any serious complications, provided it is recognized, drained and evacuated within 36 hours. Even when urine escapes into the peritoneal cavity, the irritation produced is only moderate in the early stages. Neither leakage of urine from the bladder nor stagnation of urine in the tissues should be allowed to continue after 36 hours. Finally, and most important, every precaution should be taken to avoid the introduction of infection into the traumatized area where haematoma, damage to tissues, extravasated urine and bone fragments will form the perfect nidus for the culture of any organisms.

Mode of presentation of rupture of bladder

Injuries of the bladder may be closed or open. Closed injuries usually occur following a heavy blow to the lower abdomen, or in association with a fracture of the pelvis. Open wounds result from penetration of the lower abdomen by stabbing or gunshot wounds. The penetration by the missile may be suprapubically or via the perineum or even via the anus and rectum. For the bladder to rupture, it must have been full, or nearly full, at the time of the accident. A blow to the lower abdomen can cause disruption of the wall of the bladder from a sudden increase in intravesical pressure, giving rise to an explosive burst of the viscus. The unsupported part of the bladder wall, the vault, gives way and, as this surface is covered by peritoneum, the result is intraperitoneal rupture. The tear in the bladder wall is usually a large hole. On occasion the tear may result in complete bivalving of the bladder.

When associated with a fracture of the pelvis, the rupture may be either due to penetration of the anterior wall by a spicule of bone from the pubic ramus, or it may be caused by the same blow in the lower abdomen which fractured the pelvis. In other words, an extraperitoneal rupture of the anterior bladder wall is the commonest lesion associated with a fractured pelvis, but intraperitoneal disruption of the bladder may occasionally be seen.

Associated injuries

Rupture of the bladder and rupture of the posterior urethra may be found in association with a fracture of the pelvis. Many bladder injuries may be due to road traffic accidents, where other multiple injuries are sustained. Some of these, if severe, may take treatment priority over the bladder injury.

Following any severe blow to the abdomen or serious multiple injury, the possibility of other intraperitoneal injuries must be considered. Even damage to the upper tract (kidney) as well as the lower urinary tract (bladder) have been known to occur at the same time and in the same patient – hence the need for routine excretory urography in all patients suspected of having urinary tract trauma.

369

Preoperative investigations

The diagnosis of an extraperitoneal rupture of the bladder is suspected during the first 24 hours if the patient produces no urine, develops no signs of a distended bladder and gradually shows some deterioration in general condition with increasing suprapubic pain.

Intraperitoneal rupture of the bladder presents with slowly developing peritoneal irritation and an increasing amount of free fluid in the abdomen, as indicated by steady increase in girth measurement. Needle aspiration or peritoneal lavage may suggest a diagnosis of intraperitoneal rupture.

The passage of a catheter *per urethram* is unwise, because the withdrawal of as much as 150 ml of urine does not exclude a small but significant puncture wound of the anterior wall of the bladder. At the same time, the introduction of a catheter can carry infection into the pelvic haematoma. Furthermore, there is a 10–15 per cent risk of a double injury of bladder and posterior urethra and use of the 'diagnostic catheter' would be unwise and even dangerous (*see* chapter on 'Injuries to the urethra', pp. 000–000). In an extraperitoneal rupture due to a spicule of bone the hole in the bladder wall may be very small and the bladder could still hold as much as 200 ml of urine. The patient with a small puncture wound of the bladder wall has even been known to pass urine spontaneously, with at least a trace of blood.

Any penetrating wound or gunshot wound which could involve the bladder, or perineal injury by impaling must be explored without delay. The track of the missile must be identified and injury to the bladder excluded.

Although a rupture of the urethra usually produces blood at the external urinary meatus, a clean meatus, clear of any blood, does not exclude a urethral injury. A urethrogram and a cystogram may be helpful in confirming the diagnosis. An intravenous pyelogram should also be performed to ensure the integrity of the upper urinary tract. With good concentration of contrast medium, extravasation may be seen, even from the bladder. The bladder base may also be seen to be elevated and compressed laterally within the pelvis by the perivesical haematoma and extravasated urine (the 'tear-drop' bladder).

Endoscopy should be carried out just prior to operation: first to ensure that the urethra is intact and, second, to observe the bladder wall. A tear in the bladder wall may be difficult to identify unless there is frank bleeding. Furthermore, a visible tear in the mucosa does not necessarily indicate that the rupture is through the full thickness of the muscle wall of the bladder. Finally, if there is a hole of any size, the bladder cannot be distended and no view will be obtained by cystoscopy.

Exploratory operation

Indications

With a closed injury of the bladder, exploration may be indicated by failure to pass urine without the development of a distended bladder within 24 hours of injury. By this time there will be some evidence of deterioration in the patient's condition and increased suprapubic tenderness.

There may have been a fracture of the pelvis: the anterior wall of the bladder could have been penetrated by a spicule of bone.

Alternatively, developing signs of low-grade peritonitis and the patient's general condition may suggest an intraperitoneal lesion. The only indication that this might be due to a ruptured bladder is a failure to produce urine. On the other hand, the patient may be going to the operating theature for surgery for trauma to some other unrelated structure, and the bladder injury may be discovered at laparotomy.

All penetrating wounds which may have damaged the bladder must be explored without delay in order to identify the path of the missile, to carry out a urinary or bowel diversion as necessary, to remove any foreign body such as clothing carried into the wound, and to drain the wound freely.

Preparation and anaesthesia

No particular preparation is required other than cleansing the skin of the lower abdomen and perineum. The patient should be invited to try to pass water just before going to the theatre. General anaesthesia is indicated.

The incision

The peritoneum and prevesical area are explored through a midline suprapubic incision. This can then be extended upwards if any intraperitoneal lesion is suspected.

Intraperitoneal rupture

The peritoneal cavity is opened and free urine and blood are removed by suction and mopping. A full examination should be made of the abdominal viscera, including the liver and spleen. Following a blow to the abdomen, the stomach and full length of the intestine should be examined, as well as the mesenteries. The retroperitoneal area should be inspected for haematoma.

An intraperitoneal tear following a blow to the abdomen is usually at least 4 or 5 cm long and will allow inspection of the interior of the bladder, both with a finger and subsequently by visual inspection. The rupture is closed with a continuous layer of 2/0 gauge plain catgut or polyglycolic acid (PGA). The outer layer of muscle and serosa are then closed with continuous 2/0 gauge chromic catgut, ensuring that all nonabsorbable suture material is buried within the wall of the bladder and not exposed on its inner surface so that urine can come into contact and encrust the exposed suture with phosphates. The peritoneal cavity is closed without drainage, but a small drain should be placed in the prevesical (retropubic) space. Providing there has been no blood at the external meatus (which is unlikely if the intraperitoneal rupture has been due to a blow on the abdominal wall), the bladder can be drained by an indwelling urethral catheter. If there is any suspicion of damage to the urethra at the time of injury, a urethral catheter is best avoided and the bladder should be drained by a suprapubic catheter (26 Fr Foley type).

Extraperitoneal rupture

Extraperitoneal rupture is usually associated with a fracture of the pelvis, when the anterior wall of the bladder is penetrated by a spicule of bone. The hole in the bladder wall is likely to be much smaller than in the case of intraperitoneal rupture and it may be difficult to find. Urine and blood well up from behind the symphysis pubis and the anterior wall of the bladder may be suffused with blood and difficult to identify. Under no circumstances should an instrument be passed *per urethram*, because there may be an associated but unsuspected lesion of the posterior urethra. Any blind instrumentation, such as the passage of a catheter, could aggravate the severity of the lesion (*see* chapter on 'Injuries to the urethra', pp. 000–000).

In view of the difficulty in locating the tear in the bladder wall, a formal cystotomy is advisable in order to identify the site of the rupture from inside the bladder. At the same time, the bladder neck, anterior surface of the prostate and position of the fractured pubic ramus in relation to the prostate and bladder can be decided and small tags and irregularities may be excised; but usually there is no need to trim the rupture of the bladder wall. The tear is often small and the bladder has such a good blood supply that it is uncommon for any part of the torn wall to necrose as a result of ischaemia.

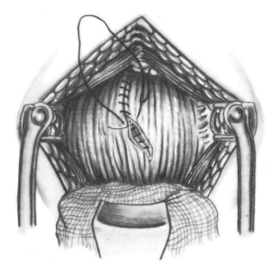

1

1 & 2

Repair of the rupture

The rent in the bladder wall is sutured in two layers, with 2/0 gauge chromic catgut being used for the outer muscle layer. If there was blood at the external meatus at the time of admission (indicating probable rupture of the urethra), the bladder should be drained by a suprapubic cystostomy for about 2 weeks until the the urethra can be inspected by endoscopy. If there was no blood at the external meatus at the time of admission, rupture of the urethra is unlikely and a catheter can be passed with reasonable safety *per urethram* and left indwelling for 4–5 days until the bladder wall has united adequately. The retropubic space is drained with a corrugated rubber drain, a Redivac or a Penrose tube drain.

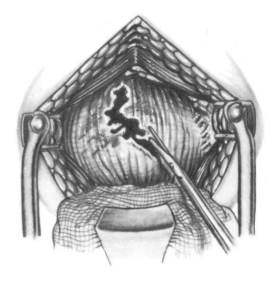

2

Postoperative care

Bladder lavage

At the close of the operation the bladder is washed out thoroughly via the indwelling urethral or suprapubic catheter to ensure that all blood clot has been removed. The catheter is connected to a closed drainage system, which need not have irrigation incorporated.

In view of the extent of soft tissue damage, the size of the haematoma and the amount of extravasated urine, it is advisable to put the patient on a broad-spectrum antibiotic for the next 10 days.

Removal of drains

The prevesical (retropubic) drain can usually be removed at 2–3 days, unless oozing of serum persists. The indwelling urethral catheter can be removed at 5 days, after which the patient should be able to pass urine normally. If a suprapubic catheter has been left in, this should be retained until the urethra can be inspected by cystourethroscopy, which is usually between 14 and 21 days after the injury.

Penetrating injuries

The bladder may be damaged by a gunshot wound or a stabbing injury. The perforation of the bladder may be only one of many severe lesions, depending on the direction of the missile, which may also have penetrated the peritoneal cavity, perforated the rectum or shattered portions of the pelvic girdle. The amount of damage to the bladder is variable. A bullet may traverse the bladder leaving only a minute entry and exit wound, while a fragment of a shell or bomb may tear a large opening and destroy much of the bladder muscle.

Examination of superficial wounds

When entrance and exit wounds are present, they provide a valuable guide to the course of the missile and to the possible structures damaged. A urethrogram can be carried out under strictly sterile precautions and will help to show whether the urethra is damaged as well as the bladder. The wound is already potentially infected, so the passage of a urethral catheter is not contraindicated on the grounds of risk of introducing infection. Nevertheless, the diagnostic value of the urethral catheter is still questionable. A ruptured bladder may have only two small perforations from entry and exit of the missile, and still retain some urine; therefore, the presence of urine in the bladder does not exclude penetration through the bladder wall. On the other hand, a dry tap with a catheter could mean either a damaged urethra, anuria or a ruptured bladder. The passage of a urethral catheter may, therefore, not be a helpful diagnostic procedure.

Exploration of wound and track

After treatment for shock is started the abdomen is explored through a midline suprapubic incision. The peritoneal cavity is opened and any free blood and urine are removed. All intra-abdominal viscera are inspected for injury, with particular reference to the small and large intestines and their mesenteries. If an intraperitoneal perforation of the bladder is present, the margins are excised and the wound closed in two layers. Where there is evidence of either intraperitoneal or extraperitoneal injury to the rectum a left iliac colostomy is established at this stage. The peritoneum is then closed without drainage. If there is evidence of an extraperitoneal wound, the bladder is opened anteriorly between stay sutures. A careful search is made for the extent of injury through the wall of the bladder; any foreign bodies or loose fragments of bone are removed.

Repair of the bladder

The subsequent course depends on the degree of vesical damage. Whenever possible the vesical wounds are excised and sutured. In civilian life, many missile perforations of the bladder may be treated by complete closure of the bladder wall, drainage of the retropubic space and an indwelling urethral catheter to drain the bladder itself. In combat situations, however, meticulous aftercare may be lacking and long-distance evacuation necessary. In these circumstances an indwelling urethral catheter is better replaced by suprapubic drainage of the bladder, using a Foley balloon catheter (26 Fr) which is brought out at the highest point of the bladder incision and at least 2 cm above the symphysis pubis. The retropubic drain may be a Redivac, a Penrose tube drain or simply a strip of corrugated rubber drain.

Wounds of the vault of the bladder usually present no difficulty for closure. The bladder wall is freely mobile and the margins may be approximated easily even after wide excision.

Injuries to the upper portions of the anterior and lateral walls may be closed easily. Difficulties arise when the wound is at the bladder neck and is accompanied by shattering of the pelvis and an open wound in the pubic or groin regions. It is often easier to repair a rent in the bladder base from inside the bladder. However, it is absolutely essential to provide a drain outside the bladder down to the site of the repair. A three-bladed Morson's bladder retractor will help provide good exposure of the bladder base. If, after introducing the self-retaining retractor, the bladder base still appears to be in folds, the incision in the bladder wall should be extended in a cephalad direction so that the centre blade, which is in the upper part of the wound, will then draw the base of the bladder into a more spherical shape. A small gauze swab under the centre blade will hold the posterior wall of the bladder so that it does not slip downwards onto the blade.

A considerable area of bladder wall may be destroyed, and contusion of the tissues and staining due to suffusion with blood may make identification of the limits of the vesical wound difficult. The base of the bladder is also relatively fixed and extremely vascular, so that difficulty may be experienced in bringing the wound margins together. In these circumstances a tense suture line will break down and allow urine (which may be infected) to leak into the perivesical tissues and around the pubic fractures causing chronic osteomyelitis. The margins of the vesical wall become adherent to the pelvic bones and a permanent urinary fistula may be established. To avoid these problems, every effort must be made to close the bladder wall without tension and to provide free drainage of urine from the bladder.

Owing to the fixity of the tissues it may be impossible satisfactorily to suture wounds of the base of the bladder and more harm than good will result from attempts to draw the bladder base together under tension. Providing a colostomy has been established and there is free catheter drainage of the bladder urine, a very high proportion of double injuries to bladder and rectum will heal spontaneously without fistula formation.

When a ureteric orifice has been damaged, it is usually unwise to attempt any wide exposure of the ureter with reimplantation into the bladder within a few hours of a penetrating injury. A catheter (polythene oesophageal catheter size 10 or 12 Fr) can be passed from the bladder up the ureter and across the site of damage into the upper part of the ureter, to act as both drain and splint. This catheter is then brought out, either through the suprapubic wound or via the urethra. If any ureteric obstruction ensues, formal operation and reimplantation may be performed later (*see* chapter on 'Ureteral injuries', pp. 307–309).

Arrangements for drainage

Suprapubic drainage is established by passing a Foley catheter (26 or 28 Fr) into the bladder, either through the upper portion of the wound when it is large, or, more commonly, through the exploratory incision in the anterior wall of the bladder. If there was no blood at the external meatus when the patient was first examined, damage to any part of the urethra is unlikely and a Foley catheter (size 18 Fr, 5 ml bag) can be passed up the urethra to drain the base of the bladder. If there is any suspicion of urethral trauma, this should be managed as described in the chapter on 'Urethral damage' (see pp. 473–479). The bladder wounds are closed as completely as possible and prevesical tissues drained.

Suction drainage

If closure of the bladder wall is inadequate or in doubt, suction drainage of the bladder may be considered. A polythene catheter should be used, as a latex or silicone catheter will collapse with suction. By attaching suction to the Foley catheter, the urine may be continuously removed. The Roberts electric pump is suitable for this purpose. When suction is being employed, it is an advantage to arrange the suprapubic tube so that it may act as an inlet vent for air. The bladder suction is then continuous and the mucosa of the bladder wall is not drawn into the eyes of the catheter by the negative intravesical pressure.

Editor's comment

It should be noted that many feel cystography plays an important role in the diagnosis of bladder injuries. A urethrogram is performed initially and confirms that there is no urethral injury. Provided the urethra is intact a small catheter is passed gently into the bladder aseptically and provides the route for instilling 150 ml of radiocontrast. A full bladder film and a post-evacuation film are obtained. If the latter is omitted, small tears in the posterior aspect of the bladder may be missed. Many minor extraperitoneal injuries of the bladder may be treated with catheter drainage alone.

Further reading

Cass, A. S., Ireland, G. W. Bladder trauma associated with pelvic fractures in severely injured patients. Journal of Trauma 1973; 13: 205–212

Culp, O. S. Treatment of ruptured bladder and urethra: analysis of 86 cases of urinary extravasation. Journal of Urology 1942; 48: 266–286

Anonymous. Wounds of the bladder. British Journal of Surgery 1950; War Injuries Supplement No. 3, 468–471

Macalpine, J. B. Wounds of the bladder. In: Bailey, H. ed. Surgery of modern warfare. Vol 2. Edinburgh: Livingstone, 1941. 247–255

Mitchell, J. P. Injuries to the urinary tract. Proceedings of the Royal Society of Medicine 1963; 56: 1046–1050

Mitchell, J. P. Injuries to the urethra. British Journal of Urology 1968; 40: 649–670

Mitchell, J. P. Trauma to the urinary tract. New England Journal of Medicine 1973; 288: 90–92

Poole-Wilson, D. S. Missile injuries of the bladder. British Journal of Surgery 1950; War Supplement No. 3, 475–477

Poole-Wilson, D. S. The treatment of injuries of the urethra and bladder. In: Rock Carling, Sir E., Paterson Ross, Sir J., eds. British Surgical practice: surgical progress. London: Butterworths, 1954: 17–41

Ross. J. C. Injuries of the urinary bladder. British Journal of Surgery 1944; 32: 44–49

Illustrations by Robert Lane and Philip Wilson

Repair of urinary vaginal fistulae

Richard Turner-Warwick   DSc, DM, MCh, FRCP, FRCS, FRACS, FACS
Senior Surgeon, The Middlesex Hospital; Senior Consultant Urological Surgeon, St Peter's Hospital Group;
Senior Lecturer, Institute of Urology, University of London, UK

It is almost always possible to close a vesico-vaginal fistula; meticulous technique is naturally essential but success with the more complicated problems depends on the ability of the surgeon to select the procedure that is best suited to the particular clinical situation and to vary it appropriately during the course of the operation, according to the findings, on the basis of a wide personal experience of the particular problems involved.

Simple traumatic vesico-vaginal fistulae can often be resolved reliably by simple closure in layers either from a vaginal or from an abdominal approach. However, even complex recurrent fistulae and those associated with tissue loss and impaired healing due to irradiation are almost invariably repairable by the addition of a vascular omental interposition graft. It follows that *any* recurrent fistula after a relatively limited vaginal approach layer closure procedure should cause a surgeon to reflect upon the technique and choice of procedure[1].

The surgical approach

A standard 'lithotomy' position is commonly used for a vaginal repair; the disadvantage of this is that it does not offer the facility of simple extension to a synchronous abdominal exploration. Consequently it is generally inappropriate because it is rarely possible to be certain before exploration that a simple vaginal repair will be successful.

1

Irrespective of whether a primary approach from the vagina or from the abdomen is planned the patient should be positioned on the operating table for a synchronous abdomino-perineal procedure[2] tilted slightly head downwards, legs widely abducted and only moderate hip flexion so that both the abdomen and the perineum are included in the one sterile operating field.

Provided a perineal ring retractor is used the synchronous abdomino-perineal position provides good exposure for vaginal surgery and one assistant is more than enough; the surgeon is seated with the scrub nurse and the instrument table immediately to his right (or left if left handed). If a vaginal approach repair proves difficult or inappropriate, the surgeon simply walks round to the abdominal approach position and the scrub nurse repositions the instrument table between the legs. It is generally unnecessary to have two surgical teams for a synchronous approach.

The same patient positioning and preparation is used for primary abdominal approach; the advantage of including the perineum in the operating field is that an orientating finger in the vagina wall greatly facilitates the separation of the vagina from the bladder around the fistula. Furthermore, a synchronous vaginal approach is also required for the creation of an appropriately wide abdomino-perineal tunnel to receive and to fix distally an adequate bulk of omental pedicle graft when interpositional support of a vesical or vesico-urethral closure proves necessary.

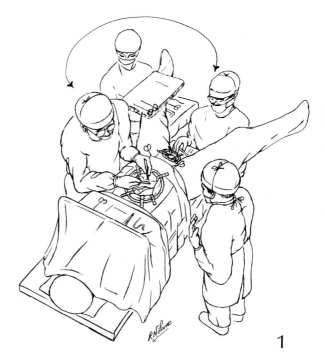

1

VAGINAL REPAIR

Good surgical access is essential for an efficient vaginal repair. It is particularly important to exclude additional fistulae. When preliminary endoscopy shows that one or both ureteric orifices lie close to a fistula it is generally advisable to insert ureteric catheters to facilitate their mobilization and to proceed to an abdominal repair.

2a

Meticulous attention to technique is a basic essential of layer closure procedures; the fistula is circumcised and the tissue plane between the vaginal wall and the bladder separated.

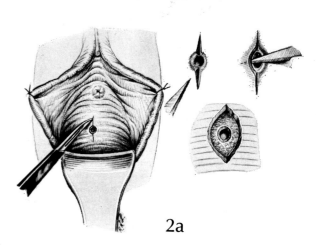

2a

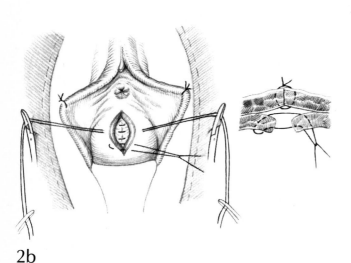

2b

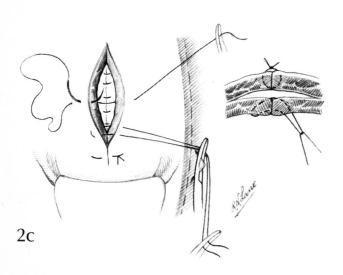

2c

2b & c

The development of low-tissue-reaction absorbable poly-glycolic acid (PGA) Dexon sutures in 1970 to replace catgut, was a landmark in the history of fistula repair that greatly increased the reliability of closure.

The bladder wall is closed by approximating the bladder with inverting 3/0 Dexon or Vicryl sutures; although Dexon sutures cause much less tissue reaction than catgut, the knots are best tied on the lumen where possible so that they can fall free.

The vaginal layer is closed with interrupted everting 3/0 sutures, carefully ensuring that the tissue bite is not strangulated by over-tightening.

Perineal interposition tissue grafts

3

If there is reason to suspect that a vaginal layer closure may not be adequate, perhaps as a result of fibrosis, poor tissue viability, or previous vaginal surgery, it is a simple matter to raise a posteriorly-based pedicle of labial tissue and to interpose this as a vascular graft between the layer closures after the technique of Martius.

Most patients with distal urethro-vaginal fistulae are continent and asymptomatic provided the bladder-neck mechanism is competent[3]; if it is not, the restoration of urethral length without re-approximation of the eccentric, anteriorly located, urethral sphincter mechanism is unlikely to restore continence at the urethral level.

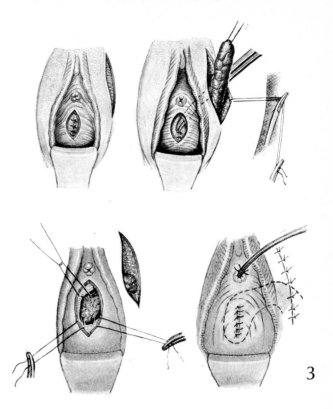

3

Instrumentation

4

The universal Turner-Warwick abdomino-perineal ring retractor set is particularly valuable.

The perineal ring has strategically placed stay suture knobs on one side with six rake blades and additional deep malleable blades that can be used posteriorly in the vagina (the reverse side of this ring is a knobless Dennis Browne infant abdominal ring).

All surfaces are finished matt black to reduce light reflection. A particular advantage of ring retractors is that the rim can be used to retain vaginal wall traction stay sutures that elevate the fistula area and greatly facilitate its repair (see Illustration 8).

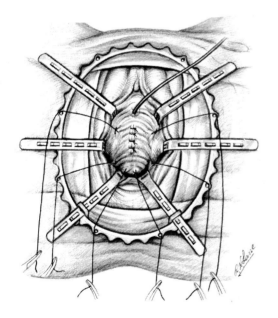

4

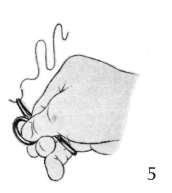

5

An angulated Turner-Warwick needle holder allows the needle to be visualized continuously when working in deep cavities, without moving the handgrip.

5

6

6

The Turner-Warwick fibrelight sucker combines two important facilities. The connections of the suction tube and the light cable provide the handle and there is an air-bleed hold to adjust the suction located immediately in front of the finger ring; another distal air-bleed helps to suck the blood-film from the base of the fibrelight face.

THE ABDOMINAL APPROACH

The abdominal approach can be used for any vesico-vaginal fistula, high or low; many surgeons find it technically easier than a vaginal approach and it is much more reliable for the repair of complicated fistulae.

The incision

A midline incision is always advisable for an abdominal approach to a vesical fistula because it is necessary to extend this up to the xiphisternum to provide access to the stomach when a formal mobilization of the gastroepiploic vascular arch is required to enable a short apron omentum to be redeployed for an interposition graft repair of a complex fistula[2].

7

However, for the scar-conscious, a vertical lower abdominal midline incision can be achieved through a horizontal suprapubic skin incision so that it is only necessary to use an upper abdominal midline skin incision when mobilization of the omental pedicle proves necessary[2]; in such cases a separate upper abdominal midline skin incision is made and the lower midline abdominal wall incision extended upwards into this.

   A Pfannensteil incision should *never* be used for an abdominal-approach fistula repair because it is ill-adapted to an upward omentum-exposing extension. In fact the relatively limited surgical access provided by a Pfannensteil incision is probably a contributing factor in the causation of a significant proportion of hysterectomy fistulae and the incidence of these could probably be reduced by adopting the suprapubic V modification as a routine because this greatly improves the pelvic exposure[4].

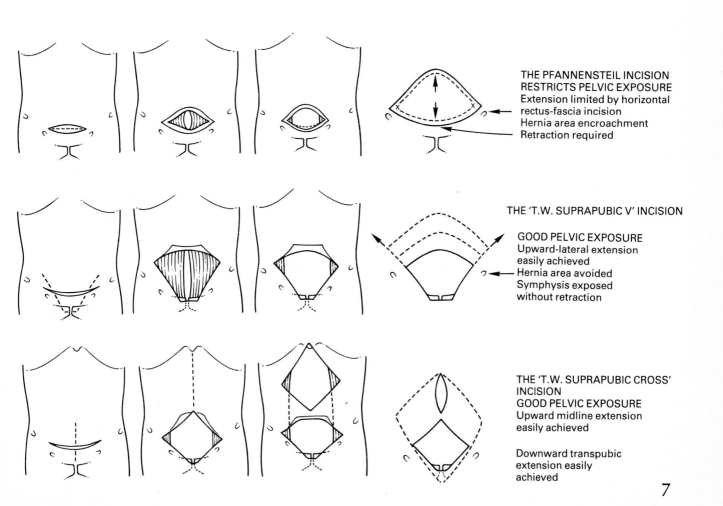

THE PFANNENSTEIL INCISION RESTRICTS PELVIC EXPOSURE
Extension limited by horizontal rectus-fascia incision
Hernia area encroachment
Retraction required

THE 'T.W. SUPRAPUBIC V' INCISION

GOOD PELVIC EXPOSURE
Upward-lateral extension easily achieved
Hernia area avoided
Symphysis exposed without retraction

THE 'T.W. SUPRAPUBIC CROSS' INCISION
GOOD PELVIC EXPOSURE
Upward midline extension easily achieved

Downward transpubic extension easily achieved

Retraction

8

The abdominal ring retractor provides maximal retraction and pelvic floor exposure without the help of an assistant. The ring is retained in position by four fully curved abdominal wall retractor blades of the appropriate size; additional deep blades between these retract the abdominal contents efficiently, a sliding clip under the inner margin of the ring locks them down to prevent them from lifting. Elevating traction stay sutures are anchored over the ring margin.

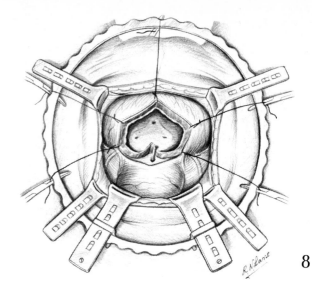

8

THE TRANSVESICAL APPROACH

9

The time-honoured simple transvesical procedure for the repair of vesico-vaginal fistulae uses a technique of tissue-plane development and separate layer-closure that is similar to that of a vaginal repair; however, the access it provides is much too limited for complicated fistulae and its use should be abandoned.

TRANSPERITONEAL SUPRAVESICAL FISTULA EXPOSURE

10

The transperitoneal posterior vesical approach is always preferable for the abdominal repair of vesico-vaginal fistulae. The initial intraperitoneal incision is made in the vesico-vaginal peritoneal fold and the posterior wall of the bladder is opened in the midline just above the fistula.

When the posterior wall of the bladder is found to be indurated and fibrotic, as it often proves to be in irradiated fistulae, it is important that the fistula-exposing incision in the posterior wall of the bladder should not be midline but curved laterally as far as possible to achieve a tension-free suture line closure of the fistula by rotating the eccentric bladder flap; in such circumstances, a midline incision in a scarred posterior bladder-wall sometimes proves difficult or impossible to close.

The separation of the vagina from the bladder around the fistula is facilitated by an orientating finger in the vaginal vault. The vaginal vault and the bladder are closed with 3/0 Dexon or Vicryl sutures.

A wide exposure of the fistula area is thus provided and a direct extravesical exposure of the terminal ureter is easily obtained if its reimplantation into the bladder is indicated. Efficient retraction is maintained by the elevating stay-sutures.

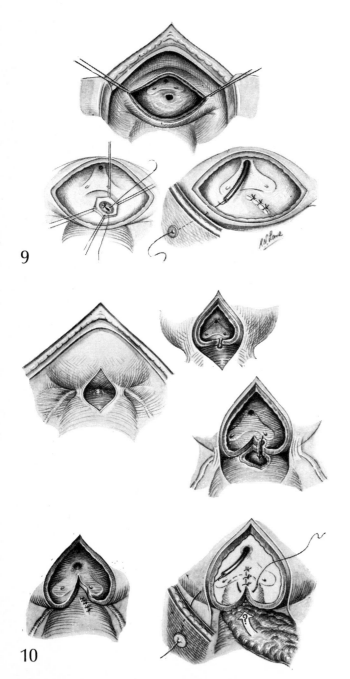

URETERO-VESICO-VAGINAL FISTULAE

The majority of lower ureteric fisulae originate at, or very close to, the terminal ureter so that continuity can often be restored by its reflux-preventing re-implantation into the bladder; the increased access provided is one of the particular advantages of the supravesical approach.

Occasionally there is a sufficient length of normal ureter distal to a simple uretero-vaginal fistula to enable ureteric continuity to be restored by a spatulated re-anastomosis to the mobilized proximal ureter, optionally supported by an omental wrap[5].

11

A simple technique for the resolution of the more complicated uretero-vaginal or uretero-vesico-vaginal fistula is to mobilize the bladder and anchor it to the psoas muscle so that the ureter can be re-implanted in a supra-iliac position; this helps to separate the fistulous track closures. The 'psoas-hitch' procedure has many other disinct advantages over the standard Boari technique[6]; not only is it easier to perform but it facilitates a reflux-preventing re-implantation of the ureter.

POSTOPERATIVE URINARY DRAINAGE

Suprapubic urinary catheter drainage should be used routinely after any vesical fistula repair: it is efficient, reliable, and less uncomfortable than a urethral catheter. Furthermore, at the conclusion of the drainage period it is easy to verify the restoration of voiding efficiency by clamping the suprapubic drainage and checking the post-voiding residual volumes before removing it; this compares favourably with the emotionally charged situation which arises when a urethral catheter has to be re-inserted repeatedly – the 'yo-yo catheter'.

An additional urethral catheter may be advisable but this must be retained by a sling-suture with a button on the abdominal wall; a balloon-retained urethral catheter is most inadvisable because inadvertent traction upon it can be disastrously disruptive.

Suction urinary drainage systems are unnecessary. Unfortunately, the calibre of the connecting tube of many standard drainage bag systems is so large that they have a tendency to retain air bubbles, and fluid levels in a hanging loop at the bedside can create a positive hydrostatic resistance to the flow of urine. If the internal diameter of the connecting tubing is small, approximating to that of the lumen of the catheter, it remains bubble free and creates a natural syphonic suction; however, unobstructed urinary drainage is all that a fistula repair requires – hence the added safety of using both suprapubic and urethral catheter drainage.

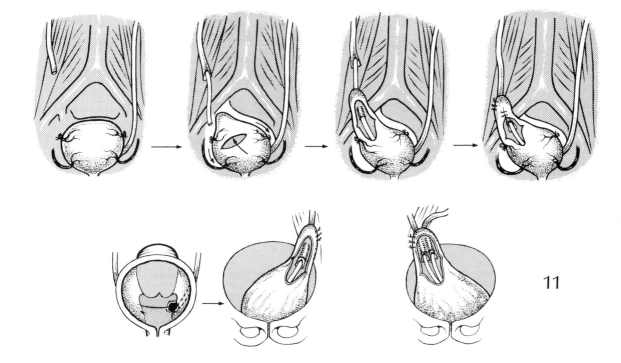

11

COMPLEX-FISTULAE

If the healing potential of the tissue margins of the fistula is compromised by scarring due to infection, previous attempts at repair or irradiation, the success rate of simple layer closure falls abruptly so that some form of viable tissue interposition is advisable.

A sizeable flap of para-pelvic peritoneum sometimes provides sufficient extra support for layer closure but the use of local tissues is contra-indicated when they are involved in scarring resulting from infection and especially from irradiation.

Pedicle grafts of skeletal muscle such as gracilis can be used but are not ideal because this tissue is ill-adapted to resist the infection and inflammation that are commonly associated with such cases.

The omentum is uniquely adapted for the resolution of local inflammatory processes; not only on account of its blood supply but also its abundant lymphatic drainage which re-absorbs inflammatory cell debris and macro-molecular protein exudates. The omentum has a well established place in complex urinary tract reconstruction in general[2, 7].

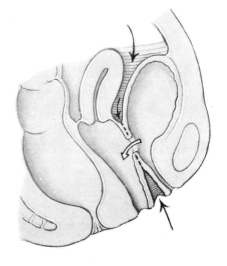

12a

Omental interposition repair of vesico-vaginal fistulae

12a & b

A wide abdomino-perineal tunnel, that will accept four fingers in the adult, is created in the tissue plane between the bladder and the vagina. The bladder and the vagina are closed with interrupted Dexon or Vicryl sutures, the knots of which lie in the respective lumina, and the omental graft is interposed, its distal margin being included in the perineal skin-closure sutures.

Provided there is an adequate bulk of well vascularized omental graft with a good overlap lateral to the suture lines, urinary fistulae rarely recur; even if the suture line of the bladder breaks down the surface of the exposed omentum rapidly urothelializes.

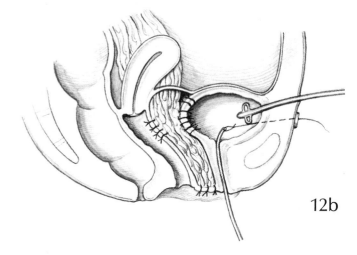

12b

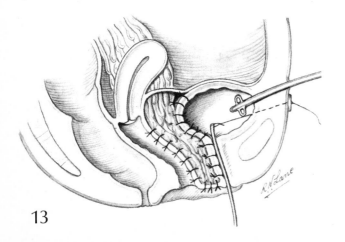

13

Omental interposition repair of vesico-urethro-vaginal fistulae

13

Complicated fistulae extending from the bladder base into the urethra can also be closed with omental support but urinary continence is, of course, dependent upon the reconstruction of either an efficient bladder neck sphincter or an efficient urethral sphincter or both; these in turn depend not only upon meticulous urethral reconstruction but also upon the functional survival of its intramural mechanism[1].

Omental interposition repair of vesico-vagino-rectal fistulae

14a–d

The omentum can be used to repair large and multiple post-irradiation fistulae, even if the rectum is also involved. The vesico-vagino-rectal fistula illustrated resulted from the treatment of a carcinoma of the cervix by hysterectomy and irradiation; the vault of the residual vagina is usually stenosed in such cases and surrounded by dense scar tissue. The abdomino-perineal tunnel is created through the vagina circumcising its wall at the upper limit of reasonably healthy tissue and developing a plane between the bladder and the rectum by synchronous abdomino-perineal dissection; it is usually impossible to identify individual tissue layers around the stenotic vaginal vault but the excess of scar tissue should be excised and the tunnel fully developed laterally, to the side walls of the pelvis, to ensure wide omental overlap of the suture lines.

Particular care must be taken to avoid leaving islands of vaginal epithelium in the region of the scarred vaginal apex because these predispose to the reformation of fistulous tracks. The bladder and the rectum are closed with interrupted 2/0 Dexon or Vicryl sutures; a large omental graft is introduced into the tunnel, its lower margin being included into the vaginal closure sutures. The defunctioning left iliac colostomy is maintained for several months.

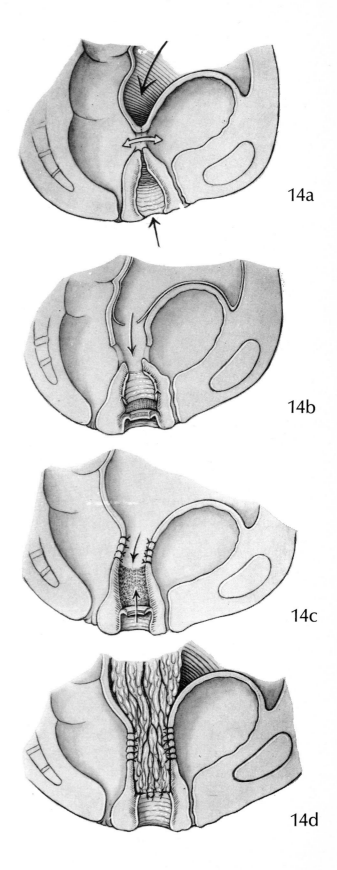

14a

14b

14c

14d

The reliability of omental interposition graft repair

The reliability of an omental pedicle graft repair depends upon achieving a large interpositional bulk with a wide lateral overlap of the closure suture lines of the bladder and the vagina – it is not just an 'omental plug'. The basic essential of the procedure is therefore the development of a 3–4 finger wide abdomino-perineal interposition tunnel and the appropriate mobilization of a sufficient bulk of omental apron to fill it.

It is also essential to appreciate that the success of the omental pedicle graft is fundamentally dependent upon an arterial blood supply that is efficiently pulsating, and upon its unimpaired venous and lymphatic drainage: any impairment of any of these diminish its potential.

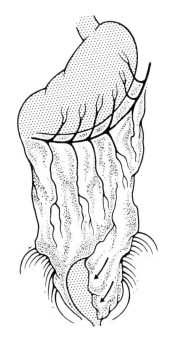

15a

15a & b

In about 30 per cent of cases the omentum apron is long enough for an adequate bulk of its lower margin to reach the perineum without definitive mobilization of the vascular pedicle; however, it should always be separated from its natural adhesion to the transverse colon and mesocolic vessels to avoid the possibility that postoperative gaseous distention of the bowel might dislocate the interposition graft.

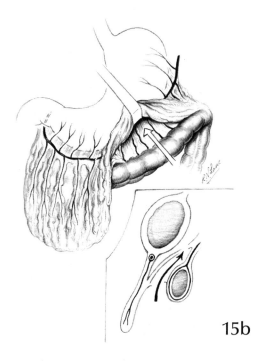

15b

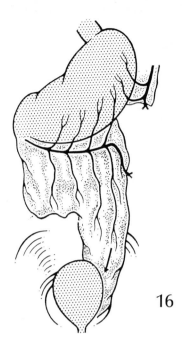

16

In about 30 per cent of cases sufficient elongation of a moderate length apron can be simply achieved by dividing the left gastro-epiploic pedicle vessels and the direct branches of the splenic vessels.

Formal full length mobilization of the right gastro-epiploic pedicle is required to enable the omentum to reach the pelvis in 30–40 per cent of patients.

16

The anatomical basis of mobilization of the omental vascular pedicle

17

Because it is necessary to elongate the vascular pedicle of the omentum in more than 50 per cent of cases to enable it to reach the pelvis, it is fundamentally important to be aware of the basic anatomical features of its vascular supply.

1. The blood supply of the omental apron is derived from vertically running vessels arising from the gastro-epiploic arch with relatively poor distal arcade communications between them. Thus when dividing the omental apron in the midline to provide a pedicle graft support for an upper urinary tract reconstruction, the two halves can often be separated between vertical vessels without the division of any collateral blood vessels sufficiently large to require ligation.

2. The main base of the gastro-epiploic vascular arcade is always on the right side; in fact the junction between the right and the left gastro-epiploic vessels that usually completes the arcade is deficient in about 10 per cent of cases at a point on the left side of the greater curvature.

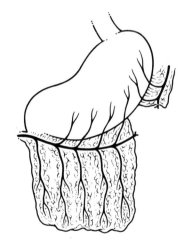

17

INAPPROPRIATE PROCEDURES FOR OMENTAL MOBILIZATION

18a & b

It follows that the omental apron should not be mobilized by a horizontal incision below the gastro-epiploic arch because this involves division of some of its vertical vessels and impairs the vascularity of the extremity of the graft.

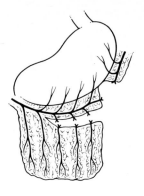

18a

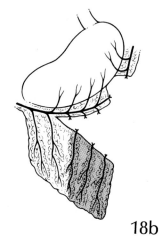

18b

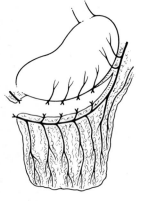

19a

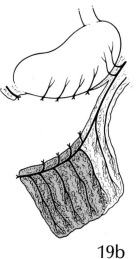

19b

19a & b

Similarly, it is generally inadvisable to mobilize the omentum on the basis of the relatively minor left gastro-epiploic pedicle as orginally advocated by Bastiaanse[8] and by Kiricuta and Goldstein[9] and others.

APPROPRIATE MOBILIZATION OF THE OMENTAL PEDICLE

20

The mobilization of a short apron should be based on the right gastro-epiploic vessels. This is fortunate for mechanical reasons because the origin of the right gastro-epiploic vessels from the gastro-duodenal vessels is much lower in the abdomen than the origin of the left gastro-epiploic vessels from the splenic vessels. When the full length of the gastro-epiploic arch is mobilized from the greater curvature of the stomach by the individual ligation division of its short gastric branches, its divided left extremity is long enough to reach the pelvis, irrespective of the length of the omental apron itself – thus the omentum can be used in children when the apron is under-developed.

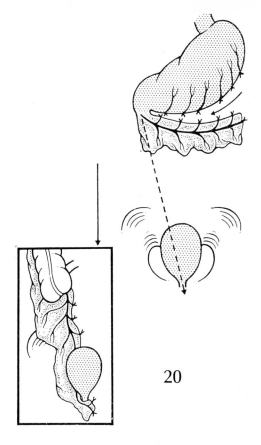

20

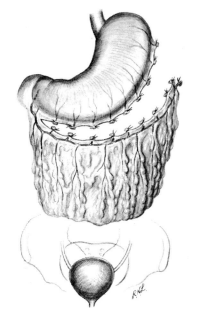

21

The technique of mobilization of the omentum

An upwardly extendable midline incision is essential.

21

The 20–30 short gastric branches must be individually ligated with absorbable suture material without damaging the main gastro-epiploic vessels.

Non-absorbable ligatures should never be used; any one could come to lie within the fistula area and cause stone formation as a result of encrustation.

22

Ligation of a bunch of several branches foreshortens the pedicle and adds to the risk that one might escape and bleed. The escape of the proximal end of any of these vessels is a potential disaster; it can rapidly create an interstitial haematoma and great care is then necessary to retrieve it for secure re-ligation without damage to the main vessels.

The proximal end of these vessels should be safely ligated in continuity before division but haemostat ligation of the gastric ends is quite acceptable because they are easy to retrieve if they escape.

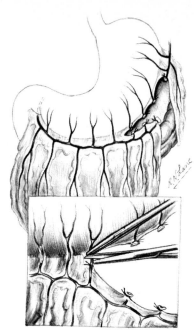

22

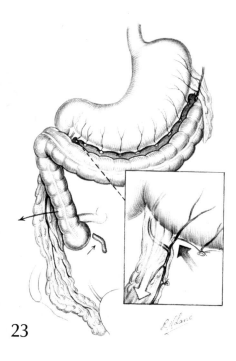

23

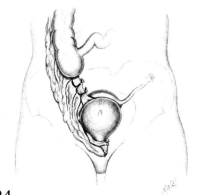

24

23 & 24

Once started, the mobilization of the gastro-epiploic arch should usually be completed to its gastro-duodenal origin otherwise there is a risk that traction on the pedicle might tear the last undivided branch.

A routine appendicectomy is advisable to avoid the possibility that a subsequent appendicitis or emergency appendicectomy might compromise the immediately adjacent pedicle.

Gastric suction for a mild intestinal ileus is often required for 3 or 4 days after an extended mobilization of the gastro-epiploic pedicle. Gastrostomy tube drainage is a humane alternative to a naso-gastric tube and, because the stomach is exposed, this is quite a simple procedure. However, a gastrostomy is prone to leak after removal of the catheter, unless an appropriate technique is used, so it is not advocated for surgeons who do not have an appropriate training in gastro-intestinal surgery.

OMENTOCAECOVAGINOPLASTY

25

In younger patients it is sometimes appropriate to reconstruct the stenosed vault of an irradiated vagina with a synchronous caeco-vaginoplasty supported by an omental wrap[10]; in such cases the suture line between the inverted ascending colon and the lower margin of the vagina usually heals quite well because they are relatively unaffected by the irradiation.

A caeco-vaginoplasty is especially valuable in the surgical management of a 'frozen' irradiation pelvis when, for instance, even after full mobilization of its pedicle, there is an insufficient bulk of omentum available to fill the 'dead space' in the pelvis after the resection of a stenotic rectum and restoration of bowel continuity by a colo-anal anastomosis. In such cases the well vascularized wall of the transposed caecum and its mucosal lining serves as a space-occupying cavity lining.

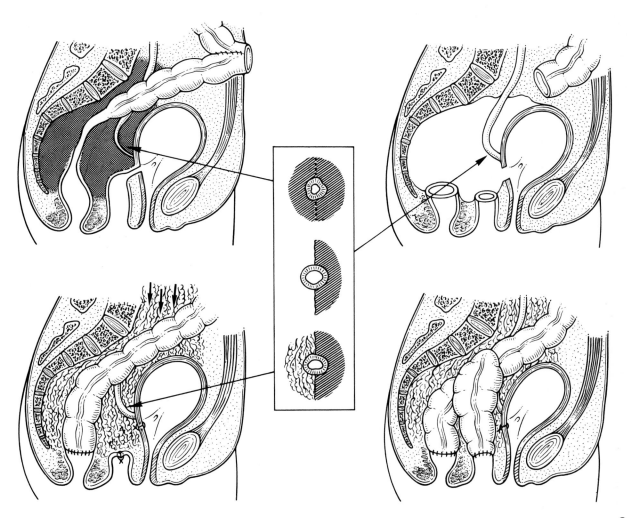

INCARCERATED 'OBSTRUCTION' OF THE LOWER URETER ASSOCIATED WITH IRRADIATION FIBROSIS

The functional drainage of the lower segment of the ureter is commonly impaired in association with extensive irradiation fibrosis. This is not always the result of a stricture – it sometimes results from fibrotic encasement of a somewhat dilated ureter which compromises the peristaltic activity of the residual muscle of the irradiated ureter. In such cases it is sometimes possible to restore functional drainage by 'hemilysis' – carefully resecting the dense fibrosis overlying its medial surface replacing this with the supple omental graft. Owing to the increased risk of necrosis it is generally inappropriate to attempt to mobilize such an irradiated ureter from its fibrotic bed, as in the management of benign retroperitoneal fibrosis, by lysis transposition and omental wrap[2,7].

The technique of hemi-omental support after the hemilysis of an irradiated ureter emphasizes the value of the omentum which, because it never 'sets solid', ensures the subsequent freedom of urodynamic movement of any urinary tract repair by preventing immobilization as a result of recurrent secondary fibrosis[2,7].

A *fenestrated* ureteric stent is generally advisable to cover the early postoperative course after hemilysis of an irradiated ureter[7].

IRRADIATION FISTULAE AND RESIDUAL TUMOUR

There is always a possibility that there are residual tumour cells in the fibrosis associated with an irradiation fistula, even when a preliminary biopsy proves negative and even if the treatment was concluded 10 or 20 years previously. The presence of a microscopic tumour in dense irradiated fibrosis is not necessarily a contraindication to the omental closure of a fistula; however, this situation requires thoughtful qualification and considered clinical judgement.

It is clearly inappropriate to attempt to close a fistula when the bulk of the induration associated with it is active recurrent macroscopic tumour. However, when a representative biopsy simply shows a few residual cells in extensive irradiation fibrosis, this may indicate that the local tumour is relatively quiescent. In these circumstances, because the prognosis is consequently poor, it is all the more important to resolve the incapacitating incontinence as swiftly and as efficiently as possible. Closure of the fistula with omental support is not only a considerably simpler surgical procedure than a uretero-ileal surface conduit but it offers patients a good chance of normal urinary voiding and control for their remaining months.

The timing of a fistula repair

It is impossible to generalize about the timing of a fistula repair: this is determined by clinical estimation of the healing potential of the local tissues of a particular case in relation to the proposed procedure.

If a repair is to be entirely dependent upon a layered closure it is obviously very important that the local tissue be in the best possible condition. It is often possible to resolve the problem of a simple traumatic or postoperative fistula by early exploration, within a few days, before a compromising degree of tissue healing reaction has developed. However, once this is established, it is usually better to wait several months until the local inflammatory response has stabilized as much as possible.

The main disadvantage of delaying a closure is the discomfort that it causes the patient – she is likely to be intractably wet until the fistula is closed; nevertheless, if this course of action is necessary it must be carried through with determination because disasters can result from impatience and premature intervention. Reasonably efficient interim collection of urine can sometimes be achieved by Foley catheter drainage of the *vagina* if the introitus is narrow enough to retain a large balloon.

Although it is obviously important to ensure that any acute inflammatory element or haematoma is resolved, the timing of a fistula repair is relatively less critical when the success of the procedure is largely dependent upon an interposed omental pedicle graft; just as this procedure has enabled repair of fistulae resulting from permanent severe tissue damage, or loss due to infection, trauma or irradiation, that were beyond the potential of a layer closure procedure, so it can also make us somewhat less time-dependent on the local tissue healing of a relatively simple fistula repair.

Thus, the timing of a repair must be considered carefully in relation to each individual fistula. It is generally unjustifiable to use a relatively major abdomino-perineal procedure involving a full length median incision for the repair of a simple fistula when, by waiting a few months, this can be simply repaired by a vaginal approach layer closure procedure. However, there are occasions when it may be quite clear that the ultimate repair is going to require the omental position anyway so that, provided any coincident infection has been reduced to a minimum and there is no haematoma mass, it may be unnecessary to wait for maximal resolution of the local tissue reaction.

References

1. Turner-Warwick, R. T. The repair of vesicovaginal fistula. In:Campbell's urology Harrison *et al* (eds: New York: W. B. Saunders 1977: 2966–2977

2. Turner-Warwick, R. T., Wynne, E. J. C., Handley Ashken, M. The use of the omental pedicle graft in the repair and reconstruction of the urinary tract. British Journal of Surgery 1967; 54: 849–853

3. Spence, H. M., Duckett, J. W. Diverticulum of the female urethra: clinical aspects and presentation of a simple operative technique for cure. Journal of Urology 1970; 104: 432–437

4. Turner-Warwick, R., Worth, P. H. L., Milroy, E., Duckett, J. The suprapubic V-incision. British Journal of Urology 1974; 46: 39–45

5. Turner-Warwick, R. T. The use of pedicle grafts in the repair of urinary tract fistulae. British Journal of Urology 1972; 44: 644–656

6. Turner-Warwick, R. T., Worth, P. H. L. The psoas bladder hitch procedure for the replacement of the lower third of the ureter. British Journal of Urology 1969; 41: 701–709

7. Turner-Warwick, R. T. The use of the omental pedicle graft in urinary tract reconstruction. Journal of Urology 1976; 116: 341–347

8. Bastiaanse, M. A. Bastiaanse's method for surgical closure of very large irradiation fistulae of the bladder and rectum. In: Gynecological urology Youssef, A. F. (ed) Springfield, Illinois: C. C. Thomas 1960: 280–297

9. Kiricuta, R. I., Goldstein, A. M. B. The repair of extensive vesico-vaginal fistulas with pedicle omentum: a review of 27 cases. Journal of Urology 1972; 108: 724–727

10. Turner-Warwick, R., H. Ashken, M. H. The functional results of partial, subtotal and total cystoplasty with special reference to ureterocaecocystoplasty, selective sphincterotomy and cystocystoplasty. British Journal of Urology 1967; 39: 3–12

Acknowledgement

The instruments illustrated here are available from the Genito-urinary Co, London; Down Bros, London; V. Mueller, Chicago; and Leibinger, W. Germany.

Exstrophy of the bladder and epispadias*

J. H. Johnston MB, FRCS, FRCSI, FACS
Urological Surgeon, Alder Hey Children's Hospital, Liverpool;
Lecturer in Paediatric Urology, University of Liverpool, UK

EXSTROPHY OF THE BLADDER

Reconstruction of the bladder

Reconstruction of an exstrophic bladder with the object of producing normal urinary control is warranted when the bladder is sufficiently large to allow the formation of an organ of useful capacity. The operation is most easily performed in the neonatal period when the bladder musculature is thin and pliable and the mucosa is smooth. Later, the vesical wall becomes fibrous and rigid and the mucosa often becomes thickened and polypoid. In such circumstances, or when the bladder is very small, effective reconstruction is not possible and urinary diversion is needed. In the female, the urethra is constructed in its entirety at the time of bladder closure. In the male, only the posterior urethra is formed; correction of the genital defect and construction of a penile urethra are carried out later, as described in the section on epispadias (pp. 397–404). Reconstruction of the abdominal wall after bladder closure is easily obtained by performing bilateral iliac osteotomies which allow approximation of the widely separated pubic bones. Otherwise, closure of the abdominal defect requires the mobilization of fascial and skin flaps. The osteotomies and the bladder reconstruction are performed at the same operative session. Since there is often considerable blood loss, a well running intravenous infusion should be in position and blood must be available for transfusion. The drawings show the technique of bladder and urethral closure in the female.

---

* This chapter has been reprinted from the 3rd edition

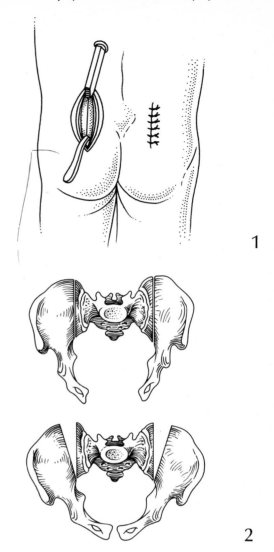

1

2

1 & 2

Iliac osteotomies

With the child prone and with a sandbag raising the pelvis, a vertical incision is made just lateral to the sacroiliac joint. The muscles are divided with diathermy down to the bone between the iliac crest and the sciatic notch. The periosteum is incised along the same line. The superior gluteal vessels and nerve emerging from the pelvis below the notch are protected by the insertion of a dissector or a malleable retractor under the periosteum; the bone is then divided from above downwards using an osteotome and hammer. The muscles and skin are sutured. The procedure is repeated on the other side. After both ilia have been divided, the two halves of the pelvis must be compressed together strongly so as to stretch ligamentous attachments which still tend to hold the pubes apart.

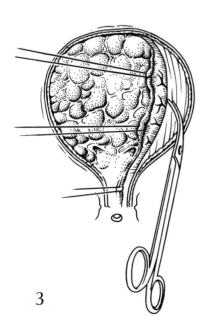

3

3

Mobilization of the bladder and urethra

With the patient supine, an incision is made around the margin of the exstrophic bladder and extended on each side of the epispadiac urethral strip. If the stump of the umbilical cord is still present it is excised, with ligation of the umbilical vessels. The bladder is freed by scissor dissection from the subcutaneous tissues, from the rectus abdominis on each side and, in the apical region, from the peritoneum. Care is needed to ensure a correct plane of dissection, especially during separation of the bladder from the recti. In the region of the bladder neck, dissection is carried out close to the deep aspect of the pubes. The ureter is seldom endangered during the dissection; if necessary it can be identified easily in the wound by passing a catheter through the orifice. The bladder must be freed sufficiently to allow its closure without tension. The edges of the urethral strip are raised from the underlying tissue on each side so that the strip can be closed into a tube.

4

Formation of the bladder neck

In order to narrow the funnel-shaped bladder neck and to lengthen the posterior urethra, a triangular area, composed of the entire thickness of the bladder wall, is excised from each side. The fibromuscular band passing from one pubic bone to the other behind the bladder neck will be exposed. The bands represent the splayed-open external urethral sphincter muscle.

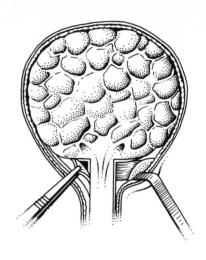

4

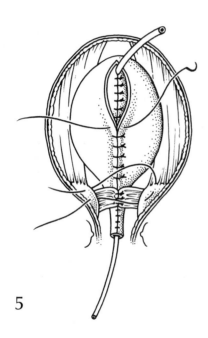

5

5

Closure of the bladder and urethra

The bladder mucosa and musculature are closed separately, using interrupted catgut or Dexon sutures. The bladder is drained by a self-retaining catheter brought out through the top of the incision. The urethral strip is closed into a tube; interrupted 5/0 Dexon sutures are employed, with the knots in the lumen so that the mucosa will be everted towards the interior. A fine catheter along the urethra during closure ensures that the correct lumenal calibre is obtained. The interpubic band is detached from the bone on each side and dissected medially; the two halves are sutured together, or overlapped, around the urethra. It is doubtful if this reconstruction of the external urethral sphincter makes any useful contribution to continence but the tissue helps to protect and support the reconstructed urethra. A 2 or 3 catgut suture, mounted on a strong cutting needle, is passed in mattress fashion through the pubic bones.

6 & 7

Wound closure

While an assistant presses each greater trochanter forwards and medially to aproximate the pubic bones, the pubic mattress suture is tightened and tied. The rectus sheaths are sutured together with interrupted catgut over the reconstructed bladder. The skin is closed with nylon, except in the vulval area where the skin is sutured to the edges of the urethral meatus. Here absorbable sutures such as Dexon are more convenient. The two clitorides can be fashioned into one by excising the epithelium on their apposing surfaces and suturing them together. The self-retaining catheter should be fixed firmly by a skin suture.

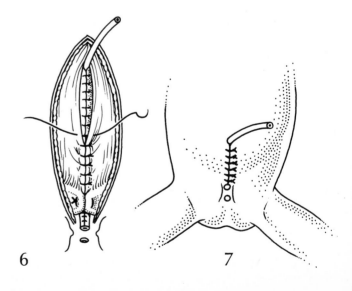

6

7

8

Aftercare

The inner aspect of each leg is padded with cellulose sponge and the legs are bound together with a crêpe bandage. Subsequently, the child is nursed supine with the legs elevated to a right angle in a gallows splint. The catheter is connected to a drainage bag. The nylon sutures are removed after 10 days. A bougie is passed gently through the reconstructed urethra before the bladder catheter is removed after 2 weeks.

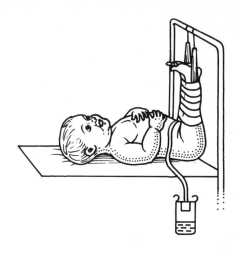

8

DISCUSSION

While the basic principles of bladder reconstruction as described above are generally agreed, different authorities have employed variations in timing, staging and technique. Williams and Keeton[1] prefer to operate later, when the child is 2–3 years of age. In the male, the penile deformity is corrected first. No attempt is made to obtain a continent vesical outlet at the initial closure operation; later, tightening of the bladder neck and ureteric reimplantation are performed. Vesicoureteric reflux is almost invariably present after bladder reconstruction. Marshall and Muecke[2] carry out ureteric reimplantation at the time of bladder closure but the procedure is more likely to be successful if performed later. The pubic bones reseparate with time, even if nonabsorbable sutures are used, and the object of iliac osteotomies is solely to allow easy wound closure. The subsequent separation of the pubes does not influence urinary control.

Early postoperative complications are mainly various degrees of breakdown of the reconstruction. These range from a temporary urinary fistula to complete wound dehiscence with reformation of the exstrophy. The most important later complication is upper urinary tract dilatation and kidney damage which results from incomplete bladder emptying, especially when associated with infection and reflux. Bladder and kidney stones may form. Frequent urine culture is needed to allow control of possible infection and intravenous urography must be carried out at regular intervals to determine the state of the upper urinary tract.

Neoplastic change in an exstrophic bladder was formerly considered to occur only as a late complication in the untreated case as a result of long-standing exposure and irritation of the mucosa. However, the complication has occurred following bladder reconstruction[3] and premalignant mucosal changes, persisting after bladder closure, can be detected histologically[4,3,5]. Regular cystoscopic examination is, therefore, advisable in the patient who obtains satisfactory urinary control.

The ideal result of reconstruction of an exstrophic bladder, namely perfect urinary control, sterile urine and a persistently normal upper urinary tract, is achieved only in a minority of patients. From a review of the literature, Johnston and Kogan[6] found that satisfactory continence had been obtained in 91 (21.9 per cent) of 415 reported cases of bladder reconstruction. However, in a considerable proportion of children with urinary control, diversion had to be performed because of upper tract and kidney deterioraton. The operation is, nevertheless, justified when the bladder is large and supple and particularly in girls, who are more likely to achieve control than boys. Secondary urinary diversion is needed if no useful control results or if there is upper tract and kidney deterioration which cannot be controlled by the elimination of infection and conservative surgical measures. When diversion is performed, removal of the bladder is indicated because of the possibility of neoplastic change.

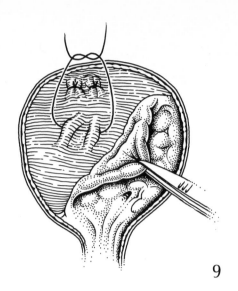

9

Excision of untreated exstrophic bladder

9 & 10

When the bladder is unsuitable for reconstruction and the child is treated by urinary diversion, removal of the unsightly and uncomfortable structure is indicated. It is not necessary to excise the bladder entirely. The mucosa is stripped off the musculature as far as the bladder neck, carefully preserving the proximal urethra in the male. The bladder muscle is plicated with catgut sutures to produce a strong, firm plaque filling the gap in the lower abdominal wall. The skin defect is closed by rotated flaps, augmented if necessary by free split-skin grafts.

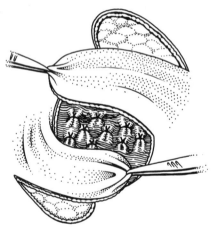

10

EPISPADIAS

Epispadias may pose two problems requiring surgical correction. In either sex the patient commonly lacks urinary control. In the male the penis is deformed.

Urinary incontinence

The degree of control shown by epispadiac children ranges from complete normality at one extreme to total incontinence with continual dribbling of urine at the other. In the incontinent case the bladder neck is wide and funnel-shaped and the posterior urethra is abnormally short. The poorly developed urethral musculature is unable to maintain a closed lumen. Urethral pressure profile measurements show that the external, voluntary sphincter is also inadequate. The bladder is often extremely small and thin-walled, since it has never been called upon to perform its normal functions of filling and emptying. Several operative procedures aimed at producing urinary control have been described. The present author's experience relates mainly to the Young-Dees[7,8] and the Leadbetter[9] techniques.

YOUNG-DEES OPERATION

This technique narrows the bladder outlet and lengthens the posterior urethra in a proximal direction. The method is applicable to the case with a relatively well-developed bladder as regards capacity and muscularity.

11, 12 & 13

Technique

The bladder is opened on its anterior wall through a vertical incision which extends into the bladder neck. The incision is held open by traction sutures. Carefully avoiding the ureteric orifices, a triangular wedge of tissue composed of the entire thickness of the bladder wall is excised from each side of the funnelled outlet. Resuturing, employing 3/0 catgut, converts the funnel into a tube and lengthens the posterior urethra. The bladder is closed with drainage.

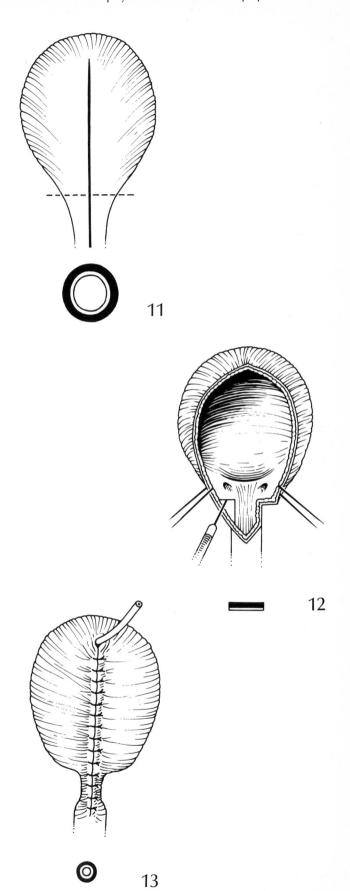

11

12

13

14

Alternative

As a modification, with the object of increasing the amount of muscular tissue around the bladder outlet, the excised triangular wedge on each side may consist of mucosa only, leaving the muscle intact. The remaining mucosal strip is closed into a tube. A transverse incision through the muscle along the upper edge of each triangle then allows the muscular flaps to be overlapped around the sutured mucosa.

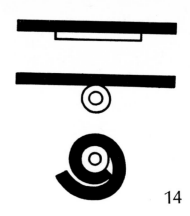

14

LEADBETTER OPERATION

The operation is similar to the Young-Dees procedure but a longer proximal extension of the posterior urethra is fashioned by constructing a neourethra from the bladder trigone. It is indicated particularly in the case in which the bladder wall is relatively thin so that the Young-Dees operation would not provide sufficient muscular tissue at the bladder outlet.

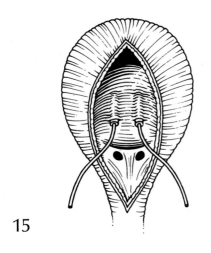

15

15 & 16

Cystotomy: reimplantation of ureters

The bladder is opened through a vertical incision on the anterior wall which extends into the bladder neck. Since the trigone is to be used for the construction of the neourethra, the ureters must be dissected free and reimplanted higher in the bladder by the Leadbetter-Politano antireflux technique[10]. When the bladder is small, the ureters are often better reimplanted transversely rather than vertically; they lie side by side within a common submucosal tunnel, each crossing to the other side of the bladder. With either technique, splinting of the ureters is advisable. A fine polythene catheter is passed to the renal pelvis on each side and brought to the exterior for drainage.

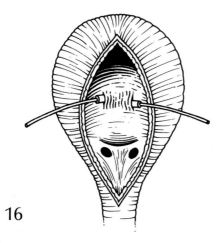

16

17

Formation of the trigonal strip

Using diathermy, a vertical incision is made on each side through the trigone to form a mucosa-lined muscular strip. Each incision extends from the original ureteric hiatus to the proximal end of the posterior urethra.

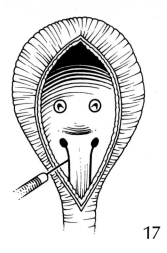

17

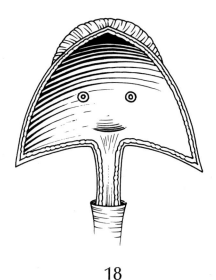

18

18 & 19

Construction of the neourethra: closure of the bladder

The bladder wall on either side of the trigone strip is raised. The strip is closed by interrupted 3/0 catgut sutures into a tube; the lower extremity is sutured to the circumference of the proximal end of the urethra. The bladder is closed with relf-retaining catheter drainage. The ureteric splints are brought to the exterior.

Aftercare

The splints are removed after 8 days. A bougie should be passed gently through the urethra and the neourethra into the bladder before the bladder catheter is removed about the 12th day.

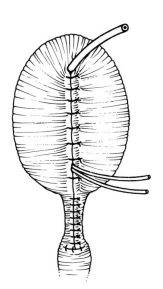

19

20 & 21

Comment: use of omentum to fill the retropubic dead space

The Leadbetter procedure as described above has the disadvantage that the bladder falls into the dead space in front of the neourethra. This causes the new internal urethral orifice to become sited high on the posterior bladder wall; difficulty in initiating micturition, a slow urinary stream and incomplete bladder emptying may result. On occasions a fistula forms through the suture lines between the most dependent part of the bladder and the lower end of the neourethra so that the latter is bypassed and its sphincter action lost. These complications can be avoided by filling the dead space with an omental graft. It is often possible to place a sufficient bulk of omentum in position without formal omental mobilization. If not, the omentum must be detached from the transverse colon and the stomach, dividing the left gastroepiploic and short gastric vessels. The omental graft is swung down to the pelvis from the pyloric region, its blood supply being derived from the right gastroepiploic vessels.

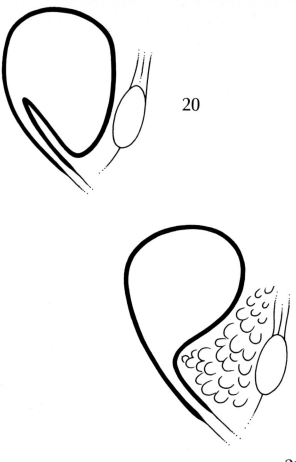

20

21

DISCUSSION

The main complication of bladder outlet reconstruction for epispadias is vesical outlet obstruction which results from an inadequate detrusor being unable to overcome the increased, but not necessarily abnormal, outlet resistance. Incomplete bladder emptying, infection, bladder stones and upper tract dilatation may result. Careful, lengthy postoperative supervision is, therefore, needed. Vesico-ureteric reflux is commonly present in epispadiac children and ureteric reimplantation is then needed during bladder neck reconstruction even when shifting of the ureteric orifices is not required for the reconstruction operation itself.

The results of bladder outlet reconstructions depend upon the quality of the tissues available. When, as is generally the case in the totally incontinent epispadiac, the bladder is very small and thin-walled, the success rate is low. Better results are obtained with a bladder of larger capacity and better developed musculature. However, immediate achievement of continence is not to be expected. Improvement in control is often slow and may progress gradually, or in steps, for many months or even years. In the male, spontaneous improvement may occur at puberty as a result of the development of the prostate. Welch[11] recorded that the control occurred at puberty in 6 of 12 epispadiac boys who had been considered operative failures until that time. In both sexes, increasing awareness of the social advantages of being dry is often an important factor in promoting continence.

The penile deformity in the male

22

The penis in boys with epispadias or exstrophy has three deformities. First, the urethra is partly, or in cases of exstrophy entirely, deficient dorsally so that the urethral meatus is abnormally sited on the penile dorsum or is non-existent. Second, there is dorsal chordee in that the penis is both tilted and curved upwards. The chordee is due largely to the short urethral mucosal strip which exerts a bowstring effect. Straightening of the penis requires that the urethra is separated from the corpora cavernosa and allowed to retract proximally.

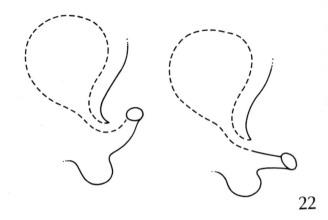

22

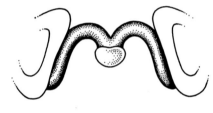

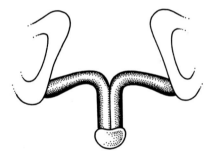

23

Third, the penis is short. This is mainly the result of the separation of the pubic bones. Each corpus cavernosum is of adequate length but much of the length is wasted between the penile body and the puboischial insertion. In order to lengthen the penis it is necessary partly to detach the crura from the bone so that the extrapenile parts of the corpora can be advanced into the shaft. Operative correction of the deformities is carried out in two stages.

23

FIRST STAGE – CHORDEE CORRECTION AND PENILE LENGTHENING

24 & 25

Skin incision and freeing of urethra

A nylon traction suture is placed through the glans penis. A V-shaped incision is made on the dorsum of the penis. The apex is anterior to the extremity of the urethral mucosal strip just proximal to the glans; the limbs of the V reach to the separated pubes. The urethra is detached by sharp dissection from the corpora to beyond their point of bifurcation and it and the triangular skin flap are held over the pubic area by a traction suture.

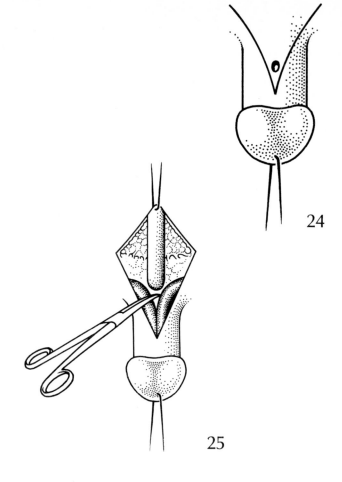

24

25

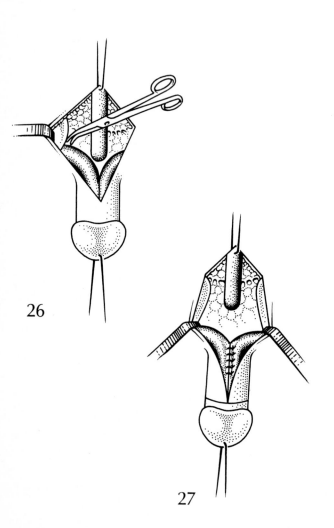

26

27

26 & 27

Detachment of the penile crura from the puboischial rami

The soft-tissue attachments passing from the corpora to the pubic area are divided and the pubic bone exposed. Using scissors, and keeping the dissection close to the bone, the fibrous attachments of the crus to the ramus are divided. The same procedure is repeated on the other side. No attempt should be made to detach the crura entirely from the bones because of the risk of damaging the neurovascular bundle entering the extremity of each crus. The tunicae of the mobilized parts of the corpora are sutured together with catgut so that they contribute to the length of the shaft of the penis.

28 & 29

Freeing skin from the penile ventrum and mobilization of the prepuce

A skin incision, joining the apex of the dorsal V incision, is made around the circumference of the penis just proximal to the corona glandis. The skin is freed entirely from the sides and ventrum of the penis. In order to increase the area of skin available, the two layers of the redundant ventral prepuce are separated by dividing the thin, retaining, fibrous adhesions between them. Care is needed to avoid damaging the longitudinally running subcutaneous vessels supplying the skin. Following the skin separation a better view is obtained of the lower parts of the crural attachments to the bones and further crural freeing may be safely carried out if necessary.

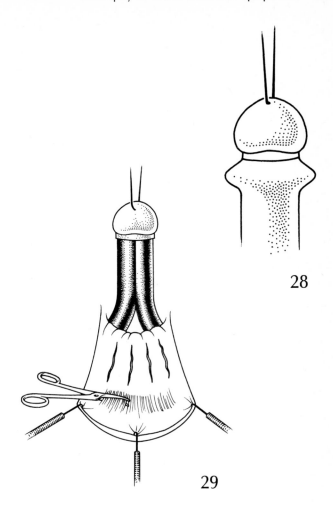

28

29

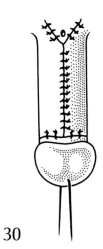

30

30

Skin closure

Using 5/0 Dexon, the mobilized skin is sutured to the edges of the fringe around the corona and joined onto the penile dorsum and to the edges of the V incision in Y fashion. The urethral meatus is at the apex of the V. In some cases, especially when previous surgery has been performed, there is insufficient penile skin to provide cover. The penis may then be covered by a relatively thick, free split-skin graft taken from the inner aspect of the thigh. Alternatively, the penis may be buried under the skin of the front of the scrotum, leaving the glans exposed. Three months later the penis is freed, at which time its ventral surface is covered with scrotal flaps. With this method it is difficult to obtain a close skin fit for the penis and the appearance is less satisfactory than with the other.

SECOND STAGE – CONSTRUCTION OF PENOGLANDULAR URETHRA

A neourethra is constructed from the skin on the penile dorsum and from the epithelium of the glans in order to advance the urethral meatus to the tip of the penis. The operation is performed about 6 months after the first stage operation.

31

Urinary diversion: outline of skin strip

A self-retaining catheter is placed in the bladder through a small suprapubic incision. A traction suture is inserted through the glans penis. A skin strip, including the urethral meatus, is formed on the penile dorsum. The width of the strip should equal the intended circumference of the neourethra. A triangular area of epithelium is excised from the glans penis on each side of the dorsal groove.

32 & 33

Tubularization of strip

The skin lateral and proximal to the strip is undermined. The strip itself should not be mobilized because of the risk of endangering its blood supply. Over a catheter inserted as a guide, the skin strip and the epithelial strip on the glans are closed into a tube, using 5/0 Dexon sutures with the knots in the lumen so as to evert the edges internally.

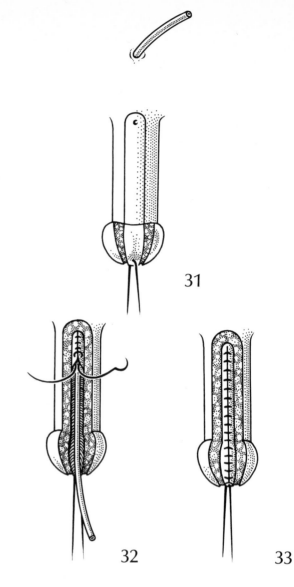

34, 35 & 36

Fascial and skin closure

Fascial layers are approximated over the neourethra. If insufficient tissue is available, a flap of the tunica of the corpus cavernosum can be raised on each side and sutured over the urethra. The raw surfaces on the glans are apposed, using vertical mattress sutures, and the skin is closed. If there is any tension on the suture line, a longitudinal relaxation incision is made on the ventrum of the penis.

Aftercare

After 2 weeks a bougie is passed gently through the constructed urethra before the bladder catheter is removed.

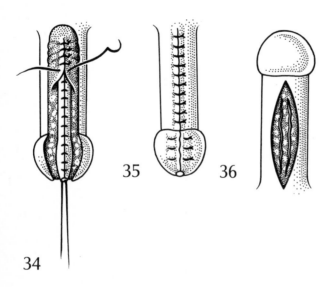

References

1. Williams, D. I., Keeton, J. E. Further progress with reconstruction of the exstrophied bladder. British Journal of Surgery 1973; 60: 203–207

2. Marshall, V. F., Muecke, E. C. Functional closure of typical exstrophy of the bladder. Journal of Urology 1970; 104: 205–212

3. Engel, R. M. E. Bladder exstrophy: vesicoplasty or urinary diversion? Urology 1973; 2: 20–24

4. Rudin, L., Tannenbaum, M., Lattimer, J. K. Histologic analysis of the exstrophied bladder after anatomic closure. Journal of Urology 1972; 108: 802–807

5. Clark, M. A., Connell, K. J. Scanning and transmission electron microscopic studies of an exstrophic human bladder. Journal of Urology 1973; 110: 481–483

6. Johnston, J. H., Kogan, S. J. The exstrophic anomalies and their surgical reconstruction. In: Current problems in surgery. 1974: August

7. Young, H. H. An operation for the cure of incontinence associated with epispadias. Journal of Urology 1922; 7: 1–32

8. Dees, J. E. Congenital epispadias with incontinence. Journal of Urology 1949; 62: 513–522

9. Leadbetter, G. W. Surgical correction of total urinary incontinence. Journal of Urology; 1964; 91: 261–266

10. Politano, V. A., Leadbetter, W. F. An operative technique for the correction of vesico-ureteral reflux. Journal of Urology 1958; 79: 932–941

11. Welch, K. J. Epispadias. In: Mustard, W. T., Ravitch, M. M., Snyder, W. H., Welch, K. J., Benson, C. D., eds. Pediatric surgery, 2nd ed. Chicago: Year Book Medical Publishers, 1969: 1333–1341

Further reading

Jeffs, R. D. Exstrophy and cloacal exstrophy. Congenital anomalies of the lower genitourinary tract. The Urologic Clinics of North America 1978; 5: 127–140

Latimer, J. K., Beck, L., Yeaw, S., Puchner, P. J., Macfarlane, M. T., Krisiloff, M. Long-term follow-up after exstrophy closure: late improvement and good quality of life. Journal of Urology 1978; 119: 664–666

Spence, H. M., Hoffman, W. M., Pate, V. A. Exstrophy of the bladder. Long-term results in a series of 37 cases treated by ureterosigmoidostomy. Journal of Urology 1975; 114: 133–137

Ilustrations by Kevin Marks

Operative management of vesicourethral neuropathy

N. O. K. Gibbon   MB, ChM, FRCS(Ed), FRCS
Consultant Urologist; formerly Head of the Urological Unit of the Royal Liverpool Hospital and
Director of Urological Studies, University of Liverpool, UK

Introduction

Surgical management of vesicourethral neuropathy is concerned mainly with the relief of retention; paradoxically, measures which are successful in this respect usually assist continence. Occasionally, specific surgical procedures may be required for the management of urinary leakage. Recent advances in vesicourethral physiology have helped provide a rational basis for investigation and treatment in this sphere, despite the fact that the mechanisms involved now seem more complex than had been supposed. With our new knowledge has come a realization that poor voiding in the cases under consideration is more commonly due to urethral obstruction than to inadequate expulsive forces. In this connection it should be stressed that an acceptable residual urine is not to be defined in terms of absolute volume or percentage of bladder capacity. Any residue which is compatible with sterility of the specimen and continued normality of annual pyeloureterograms is best left alone. Many patients tolerate residual urine of several hundred millilitres on this basis for years. More important is the presence of vesicoureteric reflux, especially if the urine is infected, which is often the case. Incompetence of the ureteric orifice is usually due to inflammatory changes; if these resolve under treatment (which may include the elimination of residual urine), the reflux ceases. When there has been much tissue destruction followed by fibrosis, or when the bladder wall is grossly trabeculated, the condition may persist and reimplantation may be called for following repeated attacks of pyelonephritis. Unfortunately, in these cases, a gross ureteritis which prejudices the result of surgical correction may be found.

The problems involved can be considered conveniently under the three main aspects of bladder function – storage, emptying and control.

STORAGE

At rest

Normal mechanism

The bladder stores urine at normal volumes, with the body supine and at rest, because of the low pressure ensured by its property of postural tone, combined with the higher resistance offered by the muscular and elastic tissue of the bladder neck.

Effect of denervation

The basic filling pressure is unaffected by central denervation at any level. The 'hypertonic' and 'atonic' bladders of the older classifications are due to infection and obstruction in the one case and overdistension in the other. Peripheral denervation usually results in a characteristic areflexic hypertonia, which develops in a few months and may produce both overflow incontinence and dilatation of the upper urinary tracts. The resistance of the bladder neck is also basically unaffected though the possibility of variations related to changes of sympathetic activity is now the subject of research. The 'wide bladder neck' as an indication of neuropathy *per se* is a myth – the determining factor is increased bladder wall tension due to overdistension or contraction, especially in association with distal obstruction.

With vesical overdistension

Normal mechanism

Increasing mural tension opens up the bladder neck; leakage is resisted by the ascending pressure gradient of the proximal urethra, which, at rest, is largely due to plain muscle under sympathetic stimulation[1]. This is reinforced by reflex contraction of the striated external sphincter, which at its height can hardly be augmented by voluntary effort.

Effect of denervation

Paralysis of the external sphincter will allow urinary leakage at an earlier stage when the bladder is overdistended. The immediate hypotonic effect of urethral sympathectomy is minimized by the development of supersensitivity of the alpha-adrenergic receptors[2].

With lower abdominal pressure increases

Normal mechanism

When the lower abdominal pressure is increased, as in the upright position or during coughing and straining, leakage is prevented by the fact that the proximal urethra in both sexes is intra-abdominal and subject to the same compression as the bladder[3,4]. This applies to the upper two-thirds of the urethra in the female and the whole of the prostatic urethra in the male. It is important with any surgical intervention on the urethra to try to preserve at least 1 cm or so of the intra-abdominal part, whether proximally or distally.

Effect of denervation

Paralysis of the pelvic floor (as in a cauda equina lesion) appears to impair reflection of the abdominal pressure increases onto the proximal urethra, which may then become incompetent allowing urinary leakage under stress, especially in the female. It is important to note that inactivity of the external urethral sphincter does not in itself cause incontinence in this situation. Stress leakage (or even continuous dribbling from an empty bladder) also occurs in the female with a spinal lesion at any level if the urethra has suffered necrosis and fibrosis from the pressure of a large and unrestrained catheter against the symphysis pubis. In this case, the urethra is incapable of watertight closure under pressure from outside. In these circumstances the patient often leaks around an ordinary catheter, but a double balloon catheter[5] may be extremely useful; anteversion of the urethra[6] may be attempted, although obesity is a common contraindication. As a last resort, ureteroenterocutaneous diversion will be required; this applies also to the female child with myelomeningocele and continuous leakage from an empty bladder. Ureterocolic anastomosis is almost always contraindicated in the neuropathic bladder because of inadequate rectal control.

EMPTYING

Normal mechanism

Detrusor contractions are mediated by the second, third and fourth sacral segments. Bladder neck opening is mainly mechanical, though some autonomic synergism has been shown which may well affect the proximal urethra too[7]. Relaxation of the external sphincter is coordinated not only in the conus but also at mid-brain level by wide-ranging circuits including the cerebellum rather than a localized 'centre'.

Effects of denervation

Sacral (lower motor neurone lesion)

In this case, the sacral reflex arcs subserving bladder contraction are interrupted, as in some cases of myelomeningocele, conus or cauda equina injuries and extensive pelvic dissections. Voiding occurs by manual compression or abdominal straining. In both instances the paralysed pelvic floor is an important factor, as it allows funnelling of the bladder neck and dissipation of abdominal pressure increases away from the urethra. Often the bladder neck does not open except when the bladder is moderately distended, and this results in residual urine. Bladder neck resection is required in both sexes if this is associated with persistent infection or progressive ureteric dilatation. The level of the obstruction should be confirmed by cystourethrography. Good results have also been reported for internal 'sphincterotomy', whether bilateral, anterior or posterior.

In the female, urethral dilatation or Otis urethrotomy (to around 40–50 Fr) may be effective, and, if bladder neck resection is done, it is wise to avoid the midline posteriorly lest a vesicovaginal fistula result and to leave a good segment of the abdominal urethra intact. In the older male, adenomatous prostatic obstruction or inflammatory bladder neck stenosis sometimes requires resection. It should be noted that although the external sphincter is paralysed, emptying of the lower motor neurone bladder is sometimes obstructed at the membranous level due to unrestrained plain muscle contraction, which is postural and under sympathetic stimulation. This is probably due to sympathetic decentralization supersensitivity. (Contrary to the usual teaching, the sympathetic neurones supplying the pelvic organs may well originate in the conus[8,9].) Diagnosis is revealed radiologically. If α-blocking agents (for example, phenoxybenzamine 10 mg t.d.s. by mouth) do not give relief without unacceptable side-effects, then internal membranous urethrotomy will be required (see 'External sphincterotomy' p. 410). If the bladder neck funnels freely or has been resected, an attempt should be made to leave a short segment of urethra intact above the urogenital diaphragm to minimize stress incontinence. In the cases referred to, some sensation of bladder fullness is retained through the sympathetic innervation and this prompts the patient to strain at suitable intervals and so minimize any tendency to incontinence. In tabes dorsalis and diabetic neuropathy, however, in addition to interruption of the sacral reflex arc, there may be total sensory denervation of the bladder and gross atonic distension may result from failure to strain at regular intervals.

Suprasacral (upper motor neurone lesion)

The upper level of sensory or motor loss is not a reliable guide to the preservation of sacral reflex activity because descending avascular necrosis may involve the conus in lesions as high as the midthoracic level. Fortunately, the state of the bulbocavernosus and anal reflexes is a reliable guide to the situation within a few hours of onset. If they are positive, then reflex bladder contractions may be expected to return after a period of spinal shock which may last from a few weeks to a year or more. During this period, as in the early stages following an acute lesion of the sacral segments when pain and recumbency prevent straining, the bladder will have to be drained, preferably by intermittent catheterization, though an indwelling plastic catheter of not more than 10 or 12 Fr is acceptable provided that blockage is watched for carefully. In the upper motor neurone cases, return of bladder reflex activity may be observed when the patient voids or it may be detected by cystometry. Emptying can then be precipitated by repeated deep sharp suprapubic tapping[10], and with a regular fluid intake a high degree of control may be attained[11]. This applies especially to women, as they cannot fall back on the use of a urinal. Unfortunately, the sacral centres are cut off from the supraspinal coordinating areas of these cases, and the

external urethral sphincter may show tonic or clonic contractions (the latter sometimes being synchronous with detrusor activity) which interfere with voiding[12]. The diagnosis is confirmed by the finding of a large residual urine and a narrow segment at the membranous urethral level on cystourethrography with dilatation proximally, which often includes the prostatic ducts. Pudendal neurotomy is sometimes successful in relieving this obstruction despite persistent doubts about the innervation of the external sphincter[13,14]. However, the operation has been virtually abandoned because impotence follows in over half the cases. Selective pudendal crush[15] may be valuable in establishing vesicourethral synergism. External sphincterotomy is the operation of choice when a permanent effect is desired, however, being both safe and effective in skilled urological hands[16]. The policy in these cases used to be to resect the bladder neck first, if emptying was unsatisfactory, and then to resort to external sphincterotomy in the failures. This is no longer appropriate. The radiological findings often indicate the need for a primary sphincterotomy. Impotence has been reported following this operation, but it is probably due to excessive incisions. In over 300 external sphincterotomies carried out at the Liverpool Regional Spinal Injuries Centre, loss of sexual potency has not been significant[17].

There is some evidence of sympathetic overactivity causing urethral obstruction in cases with lesions above the lower thoracic segments. In the membranous region this is usually overshadowed by striated muscle spasm, but it may interfere with bladder-neck opening, especially if detrusor contractions are mediocre. If cystourethrography shows poor bladder neck opening, then α-blocking agents are worth a trial. If these fail, then bladder neck resection will be required; operation will also be necessary in upper motor neurone cases for prostatic obstruction or inflammatory bladder neck stenosis.

CONTROL

Normal mechanism

Sensation, inhibition and initiation of bladder function are represented bilaterally in the frontoparietal cortex. During micturition, the flow may be interrupted quickly by voluntary contraction of the external sphincter.

Effects of denervation

Increasing cerebral compression causes retention and then involuntary voiding, perhaps because of dominance of the social instincts at lighter levels of unconsciousness. Focal lesions in the frontoparietal area may produce the classic 'cerebral micturition' – unheralded and complete bladder emptying. In hemiplegia, bladder control is rarely affected for more than the acute period because of the bilateral innervation already referred to. With suprasacral cord involvement, initiation and inhibition of micturition are impaired or lost, leading in complete lesions to spinal reflex emptying without warning.

The operations

The operations applicable to this field fall into four tiers:

1. *Operations to remove the cause of the neuropathy*, for example, a saggital sinus meningioma or a prolapsed intervertebral disc. With acute compression of the sacral segments, urgent intervention is required to forestall permanent loss of reflex detrusor activity. On the other hand, laminectomy for a patient with a complete cord lesion following fracture-dislocation of the spine is regarded by most authorities as unhelpful and sometimes dangerous.
2. *Surgical procedures designed to modify indirectly the vesicourethral disturbance*. Pudendal neurectomy for external sphincter spasticity is a typical example, though the mechanism may be indirect, as suggested above (*see* 'Emptying', pp. 407–408). Sacral neurotomy (bilateral selective section of the third sacral anterior primary ramus) may well be coming back into fashion for the 'unstable' bladder, including adult enuresis. Other measures for the treatment of this condition which are now under clinical trial are prolonged bladder overdistension[18] and transection of the bladder, with or without multiple myotomies[19,20]. Enterocystoplasty, which is known to be effective[21], is likely to be displaced by the other techniques mentioned which are considerably safer.
3. *Operations on the bladder and urethra designed to relieve retention*, the indications for which have been outlined above. Surgery may also be required for complications such as urinary calculi and urethral stricture or diverticulum. Most of these are routine urological procedures and require no detailed description here. Surgical intervention on the urethra is likely to be required in some 40 per cent of paraplegics if a rapid hospital turnover is desired, but in only about 10 per cent if unlimited time is available for the spontaneous readjustment of bladder function[22].
4. *Diversion of urine* may be indicated when attempts to achieve voiding have failed and an indwelling catheter is contraindicated, or when hopeless incontinence is present in the female. When there is gross ureteric dilatation on presentation, usualy in infants or young children, temporary ureterostomy may be invaluable. In some cases suprapubic cystostomy with a balloon catheter of about 22 Fr meets the requirements of the adult case. As drainage may continue for many years, the balloon should be inflated with only 1 or 2 ml of fluid so as to minimize the area for phosphatic encrustation. The rigidity of the suprapubic track prevents accidental withdrawal of the balloon even when of such a small size. When urinary diversion is inevitable, it will have to be carried out by an enterocutaneous method as rectal incontinence usually contraindicates ureterocolic anastomosis. Again, these procedures are all standard and described elsewhere.

Special problems arising in paraplegics during or around the time of operations include:

1. A high risk of bacteraemia during interventions on the kidney, prostate and urethra on account of the ubiquitous infection in complicated cases.
2. The fairly common occurrence of autonomic dysreflexia with severe hypertension in high lesions, especially during vesical or rectal distension. This condition responds to α-adrenergic blockade which may be prophylactic by the oral route (phenoxybenzamine 10 mg three times a day) or induced during a crisis by rapid intravenous injection (diazoxide 300 mg).

It may be thought that anaesthesia can be dispensed with in operations below the segmental level of the lesion, and this might be true in selected cases with sacral involvement. However, with suprasacral lesions, full general anaesthesia is usually required to avert troublesome flexor spasms. With complete lesions at this level, spinal anaesthesia is justifiable.

The three specialized procedures already referred to will now be described in more detail.

EXTERNAL SPHINCTEROTOMY (division of the external sphincter, internal membranous urethrotomy)

This operation can be performed with a pandendoscope and a Collings' knife, but the instrument of choice is a resectoscope with knife electrode. A near-isotonic, non-electrolytic irrigating solution is essential (e.g. 3 per cent dextrose or 1.1 per cent glycine) because of the risk of perineal extravasation and venous absorption. It is a wise precaution to use only the minimum coagulation current which will enable the knife to separate the tissues. A powerful cutting current often results in inadvertent perforation into cavernous tissue with loss of vision as well as the complications just referred to and, in the long term, impotence.

1a, b & c

An incision is made bilaterally starting at the level of the verumontanum and extending distally for 2–3 cm. The mucosa is first divided and the muscular fibres are then teased through a few at a time until they thin out, usually at a depth of around 5 mm.

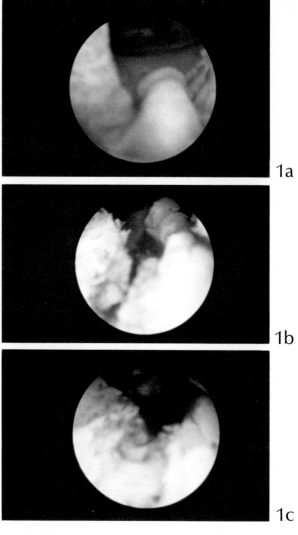

1a

1b

1c

(a) The membranous urethra on the right side (the bladder neck and verumontanum are also shown); (b) Internal membranous urethrotomy (right). The upper end of the incision is at the level of the veru; (c) The lower part of the incision alongside the crista urethralis

2

Done in this way, the operation usually produces no more than a few small arterial bleeding points which are easily dealt with using a ball electrode.

Venous bleeding cannot be controlled in this way but stops on insertion of the catheter, especially if a little pressure is applied in the perineum or per rectum. Swelling of the scrotum due to extravasation is very rare if the procedure is carried out as described, and will usually resolve harmlessly with elevation and support unless a grossly hypotonic solution has been used, when free drainage is urgently required.

A 20 or 22 Fr irrigating catheter is suitable for postoperative drainage, but this should be replaced after a few days by one of only 10–12 Fr if further drainage is required to avoid urethritis and stricture.

Successful results have also been reported from transurethral resection of the roof of the membranous urethra[23]. We have confirmed the value of the operation, especially when biopsy is desired for research purposes. This operation has been reported to be successful in cases of detrusor sphincter dyssynergia even when no striated muscle has been found in the tissue removed[24].

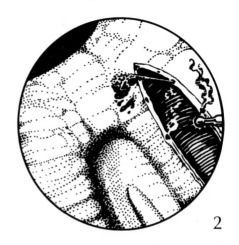

2

PUDENDAL NEURECTOMY OR CRUSH

The rationale of this operation is still far from clear (*see* 'Emptying', pp. 407–408). It is usually carried out after preliminary bilateral pudendal nerve blocks have shown improved bladder emptying.

3

The nerve is injected as it runs behind the insertion of the sacrospinous ligament, which can be palpated through the rectum or vagina. In the female paraplegic (in whom distal urethral obstruction only rarely fails to respond to overdilatation), the ligament is palpated through the vagina, in the lithotomy position. A specially guarded needle[15] is guided onto the vaginal mucosa just medial to the ischial spine. The ligament is then pierced by advancing the needle about 0.5 cm and the region of the nerve is infiltrated with 10 ml of 1 per cent lignocaine. In the male, an 8.9 cm, 19 gauge needle is introduced from the perineum and guided onto the sacrospinus ligament with the help of a finger per rectum. In a successful block, the bulbocavernosus and anal reflexes are abolished and the residual urine reduced, as measured a few hours before and about an hour afterwards.

4

For the operation, the patient is usually put in the lithotomy position, though the jack-knife position is preferable. An incision is made just medial and parallel to the inner edge of the ischial tuberosity.

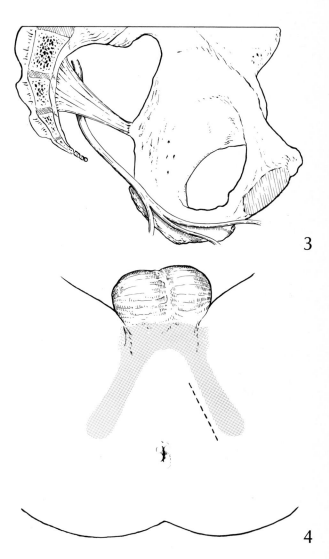

3

4

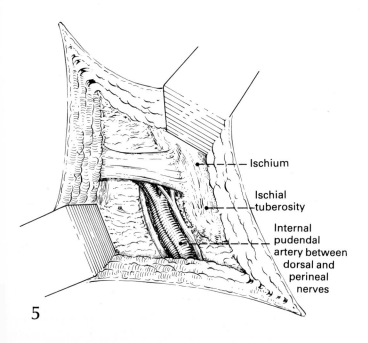

- Ischium

- Ischial tuberosity

- Internal pudendal artery between dorsal and perineal nerves

5

5

By careful dissection on the medial aspect of the bone the pudendal canal is reached and the perineal nerve and the dorsal nerve of the penis are identified with the internal pudendal vessels between them. Both nerves are dealt with, usually by crushing, as it is difficult to be sure of a complete external sphincter denervation otherwise. At this level, the inferior rectal nerve is spared, and tone is preserved in the external anal sphincter, though in fact this is not usually an important factor in rectal continence in the paraplegic. Regeneration usually occurs in 2–3 months after crushing.

TRANSECTION OF THE BLADDER

6

The bladder is exposed and opened by a transverse incision about 3 cm above the bladder neck. After coagulation or ligation of a few small arteries, the posterior wall of the bladder is picked up in the midline 2 cm above the interureteric bar, using two pairs of tissue forceps about 1 cm apart.

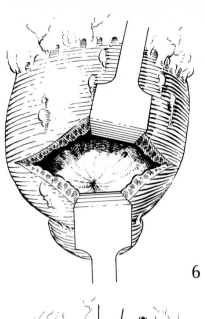

6

7

The bladder wall is divided between the forceps, opening up the plane in front of the vagina or seminal vesicles. The posterior bladder wall is then incised transversely on each side to meet the lateral end of the anterior bladder incision, keeping well above the intramural ureter which can be identified with the aid of a probe if necessary.

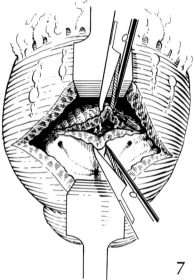

7

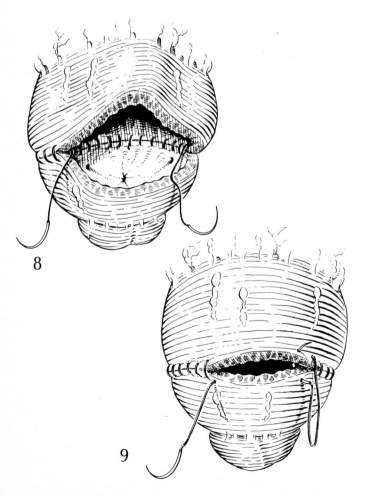

8

9

8 & 9

The two parts of the bladder are sutured together with 2/0 chromic catgut. It is convenient to use two separate eyeless sutures, commencing in the midline posteriorly and working round each side until they meet anteriorly. The wound is closed with drainage and a balloon catheter is left in the bladder for 7 or 8 days.

No attempt is made during this operation to divide any extravesical tissues, as some authors have recommended[25], since the results of both procedures are very similar, with a shift of the cystometrogram to the right and a significant improvement rate of approximately 80 per cent. Experimental evidence shows that in animals simple bladder transection results in intramural denervation as well as disruption of the detrusor syncytium[26]. In future the operation may be performed endoscopically[26].

References

1. Donker, P. J., Ivanovici, F., Noach, E. L. Analysis of the urethral pressure profile by means of electromyography and the administration of drugs. British Journal of Urology 1972; 44: 180

2. Gibbon, N. O., Parsons, K. F., Woolfenden, K. A. The neuropathic urethra. Paraplegia 1980; 18: 221–228

3. Enhorning, G. Simultaneous recording of intravesical and intra-urethral pressure. A study on urethral closure in normal and stress incontinent women. Acta Chirurgica Scandinavica 1961; Suppl. 276: 1–68

4. Enhörning, G., Miller, E. R., Hinman, F. Jr. Urethral closure studied with cine-roentgenography and simultaneous bladder urethra pressure recording. Surgery, Gynecology and Obstetrics 1964; 118: 507–516

5. Foley, J. S. Control of surgical incontinence by means of the Portsmouth valved catheter. British Medical Journal 1959; 2: 470–473

6. Griffiths, I. H. Anterior transposition of the urethra. British Journal of Urology 1960; 32: 27–31

7. Franksson, C., Petersen, I. Electromyographic recording from the normal human urinary bladder, internal urethral sphincter and ureter. Acta Physiologica Scandinavica 1953; 29: Suppl. 106: 150–156

8. Laruelle, L. La structure de la moelle épinière en coupes longitudinales. Revue of Neurologique 1937; 67: 695–725

9. Laruelle, L. Étude d'anatomie microscopique due névraxe sur coupes longitudinales. Acta Neurologica Psychiatrica Belgica 1948; 48: 189–280

10. Glahn, B. E. Manual provocation of micturition contraction in neurogenic bladders. Scandinavian Journal of Urology and Nephrology, 1970; 4: 25–36

11. Jousse, A. T., MacDonald, M., Wynn-Jones, M. Bladder control in the female paraplegic patient. Paraplegia 1964; 2: 146–152

12. Diokno, A. C., Koff, S. A., Bender, L. F. Periurethral striated muscle activity in neurogenic bladder dysfunction. Journal of Urology 1974; 112: 743–749

13. Vernet, S. G. Innervation somatique et végétative des organes genito-urinaires. Journal d'Urologie et de Néphrologie 1964; 70: 45–56

14. Donker, P. J., Droes, J. Th. P. M., Vanulden, B. M. Anatomy of the musculature and innervation of the bladder and the urethra. In: Williams, D. I., Chisholm, G. D., eds. Scientific foundations of urology, Vol. 2. London. Heinemann Medical Books Ltd. 1976: 32–39

15. Pearman, J. W., England, E. J. The urological management of the patient following spinal cord injury. Springfield, Illinois: Ch. C. Thomas, 1973

16. Gibbon, N. O. K. Division of the external sphincter. British Journal of Urology 1973; 45: 110–115

17. Jameson, R. M. The long-term results of transurethral division of the external sphincter in the neuropathic urethra with reference to potency. Paraplegia 1982; 20: 299–303

18. Dunn, M., Smith, J. C., Ardran, G. M. Prolonged bladder distension as a treatment of urgency and urge incontinence of urine. British Journal of Urology 1974; 46: 645–652

19. Gibbon, N. O. K., Jameson, R. M., Heal, M. R., Abel, B. J. Transection of the bladder for adult enuresis and allied conditions. British Journal of Urology 1973; 45: 306–309

20. Parsons, K. F., O'Boyle, P. J., Gibbon, N. O. K. A further assessment of bladder transection in the management of adult enuresis and allied conditions. British Journal of Urology 1977; 49: 509–514

21. Gibbon, N. Surgical treatment of adult enuresis. Proceedings 14th Congress International Society of Urology 1967; 2: 332

22. Gibbon, N. Management of the bladder in acute and chronic disorders of the nervous system. Acta Neurologica Scandinavica 1966; 42: Suppl. 20: 133

23. Madersbacher, H. The twelve o'clock sphincterotomy. Technique, indications, results, Paraplegia 1976; 13: 261–267

24. Rao, M. S., Bapna, B. C., Vaidyanathan, S. et al. Transurethral external sphincterotomy sans external sphincter. Paraplegia 1978; 16: 306–309

25. Mundy, A. R. Bladder transection for urge incontinence associated with detrusor instability. British Journal of Urology 1980; 52: 480–483

26. Staskin, D. R., Parsons, K. F., Levin, R. M., Wein, A. J. Bladder transection – a functional, neuro-physiological, neuropharmacological and neuro-anatomical study. British Journal of Urology 1981; 53: 552–557

Illustrations by Arthur Ellis

Transvesical prostatectomy

Warwick Macky   OBE, MS, FRCS, FRACS
Urologist, Auckland Hospital, New Zealand

Introduction

The technique of transvesical prostatectomy was first described and refined by McGill[1], Fuller[2] and Freyer[3]. Significant modifications were made by Thompson-Walker[4], Harris[5], Hryntschak[6,7], Malament[8] and others with the object of improving control of postoperative bleeding to allow primary closure of the bladder with a much lower incidence of sepsis and suprapubic fistula.

Basic considerations

The operation of transvesical prostatectomy is based on the following principles:

1. A small abdominal incision and a limited high cystotomy are used to give adequate surgical access with minimal disturbance of tissue planes.

2. Transvesical enucleation of all adenomatous tissue is effected within the concentric layers of the false or surgical capsule, avoiding interference with the highly vascular, true prostatic capsule. Coincident bladder neck obstruction is relieved.

3. Postoperative bleeding is controlled by ligature of the urethral branches of the prostatic arteries and other vessels at the bladder neck, together with reduction and tamponade of the prostatic fossa.

4. The bladder is closed either by primary purse-string or alternatively by two-layer suture with urethral catheter drainage.

In this chapter, a modified Harris prostatectomy is described with comments on the Hryntschak and Malament operations.

Preoperative

Indications

Transvesical prostatectomy is suitable for all types of intraurethral and intravesical benign enlargement of the prostate, with or without coincident bladder neck obstruction. The operation may be used to advantage when the enlargement of the prostate is associated with such conditions as calculus in the bladder or lower ureter, bladder diverticulum, ureterocele and certain bladder tumours.

A pre-existing suprapubic cystotomy may be extended for the prostatectomy. Inguinal or abdominal hernias may be repaired at the same time as prostatectomy is performed. Those patients who will not tolerate transurethral resection by reason of urethral stricture or unfavourable reactions to the passage of instruments *per urethram*, or those unable to be placed in a lithotomy position because of orthopaedic deformities, are best treated by transvesical prostatectomy.

When retropubic prostatectomy is made difficult by deformity in the bone structure of the symphysis pubis obliterating the retropubic space or by extensive vascular malformations in the anterior prostatic capsule, the transvesical approach is preferable.

Contraindications

Transvesical prostatectomy is not ideal for small fibrous glands, bladder neck obstruction due to fibrous bar, or carcinoma of the prostate. These lesions are best treated by transurethral resection. However, when transurethral resection is not feasible, transvesical resection of bladder neck obstruction gives good results.

Preoperative preparation

As transvesical prostatectomy is an elective procedure, every effort must be made to ensure that the patient is in the best possible condition for surgery. Cardiorespiratory and metabolic diseases are treated adequately and anaemia is corrected. Fluid and acid-base balance is restored.

Adequate time should be allowed for the adverse effects of such drugs as anticoagulants and antihypertensives to be corrected.

Acute retention of urine is relieved by an indwelling, self-retaining urethral catheter, 16 or 18 Fr, inserted under full aseptic precautions and connected to closed-system dependent drainage. Smaller-sized catheters are less likely to give rise to urethritis or pressure necrosis of the urethral mucosa with secondary epididymo-orchitis and late urethral stricture. If urethral drainage is impracticable, a stab suprapubic cystotomy or formal cystotomy may be needed.

When the patient is uraemic, prolonged bladder drainage should be maintained until the optimal level of renal function is established. However, surgery may be considered when renal function is seriously impaired if facilities for dialysis are available.

Urinary tract infection is treated by free drainage of the bladder urine and minimal chemotherapy. Provision is made for prompt treatment of Gram-negative septicaemia. When there is chronic retention with a vesical residue in excess of 1 litre, without uraemia, preoperative catheter drainage may be instituted in some cases, but in general urethral manipulations are avoided as haemorrhage and infection may ensue.

An intravenous pyelogram and micturating cystourethrogram may be requested when associated disease is suspected in the urinary tract, but routine pyelography is seldom warranted. Preliminary cystoscopy may be performed to exclude associated tumour, calculus or other lesions in the bladder or urethra. Provision is made for blood replacement.

Time should be taken to allay the patient's fear of the operation, and to discuss the likely effects on potency and fertility in the younger age group.

The operation

Anaesthesia

General anaesthesia with relaxation is used routinely, although a spinal or epidural anaesthetic may be preferred. Induced hypotension has been advocated by some but has not found general acceptance. Dextrose-saline solution is given intravenously during the operation and significant blood loss is replaced.

Operation time should be as short as possible to reduce the incidence of anaesthetic and cardiovascular complications.

Position of patient

The patient is placed supine on the table in the head down position to allow abdominal wall fat to drop away from the suprapubic region. Supports are placed under the tendoachillis to relieve pressure on the calf muscles. The diathermy plate is checked after final positioning.

After shaving, the abdomen, genitalia and upper thighs are painted with antiseptic solution and, if desired, adhesive drapes and an O'Connor shield are applied to the lower abdomen and perineum.

Vas ligation is not advised routinely but may be done via small scrotal incisions at this stage in selected cases.

The external urinary meatus and the anterior penile urethra are calibrated. If there is a stricture, Otis urethrotomy, meatotomy or meatoplasty with accurate 4/0 chromic catgut approximation of the penile skin and exposed urethral mucosa is effected. If this is not done, pressure necrosis of the mucosa due to the postoperative, indwelling retention urethral catheter will almost certainly aggravate the stricture.

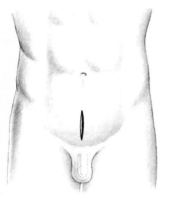

1

1 & 2

The incisions

A 5–6 cm vertical midline incision is made through skin, subcutaneous tissue and rectus fascia immediately above the level of the symphysis pubis. This short incision causes minimal disruption of tissue planes and allows adequate rapid exposure of the bladder with the Harris bladder retractor in position. It heals well without undue risk of postoperative incisional hernia. Alternatively, a transverse suprapubic creaseline skin incision 2 cm above the symphysis may be used.

The rectus and pyramidialis muscles are separated in the midline to expose the fascia transversalis and the fibrofatty tissue in the prevesical space.

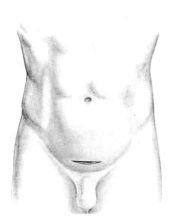

2

3

Mobilization of bladder

The extravesical fascia is incised in the midline to expose the oyster-coloured bladder muscle with a few veins coursing over the superficial aspect of the vault. If this plane is correctly exposed deep to the extravesical fascia, the peritoneum can be dissected superiorly off the vault in the midline until the dome of the bladder can be brought up to the level of the skin between Allis tissue forceps. There is no need to overdistend the bladder to facilitate this manoeuvre, which is essential to allow a high cystotomy with sufficient mobilization of the vault to ensure subsequent watertight closure.

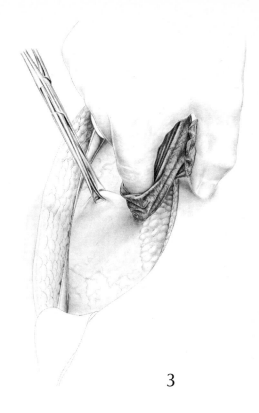

3

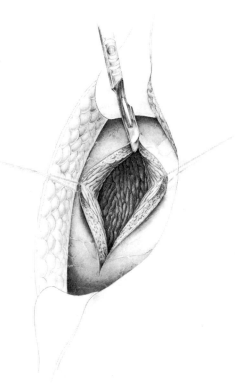

4

4

Opening the bladder

A high 3–4 cm transverse incision is made in the hypertrophied bladder muscle between Allis forceps. The bladder mucosa is seen as a 'pearly bead', which is incised, and the bladder contents are aspirated in such a way as to cause minimal trauma to the bladder mucosa. Two plain catgut stay sutures are inserted in the superior and inferior edges of the cystotomy.

The bladder and prostatic urethra are now explored digitally and any calculi removed. Associated lesions such as bladder diverticulum are best dealt with at this stage.

5

Enucleation of the adenoma

Having assessed the size, type and extent of the enlargement of the prostate bimanually, with one or two fingers of the left hand inserted *per rectum*, the enucleation is started in the urethra, at the apex of the prostate.

The correct plane for enuncleation within the concentric layers of the surgical capsule is found by rupturing through the prostatic urethra with firm pressure exerted by the index finger in the anterolateral plane near the midline on either side against the resistance of the peripheral prostatic tissue supported in turn by the bony symphysis. The separation of the apical masses is carried out circumferentially, one side at a time, until the mucosa of the prostatic urethra is separated as far as possible from that of the membranous urethra. Any residual attachments in this plane may be divided by further careful finger dissection, or with scissors, to minimize damage to the membranous urethra, a cuff of which is in danger of being avulsed by traction. This could result in incontinence, although this is rarely a problem.

If enucleation proves difficult due to fibrous tissue or unsuspected infiltrating carcinoma, it is better to stop forthwith and complete the separation of the lateral lobes by sharp dissection under vision when the retractor has been inserted. Ill-advised attempts at enucleation may result in splits of the true prostatic capsule and even rupture of the bladder with severe bleeding and extravasation of urine. When there is gross enlargement, the lateral lobes may be removed separately; on occasion, fenestrated ovum forceps may help to deliver the freed adenomatous tissue from the prostatic fossa.

Due to lack of counter-resistance, it may be difficult to enucleate well-developed subtrigonal or middle-lobe

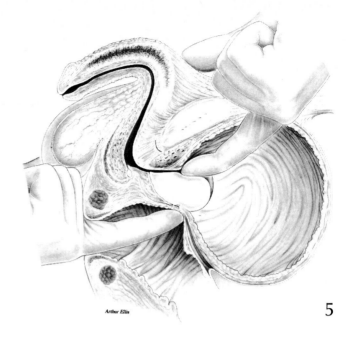

5

tissue without damaging or avulsing the trigone and bladder base. In such cases the mucosa over the base of the enlarged middle lobe is incised and the dissection completed after the bladder retractor is in position.

Finally, the prostatic fossa is carefully palpated bimanually for residual adenomata which may prolapse into the fossa after enucleation of the main adenomatous mass. These should be removed and any tags of capsule excised.

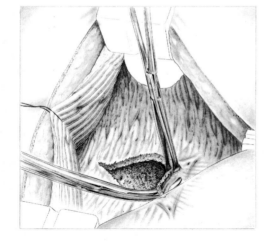

6

6

Excision of bladder neck

The Harris bladder retractor is now inserted in such a way that the vault of the bladder is supported at skin level to ensure an adequate view of the operative field. A pack placed behind the posterior blade may improve the view of the bladder neck and trigone.

The ureteric ridge and trigone are identified, and prominent fibrous bar tissue is excised *en bloc* posteriorly so that the trigonal 'shelf' is reduced in extent. Any further capsular tags, residual adenomata and mucosal remnants are excised under vision, using the curved Harris suction for additional retraction and to maintain a dry field.

7 & 8

Suture haemostasis

To secure the ureteral branches of the prostatic artery, 1/0 plain cross-mattress sutures are inserted in the plane of the bladder neck posterolaterally on each side, parallel and distal to the ureteric ridge. Harris boomerang needles facilitate this manoeuvre. Any obvious bleeding vessels in the lateral aspect of the bladder neck are similarly dealt with. One or two occluding stitches are then placed across the full thickness of the bladder neck anteriorly to reduce the prostatic fossa and support the bladder neck to prevent further extracapsular splits if traction on a bag catheter is subsequently used to tamponade the fossa. The reformed bladder neck should freely admit the tip of the index finger.

Diathermy in the prostatic fossa is not advised as the depth of tissue necrosis cannot be controlled. It is not possible to reconstitute the mucosa of the prostatic urethra by pinning down the trigone prosteriorly, as suggested by Harris.

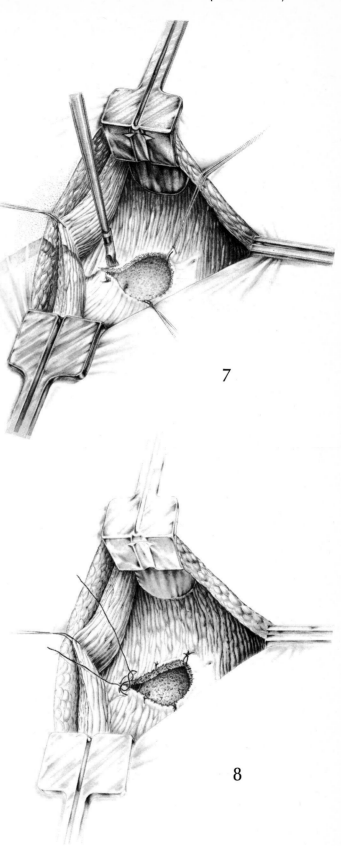

7

8

Insertion of urethral catheter

A 22 or 24 Fr three-way irrigating Foley retention catheter is passed *per urethram* and, after inflation, the bag is seated down on the bladder neck. If excessive bleeding persists, the fossa may be tamponaded by firm, gentle traction on the catheter for up to 6 hours postoperatively. When difficulty is encountered in passing the catheter through the posterior urethra, a flexible curved introducer may be used to guide the tip over any persisting trigonal shelf. The retention bag should not be inflated until the tip of the catheter is properly placed within the bladder, as overdistention of the membranous urethra may cause incontinence. The routine use of the inflated bag, positioned within the prostatic fossa for haemostasis, is not recommended. The catheter is connected to a non-return drainage bag and continuous irrigation started with normal saline at 37°C. Occasional irrigations with a sterile syringe are advisable to ensure that drainage is in fact satisfactory.

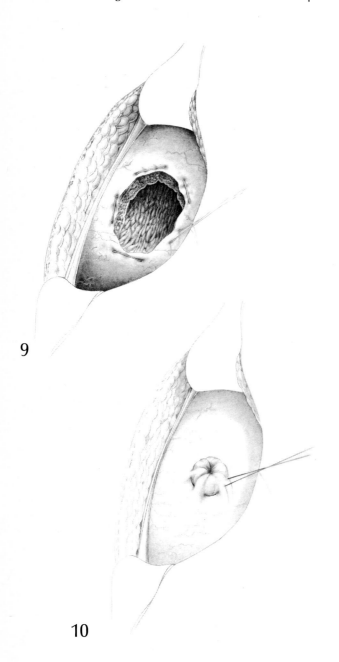

9

10

9 & 10

Bladder closure and drainage

After removal of the retractor and aspiration of any residual clots, the bladder is closed by a 2/0 plain purse-string stitch inserted deeply into the muscle so as to produce adequate inversion of the edges of the incision and to ensure watertight closure.

Alternatively, when the bladder wall is greatly thickened, two-layer closure with a deep continuous and superficial interrupted 2/0 plain catgut stitch may be used. The purse-string stitch is most effective but may be less haemostatic than two-layer closure.

A suction drain is placed in the extravesical space and the abdominal wound is closed in layers using 1/0 chromic catgut in the rectus sheath, 2/0 chromic in the subcutaneous tissue and interrupted unabsorbable stitches in the skin.

11 & 12

Hryntschak modification

In addition to the Harris stitches placed posterolaterally, Hryntschak[6,7] advocated the use of deep transverse stitches at the bladder neck, so placed as to incorporate the urethral catheter when tied. These stitches were designed to tamponade the prostatic fossa by occluding the bladder neck completely. When the catheter is removed, tension on the stitches is relieved, allowing the bladder neck to assume its normal contour.

In practice, the use of these occluding stitches has resulted in an unacceptably high incidence of bladder neck stenosis and while the method may serve to control excessive haemorrhage, its routine use is not advocated. Hryntschak also recommended purse-string closure of the bladder and he designed a useful bladder retractor.

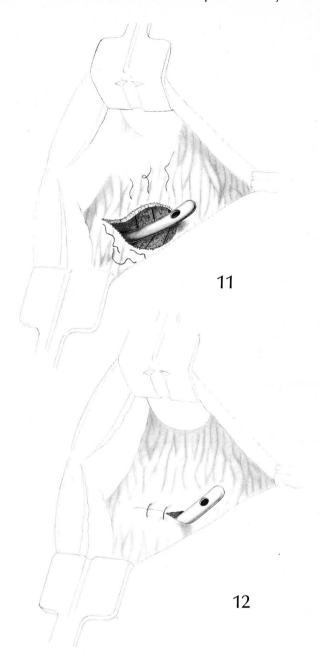

11

12

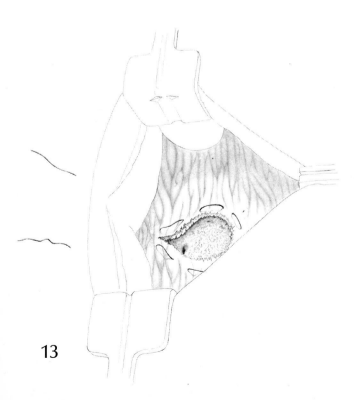

13

13

Malament modification

Malament[8] described purse-string closure of the bladder neck around an indwelling catheter as a method of tamponading the prostatic fossa. This method is undoubtedly effective in many cases and has given good results in experienced hands but may not be practicable when the bladder neck and prostatic fossa are rigid and widely patent. Attempts to close such a bladder neck may result in rupture of the capsule with additional haemorrhage and extravasation of urine.

Postoperative care and complications

In the recovery room, the patient's vital signs are closely monitored and fluid intake adjusted to ensure that blood volume is maintained. Excessive blood loss is replaced. Diuresis is promoted by intravenous fluids, supplemented if necessary by mannitol or frusemide.

The urethral catheter must drain freely at all times. If continuous saline irrigation through the three-way indwelling retention catheter is used, free drainage should be ensured by frequent small washouts with a bulb or Toomey syringe with aseptic technique. The washouts have no therapeutic effect but serve to break up and dislodge clot and debris which may accumulate about the inflated bag and over the bladder base.

If bleeding is excessive, tension on the catheter may be increased to tamponade the prostatic fossa for up to 6 hours postoperatively. In the rare case of uncommonly severe bleeding, ribbon gauze may be packed about the catheter in the prostatic fossa and brought out suprapubically so that tamponade may be made more effective. The gauze packing may be removed without disturbing the urethral catheter after 24 or 36 hours. If clot retention ensues, evacuation of the bladder is best effected *per urethram* using the cystoscope sheath and the Toomey syringe. When there is doubt as to whether the bladder is distending postoperatively, bimanual rectal examination may give useful information. The extravesical suction drain is usually removed after 24 hours.

Policy on the use of chemotherapy in the postoperative period should be flexible. When there is postoperative infection of the urine, appropriate chemotherapy or antibiotics should be given with recourse to a cephalosporin or aminoglycoside if Gram-negative septicaemia is suspected. While there may be objections to routine postoperative chemotherapy in clean cases, many urologists give suppressive doses of co-trimoxazole which may also help prevent chest infections and reduce the incidence of epididymo-orchitis. It is not unusual to give a 10–day course of suppressive chemotherapy on discharge from hospital. Symptomless pyuria and low-grade urinary tract infection may persist until healing of the prostatic fossa is complete after some weeks.

Breathing exercises and active muscle movements are supervised postoperatively. The patient should stand out of bed 12 hours after operation and walk progressively longer distances each day thereafter. Free fluids are given initially and a full diet is usually accepted a day after operation.

Continuous closed, dependent catheter drainage is maintained for 48–72 hours. The bag or plastic container should have a non-return valve and be capable of being emptied without contaminating the contents. Adherent blood clot or urethral discharge at the external meatus should be gently removed and a swab soaked in 1 per cent chlorhexidine solution placed *in situ* to reduce ascending infection.

Painful bladder spasms may be controlled by analgesics and the use of belladonna and morphine rectal suppositories. A mild laxative or suppository is given to ensure a bowel action before the catheter is removed. It is important to prevent faecal impaction at all times.

When the catheter is removed, voiding is usually frequent and painful due to urethritis and bladder spasms associated with a low-grade cystitis. On occasion, the catheter may have to be reinserted for retention, delayed bleeding or suprapubic fistula. If there is difficulty in negotiating the prostatic fossa due to a trigonal shelf, a flexible curved introducer should be used.

On discharge from hospital, the patient is encouraged to continue graded physical exercises and he should be able to resume full activity 4–6 weeks postoperatively, depending on his occupation. Fluid intake should be in excess of 2–3 litres daily and the patient should avoid constipation.

Complications

While the mortality rate of suprapubic prostatectomy of about 1.5 per cent may be higher than reported for transurethral resection, the types of cases are not strictly comparable. Death is most often due to coronary occlusion, pulmonary infarction or cerebrovascular accident, commonly seen in the older age group.

Postoperative anterior penile or bulbar urethral strictures may occur in 2–5 per cent of cases and bladder neck stenosis may be seen in about 4 per cent. Incontinence is most unusual after suprapubic prostatectomy. Late secondary haemorrhage is uncommon, but it may be severe enough to warrant readmission to hospital for evacuation of the bladder contents.

Postoperative epididymo-orchitis is also uncommon but may occur even after some weeks. Routine vas ligation does not seem to reduce the incidence of this complication. Provided all subcapsular adenomatous tissue has been removed, obstruction due to recurrent adenoma is uncommon but may be seen after 10–20 years in the younger age group. Carcinoma may develop at any time in the posterior lamella of the gland.

Most patients have some persisting urinary frequency after transvesical prostatectomy, possibly due to changes in the bladder muscle, but there is usually gradual spontaneous improvement. Suprapubic fistula is virtually unknown after one-stage suprapubic prostatectomy with adequate bladder closure. Retrograde ejaculation occurs in most cases postoperatively but there is usually minimal interference with potency. Return of potency cannot be expected in those previously impotent.

References

1. McGill, A. F. Suprapubic prostatectomy. British Medical Journal 1887; 2: 1104–1105

2. Fuller, E. Six successful and successive cases of prostatectomy. Journal of Cutaneous and Genito-urinary Diseases 1895; 13: 229–240

3. Freyer, P. J. A new method of performing prostatectomy. Lancet 1900; 1: 774–775

4. Thomson-Walker, *Sir* J. W. The Lettsomian Lectures on enlarged prostate and prostatectomy. Transactions of the Medical Society of London 1930; 53: 143

5. Harris, S. H. Suprapubic prostatectomy with closure. British Journal of Urology 1929; 1: 285–295

6. Hryntschak, T. Suprapubic transvesical prostatectomy with primary closure of the bladder by an original method; technique and post-operative treatment. Eng. transl. Rev. ed. Illinois: Thomas, 1955

7. Hryntschak, T. Suprapubic transvesical prostatectomy with primary closure of bladder: improved technic and latest results. Journal of the International College of Surgeons 1951; 15: 366–367

8. Malament, M. Maximal hemostasis in suprapubic prostatectomy. Surgery, Gynecology and Obstetrics 1965; 120: 1307–1312

Retropubic prostatectomy

John P. Pryor MS, FRCS
Consultant Urologist, King's College and St Peter's Hospitals, London;
Dean, Institute of Urology, London University, UK

Introduction

Retropubic prostatectomy is the method of choice for removing the larger benign prostate which is causing bladder outflow obstruction. Each surgeon will have his own criteria for carrying out an open operation and this will depend upon the general condition of the patient, the experience of the surgeon and the equipment that is available to him.

The operation was first described in 1908 by Van Stockum[1], but its present popularity stems from the influence of Terence Millin, an Irishman who worked in London. He first exploited the retropubic route in 1945[2] and published his monograph, *Retropubic urinary surgery*, in 1947[3]. Retropubic prostatectomy rapidly became the method of choice for removing the benign prostate, and it 'undoubtedly yielded the most impressive results in larger subcervical adenomas where the ease of enucleation, good access to the prostatic bed and preservation of an intact bladder combined to make the mortality low and convalescence rapid'[4]. The recent development of fibre-optics, surgical diathermy and the rod lens have led to a resurgence in the use of transurethral resection and have led to a decline in the use of retropubic prostatectomy by surgeons in Europe.

Preoperative

Indications

All patients undergoing prostatectomy require preliminary cystourethroscopy and the decision to perform a retropubic operation is made at that time in conjunction with the operative findings, the condition of the patient and the bimanual examination of the prostate when the bladder has been emptied. Urologists perform approximately 10 per cent of prostatectomies by the retropubic route and reserve the open operation for the larger benign prostate or when it is also desirable to move a large vesical calculus or diverticulum or to repair an inguinal hernia. A retropubic prostatectomy should not be performed if there is a concomitant bladder tumour or for a prostatic carcinoma. The size of the prostate influences the decision to perform an open operation, but other considerations, such as general fitness of the patient and the experience and equipment of the surgeon, are also important. In general, the decision not to proceed with a transuretheral resection is made when the prostate is estimated to be between 40 and 100 g in size. Occasionally heavy bleeding occurs at the commencement of trans-urethral resection – usually in the hypertensive patient – and in these circumstances it may be wiser to proceed with an open operation.

Preoperative measures

Prophylactic antibiotics are unnecessary but any urinary tract infection should be treated with the appropriate antibiotics. A period of catheter drainage is necessary if there is evidence of an obstructive uropathy and the operation should be delayed until the blood urea level approaches normal.

Routine haematological tests should include haemoglobin estimation, blood grouping, the detection of sickle cell disease and the Australian antigen status of the patient. It is safer to have 2 units of blood available for transfusion, but there is a trend to conserve blood and only crossmatch when the blood is required. This necessitates the immediate availability of a full blood transfusion service within the hospital.

Active prophylaxis against pulmonary embolism is advisable when performing a retropubic prostatectomy. Intermittent calf vein compression is effective and can be applied once the decision to proceed by open operation has been made. Low-dose heparin prophylaxis is safe but requires planning before the patient is anaethetized.

Anaesthesia

The services of a skilled anaesthetist are essential and he may choose a general or regional anaesthetic tehnique. Spinal or epidural anaesthetics are particularly useful if the patient suffers with a respiratory tract disorder. Controlled hypotension is unnecessary and is best avoided as it carries a greater risk in the elderly. It is important that the abdominal musculature is relaxed and that there should be no impediment to the venous drainage such as occurs with coughing. It is essential to commence the administration of the intravenous fluids at the start of the operation, as some degree of blood loss is inevitable.

The operation

A preliminary cystoscopy should always be performed to ensure that there is no intravesical pathology and the bladder is left empty. Small papillary carcinomas of the bladder may be resected and the base fulgurated since the operation should not be performed in the presence of a tumour.

Position of patient

The patient is placed supine on the operating table with 10° head-down tilt and the legs may also be flexed at the knee. Such a position facilitates abdominal access and also encourages venous drainage from the prostatic bed, thereby reducing haemorrhage.

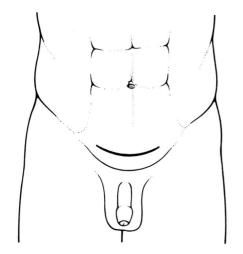

1

The incision

The skin is thoroughly cleansed with a 10 per cent povidone-iodine solution and the patient draped in such a way as to allow access to the penis once the prostate has been removed. The operation is performed through a transverse lower abdominal incision situated in the skin crease approximately 3 cm above the symphysis pubis. The incision is 10–15 cm long and depends upon the thickness of the abdominal wall fat. A right-handed surgeon stands on the patient's left, and performs most of the operation facing the patient's feet.

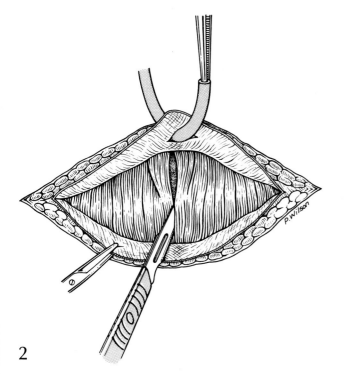

2

Separation of rectus muscles

The anterior rectus sheath is incised in the line of the skin incision and is mobilized from the underlying rectus muscles down to the symphysis pubis and upwards towards the umbilicus. It is necessary to coagulate small arteries entering the rectus sheath from the muscles. The rectus and the pyramidalis muscles are widely separated in the lower part of the incision, and it may be necessary to incise the lower part of the linea alba vertically in the upper part of the wound.

It is useful at this stage to insert a tube drain through a small incision in the midline of the lower flap of the anterior rectus sheath midway between the line of incision and the symphysis pubis. The ends of the drainage tube are clamped together with Kocher's forceps and secured to the drapes towards the patient's feet in such a way as to exert traction and obviate any subsequent need for a retractor in the inferior part of the wound.

3

Exposure of anterior surface of prostate

The retropubic fat is gently separated to expose the bladder and prostate and the blades of a Millin self-retaining retractor are inserted. Further separation of the retropubic fat exposes the anterior surface of the prostatic capsule and any haemorrhage is controlled with diathermy. At this stage it is convenient to tuck two 10 cm gauze swabs into the retropubic space just lateral to the prostate. The third blade of the Millin retractor is introduced to retract the bladder, clearly displaying the anterior surface of the prostate and adjacent bladder wall.

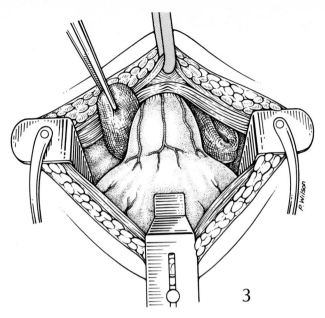

3

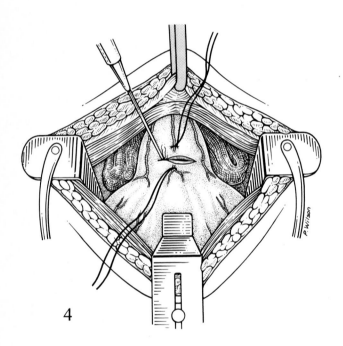

4

4

Incision of prostatic capsule

Two stay sutures (0 chromic catgut on a curved needle) are then placed through the prostatic capsule in such a way as to occlude the vein running longitudinally (a branch of the dorsal vein of the penis). The more proximal of these sutures is placed at the junction of the prostate and bladder neck. The correct situation is recognized by the longitudinal direction of the veins turning to run more laterally. These sutures are left long to facilitate identification of the incision into the prostatic capsule. A 3 cm incision is made in the prostatic capsule between the stay sutures and about 1 cm distal to the bladder neck. The incision is made through the full thickness of the capsule and stops when the white appearance of the prostate is identified. Any bleeding from the prostatic capsule should be controlled at this stage.

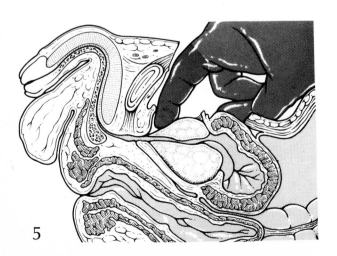

5

5

Plane of enucleation

A pair of scissors is used to commence the distal separation of the anterior surface of the prostatic adenoma from the prostatic capsule. This plane is developed by blind dissection with the pulp of the right index finger. The right lobe is freed first by separating the anterior surface, followed by the lateral and posterior surfaces from the prostatic capsule. The same procedure is repeated for the left lobe but the continuity of the urethra at the apex of the prostate is maintained. The finger dissection may be facilitated by removing the Millin retractor but this is not always necessary and it should be reinserted once the dissection is complete.

6

Division of the urethra

It is possible to insert the index and middle fingers inside the prostatic capsule in such a manner as to straddle the urethra once the lateral lobes of the prostate have been freed. A pair of curved scissors is inserted inside the prostatic capsule and, guided by the position of the fingers, is used to divide the urethra clearly in order to avoid avulsing any of the distal urethra, thereby damaging the sphincter mechanism. It is often difficult to divide the urethra under direct vision but great care is essential at this stage of the operation if postoperative urinary incontinence is to be avoided. The lateral lobes now lie freely within the prostatic capsule

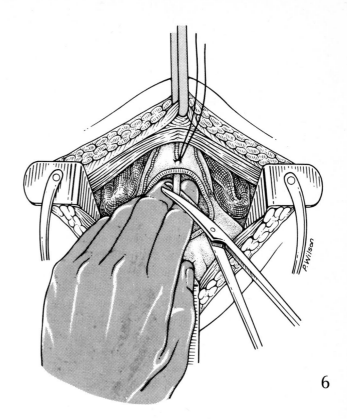

6

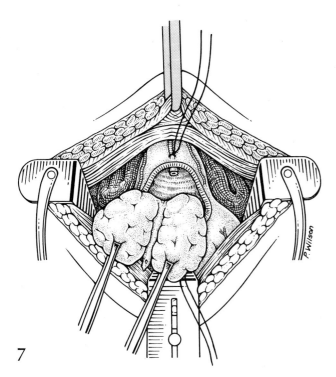

7

7

Dislocation of the adenoma

Each lateral lobe is securely gripped with a pair of volsellum forceps and dislocated anteriorly out of the prostatic cavity. The proximal end of the divided urethra is identified and a pair of scissors placed inside the urethra, which is then divided anteriorly, together with the overlying prostatic tissue, as far as the bladder neck.

8

Removal of the adenoma and control of haemostasis

A pair of bladder neck spreaders are placed inside the bladder to define the bladder neck. The attachment of the prostate to the bladder neck is then divided by sharp dissection with a diathermy point and the prostate removed. Removal of the prostate is always accompanied by bleeding, and on rare occasions this may be profuse. Immediately the adenoma has been removed it is wise to pack the prostatic capsule with gauze swabs and control any bleeding by direct pressure.

The general status of the patient is then assessed and rapid fluid replacement given if required. The packs may then be removed and the prostatic cavity carefully inspected, remnants of prostatic adenoma excised and any bleeding vessels diathermized. It is sometimes difficult to control profuse bleeding from large veins in the prostatic capsule and in these circumstances the cavity is packed and external pressure applied with a swab in a holder for 5 to 10 minutes (timed to avoid impatience). It is neither necessary nor possible to arrest the capillary oozing from the prostatic bed and this will diminish by repacking the prostatic cavity with swabs.

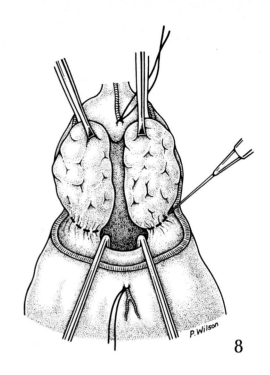

8

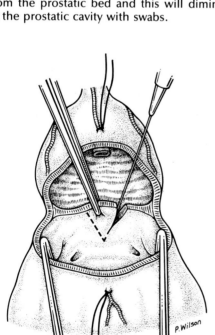

9

9

Excision of a wedge of bladder neck

Attention is next given to the bladder neck which should be sufficiently large easily to admit two fingers. If this is not possible, a wedge is excised from the bladder neck. The ureteric orifices are first identified and the middle of the bladder neck is grasped by a pair of forceps. A V-shaped wedge is then excised as shown.

10

Anchoring the bladder mucosa

It is unnecessary to suture the bladder mucosa to the prostatic bed except in those patients where the prostate extended beneath the trigone. In these circumstances it is useful to anchor the mucosa to the floor of the prostatic cavity with two or three 00 chromic catgut sutures. This technique facilitates catheterization and is of particular benefit should the urethral catheter fall out or require replacement. Persistent haemorrhage from the bladder neck may be controlled by suturing, and in these circumstances the bladder mucosa may be anchored with the same suture.

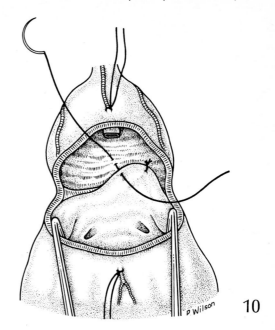

10

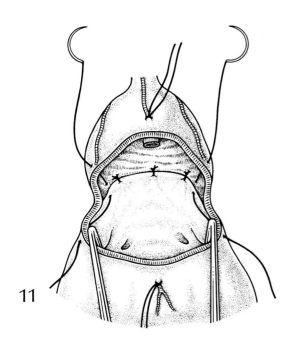

11

11

Insertion of catheter

Any swabs remaining within the prostatic capsule are removed and a marker suture (0 chromic catgut) is placed at each lateral corner of the capsular incision. These sutures act as a guide for the ends of the incision but are also haemostatic. The needle is inserted from without into the cavity of the bladder, then through the bladder mucosa and bladder neck into the prostatic cavity and finally through the prostatic capsule. Each of these sutures is tied and left long and a 20 Fr three-way Foley-type catheter is passed into the bladder. It is preferable that the catheter should be fairly rigid and have large eyes. It is seldom necessary to insert a suprapubic catheter into the bladder.

12

Closure of prostatic capsule

The prostatic capsule is closed with a continuous 0 chromic catgut suture which arrests any bleeding from the prostatic capsule and also ensures a watertight closure. It is easier to insert this suture by taking each edge of the capsule with separate bites of the needle. There may be some leakage through the prostatic capsule but it is seldom worthwhile attempting to insert any further sutures.

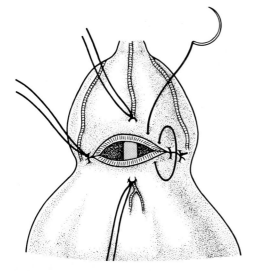

12

13

Final stages

At this stage it is useful to tie together the two initial stay sutures which were placed into the prostatic capsule. The bladder is then washed out to ensure that there is free catheter drainage. The two swabs which were placed on either side of the prostate at the start of the operation are removed and a final check is made for any bleeding from the vessels in the retropubic fat.

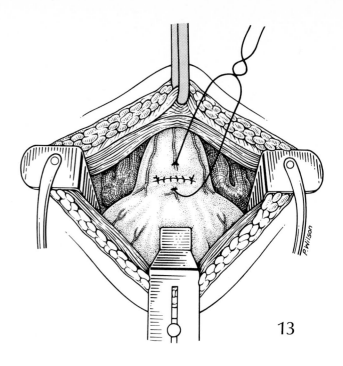

13

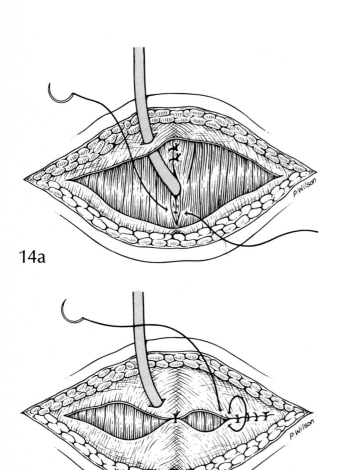

14a

14b

14a & b

Wound closure

The tubular wound drain, which, inserted at the commencement of the procedure, has acted as a retractor throughout, is then unclipped and placed down to the suture line in the prostatic capsule. The rectus muscles are approximated with interrupted 0 chromic catgut sutures and the anterior rectus sheath is closed with a similar suture material. This may conveniently be a continuous suture line. The subcutaneous tissues are loosely approximated with plain catgut sutures and the skin closed with well-spaced interrupted sutures. At the conclusion of the operation the catheter is once again checked to make sure that it is draining freely and is then connected to a closed urine collection apparatus. The retropubic drain is also connected to a closed collection bag.

ADDITIONAL PROCEDURES

It is often convenient to repair an inguinal hernia at the time of a retropubic prostatectomy but this should be deferred until the prostatectomy has been completed safely. Vasectomy is no longer performed in order to reduce the risk of epididymitis.

Postoperative care

Blood transfusion is not usually necessary except in the very large gland (greater than 250 g). Any fluid loss during the course of the operation should have been replaced by intravenous fluids and these are usually given to ensure a high urine output. In elderly patients, or in those with cardiac abnormalities, it is often wise to give furosemide 40 mg by intramuscular injection every 12 hours to minimize the risk of cardiac failure and to prevent the occurrence of clot retention. This technique is particularly useful when there has been profuse bleeding at the time of operation and the use of a three-way catheter will also help obviate the need for a bladder washout. The urine should always be collected in a closed drainage system as this is helpful in lessening the risk of urinary infection. Careful attention should be given to cleansing the penis around the catheter in the postoperative period.

The patient is encouraged to drink at an early stage and intravenous fluids are unnecessary after the first 24 hours. Early mobilization and physiotherapy are important in the prevention of pulmonary embolism and the retropubic drain is usually removed 48 hours after the operation. The urethral catheter is removed when there is no longer any risk of clot retention – usually between the 4th and 7th day.

Complications

The general risk of myocardial ischaemia, chest infection and pulmonary embolism are ever-present with an elderly group of patients undergoing surgery. These risks may be minimized by the skills of the supporting team of anaesthetists, nurses and physiotherapists. The risk of a urinary tract infection may be lessened if preoperative catheterization is avoided, and by the judicious use of antibiotics.

Prostatorectal fistulae have been reported following retropubic prostatectomy but tend to occur when the operation has been performed for an unsuspected carcinoma of the prostate. Urethral strictures are relatively uncommon after a retropubic prostatectomy but bladder neck stenosis occurs in 1 per cent of patients. Regrowth of the prostate may occur but patients rarely present in less than 10 years after the retropubic operation. The regrowth may be due to the occurrence of a prostatic cancer even though the histology of the original gland showed benign prostatic hyperplasia.

Urinary incontinence is common immediately following the removal of the urethral catheter but fortunately this only persists in approximately 1 per cent of patients.

References

1. Van Stockum, W. J. Prostatectomia suprapubica extravesicalis. Zentralblatt für Chirurgie 1909; 36: 41–43

2. Millin, T. Retropubic prostatectomy: a new extravesical technique, report on 20 cases. Lancet 1945; 2: 693–696

3. Millin, T. Retropubic urinary surgery. Edinburgh: E. & S. Livingstone, 1947

4. Sandrey, J. G. Retropubic prostatectomy. In: Innes Williams, D., ed. Operative surgery: Urology. London: Butterworths, 1977: 253–261

Illustrations by Robert N. Lane

Perineal prostatectomy

R. E. Williams   MD, ChM, FRCS(Ed), FRCS
Consultant Urologist, The General Infirmary and
St James's University Hospital, Leeds, UK

Preoperative

Indications

The particular operative technique used for the relief of benign prostatic hypertrophy depends on the surgeon's training and experience. Perineal prostatectomy provides an alternative to the other methods. There are no absolute indications but it may prove a useful method when the surgeon wishes to avoid an abdominal incision or when the anaesthetist wishes to use a spinal anaesthetic.

One advantage of the perineal approach is that frozen section microscopy can be done on biopsies from the dorsal prostate before enucleation is commenced. If adenocarcinoma is detected then the surgical procedure may be readily altered to a radical perineal prostatectomy. In some surgical units perineal prostatectomy is also undertaken in conjunction with abdominoperineal resection of the rectum for carcinoma when there is good evidence of concomitant prostatic obstruction.

Special contraindications

Some interference with sexual function may follow any prostatectomy but this is found more frequently following the perineal approach than either the transurethral, transvesical or retropubic method. While many patients subjected to perineal prosatectomy have no upset in sexual function, it is advisable to use one of the other methods if the patient is still sexually active. Another contraindication is fixation of the knee or hip joints which would prevent the patient being placed in the exaggerated lithotomy position.

Special equipment

Lowsley's modification of Young's straight and curved retractors are required, along with a boomerang needle and ligature holder. Good light, suction and diathermy are necessary.

Special preoperative preparation

This includes bladder drainage for urinary retention, the control of urinary infection and the medical management of pathological conditions affecting other systems of the body.

Anaesthesia

General or spinal anaesthesia is suitable.

The operation

1

The approach

The route through the perineum divides the rectourethralis muscle and central tendon, passes behind the transverse perineal muscles and then through Denonvilliers' fascia and the posterior prostatic capsule to reach the plane of enucleation.

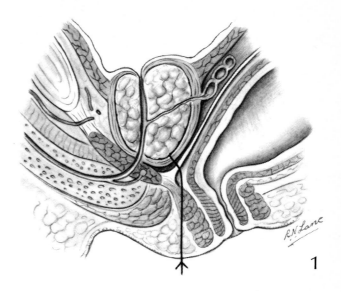

1

2

Position of patient

Good exposure is essential. After anaesthesia has been induced, the buttocks are brought down to the end of the table, the hips elevated and the legs placed in supports. An operating table with a mechanism for elevation of the perineum is helpful. Shoulder braces then force the body downward to give maximum flexion of the hips and careful padding with sponge rubber is required under the shoulder and knee joints. The table is then tilted until the perineum is nearly horizontal. Preliminary cytoscopy and bilateral vasectomy may be done at this time, if required.

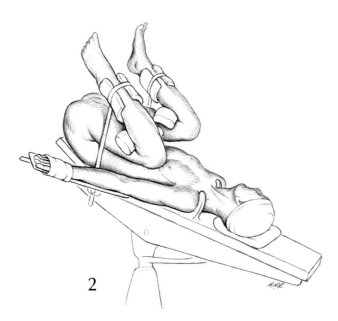

2

3

The incision

The Lowsley's curved perineal prostatectomy retractor is passed down to the membranous urethra. A semicircular skin incision is made through the perineum; care is taken that the extremities of the incision are within the ischial tuberosities to avoid a scar on this weight-bearing area. The lower skin edge is clipped to the lower perineal towel in such a way as to exclude the anus from the surgical field.

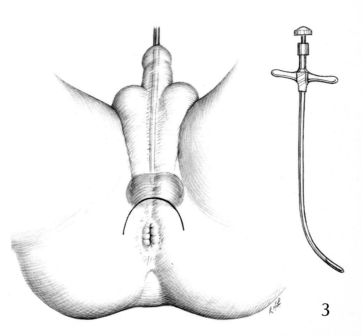

3

4

Exposure of ischiorectal fossae

The ischiorectal fossae on either side of the central tendon and rectourethralis muscle are developed by blunt dissection with the finger and handle of the scalpel, which are introduced between the transverse perineal muscles above and the levator ani muscles below. The membranous urethra with the retractor in place can be felt at this stage.

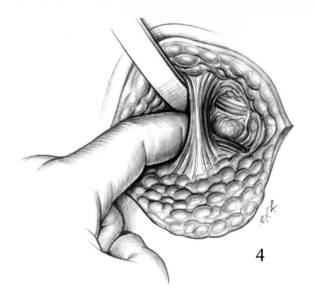

4

5

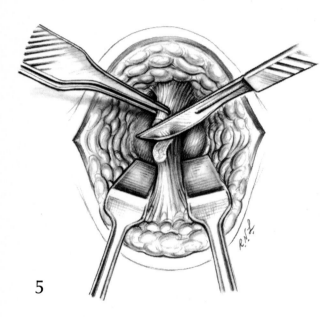

5

Division of central tendon

Lane's retractors are introduced and adjusted to stretch the central tendon and rectourethralis muscle. These structures are then divided by sharp dissection; a finger introduced between the rectourethralis muscles and the rectum will help to protect the latter. Sharp dissection is continued until the apex of the prostate is exposed. Electrocoagulation will control bleeding points but it should not be used close to the wall of the rectum.

6

Position of retractor

Lowsley's retractor is introduced into the bladder, the blades are opened and the handle depressed over the abdomen. This manoeuvre rotates the prostate into the perineal wound.

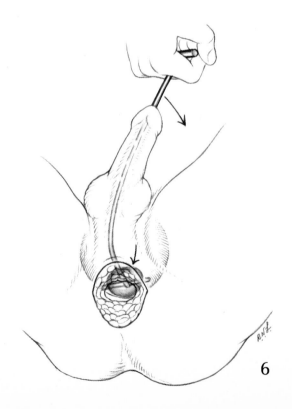

6

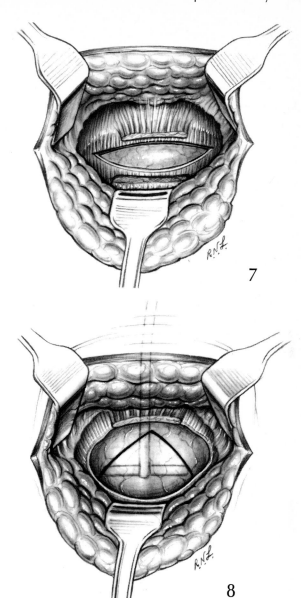

7

8

7 & 8

Incision in capsule

The apex of the prostate can be palpated under the deeper fibres of the rectourethralis muscle and dissection there exposes the posterior layer of Denonvilliers' fascia. When this layer is incised transversely, a plane of cleavage will be obtained between it and the characteristic pearly-white anterior layer. Blunt dissection carries the posterior layer backwards, taking the rectum with it, and is continued on each side to expose the lateral borders of the prostate. Deep lateral retractors expose the gland and a wide inverted 'V' incision is made through the capsule midway between apex and base.

9

Exposure of prostatic urethra

The capsular incision is carried down through the gland to open the urethra and expose the Lowsley retractor.

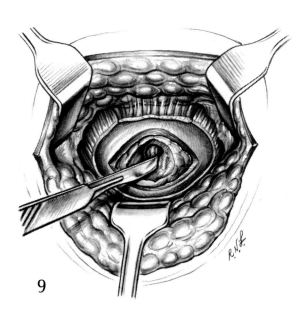

9

10

Introduction of straight retractor

The curved Lowsley retractor is then removed and a straight retractor introduced through the urethral opening into the bladder. The blades are opened and the enlarged lateral lobes are pulled downwards.

At this stage some surgeons prefer to dissect and expose the apical portions of the enlarged prostatic tissue following which they divide the prostatic urethra with the scalpel under direct vision. The straight prostatic retractor may then be inserted through the prostatic urethra into the bladder and the blades opened.

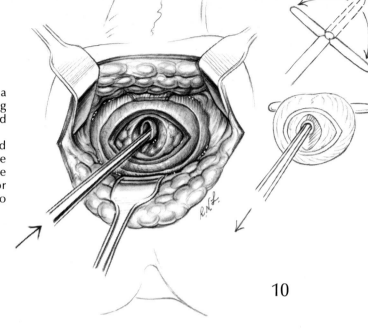

10

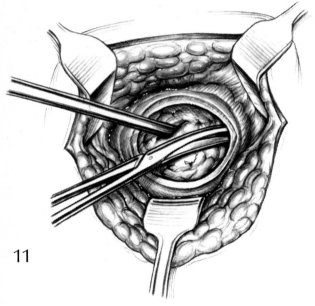

11

11

Commencement of enucleation

A plane of cleavage is developed anteriorly between the capsule and the hypertrophied lobes using dissecting scissors.

12

Enucleation with finger

The plane of cleavage is enlarged by sweeping the finger on both sides and posteriorly beneath the base of the bladder to separate the hypertrophied lobes from the capsule.

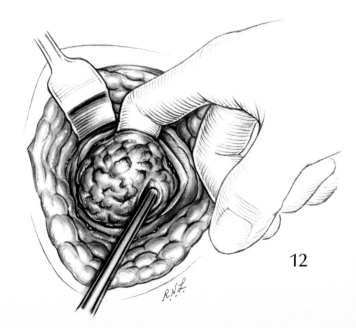

12

13

Separation from bladder mucosa

The lobes are drawn downwards by gentle retraction with the Lowsley instrument until the cuff of mucosa at the neck of the bladder is seen. This cuff is cut with scissors and the hypertrophied lobes are removed. Any remaining prostatic tissue, particularly a subtrigonal lobe, is easily enucleated. If the gland cannot be enucleated in one piece, forceps may be placed separately on each hypertrophied lobe.

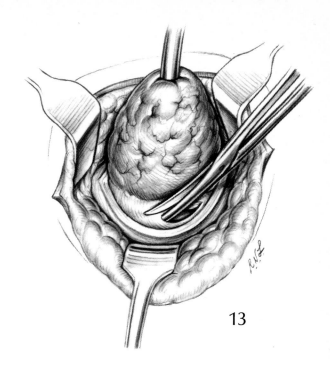

13

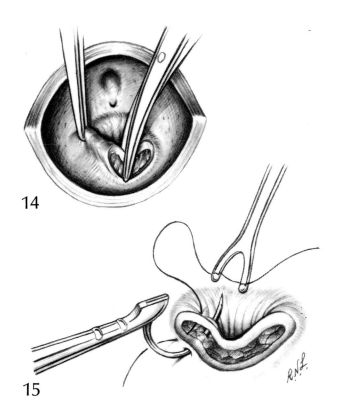

14

15

14 & 15

Excision of wedge from bladder neck

If the neck of the bladder is tight, a V-shaped wedge may be excised from the posterior margin with scissors. Bleeding round the neck of the bladder is controlled by electrocoagulation. Further haemostasis is obtained by placing sutures in the lateral edge of the vesical neck using the boomerang needle and 1/0 (No. 5 metric) plain catgut. These sutures also draw the free margin of the mucosa over the neck of the bladder.

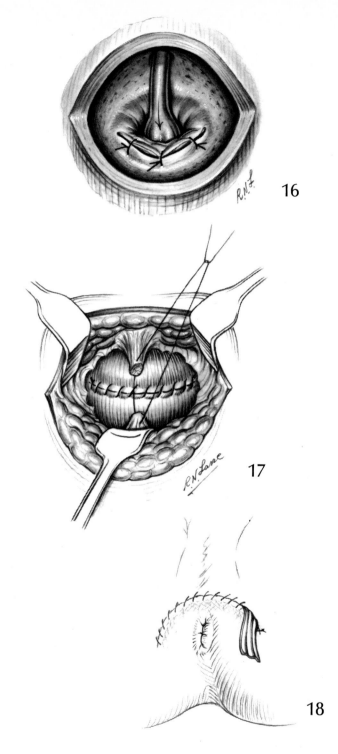

16

16, 17 & 18

Closure

A 22 Fr Foley catheter with a 20 ml bag is introduced through the urethra into the bladder, the bag is distended and continuous closed drainage is established. The posterior capsule is closed with a continuous 1/0 (No. 5 metric) chromic catgut suture – in obese patients the boomerang needle may be used for this closure. The levator ani muscles may be approximated with a single suture of plain catgut. The skin wound is closed with continuous 2/0 (No. 3 metric) chromic catgut suture with a short corrugated rubber drain on one angle. Closure may be helped by relaxing the exaggerated lithotomy position.

17

18

Postoperative care

Blood transfusion, intravenous fluids, sedatives and antibiotics are given as required. The perineal drainage tube is normally removed after 24 hours but should be left for 48 hours if there is evidence of fresh bleeding. It is advisable to leave the Foley catheter in place about 5–7 days before removal. Spontaneous micturition will then occur but if perineal leakage develops, further urethral drainage may be necessary. Daily baths help wound healing and the skin suture is easily removed at 7 days after operation. Control of continence may be slower in the days immediately following this operation than with other forms of prostatectomy, but if the operation is performed correctly the external sphincter is never damaged and permanent incontinence should not occur.

Further reading

Brendler, H. Surgery for benign disease of the prostate and seminal vesicles. In: Glenn, J. F., ed. Urologic surgery. New York: Hoeber, 1969:305–341

Hudson, P. B. Perineal prostatectomy. In: Harrison, J. H., Gittes, R. F., Perlmutter, A. D., Stamey, T. A., Walsh, P. C. Urology, Vol. 3. 4th ed. Philadelphia: Saunders, 1979:2327–2360

Illustrations by Freda Wadsworth and J. Pizer

Diagnostic procedures for carcinoma of the prostate

Geoffrey D. Chisholm ChM, FRCS, FRCS(Ed)
Professor of Surgery, University of Edinburgh;
Consultant Urological Surgeon, Western General Hospital, Edinburgh;
Honorary Senior Lecturer, Institute of Urology, London, UK

Introduction

Carcinoma of the prostate accounted for 6.5 per cent of all male cancer deaths in England and Wales in 1972[1]. It is estimated that there are 6500 new cases in the UK each year. Although the incidence varies in different countries, the frequency of its occurrence justifies a careful study of its diagnosis and management. The recorded increase in incidence in some countries may be due to better diagnostic procedures rather than to an absolute increase.

The disease is relatively uncommon before the age of 60 and the mean age at presentation in most series is approximately 70 years. The belief that the disease is more aggressive in the younger man is not supported by several recent studies. Although many older men with carcinoma of the prostate may also have other medical problems, it remains important, as with other tumours, to ensure the best quality of life that is compatible with the best choice of treatment.

It must therefore, be emphasized that accurate diagnostic procedures are essential prerequisites to proper management. It is also relevant to emphasize that there is no justification for carrying out detailed diagnostic and staging procedures if it is not intended for that information to be used in selecting appropriate treatment.

In 1978 the Union Internationale Contre Cancer made the following recommendations for the minimum requirements to classify a prostatic tumour according to the TNM system:

T – Primary tumour clinical examination, urography, endoscopy and biopsy

N – Regional and juxtaregional lymph nodes clinical examination and radiography including lymphography and urography

M – Distant metastases clinical examination, radiography, skeletal studies and relevant biochemical tests.

The investigation of a patient suspected of having a malignant prostate should be made according to the following sequence.

Rectal examination

A suspicious prostate gland should first be described and categorized according to the rectal findings. The T category is strictly a clinical assessment of the prostate.

T0

No tumour palpable

1

T1

Tumour intracapsular surrounded by palpably normal gland

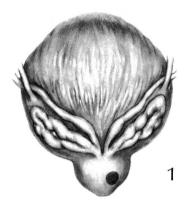

2

T2

Tumour confined to the gland. Smooth nodule deforming contour but lateral sulci and seminal vesicles not involved

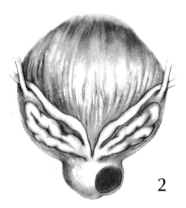

3

T3

Tumour extending beyond the capsule with or without involvement of the lateral sulci and/or seminal vesicles

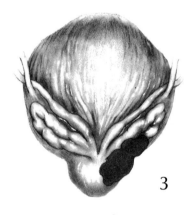

4

T4

Tumour fixed or infiltrating neighbouring structures

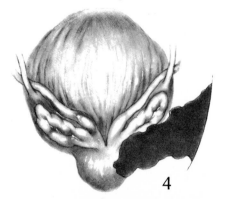

Diagnostic ultrasound

5

In recent years, ultrasound has been used in a number of centres both to screen the prostate for malignant nodules and to measure the extent of proven tumours. External scanners applied either to the suprapubic or perineal regions are generally unsatisfactory, but rectal ultrasound now offers a method of obtaining much more accurate information.

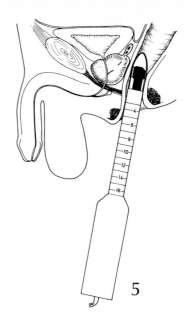

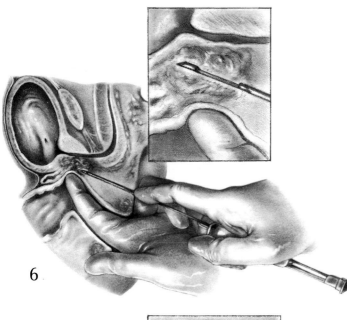

Confirmation of diagnosis

It is essential that the patient should have proof of malignancy either from a biopsy or from cytology before treatment is started.

6

Biopsy – for histological diagnosis

Under general anaesthesia, with the patient in the lithotomy position, the biopsy needle is guided across the perineum to sample prostatic tissue from an area of suspicion. In some centres it is preferred to pass the biopsy needle transrectally, directly into the area of suspicion. There is a higher incidence of infective problems with the latter procedure so that prophylactic antibiotic cover is recommended.

7

Aspiration – for cytological diagnosis

The Franzen needle is designed to be attached to the index finger which palpates the prostate *per rectum*. The needle tip is then advanced into the area of suspicion in the prostate and a sample is aspirated from the gland. The procedure is carried out without anaesthesia, either as an outpatient or inpatient procedure.

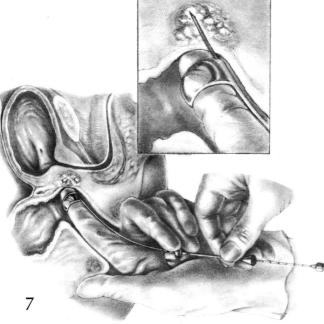

Detection of extraprostatic disease (M category)

Having confirmed the diagnosis and extent of the local disease (T category), the patient should then be assessed for evidence of extraprostatic metastases (M category). These investigations are non-invasive and should precede those described for the detection of extraprostatic disease (N category).

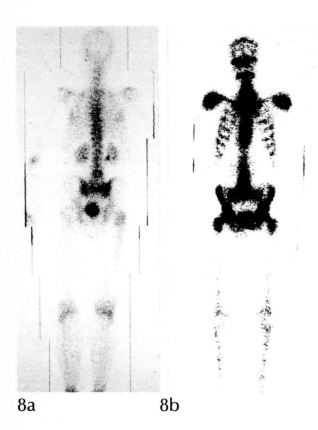

8a   8b

Serum acid phosphatase

The prostatic fraction of acid phosphatase should be measured, preferably by a radioimmunoassay technique. It is still advised that the blood should be drawn prior to a rectal examination, although several reports have suggested this may not be necessary. The proportion of patients with an elevated serum acid phosphatase shows a good correlation with the extent of the disease, but a normal value does not exclude extraprostatic spread.

Radiological bone survey

This routine examination should include X-rays of thoracic and lumbar spine, pelvis, chest (ribs) and a lateral view of the skull.

8a & b

Radioisotope bone scan

The optimum agents for bone scanning are technetium labelled compounds (e.g. technetium diphosphonate). Other radionuclides are either less reliable (e.g. strontium) or less readily available (e.g. fluorine). Approximately 20 per cent of patients with negative radiological bone surveys have a positive bone scan[3].

(a) Normal scan with symmetrical uptake of isotope (note excretion by the kidneys and accumulation into the bladder).

(b) Abnormal scan showing increased uptake, especially in the pelvis, thoracic and lumbar spine.

Detection of extraprostatic disease (N category)

If, according to the T and M categories, the disease is localized to the prostate, the urologist may consider that the patient is suitable for radical treatment, either by excision or radiotherapy. Before a final decision is made for treatment by radical prostatectomy, it is essential to stage accurately the pelvic lymph nodes. In recent years pelvic lymph node staging has shown that a significant proportion (20–40 per cent) of potentially curable early tumours (T0, T1, T2) have pelvic lymph node metastases[4]. If primary radiotherapy is selected for treatment, the need for a precise N category is not so great, since the irradiated field will include most pelvic lymph nodes.

In practical terms, staging of pelvic lymph nodes by lymphography has a high false-positive and false-negative rate, whereas pelvic lymphadenectomy, though much more accurate, has a certain morbidity and even mortality.

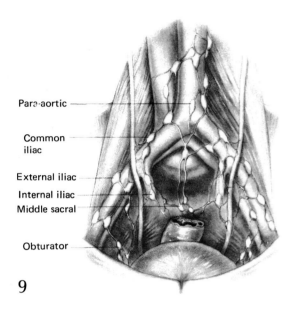

Para-aortic

Common iliac

External iliac

Internal iliac

Middle sacral

Obturator

9

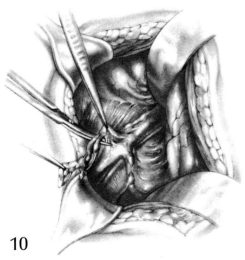

10

9

Lymphography

A lymphatic on the dorsum of each foot is detected after subcutaneous injection of Patent Blue. Lipiodol 10–15 ml is injected into a lymphatic, the dose being monitored according to the filling of the lymphatics (as illustrated) along the main vessels. This technique does not reliably demonstrate the obturator, internal iliac and lateral sacral nodes. It is possible to improve the accuracy of lymphography by fine needle aspiration of abnormal or suspicious lymph nodes.

10

Pelvic lymph node biopsy

The operative procedure consists of bilateral iliac incisions and extraperitoneal exposure of the iliac vessels. Lymph nodes are sampled from the common, external and internal iliac groups and especially the obturator groups. This procedure is preferred to either a staging laparotomy or block dissection of the pelvic lymph nodes, which may be associated with a significant morbidity especially if followed by external beam radiotherapy.

References

1. Alderson, M. R. Epidemiology. In: Duncan. W., ed. Recent results in cancer research: prostate cancer. Berlin: Springer Verlag, 1981: 1–19

2. International Union Against Cancer. TNM Classification of malignant tumours, 3rd ed., Harmer, M. H. ed. Geneva: Internation Union Against Cancer, 1978

3. Chisholm, G. D. Prostate. In: Chisholm, G. D., ed. Urology. London: Heinemann Medical, 1980: 223–246

4. Wajsman, Z. Clinical and pathological staging of prostatic cancer. In: Murphy, G. P., ed. Clinics in oncology: cancer of the prostate. London: W. B. Saunders, 1983

Radical retropubic prostatovesiculectomy

L. E. C. Franksson MD, PhD
Professor and Chairman of the Department of Surgery,
Huddinge Hospital, Caroline Institute Medical School, Stockholm, Sweden

Preoperative

Indications

Cancer originating from prostatic epithelium accounts for 97 per cent of all prostatic tumours. Other tumours occur occasionally (3 per cent[1]). The curative treatment for all malignant tumours of the prostate and seminal vesicles consists of prostatovesiculectomy.

For prostatovesiculectomy the tumour must obviously be limited to the prostate and seminal vesicles. The operation is not stressful for the patient and there is little risk of complications; therefore the indications are wide. Earlier hormone treatment is not a contraindication (*see below*).

Prostatovesiculectomy *en bloc* for malignant tumours of the prostate can be carried out perineally or retropubically. The former method carries the risk of chronic perineal fistulae and postoperative urinary incontinence. With the retropubic approach there is no risk of perineal fistulae and postoperative incontinence is uncommon. It allows inspection and dissection of the pelvic and para-aortic lymph glands and gives a good approach to the ureters and bladder if surgery is indicated. Both methods nearly always lead to sexual impotence. Because of these factors the retropubic approach is to be preferred and the author exclusively uses this method.

Preoperative preparation

The diagnosis of malignant prostatic tumours should be confirmed preoperatively by aspiration biopsy[1]. The extent of the tumour is judged by rectal palpation and bimanual palpation under anaesthetic relaxation; by urethrocystoscopy, pyelograms, computed tomography and investigations for metastases. Also during the operation the area is investigated for both local infiltration and metastases. Only then, if the tumour is judged to be confined to the prostate and seminal vesicles, is the operation carried out.

When there is prostatic enlargement with chronic retention, the bladder is drained by a urethral catheter until kidney function has improved. Clinically manifest urinary infection is treated with antibiotics and concurrent bladder lavage when there is an indwelling catheter. If hormone treatment of the tumour has been initiated it is continued during and up to a few weeks after prostatovesiculectomy.

Anaesthesia

General inhalation anaesthesia supplemented by a muscle relaxant drug is excellent. Spinal anaesthesia can also be considered.

The operation

RETROPUBIC PROSTATOVESICULECTOMY

1

The patient lies supine with a fairly firm pillow, about 5 cm thick, under the pelvis. The operating table is placed so that the patient is inclined 20° in the 'head-down' position in order that abdominal viscera can slide away from the operating field.

The patient is prepared from the navel to and including the penis and scrotum. The operative field including the penis is isolated by sterile drapes. A pliable catheter (18 Fr) is introduced via the urethra to the bladder, which is then emptied. The catheter remains in place.

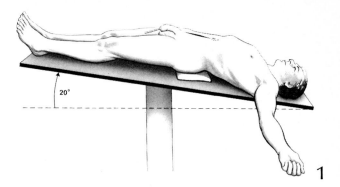

2

The arrows on the illustration indicate the course of dissection.

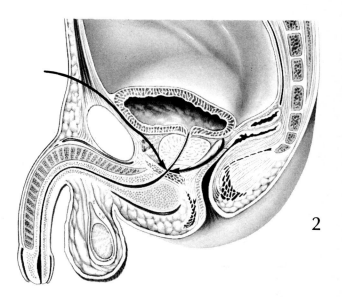

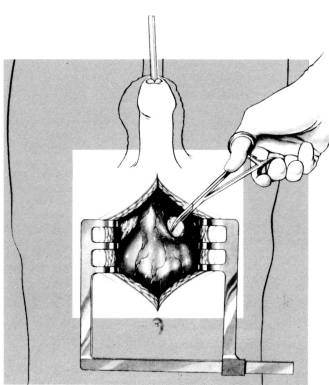

3

A midline incision is made from the symphysis to the navel. The last centimetre down to the symphysis is of particular value. The rectus muscles are separated by a self-retaining retractor. If necessary part of their attachment to the symphysis is divided. The ventral surface of the prostate is now explored. The gland is palpated and moved from side to side in order to make sure that it is not fixed to the surrounding tissues because of direct infiltration. If this is found the operation is discontinued. The peritoneum is opened for palpation of the liver and the pelvic and para-aortic lymph nodes. If metastases are found the operation is discontinued.

The tissues between the prostate and the anterior and lateral pelvic walls are freed. The loose tissue is opened by blunt dissection. The sides of the prostate are then partly free. A pad is placed down on each side of the gland. Bleeding veins are ligated. A good approach to the anterior surface of the prostate and the neck of the bladder is now available.

4

Division of the bladder neck

The ventral aspect of the bladder neck and its catheter is transected, which gives a fairly wide opening to the bladder. Bleeding vessels are ligated.

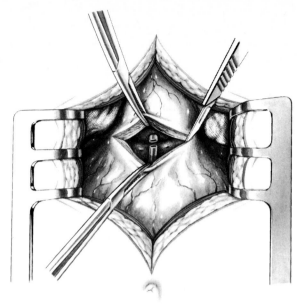

4

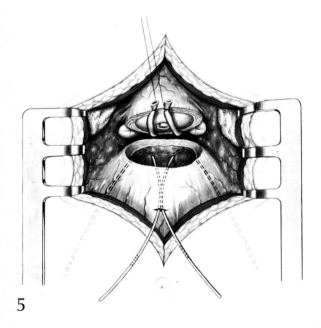

5

5

The ureteric orifices are identified and ureteric catheters are placed in the ureters, which allows them to be easily identified during the following dissection. The catheters are led out by a small incision in the dome of the bladder.

A pair of light clamps is placed on the bladder neck which is then brought forward. Because of its relative mobility it can often be lifted out to the abdominal wall. The dorsal part of the bladder neck is carefully divided so that the seminal vesicles and the vasa deferentia are exposed. The bladder is dissected free from the latter. Dorsal to the bladder, the ureters can now be palpated or even sometimes seen. The vasa deferentia are freed and transected between ligatures. By following the vasa deferentia to the prostate, the rectoprostatic septum is always entered (between the ventral and dorsal folds of Denonvilliers' fascia). The seminal vesicles are found here also and can be freed. The small vessels that supply them are divided between ligatures. When this stage is completed, the bladder is completely separated from the prostate and seminal vesicles. It is covered with a moist pad and laid back in a cephalic direction until later.

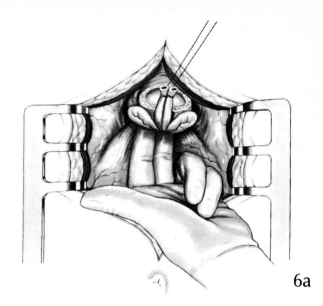

6a

6a & b

The vasa deferentia and the dorsal aspect of the seminal vesicles are followed by the finger down to the apex of the prostate. Because of the loose tissue in the rectoprostatic septum the apex is easily reached. The point where the prostate ends and the urethra begins can be identified by palpating the catheter in the urethra. Dissection should not be carried beyond this point, because of the proximity of the urethral sphincter, damage to which can lead to postoperative incontinence.

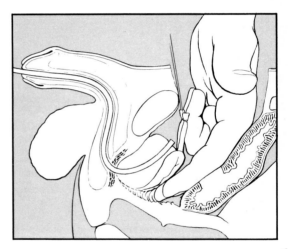

6b

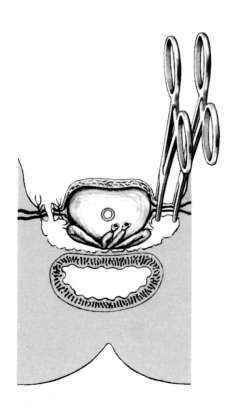

7

7

The tissue (fascia and vessels), that attaches the prostate laterally is divided between clamps and ligated on both sides with absorbable material (Dexon, catgut). Division begins at the upper part of the prostate and terminates at the apex. A few fairly large branches of the inferior vesical artery can easily slip out from the ligatures and they should then be clamped separately.

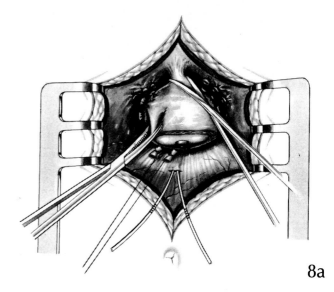

8a

8a & b

The specimen (the prostate, seminal vesicles and vasa deferentia) now remains attached only to the urethra. The latter is transected close to the apex of the prostate, completing the excision. Strong traction should be avoided, because it can cause damage to the urethral sphincter.

Bleeding from the veins around the transected urethra can sometimes be troublesome. The veins are difficult to approach. The simplest way to control haemorrhage is with the help of a retention catheter. This is introduced via the urethra and the inflated balloon is brought down on the cut end of the urethra with slight traction, e.g. by fixing the catheter with a clamp to the surgical drapes. Compression for a short time will stop much of the bleeding. Other bleeding points are ligated. The operative field must be dry before the following reconstructive part of the operation begins.

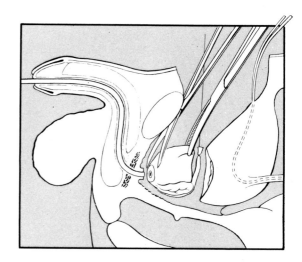

8b

9a & b

The opening at the neck of the bladder is reduced to approximately the width of the urethra. By applying traction to the ventral part of the opening it is reduced to a slit of which the dorsal part is closed with a deep row of absorbable sutures and an outer row of non-absorbable material. This results in elongation of the bladder neck. If needed, the bladder should be mobilized so that the neck reaches the urethra without tension. This can be achieved by applying traction to the neck of the bladder and at the same time loosening the tissues between the bladder and rectum with a clamp.

The balloon catheter is removed. There can still be some bleeding around the internal urethral orifice but this usually stops when the urethra is anastomosed to the bladder. Long absorbable sutures are placed around the urethral orifice (Dexon, 4/0 catgut). The urethral stump is often retracted. This can be pushed forward by a catheter or a sound which is introduced via the external urethral meatus. Slight tension on the first suture facilitates placement of the others. There is usually room for four to six sutures. The dorsal sutures are then stitched through the dorsal aspect of the neck of the bladder and tied. The neck is pulled down and fixed to the urethra.

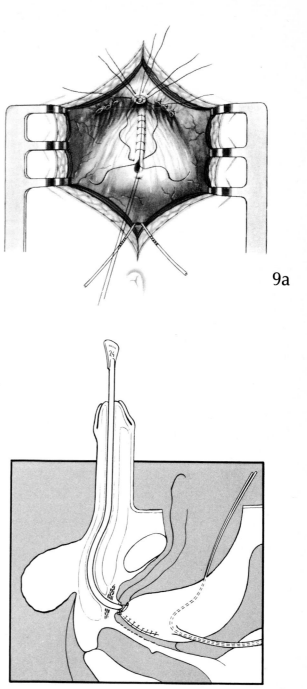

9a

9b

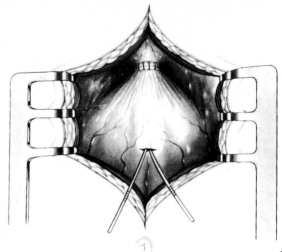

10a

10a & b

A catheter (24 Fr) with or without a balloon is introduced via the urethra to the bladder. The sutures in the ventral aspect of the urethra are stitched through the corresponding part of the neck of the bladder and tied. The bladder is then filled via the catheter with normal saline. The urethral anastomosis should tolerate moderate pressure in the bladder without leaking. If this is not the case, sutures should be placed over the leakage. Free flow of fluid in both directions should be established.

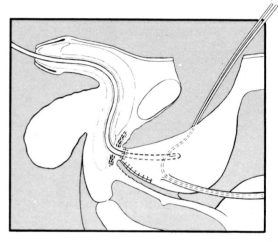

10b

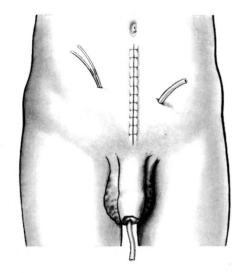

11

11

The prevesical area is drained with a 1 cm diameter drainage tube, which is brought out through a separate incision. The ureteric catheters are brought out through another incision. The abdominal wall is closed.

Postoperative care

If a retention catheter is used it is fastened so that the balloon does not press on the neck of the bladder, which can lead to ischaemia in the anastomosis. The bladder is irrigated by the urethral catheter with 100 ml normal saline a few times the first day.

The patients, who are often elderly, generally tolerate the procedure well. Many can be up on the operation day or the following day.

If there is no wound discharge, the drainage tube is removed after 3 days. The ureteric catheters can be removed after 6–7 days when the oedema in the bladder starts to recede. The urethral catheter can be removed after a few more days.

Complications

Postoperatively the bladder floor is always oedematous, which can compress the intramural parts of the ureters resulting in oliguria or anuria. Ureteric catheterization via cystoscopy during the first week is doomed to failure because the oedematous bladder bottom usually prevents location of the ureteric orifices. A temporary pyelostomy may be necessary. The complication is avoided if the ureteric catheters are introduced during the operation and allowed to remain (see above).

When the urethral catheter is removed some patients have difficulty controlling micturition. This ability, however, eventually returns. A study[2] of continence returning after catheter removal showed the following results.

Continent		5 patients
Continent	1–3 months later	7 patients
Continent	4–9 months later	5 patients
Continent	30 months later	1 patient
Slight persistent stress incontinence		2 patients

There seems to be a tendency for continence to be more satisfactory the closer to the apex of the prostate the urethra is transected.

After the procedure a number of younger patients retain a certain ability for an erection. However, it must be accepted that in most cases prostatovesiculectomy results in sexual impotence.

Recurrences

The rate of recurrence of tumour depends, of course, on how well local infiltration and metastases are diagnosed preoperatively. If the patient is investigated as described above, the cases with spread outside the prostate and seminal vesicles are excluded as far as possible. As with all tumour surgery, despite these investigations, local recurrences and/or metastases occur in a number of cases. Both local recurrences and metastases are common in highly malignant tumours. These cases, which are in the minority, should perhaps receive hormone treatment, even if the specimen seems to show radical extirpation.

All other cases are treated with hormones if the specimen shows tumour growth at the edges of the resection and also if tumour growth is evident locally or in the form of metastases. Patients should be reviewed every 3 months for the first year and then every 6 months.

With postoperative rectal palpation the urethra is pressed directly against the hard and uneven inferior border of the symphysis. This can easily be mistaken for recurrence of the tumour. The situation should be clarified by palpating with an instrument in the urethra.

Editor's comment: preservation of potency

Potency may be preserved in the majority of patients if the neurovascular bundles supplying the corpora which lie adjacent and lateral to the prostate are preserved[2]. This may be accomplished by identifying these structures prior to step shown in *Illustration 7* and completing dissection medial to them. They are identified by incising the endopelvic fascia near the apex of the prostate. They may be found immediately lateral to the urethra where it joins the apex of the prostate. Once identified, they may be traced cranially by extending the incision in the endopelvic fascia. The bundles are traced to the level of the prostatic pedicles. Having identified them at this level, the pedicles may be taken medial to the neurovascular bundle. The remainder of the operation may then proceed as described taking care not to injure either bundle in the remainder of the dissection.

Reference

1. Esposti, P.–L. Aspiration biopsy cytology in the diagnosis and management of prostatic carcinoma. Unpublished PhD thesis, Stockholm University, 1974
2. Walsh, P. C. Preservation of potency during radical retropubic prostatectomy: technique and preliminary results. American Urological Association Abstract 1983; 420

Further reading

Esposti, P.–L. Cytologic diagnosis of prostatic tumours with the aid of trans-rectal aspiration biopsy: a critical review of 1110 cases and a report of morphologic and cytochemical studies. Acta Cytologica 1966; 10:182–186

Franksson, C., Collste, L. G. Prostatovesiculectomy in 20 patients with malignant prostatic tumour. Scandinavian Journal of Urology and Nephrology 1974; 8:162–166

Paulson, D. F., Lin, G. H., Hinshaw, W., Stephani, S., Uro-Oncology Research Group. Radical surgery versus radiotherapy for adenocarcinoma of the prostate. Journal of Urology 1982; 128:502–504

Illustrations by Barbara Rankin

Radical perineal prostatovesiculectomy

L. Persky MD, FACS
Professor of Urology, University Hospitals of Cleveland, Cleveland, Ohio, USA

W. Scott McDougal MD
Professor and Chairman, Department of Urology,
Vanderbilt University Medical Center, Nashville, Tennessee, USA

Introduction

Perineal prostatovesiculectomy is executed today in much the same way as when it was described at the turn of the century by Hugh Hampton Young. However, some significant modifications were described by Belt[1]. The advantages of the perineal approach are that it gives one direct access to the prostate, affords an opportunity to avoid blood vessels anteriorly and the major nerve supply laterally, and allows easy location of the dominant arterial supply at 5 and 7 o'clock which can be divided under direct vision. It provides the opportunity to do an anastomosis between the urethra and the reconstructed bladder neck with the structures well visualized and easily reached. The operation also has the advantage of providing dependent drainage.

Preoperative

Attention must be paid to any prior orthopaedic surgery in the area of the hip joint, since this could preclude adequate positioning of the patient. Preoperative preparation should also include an evaluation of the common metastatic sites, including regional lymph nodes, bone and lungs. Prior to surgery, the patient is placed on a low-residue diet for 24–48 hours. There is usually also a 24-hour mechanical bowel preparation which helps avoid sepsis if one should inadvertently enter the rectum.

The operation

1

Position of patient

Positioning the patient properly is an essential part of the operation. The patient's buttocks should be over the edge of the table. Often the landmark used for this guide is the sacral notch. The thighs should be placed as parallel to the floor as possible. The patient should be placed symmetrically on the perineal board or modified perineal table. Preoperative preparation should include a careful shave of the perineum, scrotum and suprapubic area to the umbilicus with extension of skin preparation to the mid-thigh.

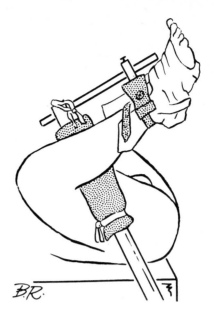

1

2

The incision

A small, arcuate incision is made between the ischial tuberosities passing anterior to the rectum at the mucocutaneous junction. The incision should be placed more anteriorly if there are significant haemorrhoidal tags or dilated veins which may cause increased bleeding and more difficult dissection.

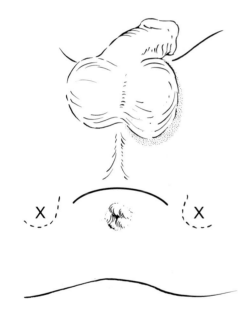

2

3

The posterior lip of the incision is retracted downwards. The median raphe of the perineum is divided by sharp dissection after Metzenbaum scissors have been spread to create a space on either side of the raphe beneath the external anal sphincter. This space allows the operator to retract and depress the rectum manually while division of the raphe is completed. It is important in this part of the operation to proceed slowly and to secure haemostasis with cautery or ligature of perforating blood vessels which can cause troublesome bleeding.

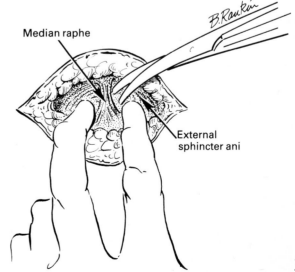

Median raphe

External sphincter ani

3

4

After the median raphe is divided, the dissection is carried down to the levators with continued traction inferiorly on the rectum. It is important to recognize that one is approaching the junction of the levators with the rectal margin. This fusion of the levators is called the rectourethralis muscle.

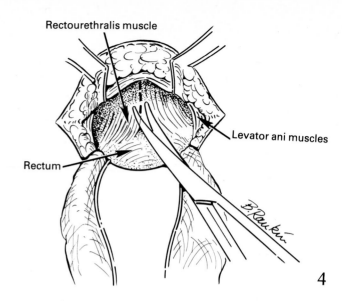

5

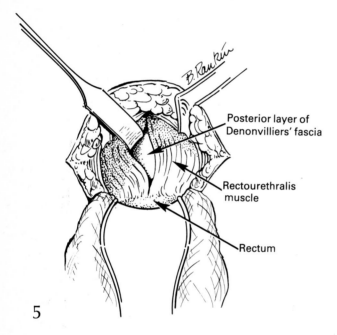

With traction downwards, either with a retractor or with continued traction over a sponge by the operator's middle, index and ring fingers, the area can be divided by sharp dissection affording exposure within the levators of the posterior layer of Denonvilliers' fascia. The rectourethralis muscle is divided by sharp and blunt dissection in a vertical manner and opens a plane within which one can insert the lateral retractors. These afford dissection and exposure of the posterior layer of fascia which is the guide to effective release of the prostate from contact with rectum posteriorly. Beneath this posterior layer, continued dissection exposes the blood supply at 5 and 7 o'clock. It is most important to secure these structures early in the operation.

6a & b

The posterior layer of Denonvilliers' fascia can be divided transversely to avoid rectal injury. With a back and forth rocking motion, one can usually see the junction of the rectum with the posterior layer of Denonvilliers' fascia. The transverse incision should be made above this junction, thereby releasing the rectum further. With careful packing with gauze and deliberate placement of the posterior retractor, the rectum is walled off out of harm's way. A long curved prostatic tractor is then placed intraurethrally. The Lowsley curved prostatic tractor is of immense help in affording exposure and control of the prostate during the subsequent dissection. A Young prostatic tractor allows equal control and manipulation of the glands. While this dissection of the fascial layer is being carried out, lateral traction of the levators affords exposure while the posterior tractor protects the rectum from inadvertent injury.

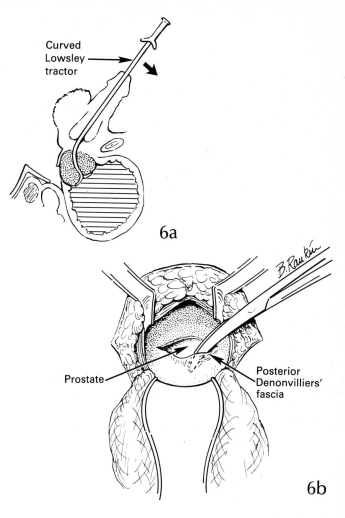

6a

Prostate

Posterior Denonvilliers' fascia

6b

7

Once the posterior layer of Denonvilliers' fascia has been reflected, dissection can be carried out at 5 and 7 o'clock to gain control of the blood vessels in this area. This is made easier by angulation of the prostate by means of the prostatic tractor. Access to the right and left side is facilitated by lateral movements back and forth. The blood supply can be freed, and clamped with right-angle clamps, divided and ligated. At this stage of the operation, the coagulating current is used to divide the vessels and to afford ready exposure without delay. This also permits fulguration of the vessels left on the gland which subsequently will be removed with the specimen.

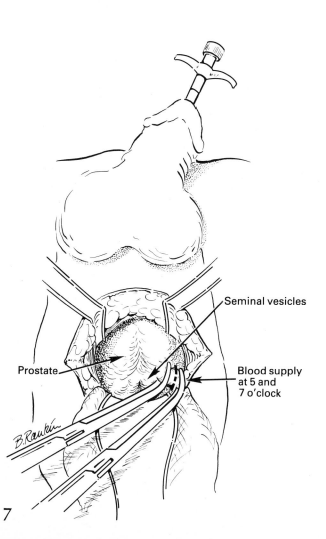

Seminal vesicles

Prostate

Blood supply at 5 and 7 o'clock

7

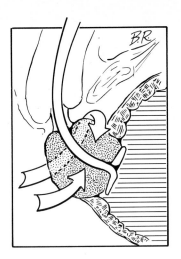

8

After the blood supply is divided, it is possible to manipulate the gland so that a finger can be placed around the prostate anteriorly to free it from investing fascia and overlying vessels. It is imperative at this point to be gentle. With care, the puboprostatic ligaments can be pushed off anteriorly, along with the blood vessels above them, thus mobilizing the gland. This makes further steps in the procedure much simpler. It is mandatory during this manoeuvre to avoid carrying one's finger into the area of the membranous urethra, since this may impair its function. Carelessness can lead to difficulty with urinary control and may ultimately result in incontinence.

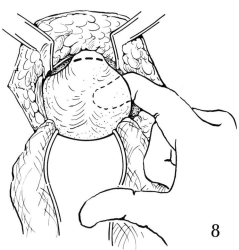

8

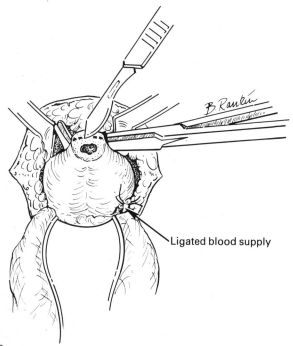

Ligated blood supply

9

9

During the dissection involving the anterior portion of the prostate, right-angle clamps (Moynihan) may facilitate separation of the investing ligaments. The junction of the urethra with the apex of the prostate is divided by scalpel dissection with a Moynihan clamp behind the junction. This permits the prostate to be dropped away distally from its continuity with the urethra. After the posterior aspect of the incision has been completed, the curved Lowsley prostatic tractor is exposed and then removed. The anterior portion of the junction can be divided by scissors or scalpel.

10

The apex of the prostate is easily secured and the straight prostatic tractor is placed in the prostatic urethra. This permits further manipulation of the prostate and helps in freeing the puboprostatic ligaments from the anterior aspects of the prostate. The puboprostatic ligaments can be clamped or divided or they can be pushed off by blunt dissection. The junction of the bladder and the prostate on the anterior surface is then easily visualized and opened.

Puboprostatic ligament

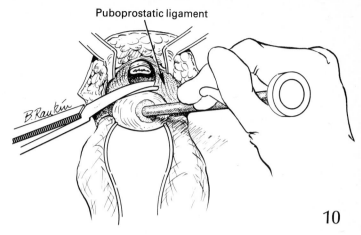

10

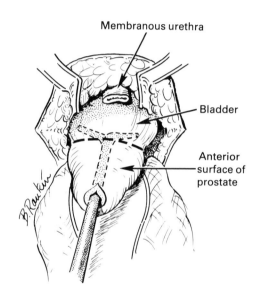

Membranous urethra

Bladder

Anterior surface of prostate

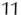

11

11 & 12

This fusion of structures can be palpated by feeling the arms of the straight prostatic tractor. Then an opening is made with scissors or a scalpel, permitting further surgical division on either side of the midline of the bladder and prostatic junction. This dissection in the right and left direction can be carried out by taking small bites with a right-angle clamp. Interrupted sutures or ligatures in the bladder muscle prevent continued bleeding from the cut margins of the detrusor. As the dissection is carried laterally on each side, the junction of the prostate and the bladder neck is visualized posteriorly. The straight prostatic tractor is removed and a pliable rubber drain or vascular loop is used to maintain traction on the prostate. It is important not to pull too hard since one can completely divide the prostate at the anterior commissure. Although this does not make the operation less successful, on occasion it requires the use of grasping Allis or Babcocks forceps on the prostatic tissue and makes the procedure a little more cumbersome.

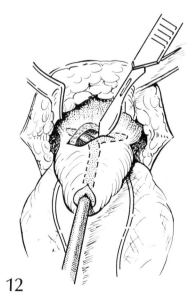

12

13

Division of the posterior bladder neck from the proximal prostate is carried out by sharp and blunt dissection to make sure that the incision is not carried too deep. Continuity of the seminal vesicles and the vas deferens should be maintained until they can be securely visualized and handled properly. Usually a good plane can be obtained during the dissection. Once this is accomplished, the prostate falls away further from the area of the bladder neck and one can see and palpate the ejaculatory ducts and the seminal vesicles, which are then easily exposed. Indigo carmine (5 ml) injected as a bolus intravenously a few minutes before the division of the posterior bladder neck, is helpful in locating the ureteral orifices, thereby lessening the chances of inadvertently injuring them.

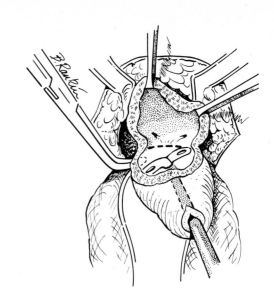

13

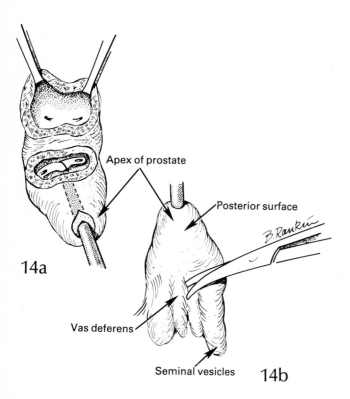

Apex of prostate

Posterior surface

14a

Vas deferens

Seminal vesicles   14b

14a & b

After the bladder has been reflected upwards and the prostate freed circumferentially, upward traction makes it possible to free the seminal vesicles and vas deferens from their investing fascial layer, and to clamp and divide the vas deferens on each side. The dissection is subsequently continued down to the apices of the seminal vesicles where clamps can be applied and the encompassing connective tissue and blood vessels can be clamped and divided. This permits the removal of the specimen with the attached seminal vesicles and prostate in continuity.

15a–d

The interior of the entire bladder can then be inspected before it is closed anteriorly in a vertical fashion with interrupted chromic catgut sutures. A 5/8 curved needle of medium size with a chromic 2/0 catgut suture is preferred. Three or four stitches placed in the bladder neck narrow it down (b) to roughly the size of a 24 Fr Foley catheter. The anastomosis (c, d) is then made over an indwelling urethral catheter. The catheter is not inserted into the bladder until the anteriormost stitch is placed through the reconstructed bladder neck and anterior aspect of the prostate. This is tied down and the two structures are approximated. The 24 Fr Foley catheter is then placed in the bladder, affording a stent over which an accurate anastomosis can be made. The first stitch is usually in the midline posteriorly and, using this as a tractor, it is possible to place several stitches on each side which go through the bladder and the membranous urethra before they are tied. These stitches must be carefully placed – penetrating not too deeply or too far into the bladder – so as not to encroach on a ureteral orifice. The suture line should be watertight, which usually requires six or eight sutures. The surgeon can determine the integrity of the suture line by irrigating gently with saline; blue indigo dye in the bladder also demonstrates ureteral integrity.

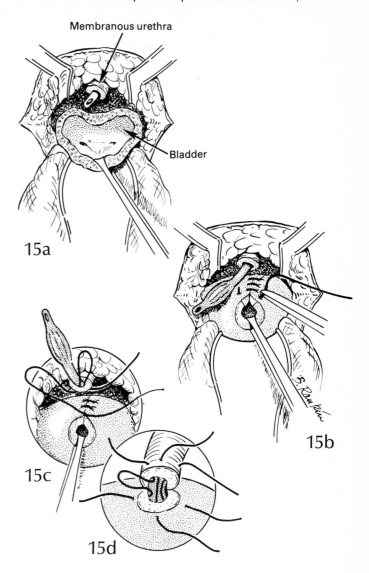

15a

15b

15c

15d

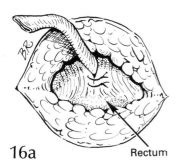

16a

Rectum

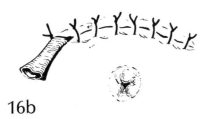

16b

16a & b

The levators are reapproximated in the midline with several interrupted chromic catgut sutures. These should be placed carefully to avoid incorporating the rectum and creating later necrosis and a rectoperineal or rectourethral fistula. A Penrose drain is brought out superiorly from the area of the prostatectomy, several subcutaneous stitches of chromic catgut are placed and the skin is closed with a row of continuous interrupted chromic catgut stitches. Subcuticular stitches may be employed to avoid the need to remove skin sutures. The patient is usually connected to continuous saline irrigation with a three-way Foley catheter. In most cases this can be discontinued in 24 hours.

Postoperative care

In the postoperative period the patient is given a low-residue diet and oral stool softeners to avoid undue pressure and pain, and to facilitate bowel movement. Sitz baths are begun. Usually after each bowel movement during the first week, it is recommended that the patient have such a perineal cleansing. Two or three such soaks are scheduled each day. Preoperative antibiotics are continued postoperatively. There is surprisingly little bleeding and postoperative pain and these patients are often ambulatory the night of surgery.

Complications

When it is recognized that the rectum has been entered early in the operation, it should be closed carefully with an inner layer of chromic catgut sutures and an outer layer of silk. The wound is closed and the localized neoplasm managed in another fashion. If the injury is recognized at the end of the operation, again it is important to close the rectal injury carefully. The anal canal is dilated in order to decrease intraluminal rectal tension. This can be done manually with several fingers. A feared late complication is the development of a rectourethral fistula which can be very difficult to manage. If the injury is missed, or if a fistula develops later, continued urosepsis may ensue, and this calls for the creation of a temporary diverting colostomy.

This operation affords excellent exposure and is indicated in selected patients with Stage A and B lesions. A high rate of impotence and a small incidence of incontinence are the major complications.

Reference

1. Belt, E., Ebert, C. F., Surber, A. C. Jr. A new anatomic approach in perineal prostatectomy. Journal of Urology 1939; 41: 482

Further reading

Jewett, H. J. The case for radical perineal prostatectomy. Journal of Urology 1970; 103: 195–199

Jewett, H. J. The present status of radical prostatectomy for stages A and B prostatic cancer. Urologic Clinics of North America 1975; 2: 105–124

Schroeder, F. H., Belt, E. Carcinoma of the prostate: a study of 213 patients with stage C tumors treated by total perineal prostatectomy. Journal of Urology 1975; 114: 257–260

Illustrations by Larry Stein

Radioactive seed implantation for carcinoma of the prostate

S. G. Mulholland MD
Professor and Chairman, Department of Urology,
Thomas Jefferson University Medical School, Philadelphia, Pennsylvania, USA

Mohammed Mohiuddin MD
Associate Professor, Department of Radiation Therapy,
Thomas Jefferson University Medical School, Philadelphia, Pennsylvania, USA

Introduction

Treatment of localized carcinoma of the prostate has been debated by urologists for decades. The decision regarding treatment of this disease is influenced by many factors. As the human male ages, his chances of developing carcinoma of the prostate increase remarkably. Also, the patient may acquire other diseases, any one of which could prove fatal. It is quite common for a patient who has had carcinoma of the prostate diagnosed to live a normal life and eventually die of another disease. Certainly more patients die with the disease than as a direct result of it.

As the urologist becomes more familiar with carcinoma of the prostate, he learns which patients should be treated aggressively. A patient with a life expectancy of 5 years or more and good health should be treated aggressively. With extensive studies on cell type and differentiation, we have learned how to predict behaviour patterns better and have come to realize that localized disease generally deserves aggressive treatment with cancer surgery or radiation therapy.

Principles and justifications

Radiation therapy has been used successfully to treat cancer of the prostate. Excellent local control of the primary tumour can be obtained, together with prolonged survival of patients[1-6]. There are several definite advantages in treating patients with radiation rather than with radical surgery. While only 10 per cent of patients are candidates for radical prostatectomy, 40–50 per cent of patients have tumours still localized to the pelvis. These can be treated adequately with radiation. The incidence of complications is somewhat lower (10–16 per cent) following radiation and sexual function is preserved in a high proportion (60–70 per cent) of patients.

There are two approaches to radiation treatment for cancer of the prostate. External beam radiation has been widely used only since the mid-1960s. Interstitial implantation of radioactive material into the prostate has been utilized for decades. In 1913, Pasteau[7] used intraurethral placement of radium to treat prostate cancer. Several others[1, 2, 8-14] have reported their experiences using radium and radioactive I^{125}. While control of local disease and survival of patients is similar, there are certain definite advantages for the use of implantation over external beam radiation:

1. Implantation is performed immediately following lymphadenectomy, as a one-stage procedure.
2. Higher tumour dose can safely be delivered to the tumour with an implant.
3. The region of high radiation dose can be localized more precisely to the exact shape and extent of the tumour.
4. The rapid fall-off of radiation dose from an implant means better sparing of surrounding normal tissue. The bladder and rectum receive 30–40 per cent less radiation dose from an implant when compared to external beam radiation therapy.
5. The bladder and rectal complications following implantation are somewhat lower than with external beam radiation (2 per cent compared with 7–28 per cent).
6. There is a lower incidence of impotence following implantation as compared to external beam radiation.

It has been shown in experimental studies that for interstitial implants, an ideal therapeutic ratio, i.e. maximum tumour cell kill with the least normal tissue damage, occurs at a dose rate of 40–60 rad per hour. This

461

dose rate can be obtained with several radioactive isotopes. In accessible sites, such as the head and neck areas, isotopes like ^{226}Rad and ^{192}Ir, with long physical half-lives and high energy of radiation emission, are preferred. These isotopes can be implanted for short periods to deliver the desired dose rate to the tumour volume. Their position and strength can be changed during the course of treatment. In less easily accessible areas of the body, such as the abdomen and thorax, only permanent implantation can be performed.

Isotopes for permanent implantation should preferably have a low energy spectrum of X-ray emission, so that there is a minimal risk of radiation exposure to physicians and nursing personnel, the patient's family and the general population. This is especially important where larger volumes of tissue are implanted, as in the prostate, for the patient carries a high activity of the radioactive isotope.

The fall-off in radiation dose from the tumour to the surrounding normal tissue is much more rapid with low energy X-ray emitters (^{125}I) than with high energy X-ray emitters (^{198}Au). Since spatial distribution of permanent implants cannot be altered once these have been completed, isotope placement of high energy X-ray emitters is far more critical and less satisfactory for larger volumes. When low energy X-ray emitters are used, isotopes with a relatively long half-life are necessary to provide biologically acceptable dose rates at the periphery of the implanted tumour volume. For these reasons, ^{125}I, with the physical characteristics as shown in *Table 1*, has become the preferred isotope among those available for implantation in prostatic cancer.

Table 1 Characteristics of isotopes used in implantation

Isotope	Half-life	Energy (MeV)	Half value layer in tissue
^{226}Ra	1604 years	0.18–2.2	10 cm
^{192}Ir	74 days	1.17–1.33	6 cm
^{198}Au	2.7 days	0.41	6 cm
^{125}I	60 days	0.028–0.035	2 cm

The implantation of ^{125}I seeds requires a surgical procedure, but most of the patients who have localized carcinoma should be staged with a pelvic lymphadenectomy. It is our feeling that if the pelvic nodes are negative at the time of pelvic lymphadenectomy, one can proceed with implantation of the gland. This procedure does not increase appreciably the morbidity of pelvic lymphadenectomy. All the treatment is given in a one-stage procedure. Implantation of seeds does not impair the individual's ability to void. Occasionally, a patient will have borderline obstructive disease; in this case, a limited transurethral resection of the prostate may be performed 2 months prior to implantation of the seeds. This is rarely necessary and should be avoided if possible.

Selection of patients

There is a definite relationship between the size of the neoplasm to be implanted and the cure rate or sterilization of the tissue of the primary tumour. The best candidates for implantation are patients with Stages B1, B2 or early Stage C disease. Stage A patients are not generally implanted. Stage A2 patients may be suitable candidates, but if an extensive transurethral resection of the prostate has been performed, an adequate implant may be technically difficult. Ideally, implants should not exceed 5 cm diameter or 30–40 ml in volume. Patients with large bulky disease, large Stage C or D1, are not suitable candidates. These patients have a high complication rate and poor local control with implants and should receive external radiation. If there is any suspicion that the tumour has invaded the seminal vesicals or adjacent viscera, external beam radiation is the treatment of choice.

Preoperative preparation

Patients are evaluated for surgery extremely carefully to ensure diagnosis of purely localized disease and significant life expectancy, and to confirm the absence of life-threatening conditions. Further evaluation includes a complete serum chemistry profile, alkaline and acid phosphatase (with prostatic fraction), bone scan, an intravenous pyelogram, chest films and cystoscopy. We do not do routine lymphangiograms because of the high false positive and false negative rates. CAT scanning of the pelvis has been shown to be of little value in this disease. Multiple transperineal needle biopsies are taken of both lobes, and carefully labelled, for anatomical description of the extent of disease.

The operation

1

The urological surgeon works closely with the radiation therapist for ^{125}I implantation of the prostate. We believe that the low lithotomy position is best for both physicians. The patient is prepared and draped in the routine manner. An O'Connor-type sheath is used to seal off the rectum properly. This allows the radiation therapist to perform rectal examination at the time of placing his needles. The bladder is catheterized at this time with an 18 Fr Foley catheter.

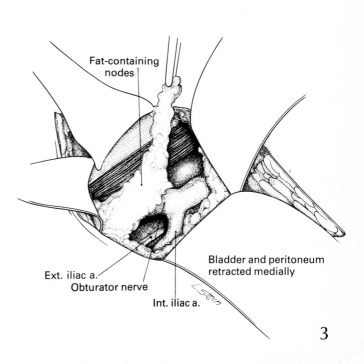

1

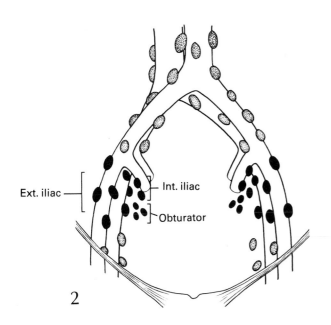

2

2

A Pfannenstiel incision is made approximately 2 cm above the symphysis pubis and carried down to the peritoneum and perivesical space. The pelvic nodes are approached first in an extraperitoneal fashion. The peritoneum is bluntly swept superiorly and medially to expose the psoas muscles and iliac vessels bilaterally. Extensive lymph node dissection is not necessary. Our dissection includes the dark shaded nodes shown in the Illustration. This is the area of primary metastases, with the highest yield of positive nodes.

Ext. iliac
Int. iliac
Obturator

3

During the lymph node dissection, all lymphatic channels must be clipped carefully with small silver clips. The obturator fossa should be identified and the nodes removed, preserving the obturator nerve. The nerve should be cleaned of nodal tissue and the obturator artery sacrificed while reflecting the bladder medially. After the lymph nodes have been removed, a 4 × 8 cm sponge is placed in the area of dissection and left until the end of the procedure. The lymph nodes are sent to the pathology department for frozen section. If they are negative, ^{125}I implantation can proceed.

Fat-containing nodes

Ext. iliac a.
Obturator nerve
Int. iliac a.

Bladder and peritoneum retracted medially

3

4

The prostate is exposed anteriorly and laterally by incising the endopelvic fascia. The dorsal vein of the penis is identified and doubly ligated. The fat and fascia are removed from the anterior and lateral aspects of the prostate so the surgeon can observe 75–80 per cent of the prostate gland. Occasionally, the puboprostatic ligaments must be partially cut. This allows the surgeon to manipulate the prostate and bladder in such a way that these can be dissected freely.

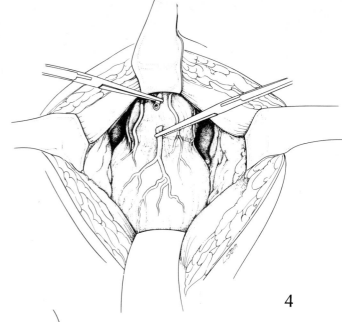

4

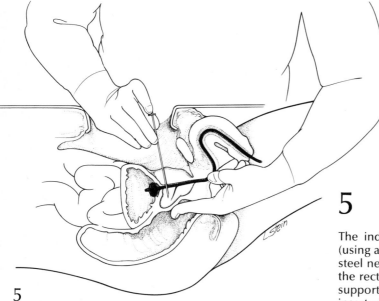

5

5

The index finger of one hand is placed in the rectum (using an O'Connor sheath) and hollow 16 gauge stainless steel needles are inserted into the prostate. The finger in the rectum is used to outline the prostate and to provide support for the tissues posteriorly as the needles are inserted. Also, it serves as a guide to determine the depth of insertion of the needles, which should not extend to the rectal mucosa. They are placed parallel to each other at a distance of 1 cm starting from the periphery of the gland and working towards the midline. Care is taken not to insert needles through the base of the bladder. The Foley catheter may be used as a guide to the location of the bladder base.

6

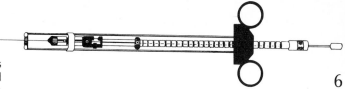

6

Once all the needles have been placed, a seed inserter is attached to each needle sequentially and then several seeds are inserted into each needle tract as the needle itself is withdrawn.

Complications

Major intraoperative complications have been reported as low (6 per cent)[15]. Occasionally excessive blood loss will occur during seed implantation (2 per cent)[15]. Injury to obturator and femoral nerves is rare. Major postoperative complications (25 per cent) include lymphocele and haematoma (10 per cent) and cardiovascular problems (10 per cent), mainly pulmonary embolus and thrombophlebitis. Mortality is exceedingly low (0.67 per cent). Late complications well beyond the operative period include voiding symptoms, which are usually limited and transient.

Calculation of iodine required activity for implantation

A planned tumour minimum dose of 16 000 rads is delivered to the prostate. In order to deliver this dose, a three-dimensional measurement of the prostate is obtained at exploration and an average volume of the gland is calculated. The number of millicuries of ^{125}I needed to deliver the desired dose to that volume is available in special tables. Total activity is divided by the available seed strength to obtain the number of seeds to be implanted. These are spaced at required distances through the implanted volume.

Postoperative considerations

The use of ^{125}I has reduced greatly the risk of radiation exposure to nursing personnel and physicians. Following implantation, patients are returned to the ward with an indwelling catheter in the bladder. The urine is collected along with all secretions from drains; all suction material is monitored with a Geiger counter on a daily basis for the presence of dislodged seeds. Any seeds that are found are returned to the department for disposal. The urine is collected for 24 hours after the catheter is removed on the 3rd day and monitored for expulsion of seeds.

Just before the patient is discharged, a plain film of the pelvis is obtained to ascertain the position of the iodine seeds. Once the patient is discharged, no special precautions are required for the spouse or the general population. However, it is recommended that, except for brief close contact, pregnant women and very young children should stay at least 6 feet away during the first 2 months post implantation.

Results

The most extensive experience with ^{125}I implantation of the prostate comes from Sloan Kettering Memorial Hospital, New York City, where patients have been treated with this technique since the early 1970s. Patient selection is a key factor in efficacy of treatment. Prostatic tumour which can be uniformly implanted so the whole of the prostate receives the minimum tumour dose has a local failure rate of 5 per cent or less and a complication rate of 12 per cent or less. On the other hand, when the dose distribution in the prostate is uneven, especially in large tumours, the local failure rate is as high as 24 per cent. Local control of tumour is also dependent on the total dose delivered to the prostate. When a minimum dose of 16 000 rad is delivered over 1 year, the local control is over 90 per cent. With smaller doses local control decreases sharply.

The response of prostatic tumour is a slow process. Most tumours may take up to 2 years for complete regression of disease. Even then positive histology on biopsy may not represent viable tumour. Only clinical evidence of progression of disease with positive biopsies indicates a true local failure. Iodine implantation has less morbidity than external beam radiation. Serious complications of rectal ulceration, urethral stenosis, fistulae, rectal or urinary urgency are seen only infrequently.

Excellent survival of implanted patients has been reported. A 5-year survival of 90 per cent for Stage B tumour (69 per cent disease-free) and 74 per cent for Stage C (46 per cent disease-free) has been reported. The presence or absence of pelvic node metastasis has a major impact on survival of patients. When multiple node metastases are present, or if the common iliac nodes are involved, survival of patients is significantly reduced[16].

References

1. Whitmore, W. F., Hilaris, B., Grabstald, H., Batata, M. Implantation of ^{125}I in prostatic cancer. Surgical Clinics of North America 1974; 54: 887–895

2. Herr, H. W. Iodine-125 implantation in the management of localized prostatic carcinoma. Urologic Clinics of North America 1980; 7: 605–613

3. Bagshaw, M. A., Ray, G. R., Pestenma, D. A., Castellino, R. A., Meares, E. M. External beam radiation therapy of primary carcinoma of the prostate. Cancer 1975; 36: 723

4. McGowan, D. G. Radiation therapy in the management of localized carcinoma of the prostate: a preliminary report. Cancer 1977; 39: 98–103

5. Perez, C. A., Bauer, W., Garza, R., Royce, R. K. Radiation therapy in the definitive treatment of localized carcinoma of the prostate. Cancer 1977; 40: 1425–1433

6. Whitmore, W. F. Jr., Batata, M., Hilaris, B. Prostatic irradiation: Iodine-125 implantation. In: Johnson, D. E., Samuels, M. L., eds. Cancer of the genitourinary tract. New York: Raven Press, 1979: 195–205

7. Pasteau, O., Degrais, P. The radium treatment of cancer of the prostate. Archives of the Roentgen Ray 1914; 18: 396–410

8. Barringer, B. S. Radium in the treatment of carcinoma of the bladder and prostate. Journal of the American Medical Association 1917; 68: 1227–1230

9. Bumpus, H. C. Radium in cancer of the prostate. Journal of the American Medical Association 1922; 78: 1374–1376

10. Bumpus, H. C. Carcinoma of the prostate: a clinical study. Surgery, Gynecology and Obstetrics 1921; 32: 31–43

11. Deming, C. L. Results in 100 cases of cancer of the prostate and seminal vesicles treated with radium. Surgery, Gynecology and Obstetrics 1922; 34: 99–118

12. Flocks, R. H., Culp, D. A., Elkins, H. B. Present status of radioactive gold therapy in management of prostatic cancer. Journal of Urology 1959; 81: 178–184

13. Carlton, C. E. Jr., Hudgins, P. T., Guerriero, W. G., Scott, R. Jr. Radiotherapy in the management of stage C carcinoma of the prostate. Journal of Urology 1976; 116: 206–210

14. Barzell, W., Bean, M. A., Hilaris, B. S., Whitmore, W. F. Jr. Prostatic adenocarcinoma: relationship of grade and local extent to the pattern of metastases. Journal of Urology 1977; 118: 278–282

15. Fowler, J. E. Jr., Barzell, W., Hilaris, B. S., Whitmore, W. F. Jr. Complications of ^{125}Iodine implantation and pelvic lymphadenectomy in the treatment of prostatic cancer. Journal of Urology 1979; 121: 447–451

16. Herr, H. W. Iodine-125 implantation in the management of localized prostatic carcinoma. Urologic Clinics of North America 1980; 7: 605–613

Pelvic lymphadenectomy

Richard K. Babayan MD
Assistant Professor, Department of Urology,
Boston University School of Medicine, Boston, Massachusetts, USA

Robert J. Krane MD
Chairman, Department of Urology,
Boston University School of Medicine, Boston, Massachusetts, USA

Introduction

Lymph node dissection of the pelvic lymphatics, including the obturator, medial chain of the external iliac, and the hypogastric lymph nodes, has led to more accurate staging of clinically localized prostate cancer. It is generally agreed that the presence of unsuspected pelvic nodal metastases has significant prognostic importance and may have direct bearing on the outcome of the treatment modality selected. Some controversy, however, still remains over the anatomical extent of the dissection and whether or not pelvic lymphadenectomy has any therapeutic role.

In the last decade staging pelvic lymphadenectomy has been embraced by urologists dissatisfied with the results of prior non-invasive techniques of evaluating the nodal status of patients with clinically localized prostate cancer. Pedal lymphangiography can often diagnose gross external iliac and para-aortic lymph node involvement but has been reported to have unacceptably high false positive and false negative rates[1–3]. Neither ultrasonography nor computerized tomography with or without guided skinny needle aspiration has had significant diagnostic impact, except in cases of gross macroscopic nodal disease. Likewise, an accurate non-invasive serum tumour marker for extraprostatic disease has yet to be discovered.

Numerous reports have appeared in the literature documenting the benefit of pelvic lymph node dissection in culling those patients with previously unrecognized lymphatic metastases [1,3–5]. In a review of 112 consecutive patients with clinically localized stages A, B, and C prostate cancer at our institution, 33 per cent were found to have pelvic lymph node involvement at surgical exploration[6]. When this figure is further scrutinized by stage, the results are quite similar to those reported at other centres. Cumulative reports reveal that approximately 25 per cent of patients with stage A2 disease, 5–15 per cent of stage B1 patients, 30 per cent of stage B2

patients and better than 50 per cent of patients with clinical stage C disease will be reassigned to stage D1 by virtue of the findings at pelvic lymphadenectomy.

The prognostic impact of pelvic lymph node involvement by prostate cancer is quite striking regardless of the subsequent therapeutic modality employed. Barzell and associates reported progression of disease as evidenced by osseous metastases in 75 per cent of upstaged patients within 5 years of initial diagnosis[7]. Pistenma et al. have noted similar results[8]. In their patients undergoing staging pelvic lymphadenectomy prior to definitive external beam irradiation, there was a significantly higher degree of tumour progression and an increased death rate in upstaged patients versus those without pelvic lymph node metastases.

It was initially reported by Barzell and associates that the degree of pelvic lymph node involvement might impact on the potential therapeutic benefit of a thorough lymphadenectomy[7]. They observed that those patients with minimal nodal disease (that is with 3 ml or less of tumour volume within the pelvic lymph nodes) would have a better prognosis than those patients with more extensive nodal disease, implying a therapeutic benefit of the operation. This presumed therapeutic impact of surgical excision has recently been retracted by the authors, who, with 10-year follow-up, have witnessed that patients with any degree of pelvic lymph node metastases are subject to the same ominous prognosis. We do not view patients with demonstrable carcinomatous involvement of the pelvic lymph nodes as candidates for curative radical prostatic surgery. Their upstaging is indicative of early systemic disease[9]. Theoretically these patients would benefit from adjuvant therapy. After local prostatic control, however, no effective systemic therapeutic regimen has to date been identified.

Pelvic lymphatic anatomy

1

Primary lymphatic drainage of the prostate is to the external iliac, obturator, hypogastric and common iliac nodes. Collectively these chains are referred to as the pelvic lymph nodes. The external iliac nodes are anatomically subdivided into three groups[10,11]. The external chain is located lateral to the external iliac artery and medial to the genitofemoral nerve. It primarily drains the lower extremity and is only secondarily involved by prostate cancer. The medial chain of the external iliac nodes is located anterior to the external iliac vein. The internal chain of the external iliac nodal group lies below the level of the external iliac vein along the pelvic side wall and probably represents the primary echelon of nodal drainage from the prostate[12]. The obturator nodes are found along the obturator fossa ventral to the course of the obturator nerve. It has been argued by some authors that these are not a separate group of nodes but rather the caudal-most extension of the internal chain of the external iliac nodes, and as such are most commonly involved with prostatic metastases.

In performing a pelvic lymph node dissection the following structures should be identified: (*a*) hypogastric artery; (*b*) external iliac artery; (*c*) ureter; (*d*) obturator nerve; and (*e*) obturator lymph node (internal chain of external iliac nodes) adjacent to obturator fossa.

Some mention should be made of the presciatic and presacral lymph nodes. While not generally considered to be in the primary echelon of nodal drainage of the prostate, Golimbu and Morales described a high degree of involvement of these nodes in patients who were subjected to extended lymphadenectomy[13]. Only 2 of their 15 patients, however, with positive presciatic or presacral nodes, had these as the sole metastases.

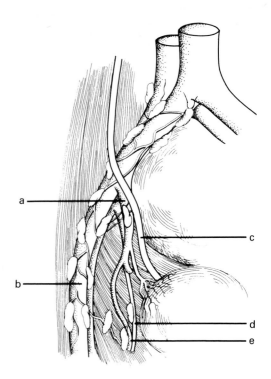

1

The operation

Pelvic lymphadenectomy may be performed as a separate staging procedure, prior to a contemplated radical perineal prostatectomy, or in concert with such definite treatment as radical retropubic prostatectomy or implantation of interstitial irradiation, using either ^{125}I or [198]Au.

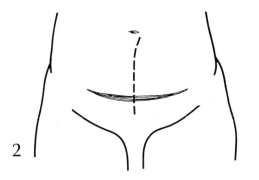

2

The patient is placed on the operating table in a modified supine position with a small degree of dorsiflexion at the pelvis provided by a roll or elevation of the kidney bar. Following skin preparation of the abdomen and genitalia a Foley catheter is passed to decompress the bladder.

2

The incision

A midline subumbilical abdominal incision (dotted line) or, alternatively, a modified transverse Pfannenstiel incision, may be employed.

The anterior rectus sheath is then incised transversely. The pelvic lymph nodes may be approached in a variety of ways, depending upon the patient's anatomy and the surgeon's preference. The rectus muscle may be split in the midline and retracted laterally to gain exposure. Some surgeons prefer to divide the muscle transversely. Our preference is to go lateral to the rectus muscle to expose the iliac vessels. Regardless of the approach taken, the dissection should be carried out extraperitoneally. With the rectus muscle retracted medially, the peritoneal envelope is swept cephalad. Care is taken to identify and avoid injury to the ureter, which is adherent to the posterior peritoneum as it crosses the common iliac artery. Once the peritoneum and ureter are safely retracted cephalad, the bladder is retracted medially along with the rectus muscle and the spermatic vessels are reflected laterally to expose the iliac vessels. The inferior epigastric vessels may be sacrificed to gain greater exposure.

Surgical dissection

3

Dissection is begun over the external iliac artery. The fibrofattylymphatic tissue is sharply incised and swept medially.

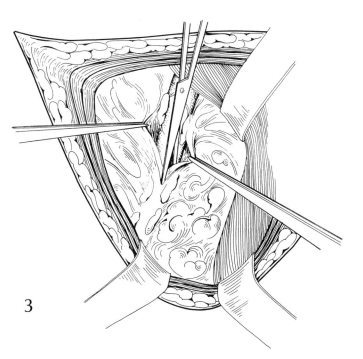

3

4

The arterial adventitia is incised from the common iliac down to the circumflex iliac artery proximal to the inguinal ligament. All nodal tissue is swept medially and the dissection performed in *en bloc* fashion. Metal haema-clips are liberally applied to the boundaries of the dissection to prevent postoperative lymphocele formation. The proximal extent of the dissection is the common iliac artery just distal to the crossing of the ureter. The hypogastric vessels define the medial border and the obturator fossa the distal-most extent. Care must be taken when sweeping tissue off the pelvic side wall towards the obturator fossa. The obturator artery and vein can be ligated with impunity but the obturator nerve must be protected. As the nodal tissue is dissected free, the obturator nerve stands out as a taut bowstring at the deepest extent of the dissection.

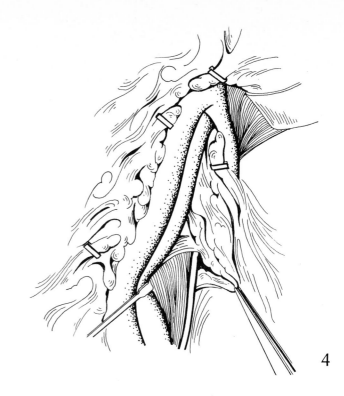

4

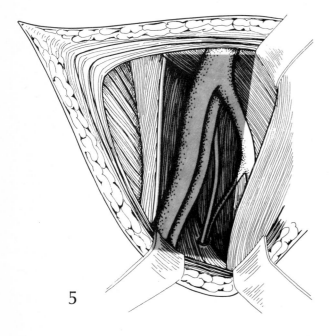

5

5

Early operative descriptions of staging pelvic lympha-denectomy emphasized the genitofemoral nerve as the lateral extent of the dissection (indicated by shaded area).

6

However, because of the increased morbidity, as manifest by scrotal and lower extremity oedema, seen especially in patients receiving pelvic irradiation after lymphadenectomy, and because of the rarity of solitary metastatic involvement of these nodes lateral to the iliac artery, without concurrent disease in the obturator or internal chain of the external iliacs, we now limit the lateral extent of our dissection to the anterior surface of the external iliac artery (indicated by shaded area).

We do not routinely employ drains after pelvic lymphadenectomy. With scrupulous attention to haemostasis and liberal use of haemaclips to ligate lymphatic channels, postoperative haemorrhage and lymphocele formation are rarely encountered.

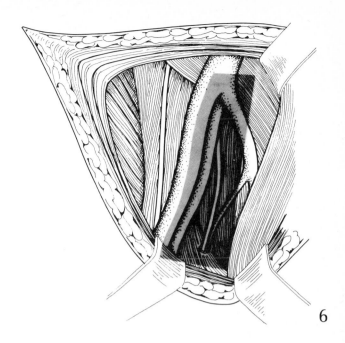

6

Complications

Staging pelvic lymphadenectomy is not without associated operative morbidity. Post-surgical complications have been reported to occur in 5–33 per cent of patients[14, 15]. In our series of 112 cases the overall complication rate was 26.7 per cent. The majority of complications involved wound infections. Other complications noted after pelvic lymphadenectomy include urinary tract infections, prolonged ileus (probably from prolonged retraction of peritoneal contents), atelectasis, deep-vein thrombophlebitis, lymphocele, and lower extremity and scrotal oedema. Since adopting the limited pelvic lymph node dissection described above, sparing dissection of the lymph nodes lateral to the external iliac artery, the operative morbidity has decreased significantly without any evident change in staging accuracy.

Future prospects

Staging pelvic lymphadenectomy has been an effective means of evaluating unsuspected pelvic lymph node involvement by prostate cancer. Although we routinely employ it prior to radical prostatectomy or interstitial irradiation, we do not feel compelled to subject patients who choose to receive external beam irradiation to such a surgical staging procedure. This is due to the fact that no clear-cut therapeutic benefit has been demonstrated by pelvic lymphadenectomy and that the presence of pelvic lymph node metastases would probably not alter the projected treatment regimen. Obviously, were an alternative adjuvant therapy available we would recommend lymphadenectomy. Because of the built-in morbidity associated with pelvic lymph node dissection, alternative, non-surgical means have been explored to obviate

surgical exploration in accurately staging patients[16]. A number of pathological grading systems have been examined for their ability to predict lymph node metastases[17, 18]. Using the Gleason grading system, Paulson found more than 90 per cent of his patients with Gleason sums of 8, 9, or 10 nodal involvement, whereas no patients with Gleason sums of 2, 3, or 4 had positive nodes on exploration[19]. This data has been refuted by Zincke and associates who reported another method known as the Mayo sum, which takes into account both pathological grade and clinical stage. In their study, the Mayo sum was consistently more accurate in predicting the status of the nodes than the Gleason grade[20]. Unfortunately, neither of these non-invasive techniques has been shown to be reproducible or accurate enough to replace surgical staging.

Another promising non-invasive technique for predicting the metastatic potential of prostate cancer was reported by Diamond and associates[21]. Using computer-assisted image analysis of histological sections, they were able to predict retrospectively the patients in whom metastatic disease had occurred – based on the nuclear area and shape. This technique of evaluating relative nuclear roundness is quantitative and reproducible and noted to be a more accurate predictive index than the Gleason grade. Although this technique is still experimental, its further refinement may have future impact.

In summary, pelvic lymphadenectomy has been shown to be a safe and accurate means of staging patients with prostate carcinoma. It has proved to be invaluable as part of any therapeutic protocol since it now allows us to stage A, B, and C disease more accurately by culling stage D1 patients, thereby allowing for more reasonable comparisons of therapeutic options.

References

1. McCullough, D. L., Prout, G. R., Daly, J. J. Carcinoma of the prostate and lymphatic metastases. Journal of Urology 1974; 111: 65–71

2. Cerny, J. C., Farah, R., Rian, R., Weckstein, M. L. An evaluation of lymphangiography in staging carcinoma of the prostate. Journal of Urology 1975; 113: 367–370

3. Loening, S. A., Schmidt, J. D., Brown, R. C., Hawley, C. E., Fallon, B, Culp, D. A. A comparison between lymphangiography and pelvic node dissection in the staging of prostatic cancer. Journal of Urology 1977; 117: 752–756

4. McLaughlin, A. P., Saltzstein, S. L., McCullough, D. L., Gittes, R. F. Prostatic carcinoma: incidence and location of unsuspected lymphatic metastases. Journal of Urology 1976; 115: 89–94

5. Wilson, C. S., Dahl, D. S., Middleton, R. G. Pelvic lymphadenectomy for the staging of apparently localized prostatic cancer. Journal of Urology 1977; 117: 197–198

6. Babayan, R. K., White, R. D., Austen, G., Krane, R. J., Feldman, M., Olsson, C. A. Benefits and complications of staging pelvic lymph node dissection in prostatic adenocarcinoma. Prostate 1980; 1: 345–349

7. Barzell, W., Bean, M. A., Hilaris, B. S., Whitmore, W. F. Jr. Prostatic adenocarcinoma: relationship of grade and local extent to the pattern of metastases. Journal of Urology 1977; 118: 278–282

8. Pistenma, D. A., Bagshaw, M. A., Freiha, F. S. Extended-field radiation therapy for prostatic adenocarcinoma: status report of a limited prospective trial. In: Johnson, D. E., Samuels, M. L., eds. Cancer of the genitourinary tract. New York: Raven Press, 1979: 229–247

9. Kramer, S. A., Cline, W. A. Jr., Farnham, R. et al. Prognosis of patients with stage D_1 prostatic adenocarcinoma. Journal of Urology 1981; 125: 817–819

10. Wheeler, J. S. Jr, Krane, R. J. Blood and lymph circulations of the prostate gland. In: Abramson, D. I., Dobrin, P. B., eds. Blood vessels and lymphatics in organ systems. New York: Academic Press, (in press)

11. Herman, P. G., Benninghoff, D. L., Nelson, J. H. Jr., Mellins, H. Z. Roentgen anatomy of the ilio-pelvic-aortic lymphatic system. Radiology 1963; 80: 182–193

12. Flocks, R. H., Culp, D., Porto, R. Lymphatic spread from prostatic cancer. Journal of Urology 1959; 81: 194–196

13. Golimbu, M., Morales, P., Al-Askari, S., Brown, J. Extended pelvic lymphadenectomy for prostatic cancer. Journal of Urology 1979; 121: 617–620

14. Fowler, J. E. Jr., Barzell, W. W., Hilaris, B. S., Whitmore, W. F. Jr. Complications of 125-iodine implantation and pelvic lymphadenectomy in the treatment of prostatic cancer. Journal of Urology 1979; 121: 447–451

15. Leiskovsky, G., Skinner, D. G., Weisenburger, T. Pelvic lymphadenectomy in the management of carcinoma of the prostate. Journal of Urology 1980; 124: 635–638

16. Paulson, D. F. and Uro-Oncology Research Group. The impact of current staging procedures in assessing disease extent of prostatic adenocarcinoma. Journal of Urology 1979; 121: 300–302

17. Gleason, D. F., Mellinger, G. T., Veterans Admistration Cooperative Urological Research Group. Prediction of prognosis for prostatic adenocarcinoma by combined histological grading and clinical staging. Journal of Urology 1974; 111: 58–64

18. Mostofi, F. K. Grading of prostatic carcinoma. Cancer Chemotherapy Reports. Part 1. 1975; 59: 111–117

19. Paulson, D. F. The prognostic role of lymphadenectomy in adenocarcinoma of the prostate. Urologic Clinics of North America 1980; 7: 615–622

20. Zincke, H., Farrow, G. M., Myers, R. P., Benson, R. C., Furlow, W. L., Utz, D. C. Relationship between grade and stage of adenocarcinoma of the prostate and regional pelvic lymph node metastases. Journal of Urology 1982; 128: 498–501

21. Diamond, D. A., Berry, S. J., Jewett, H. J., Eggleston, J. C., Coffey, D. S. A new method to assess metastatic potential of human prostate cancer. Relative nuclear roundness. Journal of Urology 1982; 128: 729–734

Illustrations by Jean Perry and Michael Courtney

Injuries to the urethra

J. P. Mitchell   CBE, TD, MS, FRCS, FRCS(Ed)
Honorary Professor of Surgery (Urology), University of Bristol, UK

Introduction

1

For the purposes of diagnosis and treatment, trauma to the urethra should be classified as to whether it is open or closed, whether it involves the male or female and, whether it is located in the anterior or posterior urethra.

The commonest cause of urethral injuries in which many other structures and systems may be involved, is road traffic accident. It should be remembered that 10–15 per cent of injuries of the posterior urethra may also be accompanied by a ruptured bladder. Furthermore, double injuries of both upper and lower urinary tract may occur.

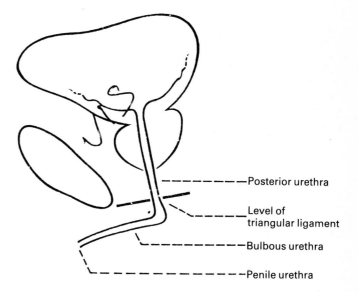

Posterior urethra

Level of triangular ligament

Bulbous urethra

Penile urethra

1

2a, b & c

Injuries of both anterior and posterior urethra are frequently partial ruptures (b): part of the wall of the urethra is torn, but the whole circumference of the urethra is not transected. Occasionally the damage to the urethral wall is only a contusion (c). Injuries at the level of the triangular ligament, however, are usually complete transections (a). The most important principle in the management of urethral injuries is to ensure that no additional damage is caused by operative or investigative procedures, which can aggravate the extent of a partial rupture or convert a contusion into a partial rupture. Every effort should be made to preserve the remaining strand or bridge of tissue which may exist between the two torn ends of urethra. This bridge of tissue can make the difference between a successful repair and a severe stricture.

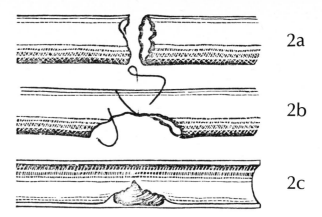

2a

2b

2c

Extravasation of urine is, in fact, unlikely to occur as the bladder neck is usually in spasm. The patient is unable to pass urine, ultimately developing a distended bladder. Even if extravasation does occur, by far the majority of patients will have sterile urine which can cause little harm within the first 24 hours. It is, therefore, safe in closed injuries of the urinary tract to give priority to the treatment of other major injuries.

OPEN INJURIES OF THE URINARY TRACT

Gunshot wounds, penetration of the perineum by sharp objects such as broken glass or being impaled, or any trauma to the penile urethra (which may be caught in machinery or involved in some sexual misadventure) must all be treated by exploration without delay. The wound of entry must be explored. If necessary the urethra can be examined by urethroscopy and the damage repaired by immediate suture over an indwelling silicone catheter, 14 or 16 Fr. The patient should be given a broad-spectrum antibiotic because infection will have been carried into the wound on the penetrating missile. Also, there is bound to be a fairly extensive haematoma and this forms a perfect nidus in which organisms can multiply.

CLOSED INJURIES OF THE URETHRA

Injuries of the perineal part of the urethra (principally bulbous urethra), transections of the urethra at the urogenital diaphragm and closed injuries of the posterior urethra associated with a fracture of the pelvis require careful management to assess the degree of damage and the localization. The diagnosis is suggested by the presence of blood at the external meatus, the inability of the patient to pass any urine and the ultimate development of a distended bladder, easily palpable above the haematoma which rises out of the pelvis. If a distended bladder is not palpable within 24 hours of admission to hospital, the possibility of an associated bladder rupture should be considered.

If an urgent diagnostic answer is required because the patient will be going to the operating theatre for other major trauma, or if he or she develops a distended bladder even though no blood has appeared at the external urinary meatus, then a urethrogram using an aqueous opaque medium will readily confirm the diagnosis and demonstrate the site and extent of the urethral rupture. If the patient's condition is such that he requires urgent surgery, and a urethrogram cannot be performed, suprapubic diversion of the urine is a wise precaution, even if only the physical sign of blood at the external meatus is present.

In no circumstances should a diagnostic catheter be passed per urethram: the information obtained can be unreliable. There is a serious risk of contaminating the haematoma at the site of injury by carrying organisms on the catheter from the external meatus: and there is a very real risk of inflicting further damage on the slender bridge of tissue that may constitute only a partial rupture of the urethra. If the diagnostic catheter draws no urine it may mean that the catheter has passed out of the urethra through the rupture. On the other hand, it may have passed into an empty bladder; it may have been obstructed at the bladder neck; the patient may be anuric; or the bladder itself may have been ruptured. Alternatively, if the catheter draws some urine, this does not exclude a partial rupture of the urethra; nor does it exclude a small puncture hole in the anterior wall of the bladder.

The operations

RUPTURE OF THE BULBOUS AND PERINEAL URETHRA

3 & 4

With the patient in the lithotomy position, the extensive haematoma in the perineum is opened. Identification of the urethra will be difficult as the tissues will be discoloured by blood. The bladder is then opened suprapubically by a vertical midline incision and a Harris, or Nelaton, catheter (22 Fr in adults, correspondingly smaller in children), is passed down the posterior urethra from the internal meatus to present in the wound. The tip of this catheter will then identify the proximal end of the ruptured urethra. A smaller sized (16 Fr) Foley catheter, preferably silicone, is then passed from the external urinary meatus, after instillation of chlorhexidine in glycerine as lubricant and antiseptic to identify the distal end of the torn urethra.

If the urethral damage is only a partial tear, a few sutures approximating the rent transversely will help to control bleeding from the corpus spongeosum. No urethral catheter is necessary as this patient may not develop a stricture because part of the circumference of the urethra is still intact. A 26 Fr Foley catheter should be left draining the bladder suprapubically.

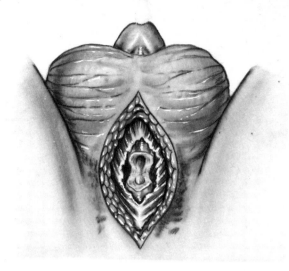

3

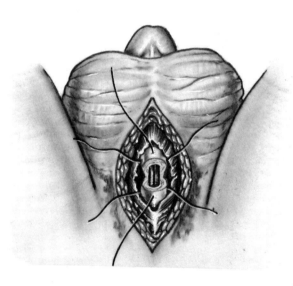

4

5 & 6

If the urethra has been totally transected, then the dorsal aspect of the two torn ends of urethra can be approximated by a few sutures of 4/0 plain catgut (or polyglycolic acid). Again, these sutures will also help to control bleeding from the corpus spongeosum. There should be no attempt at mobilizing either end of the urethra, which should approximate easily. This patient may develop a stricture and correct alignment by an indwelling catheter is essential. The tip of the Harris catheter passed down from the bladder is cut off; the tip of the smaller silicone catheter passed *per urethram* is inserted firmly into the cut end of the Harris catheter which is gently withdrawn back into the bladder, taking particular care to ensure that the mucosa of the proximal end of the urethral rupture is not invaginated. When the smaller gauge Foley catheter has reached the bladder, the balloon is distended in order to anchor it. The bladder is then closed, leaving a suprapubic Foley catheter (22 Fr) draining the bladder by suprapubic cystostomy. The wound is closed in layers with a small perineal drain.

Silicone is a completely inert material and the catheter can, therefore, be left indwelling for 2, 3 or 4 weeks. The patient should be treated with a broad-spectrum antibiotic, and the external urinary meatus should be cleansed by meatal toilet twice a day.

Later, the urethra is inspected by panendoscopy and urethrography and treated initially by endoscopic urethrotomy if a stricture develops. Ultimately the stricture may require some form of urethroplasty.

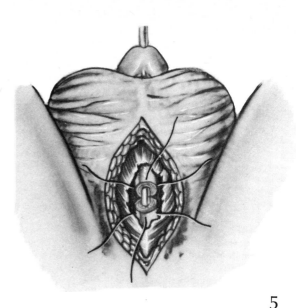

5

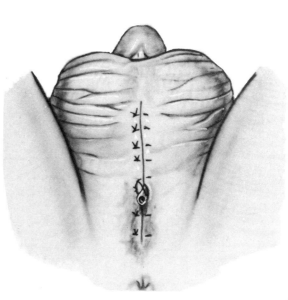

6

RUPTURE OF THE URETHRA AT THE UROGENITAL DIAPHRAGM

This type of injury is usually due to a blow in the perineum. There may be associated damage to the anus, with tearing of the perineal skin, converting the injury into an open injury. Although injury to the urethra at this site is uncommon, it is nearly always a total transection and the torn ends of the urethra retract above and below the urogenital diaphragm respectively.

Immediate repair is difficult. The proximal catheter will present in the pelvis and will then have to be threaded through the triangular ligament, as it does not readily carry the proximal end of the urethra with it. Stricture is inevitable; it is unlikely to respond to endoscopic urethrotomy because its length will probably be more than 2–3 mm. Some form of urethroplasty is usually required. In this type of injury a definitive posterior urethroplasty should be performed as soon as the local tissue reaction following the trauma has subsided i.e. within 2–3 months.

RUPTURE OF THE POSTERIOR URETHRA

This injury is almost always associated with a fracture of the pelvis and in 10–15 per cent of cases there is, in addition, a rupture of the bladder.

The patient is placed on the table in the supine position and draped with towels so that there is access to the external meatus as well as to the lower abdomen. A vertical midline suprapubic incision is made and the extravesical space opened. Blood and urine are aspirated or mopped gently from the prevesical space. It will be difficult to determine the exact site of the lesion because of the bloodstained effusion. If the bladder is distended, the lesion must be situated below the external vesical sphincter. Often the haemorrhage from the depths of the pelvis can only be stopped with packing. This should be done with great care as it is at this stage that the partial rupture can be converted into a total transection. The bladder is then identified by the direction of its muscle fibres, which may be discoloured by suffused blood, and a formal cystostomy is performed.

The damage to the bony pelvis can be felt with a finger inside the bladder and it may be possible to move a central mobile fragment into position. The surgeon then feels for the internal urinary meatus and the prostate gland to assess whether this has been grossly displaced. If the prostate gland is lying high in the pelvis, there is almost certainly a total transection of the membranous urethra and immediate repair should be performed. If the prostate does not appear to be grossly displaced, there is probably a partial rupture of the posterior urethra, in which case it is only necessary to leave a suprapubic drain (Foley catheter 26 Fr).

Immediate repair

If the prostate is lying high in the pelvis and there is no likelihood of any bridge of tissue remaining between the two torn ends of urethra, the procedure is as for open operation on rupture of the bulbous and perineal urethra.

7, 8 & 9

A Harris catheter (22 Fr) is passed from the bladder via the internal urinary meatus to present in the pelvis. This catheter should be of very soft material and should be passed with the greatest gentleness so as not to damage any other structures. After inserting 5 ml of chlorhexidine in glycerine into the external urinary meatus, a silicone catheter (16 Fr) is passed up the urethra and will also present in the depths of the pelvis. The tip of the Harris catheter is then cut off and the tip of the silicone Foley catheter is inserted into the cut end of the Harris catheter. A stitch through both catheters will ensure that they hold together. The proximal Harris catheter is then well lubricated and withdrawn, watching very carefully to see that the proximal torn end of urethra does not retract (invaginate) as the catheter recedes back into the bladder. As the silicone Foley catheter enters the bladder its balloon is inflated.

It is always tempting to try to thread the lower catheter through the proximal end of the urethra using a stilette or guide inside the catheter, all the time feeling with the finger in the bladder. The passage of this catheter may feel successful, but it is very likely to have stripped away some of the urethral mucosa, making a false passage and aggravating the future stricture.

Suturing of the urethra is unlikely to be successful as absorbable sutures will disintegrate too soon; non-absorbable sutures incur the ultimate risk of stone formation. Similarly, traction on the balloon catheter is unlikely to hold the prostate down, due to the reactive swelling of the tissues within the bony pelvis, as well as to the distortion caused by the trauma. Advice should be sought from the orthopaedic surgeon regarding realignment of the bony pelvis, as this can reduce the distortion of the intrapelvic structures. With the passage of time the reactive swelling of the soft tissues will allow the prostate to subside into the pelvis and return nearer to its normal position.

Most of these patients will develop a stricture of the membranous urethra, but with a good result this may take several years. Therefore, any rupture of the urethra should be seen for review regularly for a minimum of 5 years and a mictiograph performed to check the stream. Most of these patients will require either endoscopic urethrotomy or a posterior urethroplasty but, by using a silicone catheter, the severity of the stricture formation will probably be reduced.

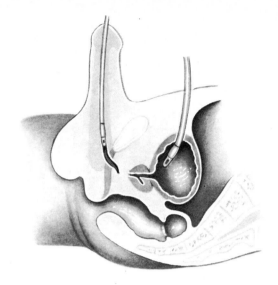

7

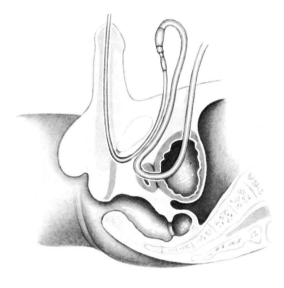

8

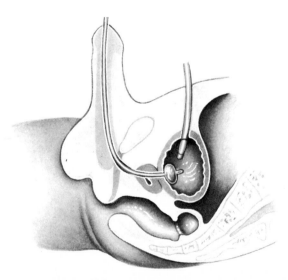

9

Delayed repair

If at the time of the initial suprapubic cystostomy the prostate is found to be almost in its normal position, indicating the probability of partial urethral damage, then a suprapubic catheter, size 22 Fr, is left to drain the bladder via the suprapubic wound. A urethral catheter is not inserted.

Depending on his general condition, the patient is returned to the operating theatre after 3 weeks and the urethra is inspected by urethroscopy. This should be carried out by an experienced endoscopist who will probably be able to find his way past the partial rupture, guided by the intact bridge of mucosa into the bladder. If the endoscopic urethrotome with the catheter guide sheath has been used it is easy to pass a catheter after withdrawing the endoscope and leaving the guide channel *in situ*. Otherwise a ureteric catheter can be left *in situ*. If the endoscopic urethrotome with its catheter guide has not been used and the rupture has been inspected by an ordinary urethroscope, after clearing the blood clot a ureteric is passed via the endoscope sheath into the bladder and left indwelling for 7–10 days. During that time the suprapubic catheter can be removed.

If endoscopy fails to find a route through, the urethra must be explored suprapubically, as for immediate repair.

RUPTURED URETHRA IN THE FEMALE

Damage to the female urethra is much less common than damage to the male posterior urethra. It is usually associated with fracture of the pelvis, but may also be due to penetrating wounds in the perineum, or to a blow to the perineum. Injuries of the female urethra usually also involve the anterior wall of the vagina and will ultimately develop a urethrovaginal fistula. Repair of a high urethrovaginal fistula can be very difficult due to extensive and firm adhesions to the posterior part of the symphysis pubis. Such cases are best treated in the combined approach by the urologist from the suprapubic area and by the gynaecologist from the perineum. Repair of the fistula in layers over a silicone Foley catheter will restore continuity, but may still leave the patient with limited urinary control.

RUPTURED URETHRA IN CHILDREN

Rupture of the urethra can be a very severe injury in children of both sexes under the age of 10. In boys the prostate has not yet developed and rupture is liable to occur just below the neck of the bladder and above the level of the external sphincter. Blood may not be seen at the external urinary meatus, even though the urethra has been torn.

Rupture of the urethra and anterior wall of the vagina seems to occur more often in little girls than in adults. Bleeding from the urethra and vagina can be so severe that the patient may have to be taken to the theatre as an emergency to pack the vagina in order to control the bleeding.

Editor's comment

Posterior membranous urethral disruptions may be treated initially with a suprapubic cystostomy and no manipulation of the urethra. The stricture which develops is repaired by a second procedure performed 4–6 months post injury. The advantage of this form of therapy is reportedly a lower incidence of impotence. The disadvantage is that all patients treated in this manner require a second operation whereas many of those who are approached as the author recommends do not require a second procedure.

Further reading

Blandy, J. P. Injuries of the urethra in the male. Injury 1975; 7: 77–83

Clarke, B. G., Leadbetter, W. F. Management of wounds and injuries of genito-urinary tract: review of reported experience in World War II. Journal of Urology 1952; 67: 719–739

Hunt, A. H., Morgan, C. N. Complete rupture of the membranous urethra. Lancet 1942; 2: 330–331

Hunt, A. H., Morgan, C. N. Complete rupture of the membranous urethra. Lancet 1949; 1: 601–602

Kidd, F. The end-results of treatments of injuries of the urethra. Rapport de la Société Internationale d'Urologie. Paris: Libraire Octave Doin, 1921

Mitchell, J. P. Injuries to the urethra. British Journal of Urology 1968; 40: 649–670

Morehouse, D. D., Belitsky, P., MacKinnon, K. Rupture of the posterior urethra. Journal of Urology 1972; 107: 255

Pasteau, O., Iselin, A. La résection de l'urethre perinéal. Annales des maladies des organes génito-urinaires 1906; 24: 1601–1644

Poole-Wilson, D. S. Injuries of the urethra. Proceedings of the Royal Society of Medicine 1947; 40: 798–804

Poole-Wilson, D. S. Missile injuries of the urethra. British Journal of Surgery 1949; 36: 364–376

Poole-Wilson, D. S., Pointon, R. C. S. The present condition of treatment of epithelial tumours of the bladder. In: Rock-Carling, *Sir* E., Ross, *Sir* J. P. eds. Surgical progress, Vol. II. London: Butterworths 1961: 62–97

Simpson-Smith, A. Traumatic rupture of the urethra. Eight personal cases with a review of 381 recorded ruptures. British Journal of Surgery 1936; 24: 309

Young, H. H. Treatment of complete rupture of posterior urethra, recent or ancient, by anastomosis. Journal of Urology 1929; 21: 417–449

Illustrations by Miss F. Wadsworth and Philip Wilson

The principles of urethral reconstruction

Richard Turner-Warwick DSc, DM, MCh, FRCP, FRCS, FRACS, FACS
Senior Surgeon, The Middlesex Hospital; Senior Consultant Urological Surgeon, St Peter's Hospital Group;
Senior Lecturer, Institute of Urology, University of London, UK

Introduction

Developments in the field of urethroplasty over the past two decades offer the opportunity of restoration of efficient voiding and freedom from follow-up instrumentation to almost every patient who has a urethral stricture.

Standards have also changed within this time. Whereas a stricture-free success rate of 75–80 per cent used to be regarded as reasonable after a definitive reconstruction now a 6–8 per cent failure rate in the long term after a substitution procedure, and almost any re-stenosis after a one-stage anastomotic repair of even complex pelvic fracture injuries, should cause a reconstructive surgeon to reflect upon the selection of the procedure or the technique of its performance.

However, restitution of a stable urethral lumen of even calibre is not an easy matter:

1. The anterior (bulbo-penile) urethra is immediately surrounded by spongy tissue and the natural spongio-fibrotic healing reaction of this predisposes to stricture formation. Consequently, even an apparently simple spatulated restorative anastomosis of a normal 'pink' spongy urethra has a peculiar tendency to re-stenose unless appropriate techniques are used to prevent this.
2. The whole length of the posterior (prostato-membranous) urethra is immediately surrounded by sphincter muscles and damage to the distal sphincter mechanism is generally irreparable.

As in other fields of urology, advances have stemmed from subspecialization; few of the reconstructive techniques that have evolved can be regarded as 'general urological' procedures – a urologist undertaking them should have considerable personal experience of the specialist techniques of plastic surgery, of video-urodynamic evaluation of functional behaviour, and, for complex traumatic pelvic injuries, of colorectal and pelvic surgery. Furthermore, success is fundamentally dependent, not only upon meticulous technique and in-depth experience, but also upon reconstructive surgical instinct to adopt and to adapt procedures according to the unpredictable findings at the time of operation.

The importance of these tenets should not be underestimated.

Internal urethrotomy is a relatively simple general urological procedure appropriate for the management of many strictures of the bulbo-penile spongy urethra; however, it is essential to recognize its limitations because its indiscriminate use can result in complications, some of which are disastrous.

Furthermore, it is most important to recognize that any failed attempt at a definitive reconstruction, however well intended and however meticulously performed, almost inevitably complicates a subsequent 'retrievoplasty'. Surgeons with a general urological training who do not have special additional experience in reconstructive procedures, and a particular aptitude for them, must be advised that 'having a go' is not in the best interest of their patients.

Within the space of one chapter it is only possible to outline some of the principal procedures that form the basis of successful urethral reconstruction.

Structural considerations and surgical anatomy

THE SPONGY (BULBO-PENILE) URETHRA

1

The unique structure of the bulbo-penile spongy urethra is a fundamental factor both in its prediposition to the formation of strictures and in their surgical treatment.

The actual wall of the bulbo-penile urethra within its surrounding spongy tissue is very thin and formed, in effect, by a layer of uro-epithelium almost directly applied to the vascular spaces of the erectile tissue; it is the healing response of this delicate spongy tissue, and consequent spongiofibrosis, that largely determines the nature of a stricture of the bulbo-penile spongy urethra[1].

In the penile area the lumen of the urethra is concentrically located within the spongy tissue which is only some 3–4 mm thick: in the bulbar area it is located eccentrically and dorsally within the bulk of the bulbar spongy expansion so that although only 3–4 mm separate it from a corpora dorsally, infero-laterally and posteriorly it may be 5–15 mm thick.

Thus throughout the bulbopenile urethra the thickness of the *dorsal* spongy tissue of both the penile and the bulbar urethra is only 3–4 mm; furthermore, in the penile area it is firmly anchored to the undersurface of the corpora in the 12–2 o'clock sector and in the narrower 11–1 o'clock sector in the bulbar area.

This uniform dorsal disposition and the sector adhesion of the bulbar spongy tissue is not only relevant to the site of internal urethrotomy (*see* p. 486), but, in the course of definitive reconstructions in the bulbar area, the eccentric bulk of it may have to be separated and redeployed in various ways (posterior spongioplasty[2,3]). The collateral blood supply of the bulbo-spongy urethra is fundamental to its surgical mobilization (*see* p. 513).

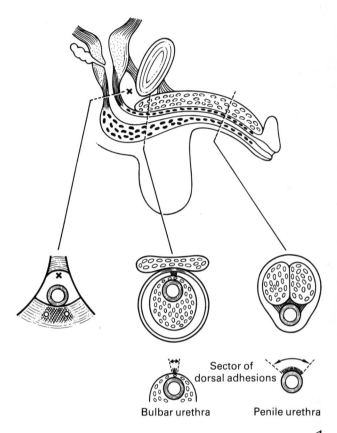

Sector of dorsal adhesions

Bulbar urethra   Penile urethra

1

THE SPHINCTER MECHANISMS OF THE POSTERIOR (PROSTATO-MEMBRANOUS) URETHRA

2

The feasibility of many posterior urethral surgical procedures, such as the resolution of prostatic obstruction and the repair of pelvic fracture urethral strictures, depends upon the independent function of the proximal and distal sphincter mechanisms; normally each of these is competent and independently capable of maintaining continence in the absence of the other, provided it has sustained no injury[4–7].

The bladder neck sphincter is functional from the internal meatus down to the level of the verumontanum and it is normally competent in the male, providing it is not rendered incompetent by unstable detrusor contractions[4,5,6].

The 3–4 cm length of the distal urethral mechanism extends from the verumontanum, down through the apical prostatic capsule, to the membrano-bulbar urethral junction; its functional occlusion is entirely dependent upon the two layers of smooth and striated muscle that form the whole 3–4 mm thickness of its wall. There is no peri-urethral 'external' sphincter mechanism 'external' to it antero-laterally and the midline fusion of the pelvic floor musculature behind it is incapable of maintaining a sustained occlusion of the urethra except in spastic neuropathy[4–6].

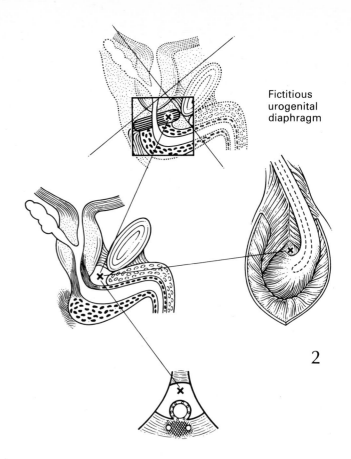

Fictitious urogenital diaphragm

2

THE SUB-PUBO-URETHRAL SPACE AND THE MYTH OF THE 'UROGENITAL DIAPHRAGM'

The common description of a 'urogenital diaphragm' enclosing a bulk of striated 'external sphincter muscle' encircling the membranous urethra is quite inaccurate. It is readily apparent in the course of bulbo-membranous urethral reconstructions that there is no significant sphincter musculature immediately anterior or lateral to the membranous urethra[1–3,5,7,8].

In the supposed location of the mythical anterior 'urogenital diaphragm' there is in fact a sub-pubo-urethral space into which, after minimal mobilization of the bulbar urethra from a perineal approach, a finger tip can be inserted between the membranous urethra and the subpubic arch, up to the level of the pubo-prostatic bundle. This pre-urethral subpubic space is particularly relevant to surgical procedures in this area, and to the variations in both the site of subprostatic urethral rupture and the extent of the associated haematoma in pelvic fracture urethral injuries (see p. 505); it can also be used for the location of the balloon of an inflatable incontinence prosthesis as an alternative to an encircling peri-urethral cuff[1,2,7,8].

Detailed anatomical studies[9] confirmed that the only muscles of the pelvic floor that relate directly to the membranous urethra are the posteriorly located pubo-urethral elements of the levator ani and the transverse perineii that insert into the perineal body adherent to its posterior surface.

Because the functionally effective muscular elements of the distal urethral sphincter mechanism are entirely located within the 3–4 mm thickness of the wall of the membranous and supra-membranous urethra, the functional competence of this is easily damaged or destroyed by longitudinal transection resulting from internal urethrotomy (see p. 487), surgical procedures such as prostatectomy and bulbo-membranous urethroplasty, and pelvic fracture injuries[4–8].

Thus, because urinary continence is entirely dependent upon the competence of the distal sphincter mechanism after functional ablation of the bladder neck mechanism during prostatectomy, great care must be taken to avoid unnecessary surgical injury to the subprostatic urethra.

The nervi erigentes, innervating the erection mechanism of the penile corpora lie in close postero-lateral relationship to the membranous urethra; injury to them may result in impotence and they are particularly at risk during sphincter-relaxing urethrotomy incisions in the 4 and 8 o'clock positions and during posterior pre-rectal surgical exposure of the membranous urethra in the exaggerated lithotomy position.

The pathogenesis of strictures of the bulbo-penile spongy urethra

3

A basic understanding of the pathogenesis of strictures, their development and the significance of spongiofibrosis, is essential to successful urethral reconstruction.

Partial loss of the uro-epithelial lining is the primary factor in the development of almost every spongy-urethral stricture, whether it is due to internal trauma, urethritis or external trauma.

The loss of any proportion of the circumference of the epithelial lining generally results in a commensurate narrowing of the lumen during healing because the margins of the residual epithelium are approximated by the natural urethral closing pressure so that the defect forms a cleft which tends to heal rapidly by cross adhesion and epithelial over-bridging. The intermittent passage of urine opens these clefts and this repeated separation and re-exposure of the vascular spongy tissue spaces leads to a gradual increase in the underlying spongiofibrosis.

Unfortunately this complex combination of slow epithelial proliferation, cleft-closure, and spongiofibrosis also results in a tendency to restenosis whenever bare areas are created by the treatment of a stricture by dilatation or by internal urethrotomy. Attempts to promote uro-epithelialization of the denuded clefts by keeping them open for a prolonged period with an indwelling catheter are generally unsuccessful.

Thus, urethral surgery must particularly take into account the inherent characteristics of urethral healing that result in a tendency to cross-adhesion of adjacent or opposing areas of uro-epithelialized tissue and suture-lines; it is for this reason that the margins of an anastomotic or roof-strip 'combination' urethroplasty should be spread apart and anchored laterally (see p. 501).

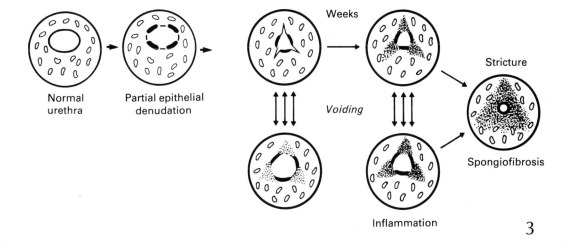

Normal urethra

Partial epithelial denudation

Weeks

Voiding

Inflammation

Stricture

Spongiofibrosis

3

Surgical significance of 'spongiofibrosis' and the 'grey' urethra

4

Proximal and distal to almost every stricture, with the exception of the rare congenital variety, the urethra is surrounded by a layer of spongiofibrosis; the degree and the extent of this varies greatly and it is particularly important to appreciate that surgically significant longitudinal extension may surround a urethral lumen which appears quite normal radiographically.

The extent of the spongiofibrosis associated with a stricture is thus an important factor that often determines both the type and the extent of the surgical procedure that is required for its satisfactory long-term resolution; unfortunately failure to appreciate the surgical significance of spongiofibrosis is still a common cause of restenosis[3,4].

To emphasize the surgical significance of a spongiofibrotic extension around a normal calibre urethra proximal and distal to a stricture we have termed it 'grey' to differentiate it from the normal urethra which appears 'pink' when it is open because the vascular spongy tissue is seen through its immediately overlying translucent uro-epithelial cover[1,2].

Surgery involving unstrictured spongiofibrotic 'grey' urethra has a high recurrent stricture potential unless appropriate precautions are taken to prevent this: re-anastomosis of the spongiofibrotic proximal and distal urethra after the excision of a 'short' stricture commonly results in recurrent stenosis and this has tarnished the reputation of anastomotic urethral repair which is much the most successful reconstructive procedure when conditions are appropriate[3]; similarly, limiting the extent of a substitution procedure to the length of the urethra that is actually strictured is a common cause of its failure[3,4,10].

Thus, in practice, both anastomotic and substitution procedures should be extended at least 2 cm into the macroscopically normal 'pink' urethra proximal and distal to the urethra abnormality and not restricted to the strictured segment.

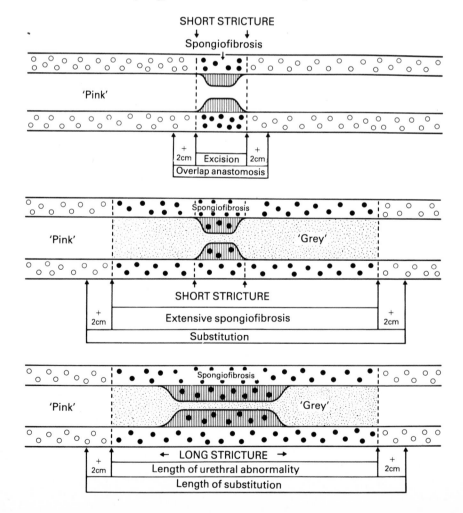

4

The three basic procedures for urethral reconstruction

Regeneration

Regeneration procedures depend upon the completion of part of the circumference of the urethral lining by the regenerative proliferation of the uro-epithelium.

The long-term success of urethral dilatation and of internal urethrotomy is entirely dependent upon this and the result depends upon whether epithelialization can occur before restenosis develops. The Dennis Brown buried strip principle depends upon induced regeneration for completion of the epithelial lining of the neo-urethra; however, although this is a most important principle as a back-up procedure in reconstructive surgery it is no longer advocated as a primary procedure for urethral reconstruction.

Excision and re-anastomosis

The only stricture procedure with an expected long-term success rate approaching 100 per cent is excision and spatulated circumferential anastomosis[2,3,11]; unfortunately, owing to the extent of the spongiofibrosis that is commonly associated with strictures of the bulbar urethra, other than those resulting from simple external trauma, few are appropriate for resolution in this way. However, 'combination procedures' have been developed to incorporate the advantages of partial circumferential restoration of urethral continuity by the formation of a redeployment fixed flat roof strip whenever possible[1,2,4].

Substitution

All epithelial substitutes and all individual techniques for their use have inherent shortcomings with an inevitable incidence of failure. Epithelium or uro-epithelium is used either on the basis of pedicled or free-patch grafts – few other substitutes have proved to be valuable alternatives.

Consensus

The inherent failure rate involved in substitution procedures means that they should never be introduced unnecessarily for the resolution of strictures that are appropriate for repair by excision and circumferential anastomosis; however, overstretching the critical criteria for an anastomotic procedure escalates the incidence of restenosis.

Furthermore, it is most important to recognize that any urethral surgery, endoscopic or open, that fails to relieve a stricture, anterior or posterior, is likely to complicate a subsequent definitive procedure – this can be critical. For instance, an iatrogenic extension of the spongiofibrotic scarring associated with a short traumatic stricture resulting from a pelvic fracture or a straddle injury may preclude a subsequent one-stage anastomostic repair; furthermore, damage to the distal sphincter mechanism is virtually irreparable.

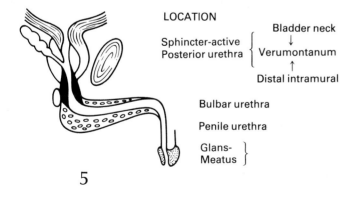

5

LOCATION

Sphincter-active
Posterior urethra { Bladder neck
↓
Verumontanum
↑
Distal intramural

Bulbar urethra

Penile urethra

Glans-
Meatus }

The four components of the urethra

5

Four regions of the urethra each present distinctly different problems of reconstruction and require quite separate consideration – the glans-meatus, the penile, the bulbar, and the sphincter-active posterior urethra.

The reconstruction or the creation of a cosmetically and functionally perfect glans-meatus requires meticulous attention to detail. The reconstruction of the penile component of the spongy urethra is relatively simple compared with that of the bulbar region which is critically demanding.

Reconstruction of the posterior prostato-membranous urethra is further complicated not only by the problem of surgical access but also by the fact that its whole length is sphincter-active: a true video-urodynamic understanding of the mechanisms and an appropriate adaptation of procedures are therefore vital to a satisfactory functional reconstruction in this area.

Internal stricturotomy

Spongio-urethral strictures

6

The basic principle of internal stricturotomy is to enlarge the urethral lumen by urethrotomy incisions carried through the spongiofibrosis that surrounds a 'stricture': when these incisions extend into a supple tissue layer, the lumen is expanded by the pressure of the irrigating fluid creating a bare area. The 'supple layer' may be either the relatively normal spongy tissue surrounding the spongiofibrosis, or the adventitial tissue outside it.

The main advantages of the Sachse endoscopic urethrotome are that it can be used when the Otis urethrotome cannot be passed and that an in-depth incision can be selectively located: the Otis urethrotome has the advantages of facility, especially in the penile area, and of achieving a uniform recalibration that can be accurately gauged. However, once achieved, the effect and the endoscopic appearances of the immediate result of a urethrotomy achieved by the two instruments are virtually indistinguishable.

The commonly advocated sector for urethrotomy is in the 12 o'clock position; however, for basic anatomical and pathological reasons a 12 o'clock urethrotomy incision in the bulbar and penile urethra may fail to find an adequately supple tissue layer to enable the lumen to expand. The dorsal spongy tissue of the bulbo-penile urethra is only 3–4 mm thick in this sector and firmly adherent to the undersurface of the corpora, and its whole depth is often spongiofibrotic as a result of the stricture process (see pp. 483–484). Thus, contrary to common advice, infero-lateral incisions in the 4 and 8 o'clock positions are more likely to enter an expandable tissue layer of supple spongiosum surrounding bulbo-spongio-fibrosis and the subcutaneous adventitia outside the penile spongiofibrosis[1,2].

The success of an internal urethrotomy depends upon whether the incisional clefts re-epithelialize before they close. Unfortunately attempts to delay cleft closure and promote circumferential re-epithelialization by the local application of steroids and urostatic distension have met with only limited success and the incidence of recurrent stenosis is not convincingly reduced by prolonging indwelling catheter-stenting from days to weeks.

With the exception of short congenital and straddle-injury strictures that are eminently suitable for simple and extremely reliable anastomotic repair there are few contraindications to a trial of urethrotomy for spongy urethral strictures. However, a urethrotomy extending posteriorly into the distal sphincter mechanism is potentially disastrous and generally contraindicated because of the risk that sphincterotomy of the 3–4 mm thickness of the intramural distal urethral sphincter will render it incompetent. This complication commonly passes unnoticed when urinary continence is maintained by the normal proximal sphincter mechanism at the bladder neck; however, incontinence is the common result after its previous or subsequent functional ablation by prostatic or bladder neck surgery[1–5] unless a definitive intra-urethral reconstructive procedure is used[11].

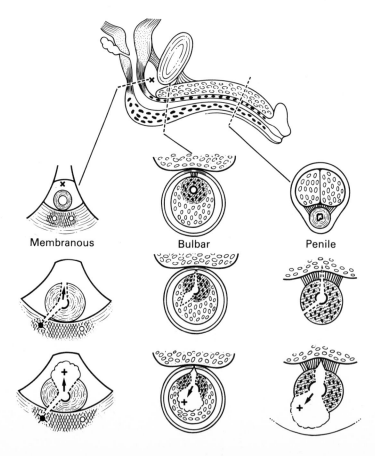

Membranous   Bulbar   Penile

6

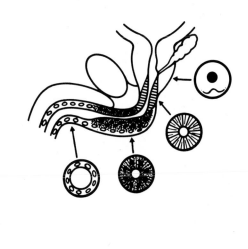

Sphincter-strictures

7

The primary consideration in the management of a sphincter stricture is the preservation of the residual sphincter function rather than the eradication of the stricture itself[1,2,5]. Thus its management by internal urethrotomy, Otis or endoscopic, carries a potentially disastrous risk to the precarious residual function of its sphincter mechanism – already damaged to a variable extent by the stricture-generating injury.

Pelvic fracture urethral defects

Urethrotomy of a sub-prostatic urethral defect resulting from a pelvic fracture is not generally contra-indicated because the distal sphincter mechanism is already damaged by the initial injury; however, for all but the most minimal injuries, it is likely to prove ineffective because, unlike spongy urethral strictures, pelvic fracture urethral defects are commonly associated with dense intervening haematoma-fibrosis through which an effective expansion of the lumen cannot be created by simple incision. Furthermore, over-enthusiastic attempts to create an inter-communicating urethral false passage through extensive intervening fibrosis may result in serious complications (see p.506).

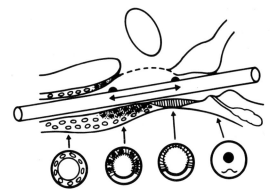

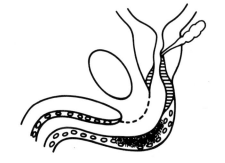

7

The principles of catheter drainage after urethral reconstruction

The use of a standard shaft catheter retained by a balloon after a urethral closure is a source of a number of predictable complications.

Catheter balloon complications

A catheter balloon may complicate a recently reconstructed urethra.

1. Balloon deflation may result in the premature removal of the catheter and this, or the need to replace it, may compromise some reconstructive procedures.
2. Partial deflation of the balloon may result in it slipping, still oversized, into the area of a reconstruction and damaging it.
3. Inadvertent severe traction may withdraw a fully inflated balloon into the reconstructed area and disrupt it.
4. Even when fully deflated, residual corrugations of an overstretched balloon surface may be sufficiently rough to disturb a skin graft urethroplasty.

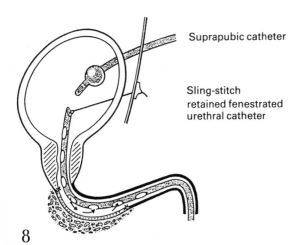

Suprapubic catheter

Sling-stitch retained fenestrated urethral catheter

8

Thus, if a urethral catheter is used it is best retained by a trans-vesical sling stitch to a crush button on the abdominal wall.

Unfenestrated catheter-shaft complications

Urethral exudates are greatly increased by urethral injury or a suture-line; if they accumulate in the urethral space they tend to become infected and may compromise healing.

Natural passive drainage of the exudates along an empty urethra occurs when urine is drained postoperatively by a suprapubic catheter; however there is a tendency for them to pool posteriorly after a bulbar reconstruction. Unless it is quite small[12], the shaft of a standard unfenestrated catheter, indwelling in the urethra tends to obstruct the free drainage of the exudates.

Fenestrated urethral catheter drainage

8

Positive drainage of the urethral lumen exudates is achieved by a fenestrated catheter[3], however, this should be regarded as a urethral drain and it should always be used in conjunction with a suprapubic catheter.

Irrigation of the peri-catheter space by the passage of urine along a fenestrated catheter does not compromise a urethral reconstruction, but appropriate management is essential; in particular, a fenestrated catheter should never be used for a 'bladder washout' after a urethral reconstruction unless its fenestrations are first pushed back into the bladder so that none lie in the urethral area – otherwise suture-line extravasation may result from the pressure of the irrigation fluid.

Postoperatively a fenestrated catheter facilitates verification of the state of healing of a reconstruction by a 'catheter-gram' – contrast introduced into a fenestrated catheter flows into the pericatheter space so that the 'water tight' healing of a reconstruction can be verified by exclusion of peri-urethral extravasation. Fenestrated catheters are best made of plastic because the lumen of these is relatively large compared with that of silicone/rubber catheters – size 16F is generally appropriate for adults. The extent of the fenestrated area of the shaft is tailored to the circumstances and does not normally extend distal to the peno-scrotal junction. Fenestrations are simply made by sharp bending a catheter and cutting off the projecting kink angle of the flattened fold with scissors.

Terminal strictures and glans-urethro-meatoplasty

With meticulous attention to detail it is possible to construct or reconstruct a glans-meatus that approximates very closely to normality – positionally, functionally and cosmetically[13].

A normal meatus is situated terminally on the glans – its lips are smooth and sharp-edged, forming a vertical slit; it is this that creates a clean spray-free voiding stream. Examination of a normal terminal urethra revealed by opening it with a ventral incision provides the format for a satisfactory reconstruction; the urethra is seen to be formed by a strip of uro-epithelium located in a deep cleft and when the glans is opened flat, the width of the glans-cleft urethral strip in an adult is about 2.5 cm = 25 mm = 25 F.

The common indications for terminal urethroplasty are hypospadiac malformations and meatal strictures including those associated with severe spongiosclerosis known as 'balanitis xerotica' – these are all associated with varying degrees of absence or less of a glans-cleft when the urethra is opened ventrally.

Ventriflexed glans

Chordee

Glans split

Scrotal rotation flap

CLOSURE

9

Two-stage glans-urethro-meatoplasty

9

Thus the creation or the re-creation of a near-normal terminal urethra requires a deep midline incision in the glans, careful separation of its anterior adhesion to the tip of the corpora and the grafting of a neo-urethral lining onto the exposed surface of the spongy tissue of the glans-cleft. A full thickness foreskin or buccal graft onto the spongy tissue of the cleft resurfaces it with a 'wet' epithelium closely simulating the normal situation of the uro-epithelium directly applied to the vascular spaces. Pedicled foreskin grafts can be used in the form of tubes or Blair-Byars flaps but the vascularizing subcutaneous tissue of these sometimes forms folds in the neo-urethra which distort the voiding stream.

There is a somewhat unexpected by-product of the mobilization involved in the deep-glans-clefting procedure when it is used for the ventri-positioned globular glans of a hypospadiac deformity – the residual attachments of the bivalved glans to the dorsal apex of the corpora reposition it remarkably effectively when it is rolled up to create the neo-urethral cleft so that the glans-meatus appears virtually normal[13].

The establishment of a full thickness fenestrated skin graft on a deep-cleft glans is facilitated by the fact that this can be spread flat; thus it is easy to fix it in this position by spreading its dorsal skin surface onto an adhesive surface, such as a suitably trimmed 'Discardo-Pad' and use this as counter pressure for a simple pressure dressing after the graft and its fenestrations have been suture anchored in position, further augmenting this by an additional ventral pressure card, forming, in effect, a 'glans sandwich'[14].

The one-stage back-to-back, double-foreskin-island neo-urethro-meatoplasty

10

The back-to-back, double-foreskin-island urethro-meatoplasty[14] is a simple modification of the Turner-Warwick island-skin pedicle flap procedure[15, 16] (*Illustration 17*) involving several distinct manoeuvres:

1. A formal subterminal repositioning glans-meatotomy – rather than a simple 'glans tunnel'. The attachments of the globular hypospadiac glans to the ventral tip of the penile corpora are meticulously separated by an undermining dissection and a midline-slit meatotomy created at an appropriate site on the dorsal repositioned glans.
2. The terminal penile urethra is mobilized, ventrally spatulated and its margins laterally anchored.
3. A two-sided island skin pedicle graft is created by unilateral mobilization of the foreskin on a unilateral pedicle.

An inner foreskin island is appropriately trimmed and tubularized to construct a neo-terminal urethra for a proximal anastomosis to the spatulated penile urethra and an invagination of its distal projection into the neo-glans-meatotomy; the dorsally located suture line of the tubularization lies deep in the spongy tissue of the glans.

The external foreskin island is extensively trimmed to replace the ventral skin defect formed by the dorsal mobilization of the glans and the penile urethral spatulation – the proximal margin of the ventral penile skin is resected so that its suture line does not immediately overlie that of the neo-urethral anastomosis and additional separation achieved by wide overlap-underlap of the pedicle-graft subcutaneous tissue.

The postoperative healing of the neo-urethral tube graft is covered by a short tube stent located with a suture.

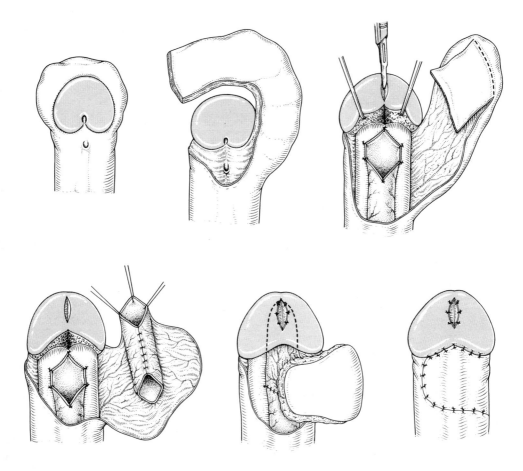

10

One-stage free skin graft glans urethro-meatoplasty

11

When a sub-terminal hypospadiac deformity is complicated by a previous circumcision, a cosmetically acceptable one-stage correction can sometimes be achieved by a free skin deep-cleft glans urethro neomeatoplasty.

This is a one-stage variation of the Turner Warwick[5] two-stage deep-cleft glans-spongio redeployment procedure (see p. 489). The fixed flat full thickness skin graft with anchored fenestrations is anastomosed to the dorsal spatulation of the mobilized distal penile urethra and a one-stage glans closure over a penile skin flip-flap completes the neoterminal urethral meatoplasty. The ventral sub-coronal skin defect is covered by a penile skin flap advancement with as much subcutaneous underlap/overlap as possible to reduce the risk of a submeatal fistula – a peno-scrotal tension-relieving incision is sometimes required to achieve this. The healing of the fenestrated neo-urethral skin patch graft is covered by a short length of a suture-retained terminal catheter stent.

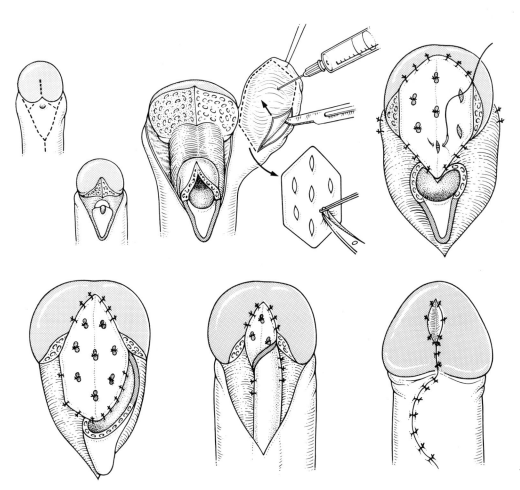

11

Penile urethroplasty

12

Reconstruction of the penile urethra is relatively simple compared with that of the glans-meatus distally and the bulb proximally – success is simply dependent upon the creation of a stricture-free tube since as it is pendulous and free draining any saccular irregularities of the reconstructed urethra do not retain urine (were it otherwise Dennis Brown's classic buried skin-strip procedure would not have achieved even passing acceptance).

Penile reconstruction is generally facilitated by the fact that the immediately overlying penile skin provides a good urethral substitute because it is relatively adaptable to a wet environment, nearly hair-free and well vascularized by its uniquely mobile subcutaneous tissue; therefore, it is easy to use as an island skin graft, simply rolled in on a long lateral pedicle extending throughout its length, either as a one- or two-stage procedure[4, 15, 17, 18].

The whole circumference of the penile urethra can be reconstructed from a 3 cm (30 mm = 30F) in-rolled strip of penile urethral skin, or any proportion of it in combination with a fixed flat residual roof strip. Thus, the introduction of an additional complication resulting from an inevitable incidence of 'failure-of-take' of a circumferential graft of full thickness skin makes it difficult to justify this option as a one-stage procedure in the penile urethra.

However, the natural mobility and reliability of the penile skin is often seriously compromised by previous surgical mobilization and the extent of this is not easy to estimate with reliability at the time of operation. For this reason, when undertaking a definitive penile urethral 'retrievoplasty' when there is a paucity of penile skin appropriate for penile urethral substitution, it is generally advisable to use the medial margin(s) of it to form a 2 cm wide fixed flat urethral roof-strip, as a full thickness graft rather than a pedicled graft, by simply removing the subcutaneous adventitial tissue relating to this area. Under these circumstances this procedure is less likely to result in a critical skin loss than the unpredictable failure of the precarious blood supply to the marginal area of pedicled inlay.

During an erection, there is little residual excess of urethral length elasticity so that one-stage anastomotic repair of a penile urethra is generally precluded, and even a limited attempt to restore roof-strip urethral continuity after the resection of a short distal penile segment is likely to result in a significant curvature-chordee. However, advancement of a mobilized bulbar urethra after resection of a short, isolated penile base structure may achieve a chordee-free approximation. In practice, penile urethral reconstruction is rarely required as an isolated procedure – it is usually a distal extension of a bulbar reconstruction or a proximal extension of a hypospadiac repair.

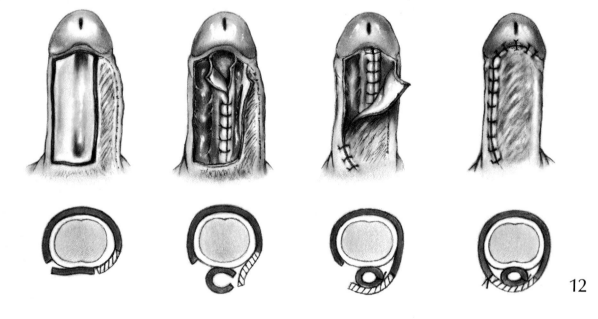

12

Scrotal-flap substitution of penile skin

13

The technical problem created by using penile skin to reconstruct the urethra is the deficiency of skin on the penile shaft that results from this. Earlier methods of resolving this by the Dennis Brown penile skin economizing procedure of burying a relatively narrow skin strip and also the Cecil scrotal burying procedure were rendered obsolete by the relatively simple replacement of the penile skin deficiency by a definitive pedicle graft of scrotal skin[4].

Although scrotal skin has serious shortcomings as a urethral substitute (*see* p. 496) it is a satisfactory substitute for penile skin; pedicle grafts can be raised in several ways:

1. A 3–4 cm wide pedicled strip of skin from one side of the scrotum can be rotated through 180° – this is a most useful procedure but careful siting of the pedicle base is required to reduce the tendency to a tethering rotation of the penis.
2. A horizontally originating scrotal pedicle strip reduces to 90° the redeployment rotation required to augment the penile skin; however, the collateral circulation across the median raphe is somewhat precarious and this occasionally results in skin loss at the extremity of the rotated flap.
3. A simple central pedicle scrotal advancement flap is appropriate for penile skin replacement when the defect is not too long; its extension can be facilitated by a midline tension relieving-incision and it has the advantage of excluding any rotational element.

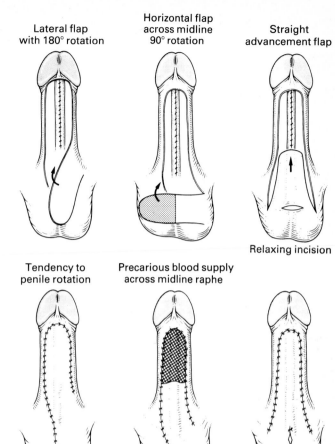

Lateral flap with 180° rotation

Horizontal flap across midline 90° rotation

Straight advancement flap

Relaxing incision

Tendency to penile rotation

Precarious blood supply across midline raphe

13

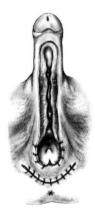
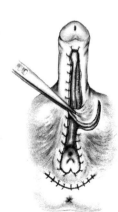

14

14

In a two-stage procedure there are advantages in rotating the scrotal flap onto the penile shaft at the first stage so that it can be trimmed for neatness rather than vascularity at the final stage; this procedure achieves a wide separation of the skin closure suture lines at the final stage of urethral closure.

The prevention of fistulae by underlap/overlap overclosure

15

The commonest complication of penile urethral reconstruction is the development of closure-line fistulae; while an incidence of this is almost inevitable after a one-stage procedure, a significant incidence after a two-stage reconstruction is unacceptable.

The most successful prophylactic procedure is wide separation of the urethral closure and overlying skin closure suture lines; the best way of achieving this is wide lateral separation of these but an extended underlap/overlap of the subcutaneous tissue layer is important, hence the width of the subcutaneous tissue of a scroto-penile overclosure flap should considerably exceed the width of the skin replacement.

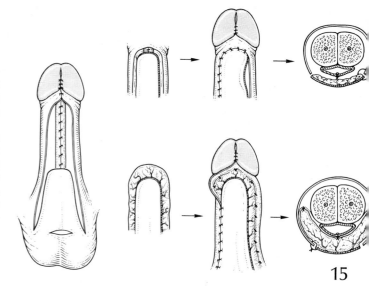

15

Bulbar urethroplasty

The options for the treatment of bulbar urethral strictures

The fundamental decision relating to the management of a bulbar stricture lies between internal urethrotomy and a definitive repair/reconstruction. Although the healing of a urethrotomy is likely to be associated with further extension of the spongiofibrosis which accompanies a stricture, this rarely compromises the subsequent definitive repair of the bulbo-penile spongy urethra except in the case of a short congenital or straddle injury stricture in which the additional length of the urethral abnormality may render it unsuitable for a subsequent one-stage anastomotic repair. The options for the definitive repair of a bulbar stricture are:

1. Excision and anastomosis
2. Substitution procedures
3. 'Combination' procedures.

Patient positioning and surgical approach for bulbo-membranous and penile surgery

A simple midline perineal incision with the patient in a standard lithotomy position provides excellent exposure for bulbo-membranous surgery; if an observational scroto-urethral inlay proves necessary it is easily achieved by the Turner Warwick drop-back procedure (see p. 498)[4, 19]. No surgical assistants are required if an appropriate ring retraction system is used (see p. 519) and certainly none should intervene between the seated surgeon and the low instrument table and seated scrub nurse.

When there is any possibility of a need for a synchronous abdominal approach the position is appropriately modified (see p. 509). The exaggerated lithotomy position has no advantage for an anterior approach to the prostato-membranous urethra (see p. 508) through the subpubo-urethral space and generally requires a surgeon to stand for a synchronous penile procedure. The posterior approach to the prostato-membranous urethra involves some risk to potency.

The classic posterior horseshoe incision limits the anterior exposure, is awkward to extend and compromises an observational inlay graft unless it is formally modified to a posteriorly based scroto-perineal flap (see p. 498)[20, 21], which is unnecessarily complicated unless a prior decision has been made to use a scrotal skin substitution procedure in spite of the inherent shortcomings of this.

The technique of bulbo-bulbar anastomosis

16

The feasibility of a circumferential anastomotic repair of a radiographically 'short' bulbar urethral stricture is dependent upon a critical assessment of the extent of the associated spongiofibrosis at the time of operation.

The factor limiting the length of a bulbar urethral abnormality that can be resolved by anastomosis is the extent of the elastic lengthening that can be obtained by mobilizing the residual bulbar urethra proximal and distal to the stricture; this tends to be somewhat compromised by scarring resulting from the stricture injury so that in practice it is rarely possible to excise a bulbar stricture longer than about 1.5 cm and still obtain a 2 cm overlap anastomosis without risking chordee.

The bulbar urethra is exposed through a midline incision. A sound in the urethra identifies the distal limit of the stricture and provides 'internal retraction' to facilitate mobilization of the bulbar urethra from the base of the penis back to the subpubo-urethral space. The urethra is opened *inferiorly* over a distance of 2–3 cm immediately *distal* to the stricture, and retracted by stay sutures and both its lining and the cut edge of the spongy tissue inspected critically to determine the anterior extent of the associated spongiofibrosis. The appropriate siting of the incision into the bulbar urethra proximal to the stricture is dependent upon this finding. If the anterior extent of the spongiofibrosis is minimal the spatulating incision into the proximal bulbar urethra should be *superior* so that a spatulated posterior and anterior overlap anastomosis can be achieved if the proximal extent of the urethral abnormality is minimal (other than the common prestricture leucoplakic appearance of the uro-epithelium which is irrelevant). If, however, the extent of the spongiofibrosis distal to a short bulbar stricture precludes a circumferential anastomotic repair, the urethra proximal to it is spatulated inferiorly for the creation of a redeployment fixed flat roof strip of a 'combination' urethroplasty (*see* p. 502). To avoid cross adhesions and restenosis, the lateral margins of a spatulated antero-posterior anastomosis are spread-fixed laterally to the under surface of the penile crura after exposing them by detaching the dorsal midline origin of the circumferential bulbo-spongiosis muscle which otherwise impairs a firm anchorage (*see* p. 503).

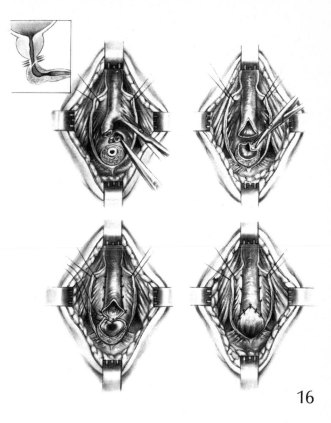

16

Penile curvature-chordee is prevented by avoiding mobilization of the penile urethra and angulation chordee reduced by relaxing the suspensory ligament exposed by a minimal extension of the dissection around the base of the penis. Tension-relieving sutures along the lateral margins of the mobilized bulbar urethra avoid erection-traction on the anastomosis postoperatively.

An overclosure posterior redeployment spongioplasty supports the anastomosis. The bulbospongiosis muscle is overclosed in an endeavour to preserve the normal urethral emptying mechanism. The wound is closed with dead space encircling sutures which subdivide it into vertically draining compartments so that no wound drain or separate subcutaneous sutures are required (*see* p. 500)[4].

Postoperatively a combination of suprapubic catheter urine drainage and sling-stitch retained fenestrated urethral catheter drainage of the urethral exudates is advised (*see* p. 487).

The principles of substitution urethroplasty

No substitute for the urethra is as good as the urethra itself – all substitution procedures have inherent short-comings and consequently an incidence of restenosis. Thus, a substitution procedure is generally inadvisable for the resolution of a stricture that is truly appropriate for excision and anastomosis.

'Wet' and 'dry' skin

Not all skin areas are equally appropriate for urethral substitution. 'Wet' epithelial surfaces such as those of the urethra, the foreskin, the mouth, the vagina and the labia are particularly adapted to a moist environment; 'dry' skin, such as that of the scrotum, the thigh and the lower abdomen tends to become inflamed and eczematous when constantly urine-soaked; penile skin is a relatively moisture-resistant 'dry' skin and generally satisfactory for urethral substitution.

Free grafts versus pedicle grafts

The survival of a pedicled skin graft with an adequate blood supply is naturally more reliable than that of a free skin graft which has an inevitable incidence of a partial failure-of-take; thus when a pedicle graft of appropriate skin is available it has clear advantages over a free graft.

However, when a pedicle graft of an appropriate skin cannot be mobilized sufficiently to reach, or when previous surgery has critically impaired its blood supply or extent, free grafts have the advantage that appropriately 'wet' or 'moist' skin can be used and this is often preferable to an easily available pedicle graft of scrotal skin.

17 & 18

Pedicle grafts

1. Penile and foreskin The unique mobility of the penile skin and the pattern of its blood supply usually enables a well vascularized island pedicle flap to be mobilized to reach the bulbar urethra and sometimes as far as the bulbo-membranous area, either as a rotation flap or as a skin island procedure[15] (*see Illustrations 17 and 18*). Thus, coupled with a scrotal skin substitution of the consequent penile skin deficiency (*see p. 492*) the peno-scrotal 'exchange-pedicle graft' procedure[15] is often useful as a two-stage, and sometimes as a one-stage bulbar urethral substitution procedure.

2. Pedicled scrotal skin substitution Although the mobility of the scrotal skin facilities its use as a pedicled inlay, scrotal skin has two major inherent shortcomings which compromise its use as a urethral substitute: (*a*) it is hair bearing; (*b*) it is a dry skin and prone to develop an eczematous inflammatory reaction when urine-soaked; this reaction is sufficient to preclude its use in occasional cases.

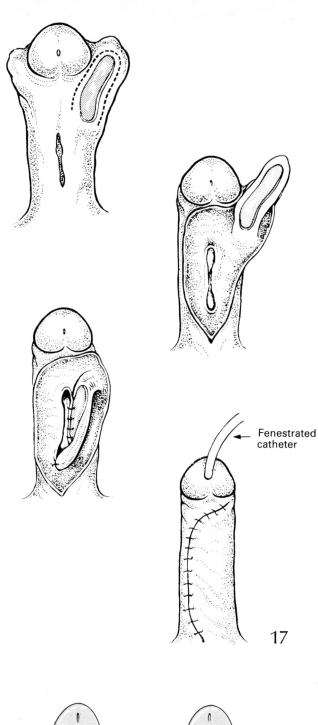

← Fenestrated catheter

17

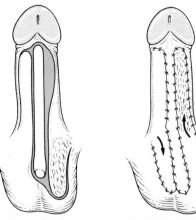

18

However, a scroto-urethral inlay provides excellent access for the direct observation and revision of a first-stage 'combination' bulbar urethral reconstruction (*see* p. 502).

If hair-bearing skin is used to reconstruct the urethra it is always advisable to epilate the neo-urethral area meticulously during the interval stage of a two-stage procedure (*see* p. 504); inability to do this in children before pubertal hair development results in a significant incidence of late complications when scrotal skin is used for perineal hypospadiac urethral reconstruction. Furthermore it seems generally inadvisable to use scrotal skin as a circumferential replacement for the urethra and certainly its use as a one-stage skin island pedicle graft provides no opportunity to rectify its shortcomings.

Island-skin pedicle-graft urethroplasty

The preservation of its vascular pedicle naturally increases the chance of survival of a skin patch graft; this technique is particularly suited to the penile skin, island-skin pedicles of which will readily reach the anterior, and sometimes the posterior bulbar urethra[15].

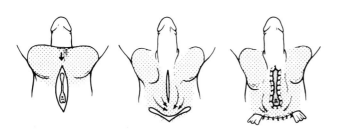

Turner Warwick 1959

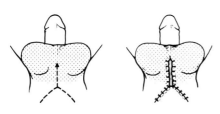

Leadbetter 1960

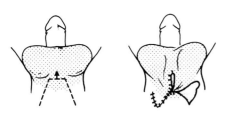

Gil Vernet 1966: Blandy 1969

19

Principles of two-stage scroto-urethral inlay urethroplasty

19

The wide, posteriorly-placed scroto-urethral funnel was developed[19] to overcome the disadvantages of Johannson's sub-perineal scrotal invagination tunnel procedure which failed to provide direct access to overcome the inherent shortcomings of scrotal skin as a urethral substitute.

A wide posteriorly placed scroto-urethral inlay can be achieved either by a scrotal drop-back procedure[4, 19], or by a posteriorly-based perineo-scrotal flap[20, 21] which was a development of Leadbetter's posteriorly based perineal skin inlay[22].

In most cases the choice between the drop-back and the posterior flap procedure for a scroto-urethral inlay is simply a matter of surgical preference because the management of the interval stage, the incidence of complications arising from the deficiencies of scrotal skin urethral substitution, and the procedure of the final stage closure, are all virtually identical.

A particular advantage of the Turner Warwick drop-back procedure is that it is based on a midline incision which provides the simplest exposure and closure for bulbar urethral surgery; it thus provides the option of a first-stage scroto-urethral inlay whenever the operative findings indicate the need for this; it is the only option when perineal skin is compromised by chronic infection and fistulae.

However it is achieved, a definitive circumferential scroto-urethral inlay substitution procedure has been largely abandoned in favour of one of the variety of options offered by one of the Turner Warwick augmented roof-strip 'combination urethroplasty' procedures which have proved more reliable in the long term (*see* p. 502). Nevertheless, there are few remaining indications for a simple scroto-urethral inlay, particularly after the *en bloc* excision of the spongy urethra and its surrounding tissues required for the classic 'water can' stricture associated with infection and fistulae.

The Turner Warwick scrotal drop-back procedure

The drop-back of the scrotum which ensures direct vision/access to the prostato-membranous urethra is achieved by incising the obstructing perineal skin in the midline and closing this horizontally. It is particularly important to ensure that the bulk of the inter-testicular subcutaneous tissue behind the peno-scrotal junction is mobilized by appropriate relaxation so that it drops back behind the inlay to provide a well-vascularized skin bridge posteriorly. A secondary incision into the invaginated scrotal drop-back is appropriately sited and sutured with 3/0 PGA sutures.

Trans-sphincter scroto-urethral inlay and distal sphincter preservation

When an appropriate posterior extent of a combination procedure roof-strip requires a *subsphincter* scrotal drop-back inlay, the suturing of this is readily achieved with standard instruments.

However, the spongiofibrosis associated with many posterior bulbar strictures extends to the distal margin of the distal sphincter mechanism so that it is often necessary to proceed to a trans-sphincter inlay to a point just below the verumontanum to reach an appropriate length of normal proximal urethra[4].

Our experience over many years is that a *normal* distal urethral mechanism remains competent after recalibration to 36–38 F and a trans-sphincter substitution inlay; however, appropriately specialized instruments are required to achieve this because an over-relaxation of the distal sphincter that enables the apical sutures of a posteriorly based inlay flap to be inserted with standard instrumentation carries a considerable risk of rendering it incompetent.

20

Special instruments are required to suture a scrotal inlay or a free skin graft into a trans-sphincter position within a calibre of 36 F. Speculum retraction can be achieved by: (*1*) the tapered groove of a Teal's probe-pointed gorgette: particularly useful for the insertion of antero-lateral sutures; (*2*) a self-retaining fibrelight calibrating Turner Warwick posterior urethral retractor greatly facilitates the insertion of the postero-lateral sutures: the blades of this are 9 mm wide so that when they are separated by an equivalent distance the posterior urethra calibrates to 4 × 9 mm = 36 F.

The insertion of interrupted 3/0 PGA sutures within a calibre of 36 F is facilitated by:

1. A fully curved Turner Warwick posterior urethral needle designed so that it can be rotated within the blades of the posterior speculum. It is pre-threaded and after a bite of a posterior margin of the inlay

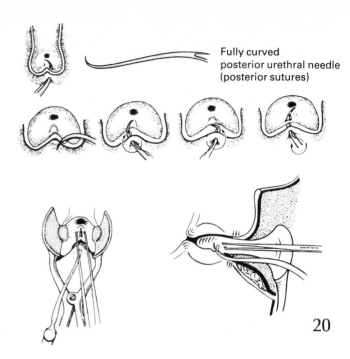

Fully curved posterior urethral needle (posterior sutures)

20

incision in the scrotal skin has been taken, the needle is advanced and a further deep bite of the prostatic urethral margin is taken by a rotation advancement movement; the suture is picked off the tip with fine forceps and the needle withdrawn and five or six sutures are placed posteriorly before any are tied.
2. Posterior inlay sutures can also be inserted by Chalmer's technique, using an atraumatic needle bent into a spoon-shape which is pushed up the urethra and withdrawn backwards after the suture bites have been taken.
3. The appropriately curved Turner-Warwick fibrelight sucker (*see Illustration* 42).

The management and duration of the 'interval' stage

The term 'two-stage' applied to a scroto-urethral inlay is technically a misnomer because it fails to emphasize that the key to the success of a reconstruction of the more complex bulbar membranous strictures is the meticulous management of the *interval* stage; the prime purpose of such an inlay is to provide access for:

1. Direct observation of the healing of the fixed flat roof strip of a 'combination' procedure (*see* p. 502).
2. The local rearrangement of the inlay or regrafting of the roof strip.
3. Hair follicle destruction in any part of the inlay which is required for the closure completion of the circumference of a 'combination' urethroplasty.

The duration of the interval between the first stage and the final closure is dependent upon the time that it takes to establish a stable time proven stricture-free inlay; long-term success is fundamentally dependent upon this.

Closure of a scroto-urethral inlay

21

The successful closure of a scroto-urethral inlay urethroplasty requires meticulous attention to detail. It should be covered by a combination of suprapubic urinary and fenestrated urethral catheter drainage (see p. 487).

The scroto-urethral inlay funnel is circumcised, taking care not to cut the skin 'on the stretch' and thus leave a neo-urethral strip that is less than 3 cm wide (30 mm = 30 F). In practice it is best to incise the inlay skin on one side and to separate it completely before proceeding to the other.

Because a scroto-urethral inlay is invaginated through the incised margins of the bulbospongy tissue and muscle, to preserve these for overclosure, they must be carefully separated from the inlay funnel by *upward* and *outward* rather than inward, dissection.

After the suprapubic and fenestrated urethral catheters have been inserted the neo-urethral skin strip is trimmed to size. In the penile area, the neo-urethra is tube closed with a loose continuous 4/0 PGA suture approximating the subdermal tissues rather than the skin margin itself; however, in the bulbar area, when there is sufficient spongy tissue for effective overclosure, the margins of the neo-urethral tube are simply approximated by including the subdermal tissues in the bite of interrupted 3/0 PGA spongio-overclosure sutures.

The bulbo-spongiosus muscle is overclosed in an endeavour to restore bulbar urethral evacuation. The closure of the perineal subcutaneous tissue is achieved by dead-space encircling sutures which divide the subcutaneous tissue space into compartments, each of which drains efficiently onto the surface so that no drainage tubes are required.

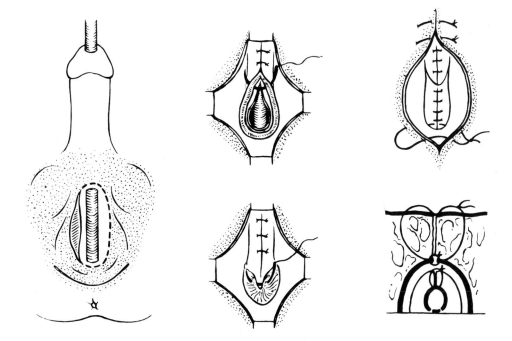

21

The principles of full thickness skin-graft urethroplasty

22

The pioneer work of Devine and Horton[23] confirmed that grafts of full thickness skin are superior to split-skin for urethral substitution.

Free skin grafts can be used either as a partial circumference patchplasty or as a circumferential tube-plasty. In simple patch procedures they are 'unsupported' basing the graft on the peri-bulbar tissues. However, normal spongy tissue provides a particularly good graft bed and the end result approximates to normal 'pink' urethra in which the epithelium is virtually directly based upon spongy tissue (see p. 482). Skin-patch spongioplasty is particularly appropriate for glans-meatoplasty[1,7] and as a component of the augmented roof-strip procedures (see p. 502).

When a free graft is used as a one-stage procedure success is dependent upon 100 per cent survival of the graft because a partial loss involving any proportion of the circumference of a neo-urethral graft results in a commensurate diminution of the calibre of the reconstructed lumen in that area – and consequently a proportional restricture. Thus, long one-stage full-thickness epithelial grafts are naturally less successful than short ones because, if the length of a graft is doubled, the risk of significant partial 'failure-of-take' must increase proportionally; furthermore, free grafts are naturally less successful when bed tissue is fibrotic or infected.

Donor site and preparation

Foreskin or anterior penile skin is the generally preferred donor site[23]. However, buccal skin is particularly useful for relatively small areas such as hypospadiac glans meatoplasty corrections as is bladder urothelium[13].

The meticulous dissection removal of the subdermal adventitia is important to reduce the thickness of the tissue intervening between the graft bed and the basal epidermal cells to a minimum; technically this is facilitated by spreading the graft on an adhesive surface such as that of a scrub nurse's Sharps-disposal 'Discardopad'.

When there is a paucity of penile skin and a long graft is required a full thickness graft from the groin or from the inner aspect of the arm can be used, but because the dermis is thicker and the underlying tissue is fat laden, subdermal cleaning must be particularly meticulous and close fenestration or 'tessellation' of the graft is especially important. The Turner Warwick technique of spongio-supported skin patch urethroplasty differs in significant detail from Devine's unsupported tube patch plasty; it is, however, most reliable when it is used in 'combination' with a fixed flat roof strip and a definitive redeployment spongioplasty (see pp. 503–504).

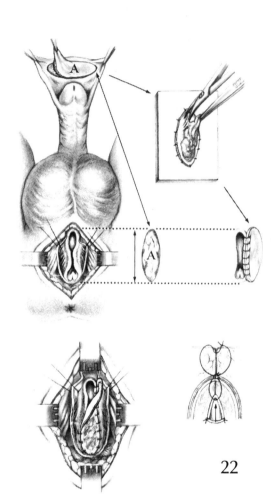

22

The Turner Warwick 'Augmented Roof-Strip' procedures

23

To reduce the incidence of restricture after circumferential urethral reconstruction by both one-stage full thickness skin graft urethroplasty and two-stage pedicled scroto-urethral inlay procedures, Turner Warwick[4, 8], developed a variety of one-stage and two-stage augmented roof-strip 'combination' procedures, avoiding circumferential urethral substitution either by scrotal skin or full thickness skin grafts, restricting each to half of the urethral circumference in any area.

The creation of a roof-strip

The basic principle of 'combination' urethroplasty is the creation of an epithelialized roof-strip that is 1.5–2 cm wide; this roof-strip creates at least 50 per cent of the neo-urethral circumference and its contraction is prevented by lateral sutures anchoring its margins to the undersurface of the crura. The 'fixed flat roof-strip' may be created in several ways:

1. Rearrangement of the residual urethral element by side-to-side overlap anastomosis after appropriately extensive mobilization.
2. Lateral augmentation of the width of the bulbar urethral element by strategic longitudinal fenestrating incisions which are held open by lateral fixation so the defects heal by epithelial regeneration.
3. Augmentation of the urethral roof strip with a free patch graft when necessary.
4. Complete replacement of the urethral roof-strip by a free patch graft.

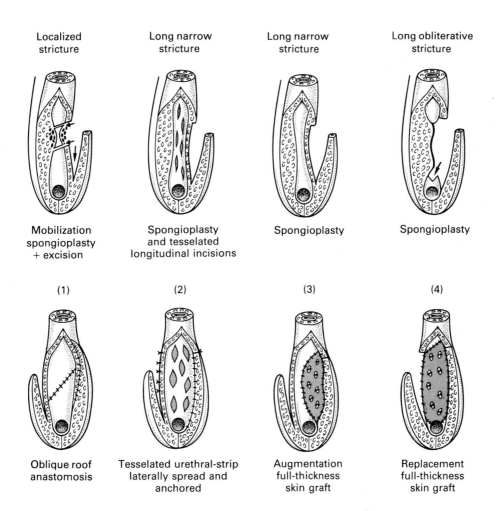

Localized stricture	Long narrow stricture	Long narrow stricture	Long obliterative stricture
Mobilization spongioplasty + excision	Spongioplasty and tesselated longitudinal incisions	Spongioplasty	Spongioplasty
(1)	(2)	(3)	(4)
Oblique roof anastomosis	Tesselated urethral-strip laterally spread and anchored	Augmentation full-thickness skin graft	Replacement full-thickness skin graft

23

24

Redeployment lateral spongioplasty

To create a fixed flat roof-strip by redeployment of the residual bulbar urethra after excision of a stricture it is necessary to separate and to redeploy the excess postero-lateral bulk of the bulbospongy tissue (*see* p. 480).

After the whole length of the bulbar urethra has been carefully mobilized from the membranous urethra to the base of the penis and opened, posteriorly based flaps of the excess spongy tissue are reflected by sharp dissection; any areas of spongiofibrosis within these spongy flaps must be carefully excised but any normal supple spongy tissue that remains can be preserved on the basis of its main posterior blood supply and redeployed lateral to the fixed flat roof-strip for subsequent overclosure support – 'lateral redeployment spongioplasty'[24] – a variation of 'posterior flap spongioplasty' (*see* p. 517)[3].

In appropriate cases, when the urethral abnormality is sufficiently short, this can be excised and the residual spongio-supported urethra redeployed with side-by-side overlap to create a roof-strip. This redeployed roof-strip is anchored laterally to the surface of the penile crura to spread it to its maximum width; to provide firm crural anchorage these must be exposed by reflecting the overlying bulbo-spongiosis muscle which is separated from its origin in the midline. The lateral roof-strip anchoring sutures include the inner margin of the redeployment spongioplasty flaps and the detached bulbo-spongiosis muscle.

Furthermore, there is an important manoeuvre that reduces the risk of posterior stenosis when a bulbar stricture extends close to the sphincter mechanism. The incision separating the spongioplasty flaps is extended posteriorly and the bulbo-membranous junction is 'funnelled open' by two antero-lateral fixation sutures, and an additional one in the posterior midline is inserted from the posterior surface of the bulb and back again.

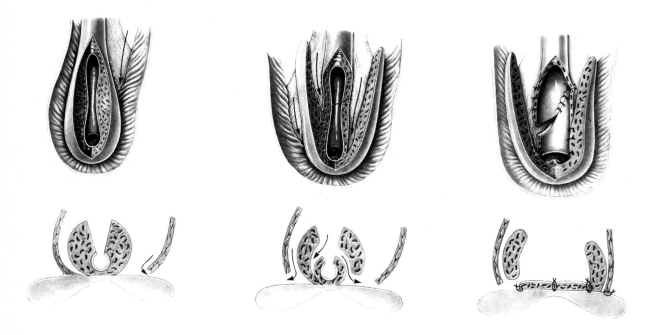

24

25a, b & c

The augmentation of a roof-strip 'combination' urethroplasty

The remaining 50 per cent of the neo-urethral circumference overclosing the roof-strip can be completed either as a one-stage procedure or deferred as a second-stage procedure.

Whether a one-stage completion, using a patch of pedicled or full thickness skin or scaffold material (lyophilized dura, PGA mesh, etc.) is appropriate depends upon whether a really satisfactory roof-strip has been created by redeployment of the residual bulbar urethra; if this is substandard, or the creation of the roof-strip has already required skin graft augmentation, a scrotal skin 'drop back' is inlaid to the margins of the roof-strip so that the progress of its healing can be directly observed – and readjusted if necessary.

Even if part of the full-thickness graft of a one-stage overclosure of the roof-strip, or the scrotal skin margins of a two-stage overclosure, should fail, it is relatively unlikely to result in restenosis because the defect opposing a well-established laterally anchored roof-strip is likely to re-epithelialize on the Dennis Brown principle.

Considerable advantages accrue from the use of one of the two-stage 'combination' procedures for the reconstruction of complex bulbar urethral strictures, particularly those associated with extensive spongiofibrosis, because the success of the procedure depends upon the verified establishment of a satisfactory roof-strip; the scroto-urethral inlay provides direct observation and access to ensure this:

1. Because the roof-strip of a 'combination' procedure is fixed flat it should not contract once it is established.
2. Restricturing due to partial failure-of-take of a full-thickness skin graft roof-strip is obviated because any defect is directly visible through the observational inlay and easily regrafted.
3. Closure can proceed as soon as healing is satisfactory because only a small margin of scrotal skin is used to complete the circumference so that the time-proven quality of this is less important to success, so the duration of the interval stage can be reduced.

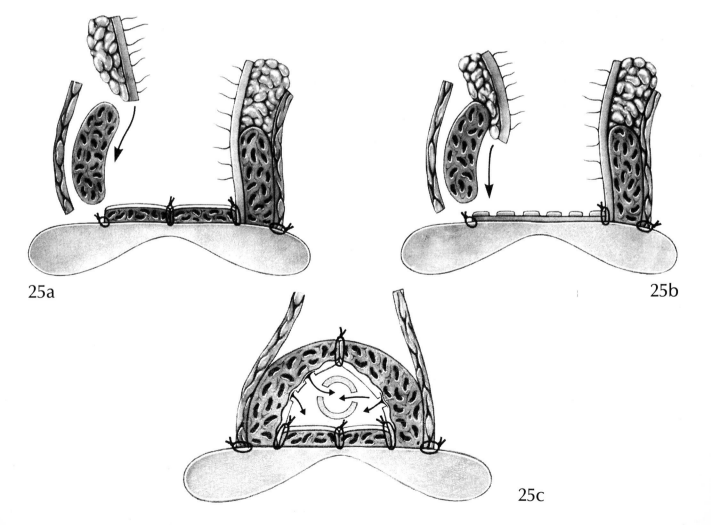

25a

25b

25c

The principles of the management or post-prostatectomy sphincter-strictures

Post-prostatectomy strictures involving the distal sphincter mechanism are the most difficult of all strictures to resolve satisfactorily because they are located in the only sphincter mechanism that remains after prostatectomy, whether transurethral or enucleation. The unsatisfactory prostatectomy that creates the stricture by damaging the sphincter-active urethra also damages its functional competence to a varying extent. Strictures in the sphincter-active area tend to recur particularly rapidly and all forms of management carry some risk of further impairment of sphincter function – some more than others.

The prime consideration in the management of post-prostatectomy strictures in the distal mechanism must be the preservation of its residual sphincteric function rather than the definitive resolution of the stricture itself[5,7].

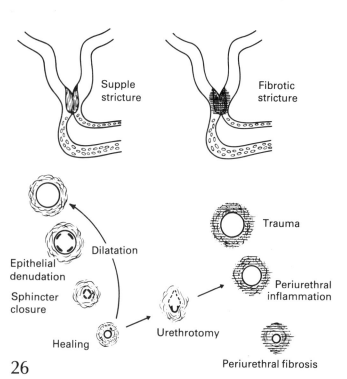

26

26

THE SIGNIFICANCE OF THE DISTINCTION BETWEEN 'SUPPLE' AND 'RIGID' SPHINCTER-STRICTURES

There is a wide variation in the extent of sphincter-damage associated with sphincter-strictures. On the one extreme the sphincter mechanism may be almost undamaged and supple, the stricture being the result of simple denudation of the epithelial lining. On the other hand, densely fibrotic sphincter strictures are associated with severe sphincter damage; there are, of course, all variations between these[24].

Even a minimal recalibration of a rigid sphincter stricture to 16–18 F by the passage of dilators may be sufficient to render it incompetent and a patient incontinent – on the other hand the oversized dilatation of a 'supple' stricture associated with minimal sphincter damage to a calibre of 36 F results in no significant diminution of urinary control.

The safest method of treating the more rigid sphincter-deficient stricture is by simple frequent small-calibre dilatation; often this is best achieved by teaching the patient to pass a soft olive-tipped plastic dilator once or twice a week.

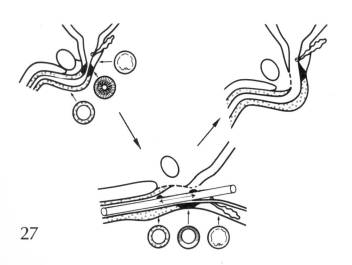

27

27

The potential disasters of treating a post-prostatectomy sphincter stricture by internal urethrotomy are obvious – if the patient is not immediately rendered incontinent as a result of transecting the thin intramural sphincter mechanism, secondary fibrosis is likely to convert a supple mechanism into a rigid one.

The evaluation of urethral stricture surgery calibration vs uroflow rate

Two distinct criteria are used for the evaluation of the results of operative procedures for urethral strictures.

A truly successful urethral reconstruction should recreate a tube of even calibre normal diameter (22–24 F). Such a state of affairs cannot be proven urodynamically because, while a recording flowmeter is an important instrument for the evaluation of patients both before and after urethral reconstruction, it is only a screening test for the identification of bladder outlet obstruction; a rigid stricture can stenose to a calibre in the region of 10 F before it significantly impairs the voiding flow rate[25]. Furthermore, a patient's stricture may not be the only cause of outlet obstruction – many patients attending stricture clinics are dilated with increasing frequency for an obstruction which is in fact the result of increasing prostatic enlargement and a few patients with long-standing dysynergic bladder neck mechanisms prove never to have had a urethral stricture at all[5,11]. This emphasizes the importance of retrograde urethrography in the diagnosis and the follow-up and also of video voiding cystourethrography, especially when flow studies identify a significant outlet obstruction in the absence of a rigid urethral stenosis calibrating to less than about 14 F.

Urodynamic criteria are often adopted for evaluating the results of endoscopic urethrotomy; this is acceptable so far as a particular patient's management is concerned but they are not valid measurements for comparison with 'calibration-success'.

A patient who is reported as having a normal flow rate 2 years after a urethral procedure may in fact have borderline restenosis and a prognosis that is considerably less good than one who has had a urethral reconstruction through which a soft 22 F catheter will pass easily.

PELVIC FRACTURE URETHRAL INJURIES

The urethra is damaged in about 10 per cent of pelvic fracture injuries; this communication is based on a personal experience of the repair of more than 300.

The site of urethral injury

The usual location of urethral rupture in the adult is within the 2 cm length of the sphincter-active sub-prostatic urethra. In childhood, before the prostate matures and mechanically protects the urethra within it, the site of injury is less predictable so that it is not unusual for the bladder neck mechanism to be involved.

The 2 cm of urethra below the prostate relate anteriorly to the sub-pubo-urethral space, not to an imaginary 'external sphincter' or 'urogenital diaphragm'[1,2]. The rupture may occur at any point within this relatively unsupported 2 cm; most commonly, it is located close to the prostate and in our experience it is unusual to find more than 1 cm of intact urethra distal to it and usually only a few millimetres remain.

Urethral injury stenosis

Partial injuries of the urethral circumference may or may not result in a urethral stenosis – circumferential urethral rupture almost always results in the formation of either a stenosis or a prostato-bulbar urethral distraction defect.

Haematoma and haematoma fibrosis

When the sub-prostatic urethra is torn across in association with a pelvic fracture injury the immediate consequence is the development of a haematoma between the distracted urethral ends, the extent of which varies from minimal to massive.

The natural resolution of the haematoma is a combination of urethral drainage, absorption, and organization in unpredictable proportions: the end result is a considerable reduction in haematoma volume but almost always with the formation of a significant extent of dense haematoma-fibrosis. The time that this resolution process takes to complete varies from a few months to a year or so, according to the size of the haematoma. This haematoma-fibrosis is a complicating feature of almost every urethral reconstruction.

Sphincter damage

1 The distal sphincter Because there is no circumferential sphincter-mechanism 'external' to the membranous urethra, the functional efficiency of the distal sphincter is wholly dependent upon the sphincter muscle mechanisms that are located with the 3–4 mm thickness of the 1.5–2.0 cm length of the sub-prostatic 'membranous' urethra that relates to the sub-pubo urethral space (see p. 482)[1,2]: it is not surprising, therefore, that a circumferential injury to the sub-prostatic urethra generally destroys the functional competence of the distal mechanism so that subsequent urinary incontinence is entirely dependent upon the bladder neck mechanism located proximal to the verumontanum.

2 The bladder neck sphincter The normal mechanism of an uninjured bladder neck sphincter is reliably competent and fortunately, in the adult, it is relatively unusual for this mechanism lying proximal to the verumontanum to be damaged at the time of accident.

The normal functional competence of an uninjured bladder neck may be rendered secondarily incompetent by the natural shrinkage replacement of an extensive pelvic floor haematoma by haematoma-fibrosis which prevents its occlusive contraction by outward circumferential retraction. This is in fact the commonest cause of an incompetent bladder neck dysfunction after pelvic fracture injury.

In such cases its functional competence is usually restored by lysis – meticulously removing the anchoring retropubic fibrosis anteriorly and laterally; the reliability of this procedure is dependent upon preventing secondary fibrotic immobilization by filling the resulting paraprostatic fibro-osseus dead space cavity with a supple omental pedicle graft which ensures the continued functional mobility of the bladder neck mechanism.

The bladder neck mechanism itself may be damaged by coincident injury at the time of the pelvic fracture or iatrogenically as a result of:

1. Balloon catheter traction reduction of the initial displacement.
2. The misguided passage of urethral dilators.
3. Overadventurous optical urethrotomy.
4. Erroneously conceived endoscopic loop resection.

The end result of the healing of pelvic fracture urethral injuries

28

When the primary healing reaction to a sub-prostatic urethral injury is complete, 4–12 months after a pelvic fracture, the results are many and varied.

Some minimal injuries, especially partial circumference, heal without either stenosis or distal sphincter injury.

Occasionally the functional competence of the distal sphincter mechanism may be lost without the development of a stricture, a disability which may be pre-identifiable but may not become apparent until a patient becomes incontinent after a subsequent prostatic resection which destroys the only remaining sphincter mechanism at the bladder neck.

The commonest result of a sub-prostatic urethral injury is the development of a relatively short prostato-bulbar urethral gap, 1.0–1.5 cm in length, with or without lumenal communication. When a narrow prostato-bulbar communication forms it is commonly referred to as a 'urethral stricture' but in reality it is simply a false passage through the intervening haematoma fibrosis.

A short 1.0–1.5 cm prostato-bulbar urethral gap lesion can usually be resolved by a relatively simple one-stage bulboprostatic anastomosis achieved through a perineal approach if it is not associated with a compromising extent of haematoma fibrosis. Such a 'stricture' is appropriately referred to as 'simple'.

No sphincter damage

No stricture

Sphincter damage

No stricture

Sphincter damage

SIMPLE stricture

COMPLEX strictures

28

'Complex' pelvic fracture urethral injuries

A 'complex' pelvic fracture urethral injury requires a lower abdominal approach to resolve one or more of its features[3]:

1. a long prostato-bulbar defect;
2. extensive retropubic haematoma fibrosis;
3. side-tracking false passages into retropubic or osteomyelitic cavities;
4. fistulae into the rectum, the bladder base, the perineum or suprapubic areas;
5. overt incompetence of the sphincter mechanism at the bladder neck demonstrated by preoperative cysto-urethrography.

The preoperative evaluation of pelvic fracture urethral injuries

SYNCHRONOUS CYSTO-URETHROGRAPHY

A synchronous cystogram and retrograde urethrogram – the 'up-and-downagram' is an essential pre-repair investigation of urethral injuries because it may reveal abnormalities such as fistulous tracks and false passages that are highly relevant to the extent of the reconstructive procedure; some of these may be difficult or even impossible to identify at operation, particularly in the case of an apparently short-gap defect which might otherwise be deemed suitable for a perineal-approach repair.

Cystographic failure to demonstrate the prostatic urethra is reassuring evidence of bladder neck competence (provided of course it is not stenotic as a result of a coincidental injury); the demonstration of a patulous bladder neck mechanism that remains open at all stages of bladder filling clearly indicates that it is incompetent, either as a result of intrinsic damage or traction tethering by an extensive retropubic haematoma-fibrosis.

Thus, a preoperative 'up-and-downagram' reveals most of the features that identify a pelvic fracture urethral injury as 'complex' and consequently requiring an abdominal approach repair.

However, it is fundamentally important to appreciate that *the radiographical demonstration of a short-gap urethral defect is not a valid basis for the assumption that it is appropriate for a simple perineal approach repair*; this can only be accurately determined by the operative findings at the time of reconstruction. Short gap pelvic fracture urethral defects are sometimes associated with an unpredictable extent of local haematoma-fibrosis that not only compromises the continent, stricture-free result of a perineal-approach anastomotic repair but sometimes makes this virtually impossible when the prostate is found to be encased in 'retropubic concrete' so that the procedure is abandoned: *these are surgical disasters*.

'Gapometry' – measuring the distance between the prostatic and the bulbar urethral contrast or between the tips of retrograde and antegrade sounds – is rarely very helpful and is potentially misleading if the result encourages a surgeon with inadequate experience of repair of complex strictures naively to suppose that a short gap stricture is appropriate for a simple perineal approach and thus fail to make contingency plans for an extended procedure. In practice the gap is of no consequence if an appropriate progression-approach procedure is used.

Options for the management of pelvic fracture urethral defects

The hazards of simple dilatation

If a curved metal dilator is used at an early stage of healing in an attempt to maintain the passage between the distracted ends of the urethra, it may enter the intervening cavity and pass up in front of the prostate; it is then remarkably easy to create an anterior false passage into the bladder base when its wall is softened by the process of healing inflammation.

The hazards of internal urethrotomy

A trial of internal urethrotomy may be appropriate for minimal sub-prostatic pelvic fracture urethral injuries; however, it is unrealistic to suppose that a simple incision into dense haematoma fibrosis will not close immediately. Urethrotomy can only succeed if the incision can extend into a supple expandable tissue plane (*see* p. 6) and the problem with all but the most minimal pelvic fracture urethral injuries is that the sub-puboprostatic space is characteristically obliterated and filled with dense haematoma-fibrosis.

The essential aim of a trial of internal urethrotomy is to avoid inappropriate endeavours that can result in complications:

1. Postero-lateral incisions are generally contraindicated by the proximity of the nervi erigentes in this sector and the consequent risk of secondary damage to potency if this has survived the primary injury.
2. Distal extensions of an incision into the bulbar spongy urethra commonly compromise a subsequent anastomotic repair by foreshortening its length available for overlap anastomosis by an extension of the spongio-fibrosis.
3. Blind 'dead reckoning' endoscopic incisions in search of the distal end of the prostatic urethra embedded in a solid mass of fibrous tissue are particularly hazardous because they may:
   (a) enter the mid-prostatic urethra, compromising a subsequent sub-verumontanal bladder-neck preserving anastomotic repair;
   (b) directly damage the only residual sphincter mechanism at the bladder neck by creating a proximal false passage into the bladder through it;
   (c) create a bladder base false passage fistula which short circuits the bladder neck mechanism and results in incontinence.

The shortcomings of substitution procedures

It is generally unjustifiable to introduce the inherent complications resulting from the shortcomings of substitution procedures (both free patch and pedicled scrotal skin grafts) unless there is a really cogent reason for accepting this risk in an individual case. Occasionally, however, a pelvic fracture urethral defect is associated with an abnormality of the bulbar urethra resulting either from the accident, from an incidental lesion. or more commonly from failure of a previous attempt at its surgical resolution – such a case requires appropriate modification and combination procedures, some of which involve substitution grafts and among these the urothelial-island pedicled bladder flap is particularly useful[15].

The anastomotic repair of urethral distraction injuries

Inspite of the severity of the many and various complicating features that render a pelvic fracture urethral injury 'complex', and irrespective of the length of the prostato-bulbar gap, it is almost invariably possible to achieve a long-term stricture-free restoration of urethral continuity by a one-stage bulbo-prostatic anastomotic repair *provided* both the bulbo-penile spongy urethra and the prostatic urethra are normal[1-3, 27]. Additional injury resulting from failures of previous surgery is unacceptable.

Irrespective of the surgical approach required the long term stricture-free success of a definitive one-stage anastomotic procedure for the restoration of urethral continuity after a pelvic fracture injury is dependent upon:

1. meticulous excision of the peri-urethral and retropubic haematoma-fibrosis together with any fistulating tracks or pockets of infection with it;
2. mobilization of the bulbar urethra to achieve a tension-free approximation of a well-vascularized spatulation of its proximal end to the prostate;
3. meticulous prostato-bulbar anastomotic technique;
4. prevention of the potential complications resulting from a 'dead space' around the anastomosis by filling any fibro-osseus cavity resulting from excision of the haematoma-fibrosis with a mobilized omental pedicle graft.

Because urinary continence is entirely dependent upon the only residual sphincter mechanism at the bladder neck, appropriate additional synchronous procedures are required when the occlusive function of this has also been impaired.

The timing of repair

A definitive repair is best deferred until the healing reaction to injury is virtually complete; the time that this takes is largely dependent upon the size of the pelvic floor haematoma. The haematoma associated with minor injuries is usually minimal so that they are usually ready for repair after about 3 months; a sizeable haematoma may take 4–8 months to resolve and a massive one up to a year. In spite of contrary opinion, when an extensive urethral distraction injury is treated simply by suprapubic catheter drainage without a urethral catheter, it nevertheless results in a significant, and sometimes very extensive mass of dense haematoma-fibrosis and the development of a 'complex' urethral distraction injury.

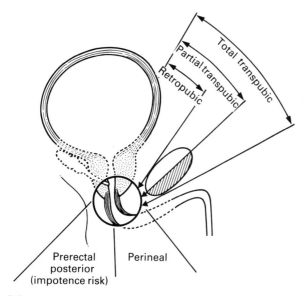

Prerectal posterior (impotence risk)   Perineal

The surgical approach options for the repair of sub-prostatic urethral defects

29

Surgical access for the repair of sub-prostatic urethral defects is complicated by its retropubic location. A number of options are available.

29

The deficiencies of the two-option perineal vs pubectomy approach procedures

There are serious disadvantages in the common urological practice of restricting the surgical approaches to a pelvic fracture urethral injury repair to a choice between the simple perineal and the formal total pubectomy 'Transpubic' without intermediate options that avoid the need for an extensive bone resection.

These disadvantages are greatly augmented when entirely different patient positions are used for these procedures because it is difficult to change an 'exaggerated lithotomy' into a 'frog-leg' in the course of an operation; thus, a surgeon is required to make an arbitrary decision which to use preoperatively.

In marginal cases, the facts upon which the approach decision should be based can only finally be determined at the time of operation. The preoperative decision to confine the repair procedure of a 'short' urethral defect to a perineal-approach procedure can result in an unacceptable incidence of complications that could have been avoided by an extended procedure; these range from incontinence (resulting from failure to pre-identify a coincident incompetence of the bladder neck mechanism), restenosis (resulting from a compromising extent of unsuspected retropubic haematoma fibrosis or para-anastomotic dead space cavity complications) and even to abandonment of the anastomotic repair or procedure to a sub-stricture inlay.

The advantages of the Turner-Warwick Progression-Approach perineo-abdominal procedure

30

The inability accurately to predict the extent of the approach required for a really reliable anastomotic repair of a short gap urethral defect was the prime consideration in the development of the progression-approach anastomotic repair (PAAR) procedure[3]; this facilitates transition from a perineal to a perineo-abdominal approach, with or without partial or total resection of the pubic bone according to the per-operative findings. The patient is positioned with a single perineo-abdominal operating field equally appropriate for any procedure required for the resolution of both 'simple' and 'complex' urethral injuries.

The routine use of the abdomino-perineal position for apparently simple perineal approach repairs has obvious advantages over the exaggerated lithotomy position in as much as it provides the easy option for an abdominal extension of the procedure when the retropubic fibrosis proves unexpectedly extensive. It also has advantages over the 'frog-leg' position for the repair of 'complex' injuries because comfortable access for a perineal approach facilitates the preliminary mobilization of the bulbar urethra and a synchronous perineo-abdominal approach obviates the necessity for a total pubectomy access.

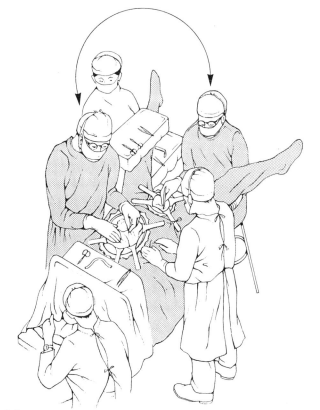

30

The progression approach anastomotic repair procedure

31

An elective definitive repair of a complex pelvic fracture urethral injury is a multi-major-procedural operation which, even with considerable experience, takes at least 3–4 h and sometimes twice this time. Even with excellent haemostatic anaesthesia, a blood loss of 300–500 ml/h must be budgeted for and this presents special problems in children whose circulating volume is relatively small.

The operation cannot be staged, the various individual major components of it are necessarily interrelated. Furthermore, the operation cannot be described as a single procedure because it is in reality a variable combination of a series of distinct surgical procedures appropriately adjusted according to the findings at the time of operation – a TITBAPIT (Take It To Bits And Put It Together) procedure that may involve most if not all of the following procedures.

1. Abdomino-perineal positioning of the patient.
2. Perineal mobilization of the bulbar urethra and excision of the distal stricture scar tissue.
3. Midline lower-abdominal exposure for resection of retropubic haematoma fibrosis.
4. Partial pubic resection access for excision of sub-prostatic haematoma fibrosis and fistulous tracks.
5. Vesicostomy for unequivocal identification of prostatic urethra, examination of bladder neck and removal of coincident bladder stones.
6. Restoration of urethral continuity by spatulated bulbo-prostatic anastomosis.
7. Total resection of pubic bone if supracrural transpubic rerouting of the mobilized bulbar urethra is required to achieve tension-free anastomosis to a high-lying prostatic dislocation.
8. Suprapubic catheter and fenestrated urethral catheter drain.

9. Mobilization of omental graft with extension of midline incision for pedicle mobilization if required, with colonic mobilization, appendicectomy and temporary gastrostomy. Additional synchronous procedures may be required.
10. Excision of osteomyelitic pubic abscess cavities, and fistulous tracks into the rectum.
11. Separation of bladder neck compromising fibrotic adhesions for definitive bladder neck sphincteroplasty.
12. Inlay urethroplasty for coincident anterior urethral stricture.

Thus, a progression-approach anastomotic repair procedure should not be underestimated. The full potential of its success depends upon appropriate subspecialist training, an in-depth experience of the many challenging situations that can arise in the course of a long operation, and sophisticated postoperative care facilities. However, there can be no doubt that it can be one of the most time/cost effective major procedures in the field of surgery. A patient who enters hospital as a urological cripple should have an exceedingly high chance of leaving a few weeks later voiding freely with reasonable urinary control and an expectation of a stricture-free result in the long term without the need for regular urological supervision.

However, because the distal mechanism is destroyed by the original sub-prostatic injury and replaced by a bulbo-prostatic anastomosis with an increased calibre, continence is entirely dependent upon the only remaining sphincter mechanism at the bladder neck. The treatment of any subsequent prostatic obstruction by a transurethral resection inevitably destroys the function of the bladder neck mechanism so that a prostatic obstruction-relieving procedure should be deferred until it is inevitable and then undertaken only by a sphincter-preserving reconstructive procedure[11].

Unfortunately, many patients with complex urethral injuries are impotent; this is a separate consideration and its resolution by the insertion of a penile prosthesis should be deferred until the healing of the urethral reconstruction is complete and its success time-proven.

Simple short stricture
Minimal fibrosis

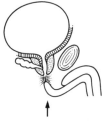

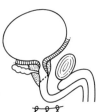

Perineal bulbo-prostatic
anastomosis

Simple stricture
More extensive fibrosis

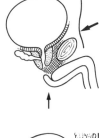

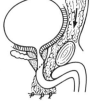

Perineal anastomosis
+ retropubic excision of
fibrosis + omental support

Complex stricture: long with extensive fibrosis
± fistulae ± bladder neck incompetence

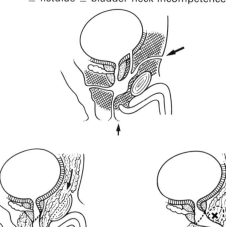

Partial transpubic excision
of fibrosis + bulbo-prostatic
anastomosis + omental support

Total transpubic excision with supra-crus
urethral re-route to bulbo-prostatic
anastomosis + omental support

31

Access and excision of haematoma fibrosis fistulous tracks and abscess pockets

Meticulous and complete excision of all para-urethral and retropubic fibrosis is an essential component of a reliably successful restoration of prostatobulbar urethral continuity after a pelvic fracture injury.

If the para-urethral fibrosis associated with a short gap urethral defect is minimal it can be removed and the prostato-bulbar anastomosis completed from a perineal approach without leaving a significant rigid walled 'dead space' surrounding it – otherwise progression to a synchronous perineo-retropubic approach with omental pedicle graft support of the reconstruction within the cavity is important for the reliable prevention of recurrent stenosis.

When there is extensive retropubic fibrosis a synchronous perineo-retropubic approach is essential for its removal. A midline incision is always used for an abdominal approach so that it can be extended up to the xiphisternum when necessary, to obtain upper abdominal access for the full length mobilization of the gastro-epiploic pedicle when the omentum is short, to enable it to be repositioned to obliterate the dead space and to support the retropubic reconstruction (see p. 510).

32

Because the rectus abdominus tendon is not attached to the pubic crest but extends down in front of it to the inferior margin of the pubis, it can be separated from the front of the pubic bone by sharp dissection and reflected laterally without detaching it; and this greatly improves the width of the retropubic exposure (see Illustration 31)[28]. Access for the removal of the sub-prostatic fibrosis and for anastomosis of the spatulated end of the mobilized bulbar urethra usually requires resection of the upper half of the back of the pubis. This is best achieved with a Capener double curved bone gouge (see Illustration 40). Infected tracks within the haematoma-fibrosis are removed with the block of haematoma-fibrosis. An omental pedicle graft is generally sufficient to resolve any coincident fistulous communication with the rectum (covered of course by a colostomy) or osteomyelitic cavities within the pubic bone after they have been marsupialized into the cavity.

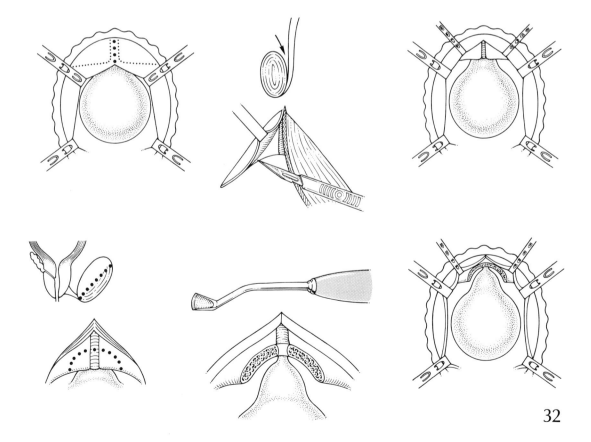

32

Tension-free bulbo-prostatic urethral approximation

33

After division of the urethra at the bulbo-membranous junction, mobilization of a normal bulbar urethra distally to the base of the penis achieves 4–5 cm of elastic lengthening, sufficient to achieve a tension-free 2 cm overlap anastomosis with the apical prostatic urethra after bridging a gap of 2.0–2.5 cm or so. After the anastomosis is completed, tension-relieving sutures between the lateral margins of the mobilized anterior bulbar urethra and the crura on either side are placed to avoid anastomotic distraction by erections during the healing period.

When the prostato-bulbar gap is longer than 2–3 cms as a result of an established major upward dislocation of the prostate, or when the available elongation of the mobilised bulbar urethra has been foreshortened by damage due to previous surgical failures, it may be necessary to re-route the mobilised bulbar urethra transpubically over the crura on one side, to enable it to reach the high-lying prostate – this requires a total resection of the pubis to prevent secondary osseus incarceration – especially in children before bone growth ceases.

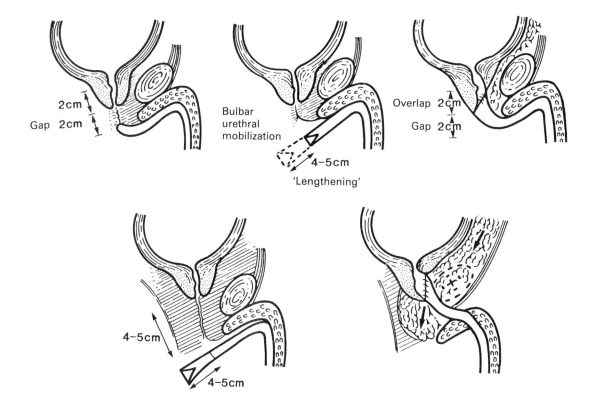

The principles of bulbar urethral mobilization

Care is required to achieve maximum mobilization of the distal spongy urethra in order to obtain a tension-free approximation of its proximal spatulation end to the spatulated distal prostatic urethra without critically impairing its blood supply or creating a penile chordee.

In practice, the maximum available elongation of the anterior spongy urethra is obtained by mobilization of the bulbar urethra – attempts to achieve additional elongation by mobilizing the penile urethra risk both impairment of the blood supply of its proximal end and penile-curvature chordee.

34

The blood supply of the posteriorly mobilized bulbo-spongy urethra

The bulbo-spongy tissue normally receives most of its blood supply from the bulbar arteries posteriorly; when these are divided by proximal urethral transection the retrograde blood flow along normal bulbo-penile spongy tissue derived from its distal vascular communications in the penile area is generally sufficient. However, this may be critically impaired by:

1. over-extensive mobilization of the urethra onto the penile shaft;
2. the coincidence of a hypospadiac deformity in which there is no continuity of the penile spongy urethra with that of the glans;
3. extensive spongiofibrosis resulting from previous urethritis or urethral surgery.

Chordee

35

Because the available longitudinal elasticity of the penile urethra is stretched during an erection, any attempt to gain extra urethral length by mobilizing the penile urethra is likely to result in curvature chordee of the penile shaft.

When the suspensory ligament of the penis is tight, mild tension on a mobilized urethra may result in angulation chordee; this effect can be minimized by dividing the ligament so that the peno-scrotal junction slides back a little rather than acting as a fulcrum – no significant disability results from this. Division of the suspensory ligament is a natural consequence of a pubectomy and is easily achieved through the lower end of a midline incision during a retropubic or partial transpubic procedure; it is equally easy to achieve through the anterior end of a midline perineal incision by simple dissection around one side of the root of the penis.

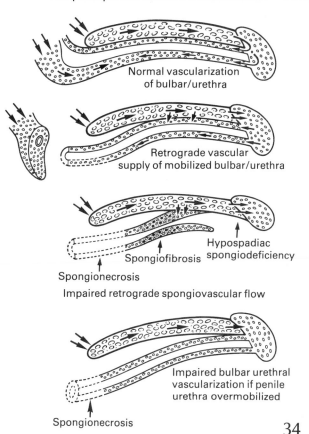

Normal vascularization of bulbar/urethra

Retrograde vascular supply of mobilized bulbar/urethra

Spongionecrosis Spongiofibrosis Hypospadiac spongiodeficiency

Impaired retrograde spongiovascular flow

Impaired bulbar urethral vascularization if penile urethra overmobilized

Spongionecrosis

34

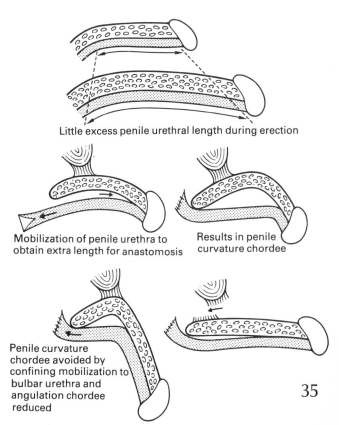

Little excess penile urethral length during erection

Mobilization of penile urethra to obtain extra length for anastomosis

Results in penile curvature chordee

Penile curvature chordee avoided by confining mobilization to bulbar urethra and angulation chordee reduced

35

The spatulated bulbo-prostatic anastomosis

36

In the adult, the normal calibre of both the apical prostatic urethra and the posterior bulbar urethra is at least 25 F and so the calibre of a proficient overlap anastomosis should be 25 + 25 = 50. This short segment of augmented calibre persists as a small localized dilatation on follow-up urethrography, positively excluding any recurrent stenosis.

The distal end of the prostatic urethra is surrounded by apical prostatic tissue. Thus, when the distal 2 cm below the verumontanum is opened by an anterior incision a wedge-resection of the antero-lateral apical prostatic tissue is required on either side; this allows the lateral margins of the spatulated apical urethra to be opened outwards in such a way that they can be laterally anchor-sutured to the prostatic capsule and thus present a flat surface more than 2 cm wide for anastomosis to the bulbar urethra.

Whatever the surgical approach, the anastomotic spatulation of the apical prostatic urethra should be located anteriorly because a meticulous anterior approach bulbar prostatic anastomosis is relatively unlikely to affect potency if this has fully survived the original accident; however, unpreditable variations sometimes occur after repair when the erection mechanism has been partially affected by the accident.

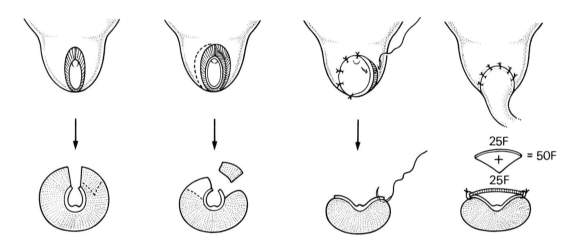

Wedge resection of anterior apical prostatic tissue → required to achieve → fixed flat spatulated anastomosis

36

Omental pedicle graft support

Removal of extensive retropubic fibrosis and any proportion of the back of the pubis required to achieve good access for an abdominal approach bulbo-prostatic anastomosis leaves a sizeable rigid-walled dead space cavity around it. In the author's opinion, the reliable success of the anastomotic repair of a complex pelvic fracture urethral defect is fundamentally dependent upon the routine obliteration of this space and this is best achieved with an omental pedicle graft[3]. The omentum is uniquely adapted for the resolution of local inflammatory processes, not only because of its blood supply, but also because of its abundant lymphatic drainage which absorbs inflammatory cell debris and macro-molecular protein exudates that would otherwise result in purulent accumulations. Furthermore, once an inflammatory situation has resolved, the omentum always regains its suppleness and consequently ensures that the freedom of the functional movement of any part of the urinary tract that it envelops is not impaired by the secondary fibrosis that commonly develops in peri-ureteric and retropubic fat – omental wrapping is often fundamental to the urodynamic success of complex refunctional procedures such as sphincteroplasty and reduces the incidence of complications after the surgical repair and reconstruction of the urinary tract[29, 30].

The principles of omental redeployment

37

The lower margin of the omental apron is long enough to reach the pelvic floor and the perineum without mobilization of its vascular pedicle in about 30 per cent of cases; however, it should always be separated from its natural adhesion to the transverse colon and mesocolic vessels to avoid postoperative gaseous distension of the bowel which may cause traction and dislocation of the interposition graft.

In about 30 per cent of cases sufficient elongation of a moderate length apron can be achieved by dividing the relatively small contribution to its blood supply from branches of the splenic vessels on the left. Meticulous full length mobilization of the whole length of the right gastro-epiploic pedicle is required to enable the omentum to reach the pelvis in about 30 per cent of patients[29, 30].

The blood supply of the omentum

The preservation of the 'magic' of the omentum during its mobilization is dependent upon the preservation of the 'pulsating efficiency' of its vascularization and naturally therefore upon an accurate knowledge of the anatomical features of this. Unfortunately, many of the mobilization procedures illustrated in surgical and gynaecological text base this upon the minor vascular pedicle on the left or simply elongate the apron by horizontal incisions:

1. The blood supply of the omentum is derived from vertically running vessels arising from the gastroepiploic arch with relatively poor arcade communications between them; thus, when providing graft-support for

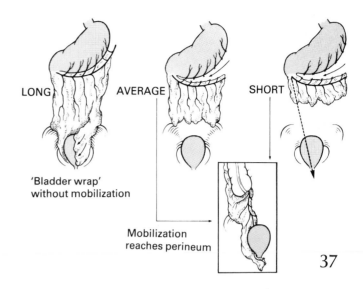

'Bladder wrap' without mobilization

Mobilization reaches perineum

37

an upper urinary tract reconstruction on one side, the two halves of the omental apron can often be separated in the midline without providing a collateral blood vessel that is sufficiently large to require ligation. It follows that elongation of the omental apron by a horizontal incision below the gastro-epiploic arch involves the division of a number of its vertical vessels which, to some extent, impairs the efficiency of the vascularization of the extremity of the graft.

2. The main origin of the gastro-epiploic vascular arcade is always from the right side; in fact, the junction between the right and the left gastroepiploic vessels that usually completes the arcade is deficient in about 10 per cent of cases at a point on the left side of the greater curvature of the stomach. It follows that mobilization of a short apron omentum must be based on the right gastro-epiploic vessels, not the left; this is fortunate for mechanical reasons because the origin of the right gastro-epiploic vessels from the gastro-duodenal vessels is much lower in the abdomen than the origin of the left gastro-epiploic vessels from the splenic vessels, so that when the full length of the gastro-epiploic arch is mobilized from the greater curvature of the stomach by meticulous individual ligation division of its 30–40 short gastric branches after division of its left pedicle, its extremity is long enough to reach the pelvis irrespective of the vertical length of the apron; thus, the omentum can be used in children when the apron is underdeveloped.

Technical details of omental mobilization

A midline abdominal wall incision must always be used whenever there is any possibility that a reconstruction in the pelvis may require omental support; it can be extended upwards to provide appropriate surgical access to the stomach for the meticulous mobilization of its pedicle vessels when necessary.

Technical details of omental mobilization are described in the chapter on 'Repair of urinary vaginal fistulae', pp. 374–391.

The restoration of bladder neck sphincter function

The cystographic demonstration of an incompetent bladder neck mechanism is in itself, a definitive indication of the need for a lower abdominal exploration even if the urethral defect is otherwise suitable for a perineal repair.

The commonest cause of incompetence of the bladder neck mechanism after a pelvic fracture urethral injury is outward tethering by retropubic haematoma-fibrosis; the endoscopic appearances are those of a fixedly open but otherwise normal circular bladder neck mechanism and simple lysis by resection of the fibrosis anteriorly and laterally, and its replacement by a supple omental graft, is usually all that is necessary to restore its competence (see p. 510).

Cystographic evidence of this type of bladder neck incompetence is particularly important when the retropubic fibrosis is the result of a separate pelvic floor haematoma which is not in continuity with minimal fibrosis associated with a short-gap urethral lesion, so that its critical extent might not be recognized during a simple perineal repair; however, much more commonly, they are in continuity so that the upward extent of the fibrosis requiring an extension to a retropubic approach is readily apparent on perineal exploration (see p. 482).

Incompetence of the bladder neck resulting from a segmental injury of the mechanism itself is generally indicated by the endoscopic identification of a notched scar in one sector of its circumference, the location of which varies according to its cause.

When this lies anteriorly a reduction-sphincteroplasty is not a particularly intricate procedure and the results can be remarkably satisfactory[31].

A formal bladder neck reduction-sphincteroplasty should not be undertaken simply because transvesical examination of the lax bladder neck allows entry of the finger tip; many such mechanisms prove to be functionally competent and if they do not a sphincteroplasty can be undertaken at a later date, a re-exploration which is greatly facilitated by routine omental wrapping of the primary procedure.

Perineal bulboprostatic spatulated anastomosis

38

The bulbar urethra is exposed through a midline perineal incision. The posterior bulbar spongy tissue lies predominantly behind the urethra so it is useful to leave it *in situ* as a posterior flap. The bulbar urethra is fully mobilized to the penoscrotal junction; the membranous urethral stricture is dilated and any areas of dense fibrosis carefully resected to create a supple-walled tunnel to the apex of the prostatic urethra which is opened anteriorly below the verumontanum. The lateral apical prostatic tissue is wedge-resected so that the spatulated distal prostatic urethra can be spread open and suture-anchored laterally to present a flat surface for anastomosis to the invaginated spatulated bulbar urethra after the excess of spongy tissue has been trimmed from it; the insertion of these 3/0 Dexon sutures is facilitated by the fibrelight posterior urethral retractor and the posterior urethral needles (see *Illustration* 20).

At the conclusion of the anastomosis the flap of posterior bulbar spongy tissue is sutured to the bulbar urethra to overclose the suture line and hold it in an invaginated position; push-in tension-relieving sutures also anchor the lateral margins of the mobilized bulbar urethra to the membrane.

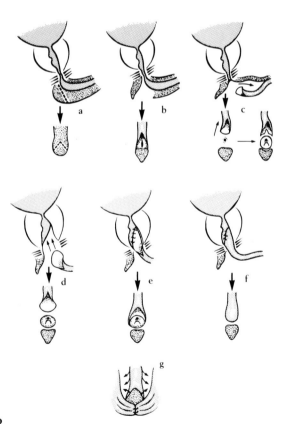

The perineo-abdominal repair of a complex pelvic fracture urethral distraction injury

39

Good access is provided by a partial-pubectomy approach. The fibro-osseous cavity surrounding the prostato-bulbar anastomosis that results from the excision of the extensive haematoma-fibrosis and the fistulous tracks within it is occluded with a mobilized omental pedicle graft. A coincident rectal fistula does not greatly complicate such a repair but it should, of course, be covered by a temporary colostomy.

Instruments for urethroplasty

40 & 41

All perineal operations, and urethral reconstructions in particular, are facilitated by the self-retaining ring retractor with stay-suture directional guide knobs and six blades; the edges of the 'perineal' side of the smallest ring are bevelled so that the retractor blades can dip in to align automatically. This is one element of the universal Turner Warwick abdomino-perineal ring retractor set.

The Hey-Groves half-circle sound (*see Illustration* 40a) with a subterminal suture hole; introduced retrogradely, this facilitates the accurate introduction of a suprapubic catheter; passed transvesically into the prostatic urethra, it facilitates the perineal repair of a pelvic fracture urethral defect.

The Capener double curved bone gouge (*see Illustration* 40b), designed for hip surgery, is ideal for partial or total resection of the pubic bone required for the abdomino-perineal repair of pelvic fracture urethral defects.

42

The Turner Warwick fibrelight sucker combines two important facilities. The connections of the suction tube and the light cable provide the handle; there is an air bleed hole immediately in front of the finger ring to adjust the suction pressure and another distal air bleed to reduce the blood film on the fibrelight face. This instrument is essential for posterior urethral inlay sutures and the perineal anastomotic repair of pelvic fracture urethral defects.

43

The Turner Warwick angulated needle holder allows suture needles to be visualized continuously while working in deep cavities without the hand obstructing the line of vision.

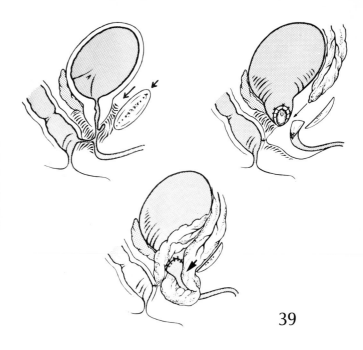

39

44

The blades of the self-retaining Turner Warwick fibrelight posterior urethral retractor are calibrating; they are 9 mm wide so that when they are opened to an equivalent amount, the calibre of the posterior urethra is 4 × 9 mm = 36 mm/F.

The Turner Warwick posterior urethral needles are supplied with three curves; the fully curved needle is shaped so that it can rotate within the blades of the posterior urethral speculum (*see Illustration 20*).

45

Teal's probe pointed gougette, designed last century for perineal vesical lithotomy, requires no modification to facilitate the insertion of antero-lateral posterior urethral sutures.

46

Six double-ended Canny-Ryall meatal dilators conveniently span the range of 3–36 F required for per-operative urethral probing, dilating and calibrating.

To eliminate unnecessary light reflection, the surfaces of all Turner Warwick instruments are finished matt black, with the exception of the tip of the posterior urethral needles and the inner surfaces of the retractor blades.

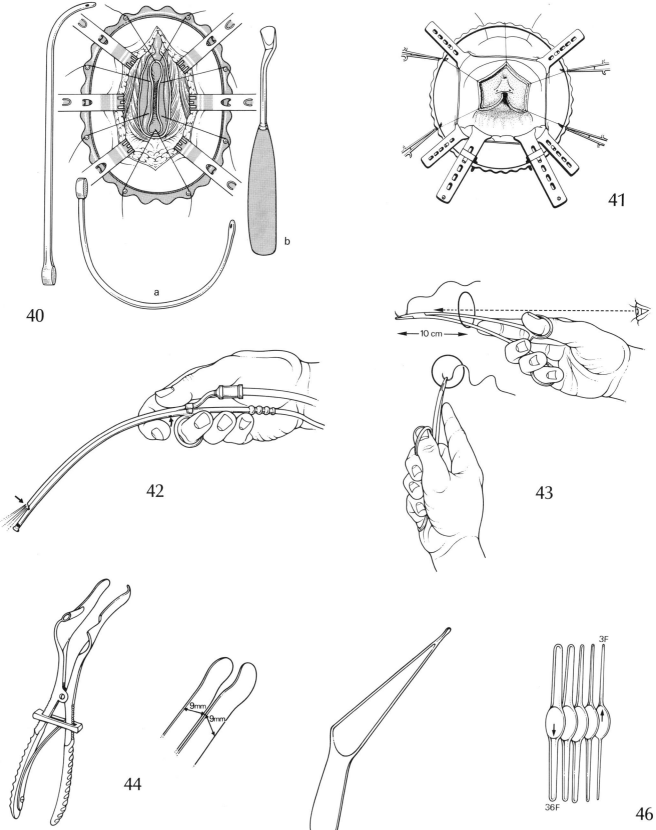

Conclusion

While some techniques for the resolution of urethral strictures such as urethral dilatation and internal urethrotomy can be regarded as general urological procedures, the problems involved in definitive urethral reconstruction should not be underestimated. It is essential to appreciate that any operative procedure that fails, however well intentioned and well performed, inevitably complicates a subsequent retrievoplasty and damage to the distal urethral mechanism is virtually irrepairable.

While there can be no question of a particular 'right' way of doing any surgical procedure, there are certainly many 'wrong' ways. The avoidance of complications is the essence of good surgery and essentially a personal matter because many contrarily conceived procedures work quite satisfactorily in the hands of others. Consequently many of the views expressed in this chapter are essentially personal and references to personal publications are made to substantiate statements; however no one is more conscious than I am of the contributions of many friends and colleagues across the world who are interested in this most intriguing field of surgery. I am also particularly grateful to the many who have most generously referred the patients and who thus created the series of several thousand operations upon which this communication is based.

References

1. Turner Warwick, R. The principles of functional reconstruction of the lower urinary tract. In: Bevan, P. G. ed. Reconstructive procedures in surgery. Oxford: Blackwell Scientific Publications, 1982: 193–233

2. Turner Warwick, R. Urethral stricture surgery. In: Glenn, J., Boyce, G. eds. Urologic surgery, 3rd ed, Philadelphia: Lippincott, 1983: 689–719

3. Turner Warwick, R. T. Observations on the treatment of traumatic urethral injuries and the value of the fenestrated urethral catheter. British Journal of Surgery 1973; 60: 775–781

4. Turner Warwick, R. T. The repair of urethral strictures in the region of the membranous urethra. Journal of Urology 1968; 100: 303–314

5. Turner Warwick, R. Clinical urodynamics. Urologic Clinics of North America, 1979; 13–30

6. Turner Warwick, R. Clinical problems associated with urodynamic abnormalities with special reference to the value of synchronous cine/pressure/flow cystography and the clinical importance of detrusor function studies. In: Lutzeyer, W., Melchoir, H. eds. Urodynamics: upper and lower urinary tract. Berlin: Springer Verlag, 1973; 237–263.

7. Turner Warwick, R. The sphincter mechanisms: their relation to prostatic enlargement and its treatment. In: Hinman, F. ed. Benign prostatic hypertrophy. New York: Springer Verlag 1983; 809–828

8. Turner Warwick, R. The sphincter mechanism – the avoidance of post-prostatectomy incontinence. In: Weber, W., Jonas, D., eds. Die Post Operative Harninkontinenz des Mannes. Internationales Symposium, Frankfurt an Main 1979. Stuttgart: Thieme; 1981: 17–33

9. Chilton, C. The distal urethral sphincter mechanism and the pelvic floor. In: Munday, A. R., Stephenson, T. P., Weir, A. J., eds. Urodynamics: principles, practice and application. Edinburgh: Churchill Livingstone 1984: 9–13

10. Turner Warwick, R. Repair of urethral strictures in the male. In: Rob. C., Smith, R., eds. Operative Surgery: urology 3rd edn, London: Butterworths 1977: 315–342

11. Turner Warwick, R. T. Bladder outflow obstruction in the male. In: Mundy, A., Stephenson, T. P., Wein, A., eds. Urodynamics; principles, practice and application. Edinburgh: Churchill Livingstone 1984: 183–204

12. Gibbon, N. A new type of catheter for urethral drainage of the bladder. British Journal of Urology 1958; 30: 1–7

13. Turner Warwick, R. Observations upon techniques for reconstruction of the urethral meatus, the hypospadiac glans deformity and the penile urethra. Urologic Clinics of North American 1979; 6: 643–655

14. Turner Warwick, R. The back-to-back double sided foreskin tube-flap glans urethro meatoplasty. British Association of Urological Surgeons Meeting 1985 (To be published in the British Journal of Urology)

15. Turner Warwick, R. T. The use of pedicle grafts in the repair of urinary tract fistulae. British Journal of Urology 1972; 44: 644–656

16. Duckett, J. W. The island flap technique for hypospadias repair. Urologic Clinics of North America 1981; 8: 503–512

17. Orandi, A. One-stage urethroplasty; four year follow-up Journal of Urology 1972; 107: 977–980

18. Duplay, S. Sur le traitement chirurgical de l'hypospadias et de l'episadias. Archives générales de médecine. 1880; 145: 257–274

19. Turner Warwick, R. A technique of posterior urethroplasty. Journal of Urology 1960; 83: 416–419

20. Gil Vernet, J. M. Un traitement des sténoses traumatiques et inflammatoires de l'urètre postérieur. Nouvelle méthode d'uretroplastie. Journal d'Urologie et de Nephrologie. 1966: 72: 97–108

21. Blandy, J. P., Singh, M., Tressider, G. C. Urethroplasty by scrotal flap for long urethral strictures. British Journal of Urology 1968; 40: 261–267

22. Leadbetter, G. W. A simplified urethroplasty for strictures of the bulbous urethra. Journal of Urology 1960; 83: 54–59

23. Devine, C. J., Horton, C. E. One-stage hypospadias repair. Journal of Urology 1961; 85: 166–172

24. Turner Warwick, R. Post-prostatectomy strictures. In: Hinman, F. ed. Benign prostatic hypertrophy. New York: Springer Verlag, 1983

25. Smith, J. The measurement and significance of the urinary flow rate. British Journal of Urology 1966; 38: 701–706

26. Turner Warwick, R., Pitfield-Marshall, J. Outpatient evaluation of lower urinary tract function and dysfunction. In: Kaye, K. W. ed. Outpatient Urologic Investigation, 1983: pp. 92–108

27. Turner Warwick, R., Thomas, D., Pengelly, A. W. The results of pelvic fracture urethral distraction strictures. British Association of Urological Surgeons Meeting 1984 (To be published in the British Journal of Urology)

28. Turner Warwick, R. Improving the access to retropubic space. (To be published in the British Journal of Urology)

29. Turner Warwick, R., Wynne, E. J. C., Handley Ashken, M. The use of the omental pedicle graft in the repair and reconstruction of the urinary tract. British Journal of Surgery 1967; 54: 849–853

30. Turner Warwick, R. The use of the omental pedicle graft in urinary tract reconstruction. Journal of Urology 1976; 116: 341–347

31. Turner Warwick, R., Nesbitt, T., Kirby, R., Fitzgibbon, H. The role of the bladder neck mechanism in the control of urine after pelvic fracture urethral injuries – and its surgical resurrection. British Association of Urological Surgeons Meeting (To be published in the British Journal of Urology)

Illustrations by Robert N. Lane

Operations on the urethra

P. H. L. Worth   MB, BChir, FRCS
Consultant Urologist, University College Hospital and St Peter's Hospital, London, UK

Introduction

For all operations on the female urethra the patient should be in the lithotomy position. A posterior vaginal retractor will provide simple weight retraction and help vision and access. All sutures used should be absorbable and those used adjacent to the urethral epithelium need not be stronger than 3/0 chromic catgut or its equivalent.

In the male the position will depend on the anatomical site of the problem. Anterior urethral surgery can be done with the patient lying flat, but for operations on the bulbar urethra the full lithotomy position is required.

The operations

URETHRAL OBSTRUCTION IN THE FEMALE

The diagnosis can only satisfactorily be made by cystography together with flow studies. Urethroscopic appearances can be misleading, and the absolute size of the urethra is irrelevant. Obstruction, other than at the bladder neck, can be treated by dilatation or internal urethrotomy. When urethrotomy is done the urethra is calibrated with an Otis urethrotome. The calibration is increased by 10 points and an incision is made at 12 o'clock.

CARUNCLE

A caruncle is a polypoidal growth visible without instrumentation on part of the circumference of the external urinary meatus. It can be treated by simple diathermy or by local excision. Stay sutures are inserted lateral to the lesion and a small portion of normal epithelium adjacent to the lesion is excised. The defect is closed with interrupted sutures.

URETHRAL PROLAPSE

This is a circumferential eversion of the mucosa. If the patient presents with an irreducible prolapse she should be kept in bed with the foot of the bed elevated and treated with an indwelling urethral catheter and cold compresses. Surgical excision should be done as an elective procedure.

1

Four stay sutures are inserted adjacent to the prolapse and the epithelium is separated from the underlying muscularis. When sufficient epithelium has been mobilized an incision is made in one quadrant into the lumen of the urethra. The urethral epithelium should be held gently with non-crushing forceps to prevent it from retracting. The incision is then continued around the circumference of the urethra.

2

Four to eight sutures are inserted to approximate the urethral and vaginal epithelium. If anterior vaginal wall prolapse is also present, an anterior colporrhaphy should be carried out at the same time. Catheter drainage is required for 5 days.

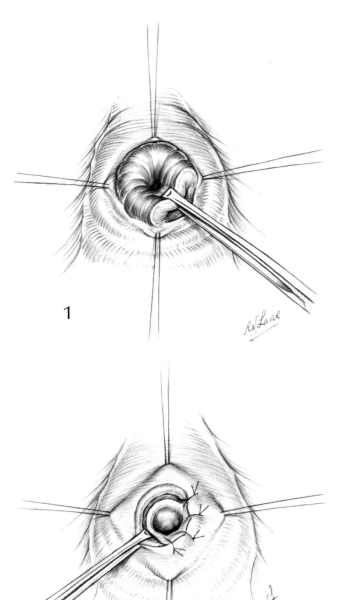

1

2

PERIURETHRAL ABSCESS

This is very rare in the female and should be treated by incision and drainage. The possibility of an associated urethral diverticulum should be considered; if present, it must be treated.

In the male a periurethral abscess is usually related to a urethral stricture. The abscess should be drained adequately and the wall biopsied to exclude tuberculosis or tumour. A formal suprapubic cystostomy should be carried out to drain the bladder until the inflammation settles. A stricture, when present, should then be treated in the appropriate manner.

URETHRAL DIVERTICULUM IN THE FEMALE

Symptoms range from difficulty and discomfort when passing urine to a purulent discharge. The overall incidence is about 3 per cent. Diverticula are usually acquired and are often symptomless, and should not be treated unless they cause trouble. On examination there may be localized urethral tenderness, and a mass may be present.

The diagnosis is probably best made on voiding micturating cystography, rather than urethrography. This will given useful information about the competence or otherwise of the bladder neck. At operation the site of the opening of the diverticulum should be identified through a panendoscope. It sometimes helps to pass a ureteric catheter into the lumen of the diverticulum.

Formal excision

3, 4 & 5

The incision may either be U-shaped, based inferiorly or laterally, or longitudinal and made directly over the diverticulum. The dome of the diverticulum is identified and separated from the surrounding adventitia. The neck is cleared and divided and the urethral defect is closed transversely. The vaginal epithelium is closed in 2 layers with 2/0 chromic catgut.

Alternatively the urethra can be opened by cutting from the external meatus to the opening of the diverticulum, which is then freed and excised. The urethra is reconstructed with interrupted sutures (3/0) and the vagina closed.

Marsupialization of the diverticulum

A longitudinal incision is made over the diverticulum, which is then opened. No attempt is made to excise it, but the edges are sewn to the vagina. This technique can only be used if the bladder neck is known to be competent.

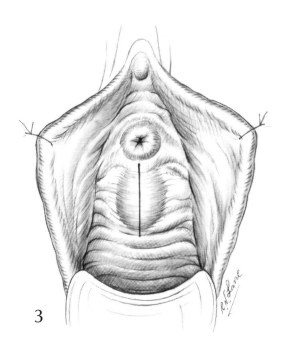

3

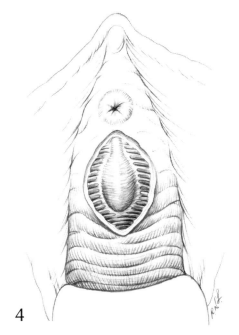

4

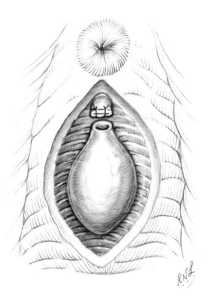

5

6

Alternatively the urethra can be split from the meatus to the opening of the diverticulum. The excess tissue is excised and the back layer of the diverticulum is sewn to the vagina, leaving a female hypospadias.

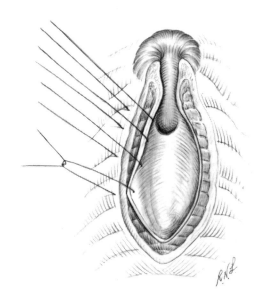

6

URETHRAL CARCINOMA IN THE FEMALE

When this involves the lower third of the urethra local excision may be adequate. The technique used is similar to that for excising a mucosal prolapse. If the proximal part of the urethra is involved, radical cystourethrectomy with radiotherapy is necessary.

URETHRAL DIVERTICULUM IN THE MALE

Congenital diverticula are found in the anterior urethra and may cause obstruction by compressing the urethra. Small diverticula in the bulbar urethra may cause postmicturition dribble. Large diverticula may develop following the treatment of a ruptured urethra when traction has been applied to a urethral catheter.

The diagnosis and anatomical site is made by a micturating cystourethrogram. Do not confuse a diverticulum with a baggy urethra after urethroplasty. The diverticulum should be identified endoscopically. An incision is made over it. The bulbocavernosus is separated from it. The excess epithelium is excised and the urethra closed with interrupted 3/0 sutures over a 16 Fr catheter. The muscle and skin are closed separately. The catheter is left for 10 days.

FEMALE URETHRAL RECONSTRUCTION

If the urethra has been damaged either surgically or traumatically a stricture may develop; this may be associated with a fistula. If the adjacent urethra is normal the damaged segment can be excised and an end-to-end anastomosis performed using 3/0 sutures. With more extensive damage the repair can be supported by a Martius graft (*see* chapter on 'Repair of urinary vaginal fistulae', pp. 374–391). If the proximal urethra and bladder neck have been damaged and primary repair is impossible, either a Tanagho anterior bladder flap or a Leadbetter trigonal tube can be fashioned (*see* chapter on 'Exstrophy', pp. 392–405, for a description of the latter technique).

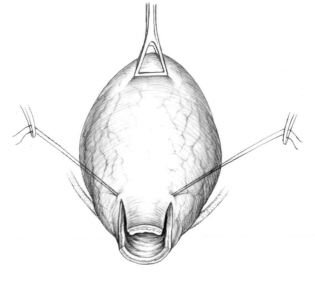

Tanagho anterior bladder flap

7 & 8

The bladder neck is identified through a suprapubic approach. A flap 2.5 cm long and 2.5 cm wide is marked out on the anterior bladder wall with stay sutures. The bladder is opened transversely at the level of the bladder neck and the incision carried posteriorly until the bladder is totally separated from the urethra. The posterior wall of the bladder is mobilized for a short distance. The flap is cut and closed around a 14 Fr catheter with interrupted 3/0 sutures (catgut or Dexon). The apex of the trigone is sewn to the base of the flap and the lateral defects are closed with interrupted sutures. The tube is anastomosed to the distal urethra, when present, or to the epithelium at the site of the urethral meatus with 6–8 interrupted sutures.

The bladder is held up to the retropubic space by attaching the top of the new urethra to the back of the symphysis with 2/0 sutures. If there is a lot of scarring it may be wise to consider formal mobilization of the omentum to fill the cavity and support the new urethra and bladder neck.

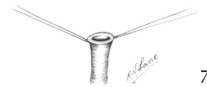

7

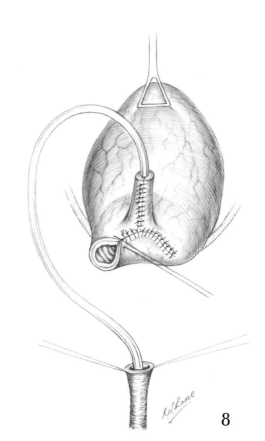

8

Further reading

Spence, H. M., Duckett, J. W. Diverticulum of the female urethra, clinical aspects and presentation of a simple operative technique for cure. Journal of Urology 1970; 104: 432–437

Woodhouse, C. R. J., Flynn, J. T., Molland, E. A., Blandy, J. P. Urethral diverticulum in females. British Journal of Urology 1980; 52: 305–310

Tanagho, E. A. Bladder neck reconstruction for total urinary incontinence: 10 years of experience. Journal of Urology 1981; 125: 321–326

Illustrations by Barbara N. Rankin

Urethrectomy

W. Scott McDougal MD
Professor and Chairman, Department of Urology,
Vanderbilt University Medical Center, Nashville, Tennessee, USA

Introduction

The indications for urethrectomy invariably involve the presence of a malignancy within the urethra or the potential for developing one. Approximately 12.5 per cent of patients undergoing cystectomy for bladder malignancy have either concurrent microscopic evident of carcinoma in the urethra or marked cellular atypia[1]. Moreover, 4–12 per cent of patients develop a malignancy in the retained urethra following cystectomy[1, 2, 3]. Not only is the urethra frequently involved in malignant or premalignant lesions, but the meatus has also been reported as the site of recurrent disease, particularly in patients in whom gross evidence of a urethral malignancy is in evidence at the time of urethrectomy[4]. If a patient undergoing cystectomy for bladder cancer has a urethra with carcinoma *in situ*, neoplasia or concomitant prostatic involvement, then an *en bloc* cystoprostatourethrectomy should be performed. Where the urethra is left in place following radical cystectomy for malignant disease, patients should be examined at regular intervals, with cytological washings of the retained stump, urethroscopy and biopsy when indicated. If the bladder has already been removed, the technique described below for *en bloc* cystoprostatourethrectomy may be used with the following modifications: the patient is placed in lithotomy rather than supine position, and no abdominal incision is required.

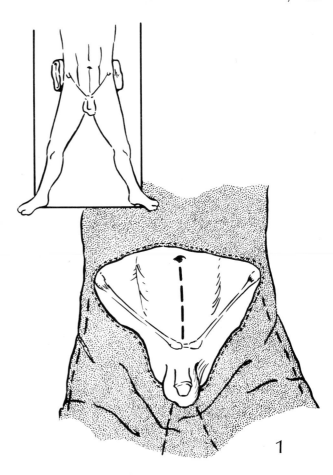

1

The operation

1

The patient is placed in the supine position with a 10 cm roll beneath the buttocks and the legs spread slightly apart. Drapes are placed to expose the abdomen, penis, scrotum and half the perineum (the rectum is excluded) and a Foley catheter is introduced into the bladder through the urethra.

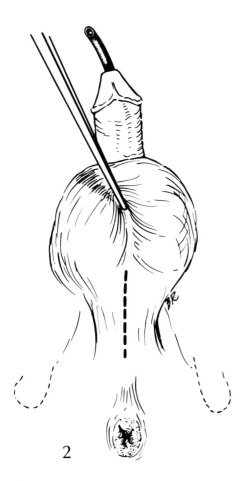

2

Following the pelvic lymphadenectomy, the bladder and prostate are mobilized in the standard radical manner; however, the puboprostatic ligaments are left attached. A 4–5 cm vertical incision is made, centred over the base of the scrotum.

3

The bulbocavernosus muscle is incised and the corpus spongiosum urethra identified and encircled with an umbilical tape. A Moynihan clamp is placed on the Foley catheter at the meatus and the catheter is transected distally. The corpus spongiosum urethra is dissected in a distal direction from the adjacent corpora cavernosa and Buck's fascia. Multiple small vessels are transected in the process and bleeding is easily controlled with the electrocautery unit. During the dissection, the penis inverts keeping the operative field within the confines of the perineal incision. The dissection is carried distally to the fossa navicularis. The penis is returned to its normal position and a circular incision is made on the glans, around the catheter, down to the level of the freely dissected urethra.

4

The urethra and meatus are thus freed from the perineum to the glans and can be gently brought out through the perineal wound. Care must be taken not to pull too hard on the urethra which is easily torn. Attention is then directed towards the perineum. Using sharp dissection, the urethra is freed to the urogenital diaphragm. Several arteries to the bulbocavernosus muscle are identified, ligated and transected. The urethra is freed circumferentially from the urogenital diaphragm. At this juncture the puboprostatic ligaments are approached through the abdominal incision and transected.

One finger enters the pelvis through the suprapubic wound. With a second finger in the perineal wound all remaining attachments are freed by blunt finger dissection and the entire specimen is removed intact through the abdominal incision.

It is important to keep the urethral Foley catheter in place throughout the entire dissection to prevent inadvertent disruption of the specimen. The perineal wound is closed in layers with reabsorbable sutures and no drain is required in either the meatus or the perineal wound.

Postoperative course

Following urethrectomy, particularly when the *en bloc* cystoprostatourethrectomy method is used, penile oedema often results as well as scrotal and penile ecchymosis. The oedema resolves in 3–4 days and the ecchymosis by 7–10 days. There is minimal blood loss with this technique, and when the *en bloc* cystoprostatourethrectomy is utilized operative time is not greatly increased.

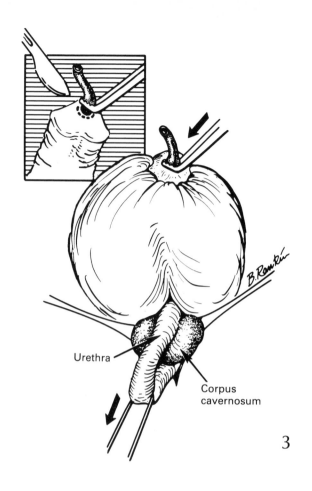

Urethra

Corpus cavernosum

3

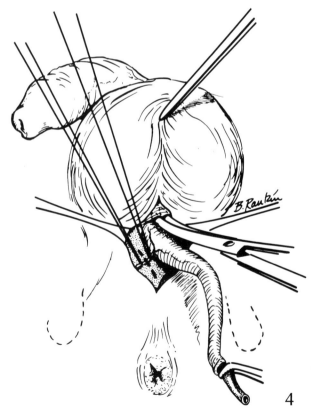

4

References

1. Schellhammer, P. F., Whitmore, W. F. Transitional cell carcinoma of the urethra in men having cystectomy for bladder cancer. Journal of Urology 1976; 115: 56–60

2. Poole-Wilson, D. S., Barnard, R. J. Total cystectomy for bladder tumors. British Journal of Urology 1971; 43: 16–24

3. Cordonnier, J. J., Spjut, H. J. Urethral occurrence of bladder carcinoma following cystectomy. Journal of Urology 1962; 87: 398–403

4. Schellhammer, P. F., Whitmore, W. F. Urethral meatal carcinoma following cystourethrectomy for bladder carcinoma. Journal of Urology 1976; 115: 61–64

5. Whitmore, W. F., Mount, B. M. A technique of urethrectomy in the male. Surgery, Gynecology and Obstetrics 1970; 131: 303–305

Congenital urethral abnormalities in children

Herbert B. Eckstein   MD, MChir, FRCS
Consultant Paediatric Surgeon, Hospital for Sick Children, Great Ormond Street, London, UK

Introduction

Whether some of these lesions are regarded as rare or common tends to depend more on the personal points of view of the surgeon and his colleagues than on scientific fact. The relevance of this introductory remark will be discussed in the various sections of this chapter.

1

Three tracings of different cystourethrograms in girls, all of which should be regarded as normal. Note the variable distensibility of the female urethra within different individuals

Urethral stenosis

Urethral stenosis is a very unusual finding as an isolated abnormality. Stenosis following exstrophy or epispadias repair is a different matter and will be discussed elsewhere. There are no clear-cut symptoms in relation to urethral stenosis, although the condition has been blamed for urinary tract infection secondary to turbulence of the stream or to residual urine.

1

The diagnosis is invariably established radiologically and a cystourethrogram is the key mode of investigation. Cystomanometry and a urethral pressure profile may provide additional information but are no substitute for careful radiological study. The difficulty in making the diagnosis is the enormous variation in size (width), and above all in distensibility, of the urethral wall during micturition and this in turn is dependent on the laxity and quantity of the para-urethral tissues. A lax urethra may distend easily and apparently excessively so that there may be a relative narrowing of the distal third of the urethra (which always has a firmer supporting wall than the proximal two-thirds) and this is mistaken as a 'distal' urethral stenosis.

The treatment (if necessary) is urethral dilatation and it is of note that it is definitely unusual to confirm a mechanical stenosis with urethral sounds passed under general anaesthesia. While urethral dysfunction should certainly be treated by urethral dilatation, it is not right to assume that the cause of urethral dysfunction is urethral stenosis.

Meatal stenosis

2

Meatal stenosis refers only to the terminal few millimetres of the urethra. The size of the urethral opening can be assessed by careful clinical examination and confirmed by the passage of graduated sounds or, better still, by 'bougie à boule'. On withdrawing the bougie a stenotic ring may be demonstrated.

The symptomatology is usually vague and often related to urinary tract infections, or there may be episodes of frequency and dysuria even in the absence of urinary infection. Difficulty with micturition is an unusual symptom in little girls, even when the urethral meatus appears to be genuinely tight, but hesitancy during micturition is a not infrequent symptom. This has, however, to be asked about as spontaneous mention by the child herself is unusual.

The approximate sizes of the urethra are given as follows[1]: 0–4 years (15 Fr); 5–9 years (17 Fr); 10–14 years (21 Fr). Dilatation to 22 Fr is often possible at any age over 2 years.

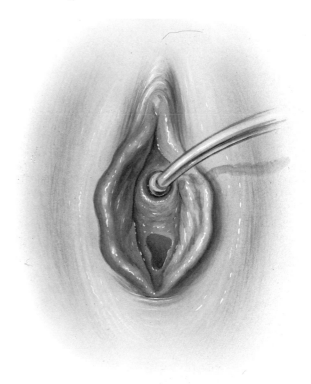

2

3a, b & c

If progressive dilatation (with rupture of some of the circular fibres) fails to relieve the stenosis, a meatotomy should be performed. The Otis urethrotome (a) is suitable for older girls while the Storz-Hertel urethrotome (b and c) can be used at any age.

Following urethrotomy, catheter drainage of the bladder is recommended for 24–48 hours.

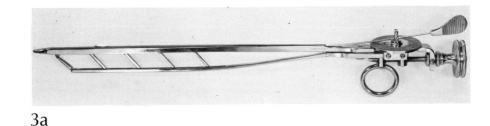

3a

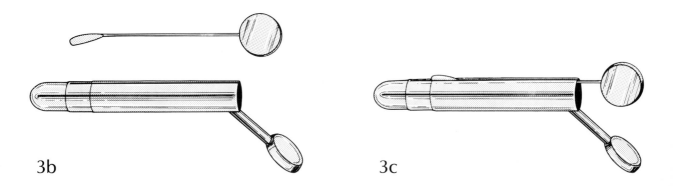

3b   3c

Urethral prolapse

4

Urethral prolapse is unusual in children. It may present with dysuria, urethral bleeding or discharge or contact pain and the diagnosis is self-evident at clinical examination. The lesion is usually annular but may affect one segment of the urethral opening only. It is important to consider a rhabdomyosarcoma in the differential diagnosis, especially if the lesion is not annular.

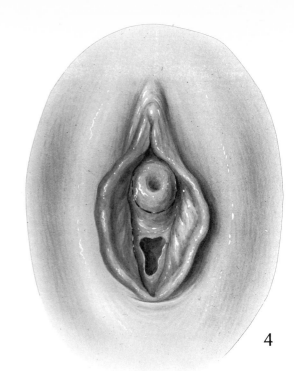

4

5

The lesion may respond to local therapy (using anti-inflammatory drugs) or to Sitz-baths but, should these fail, surgical treatment is needed. In mild cases, radial incision with diathermy coagulation may be used to reduce the bulk of the prolapsed tissue.

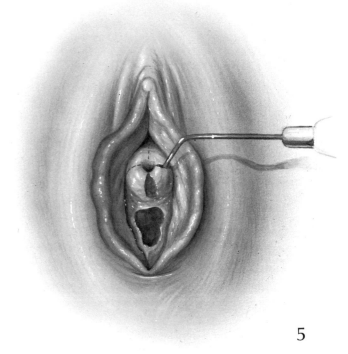

5

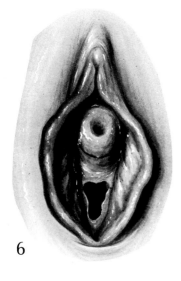

6

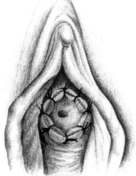

7

6 & 7

In the more extensive case, the prolapsed urethra should be resected and the defect repaired with interrupted absorbable sutures. Excessive shortening of the urethral mucosa must be avoided.

Postoperative catheter drainage for 48 hours is recommended after both procedures. It is of note that meatal stricture following these procedures is exceedingly uncommon.

Urethral duplications

Urethral duplication as an isolated congenital abnormality is very rare and may at times pose very difficult problems where treatment is concerned. On the other hand, limited degrees of urethral duplication are commonly associated with hypospadias and can usually be corrected at the time of the hypospadias correction procedure[2].

8

The accessory urethra is invariably dorsal to the functioning one and the orifice of the accessory urethra is always more distal in position on the shaft of the penis or the glans in patients with hypospadias than is the meatus of the functional urethra. The accessory urethra usually extends for a few centimetres only in a proximal direction and virtually never communicates with the urethra at a higher level or with the bladder.

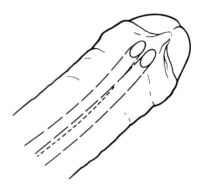

8

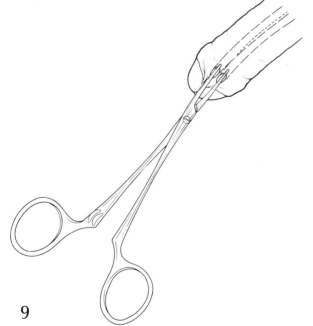

9

9

A short segment of duplication (2–3 cm) is best dealt with by inserting a narrow fine straight haemostat in such a way that one of its blades is in the urethra proper while the second blade is in the accessory urethra. Preliminary dilatation of the accessory urethra may be necessary.

10

The haemostat is then closed and locked so as to crush the intervening septum. Some 3 min should be allowed for this. The haemostat is then carefully opened and withdrawn and, using small, straight, blunt-ended scissors, the crushed septum between the two urethras is carefully incised down the centre so that no bleeding occurs. It is important that no instrument or catheter is passed through the urethra after this procedure has been carried out.

Duplications of the urethra in association with hypospadias which extend beyond the range of the above technique are unusual and do not usually require surgical correction.

Urethral duplication as an isolated abnormality is unusual and may be partial, in which case the urethra terminates in a proximal direction as a blind tract, or duplication may be complete so that the accessory urethra communicates with the bladder directly. In this event, the communication may be into the prostatic urethra, at the bladder neck region, or rarely well above and anterior to the bladder neck. It is essential to determine the exact anatomy and pathology of this abnormality by the passage of sounds, by endoscopy, urethrography and cystourethrography. Incomplete duplications can be excised through a longitudinal incision on the penis and there is normally no risk of damaging any vital structure. The excision of complete duplications, and especially of those that terminate in the prostatic urethra or the bladder neck, are technically difficult and indeed hazardous to correct and the possibility of interfering surgically with the sphincter mechanism must be considered. It is advised that this procedure should be done only by a paediatric urologist. Division of the symphysis pubis may be useful to provide good surgical exposure of the prostatic urethra and bladder neck.

Megaurethra

By definition the term megaurethra is restricted to patients with dilated and tortuous urethras in the absence of any obvious outflow (urethral or meatal) obstruction. In clinical practice, megaurethra is most often associated with the prune belly syndrome and indeed the majority of boys with prune belly syndrome also have a megaurethra. Presumably the mesenchymal abnormality of the renal pelvis, ureters and bladder affect the urethral musculature likewise.

The diagnosis is established by clinical inspection. A urethrogram, cystourethrogram and endoscopy are essentially confirmatory investigations. In the classical case of prune belly syndrome with its insipient renal failure no active treatment of the megaurethra is indicated or necessary.

On the other hand, megaurethra may occur as an isolated congenital abnormality in otherwise normal male infants and toddlers. These patients tend to be referred for specialist opinion because of apparent urinary incontinence. Careful questioning will reveal that the boy empties his bladder normally but that he continues to dribble for a long time after proper micturition has

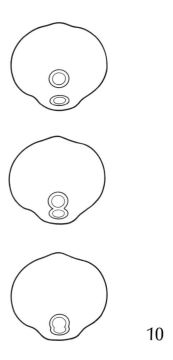

10

ceased. Physical examination shows a large and flabby penis which, on compression, yields a fair quantity of urine.

If the diagnosis of 'idiopathic' and isolated megaurethra is suspected on clinical grounds, the possibility of a meatal or urethral stricture should be considered. This should be investigated radiologically (urethrogram or cystourethrogram) or by instrumentation and/or endoscopy. Obviously any stricture found should be treated on its merits. In the absence of obstruction the treatment of megaurethra should be conservative and the boy (and perhaps his parents) should be taught to squeeze or 'milk' the penis at the end of micturition so as to expel all the urine within the capacious urethra. In the majority of patients this regime will result in acceptable dryness and continence.

A longitudinal plication of the corpus spongiosum and the urethral wall can result in a gratifying radiological improvement after such cosmetic surgery but the procedure is unlikely to improve the symptoms in the long term and urethral dilatation is likely to recur as the primary developmental defect has not been corrected. Cosmetic urethral reduction is therefore not recommended.

Acknowledgement

Illustrations 6 and 7 have been reproduced from Williams[1] by courtesy of the Publishers.

References

1. Williams, D. I. In: Eckstein, H. B., Hohenfellner, R., Williams, D. I., eds. Surgical pediatric urology. Stuttgart: Thieme, 1977: 444

2. Williams, D. I. Urethral duplications. In: Williams, D. I., Johnston, J. H., eds. Paediatric urology, 2nd ed. London: Butterworths, 1982: 244

Illustrations by Kenneth Louis Clark

Posterior urethral valves

R. Dixon Walker MD
Professor of Surgery and Pediatrics and Director of Pediatric Urology,
University of Florida College of Medicine, Gainesville, Florida, USA

Introduction

Posterior urethral valves are leaflet valves developing as a congenital anomaly from structures which are normally present but not obstructive. Posterior urethral valves arise from the lateral or ventral wall of the male prostatic urethra, close to the membrane, and sweep towards the verumontanum. When they arise entirely from the ventral wall they are more obstructive and may actually form an iris diaphragm when they fuse ventrally. Those arising from the lateral walls are smaller and may be less obstructive.

Although posterior urethral valves were identified before development of roentgenograms, in those days most diagnoses were made at autopsy. Today the voiding cystourethrogram is the radiological procedure which allows us to diagnose posterior urethral valves most accurately. In the early days of cystourethrography, posterior urethral valves were frequently misdiagnosed as bladder neck obstruction. This mistaken diagnosis caused many children to have bladder neck revisions, which did not improve the clinical condition. These errors were rapidly avoided as techniques and our knowledge of the anatomy improved. Almost all the recent advances in treatment of posterior urethral valves have been due to improved techniques of surgical management.

Initially, posterior urethral valves were treated by open surgery. The first resectoscopes developed for use in small children had incandescent bulbs and poor optics so that visualization and endoscopic destruction of the valves were difficult. Development of fibreoptic systems has allowed smaller instruments to be devised and many such instruments are now available in sizes 10–13 Fr. The resectoscope can be used with a traditional loop or a hooked electrode. One can also use a 10 Fr pandendoscope with an insulated hook passed down the catheter port of the scope. This hook is made by fashioning a bend in the end of a wire catheter guide for a 3 Fr ureteral catheter and using the catheter as the insulator. The same apparatus can be passed alongside an 8 Fr pandendoscope and the valve destroyed in this manner. Last, a 3 Fr Bougby electrode has been used with either an 8 or 10 Fr instrument to destroy valves.

Principles and justification

If posterior urethral valves can be identified on a voiding cystourethrogram, they should be destroyed endoscopically. The voiding cystourethrogram is indicated in male neonates who have difficulty voiding, have distended bladders or palpable kidneys, who fail to thrive or have urinary tract infection. In older boys this procedure is usually performed if they have voiding problems, incontinence or urinary tract infection. Voiding problems which are particularly important and which should alert one to the need for a voiding cystourethrogram are a weak, dribbling or intermittent stream or straining to void.

If a posterior urethral valve can be identified, the patient should have both an intravenous pyelogram and renal functional evaluation. The characteristic voiding cystourethrogram shows an elongated dilatated posterior urethra with the valve leaflets seen coming from the ventral position. There is almost always a secondary bladder neck obstruction. The posterior urethral valve needs to be distinguished from the prune belly urethra or from the urethra with a spastic sphincter. The bladder with posterior valves may be trabeculated or have diverticula and often there is a significant degree of reflux. Reflux may well indicate severe renal dysplasia and one should not be surprised if the intravenous pyelogram shows that the refluxing kidney does not function. The intravenous pyelogram will most often show hydronephrosis and dilated ureters, unless severe dysplasia is present, in which case the involved kidney may not function. Non-functioning dysplastic kidneys, particularly associated with infection, probably should be removed. Reflux should not be repaired in the infant or older boy until after the valve is resected. Frequently, the reflux will improve or resolve with time.

The infant who has a posterior urethral valve needs to have either the valve primarily destroyed or a cutaneous vesicostomy with delayed valve destruction. The author prefers the latter course, since the instruments presently available may still be too large for many neonatal urethras, and urethral strictures can develop from injudicious use. However, some authorities advocate the other position and either course can be followed. Early diversion and late valve destruction is probably the safest course for the inexperienced urologist.

Total reconstruction of the urinary tract as advocated by Hendren[1] is much more controversial. Hendren actually reserves this procedure for only a few infants, and, although it works well for him, total reconstruction is too complicated to be undertaken by the average practitioner. The long-term results of patients treated by total reconstruction do not appear to differ greatly from those treated by more conservative means.

On rare occasions, temporary cutaneous vesicostomy will not relieve the obstruction, and the kidneys will continue to deteriorate. If this happens, one must proceed to either nephrostomy or ureterostomy. The author prefers tubeless diversions, and, if ureterostomy is indicated, uses the ring ureterostomy developed by Williams and Cromie[2]. Reconstruction is much simpler with this than with other forms of ureterostomy, and, if a reimplant of the lower ureter is needed, it can be accomplished with less risk to the blood supply of the intervening ureter.

A few urologists may identify valves during cystoscopy that were not visible on a voiding cystourethrogram. The diagnoses in these cases are tenuous and unquestionably normal structures are sometimes destroyed. One has to be very careful in making a diagnosis in this manner. The likelihood is that any valves that are not visible on a voiding cystourethrogram are insignificantly small and injudicious instrumentation could result in the formation of a stricture.

Preoperative

Newborn infants with suspected posterior urethral valves should have a 5 Fr feeding tube inserted into the bladder and taped in place until the diagnosis is established by a voiding cystourethrogram. After cystography, the catheter is left in place until appropriate therapy is determined. During the hours between diagnosis and surgery, electrolyte and acid-base balance should be restored to normal. If severe uraemia is diagnosed, peritoneal dialysis may need to be performed. All patients are given antibacterial therapy.

In older children, particularly those with smaller valves, a catheter does not need to be left in place, although it is often wise to do so. Again, one should proceed expeditiously toward resection of the valves.

Anaesthesia

In the neonate, preoperative medication usually consists of appropriate doses of atropine alone; atropine and pentobarbitol are preferred for older children. Maintenance intravenous fluids of D5-1/4 of normal saline are given during the procedure and in the immediate postoperative period. During surgery the heart, temperature, blood pressure and pulse rate are monitored. The anaesthetic most commonly used is halothane and the patient is kept in Stage III anaesthesia. A decision regarding intubation is made depending on the length of time estimated for the procedure.

The operation

The patient is placed in the lithotomy position. A newborn infant may be placed in the frog-leg position to give adequate exposure of the penis. After the patient is prepared and draped, the urethra is calibrated with a soft rubber or plastic catheter, rather than by the use of sounds. Dilatation of the urethra with sounds is ill-advised because of possible stricture formation. In the neonate, the urethra must accept a 10 Fr catheter with ease in order to accept either a 10 Fr resectoscope or an 8 Fr pandendoscope with lateral catheter and hook. A generous meatotomy is acceptable if the catheter is obstructed at this point. The author prefers not to do a perineal urethrostomy if either of the instruments does not pass through the anterior urethra easily. Instead, a cutaneous vesicostomy is performed and valve resection is postponed until after the patient is a year old. In children older than one year, the 10 Fr resectoscope is easily accommodated by the urethra.

Meatotomy, if necessary, is performed by crushing the ventral meatal tissue with a straight clamp into the area of the fossa navicularis. After 5 minutes the clamp is removed and the tissue divided with iris scissors. The cut edges, and particularly the apex of the meatoplasty, are approximated with 6/0 Dexon suture.

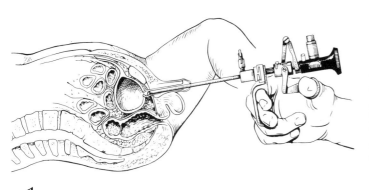

1

Once it is determined that the urethra is sufficiently large, the instrument is liberally lubricated with water-soluble lubricant and introduced through the urethra and into the bladder under direct vision. The instrument preferred by the author is the 10 Fr Stortz resectoscope with the hook electrode. The bladder is first examined and the position of the ureters and degree of trabeculation noted.

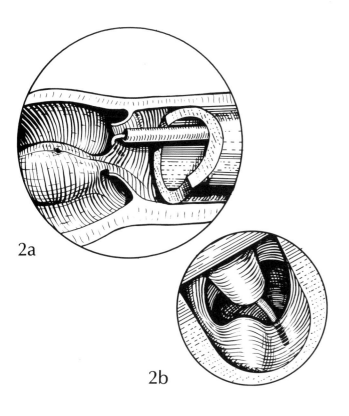

1

2a

2b

2a & b

The instrument is withdrawn into the prostatic or posterior urethra. The hook electrode can be used to engage the valves in the 3 and 9 o'clock positions and to draw the valve into the lumen. With a quick burst of cutting current, the valve is easily destroyed on each side.

Extensive coagulation and resection with a loop electrode should be avoided as should any resection at the bladder neck level. It is better to leave a small amount of valve tissue than to do too extensive a resection. Although some surgeons also advocate cutting the valve at 12 o'clock, the author has found this unnecessary. The proximity to the external sphincter should be carefully noted and every effort made to avoid resecting in that area. Occasionally the valve will extend distally, so that it must be destroyed either right at, or even distal to, part of the external sphincter. Extreme care is necessary when this is done. In particular, one needs to be careful to keep the hook electrode well within the lumen of the urethra when applying the cutting current.

After the valve is destroyed and the urethra re-examined, an 8 or 10 Fr Silastic Foley catheter is left in the bladder.

Postoperative care

In neonates or infants with severe obstruction the most important postoperative steps are to manage the associated uraemia, the fluid and electrolytes and acid-base balance, and to prevent infection. Initially newborn infants should be kept in an intensive care unit until they are stable. Paediatric nephrological consultation is strongly advised.

The Foley catheter is usually removed 48 hours postoperatively. The child's voiding should be observed closely. A continued obstructive pattern may indicate that the valve was inadequately destroyed. Studies of pre- and postoperative flow are a more objective way to judge results in older children. Increased blood urea nitrogen and creatinine, in spite of improved flow, may indicate secondary obstruction of the ureters and judgement will be required as to whether reimplantation, ureterostomy, or nephrostomy is advisable.

An intravenous pyelogram is obtained with a voiding film 3–6 months after destroying the valves. This gives the surgeon the necessary anatomical information about the kidneys and ureters. It also shows the completeness of valve destruction and whether or not a stricture has developed. If reflux was present preoperatively, then voiding cystourethrography should be repeated approximately a year after surgery to reassess the reflux. Most often, reflux does not require surgical repair, but can be conservatively treated.

Long-term follow-up depends on the degree of renal impairment. Children with a normal or near-normal postoperative intravenous pyelogram and renal function studies need yearly functional and anatomical reassessment for several years; if stable, they can be discharged from the clinic. Children with mild structural change or mild renal impairement should have blood pressure and renal function evaluations at 6-monthly intervals, and renal structure evaluation by intravenous pyelogram yearly, at least through adolescence. Children with moderate to severe renal impairment must be closely observed for hypertension, failure to grow and other signs of chronic renal failure. They should be evaluated at least every 3 months and preferably followed up with paediatric nephrological assistance.

Results

Because posterior urethral valves are uncommon, children with this disorder are most often seen in major centres. Between 1970 and 1980, the author saw 44 infants and children with posterior urethral valves. In 16 of these the valve had been resected elsewhere, and they were referred for secondary surgery or management of renal failure. Six of the 44 children have had renal transplantation. The author has resected valves in 28 of these children – 14 of whom were more than a year old at the time – and all of these have done well. The 14 cases where the valve was resected at less than one year had a high incidence of stricture formation, probably related to the size of the instrument used for the small urethra. None of the children who had had cutaneous vesicostomy and delayed valve resection have formed a stricture. There have been two deaths in the early years from renal failure and acidosis in neonates with posterior urethral valves, but none since our transplantation programme has been active over the last 4 years. Because of the high prevalance of strictures in neonates, the author's current approach is to perform cutaneous vesicostomy in almost all cases, and to delay valve resection until after the infant reaches one year of age.

References

1. Hendren, W. H. A new approach to infants with severe obstructive uropathy: early complete reconstruction. Journal of Pediatric Surgery 1970; 5: 184–199
2. Williams, D. I., Cromie, W. J. Ring ureterostomy. British Journal of Urology 1975; 47: 789–792

Illustrations by Robert N. Lane

Traumatic injuries of the external genitalia

W. Scott McDougal MD
Professor and Chairman, Department of Urology,
Vanderbilt University Medical Center, Nashville, Tennessee, USA

Proper care of the patient with an injury of the external genitalia requires a thorough knowledge of the principles of urological and plastic surgery, as well as sensitivity to the patient's psychological needs. Occasionally, patients with these injuries will present to the hospital in hypovolaemic shock. However, more commonly they are haemodynamically stable but in emotional shock and are reluctant to express their concern over the possible loss of sexual potency and reproductive ability. It is, therefore, most important that the urological surgeon has a thorough knowledge of what can be accomplished so that after initial inspection of the wound the patient may be given realistic expectations and provided with the proper counselling and support from the outset.

These injuries pose special problems due to the anatomy of the overlying skin and to the proximity of the urinary and faecal streams. Initial evaluation of the injury must not only include an appraisal of the extent of perineal soft tissue and cutaneous loss, but the competency of the urinary and rectal sphincters as well as the integrity of the urethra and rectosigmoid colon. Urethral and/or rectal injuries may require urinary or faecal diversion prior to definitive management of the perineal injury.

Marked oedema formation is a commonly encountered problem in these injuries, since the very thin dermis of the skin with the loose areolar tissue beneath allows for the accumulation of large amounts of fluid, resulting in appreciable swelling following trauma. These tissues do not hold sutures well, and when oedema causes tension wounds are likely to disrupt. Moreover, the loose areolar tissue allows for extensive haematoma formation when bleeding is uncontrolled. Erections may also cause tension on suture lines, and must be controlled with oral administration of stilboestrol or inhalation of amyl nitrite.

LOSS OF THE GENITAL SKIN

Extensive loss of the scrotal and penile skin may be due to either trauma or infection. Traumatic losses are usually due to a degloving type injury in which the loose skin is caught with the clothing in a device which tears both from the patient. A moving belt on farm machinery is often the culprit. Separation of the skin from the penis occurs at the level of the loose areolar tissue just superficial to Buck's fascia, and in the scrotum separation occurs immediately beneath the dartos muscle.

Loss of skin due to infection is usually the result of a necrotizing gangrenous process (Fournier's gangrene). Although originally described as a synergistic infection caused by Gram-positive organisms, today the condition is mostly attributed to Gram-negative organisms. Indeed, recent evidence indicates that anaerobes play a major role in this type of necrotizing gangrene.

Patients who have sustained traumatic avulsions are generally not in shock at the time of presentation, in contrast to those presenting with necrotizing fasciitis, who invariably present in septic shock. The mortality for the infective lesion is 38 per cent; the mortality increases to 63 per cent if the patient is also a diabetic.

1a–d

Avulsion injuries

Proper treatment of avulsion injuries involves debridement of the skin to viable tissue. On the penis, however, if the defect is circumferential at the base, the remainder of the skin on the penile shaft is debrided to within 1–2 mm of the corona (a). If this is not done, brawny oedema of the distal penile skin will occur, producing an unacceptable cosmetic and functional result. The wounds should be thoroughly cleansed and loose skin and necrotic debris removed. If enough scrotal skin can be mobilized, the wound is closed primarily. If there is insufficient remaining scrotal tissue, then a split-thickness graft meshed 1½ to 1 provides a very satisfactory covering and results in immediate wound closure. If large losses of scrotal skin have occurred and the testicles are viable, they may be sutured together in the midline (a) and covered with split-thickness graft meshed 1½ to 1 (c), with a reasonable expectation of an excellent cosmetic and functional result. It is important to note that the testicles must be kept at a temperature 1–2°C below that of the body core if fertility is to be preserved. A thin covering provided by split-thickness graft accomplishes this purpose. The grafts are stented (d).

If the testicles do not appear viable, they are implanted at asymmetric levels into medial thigh pockets. The implantation should be performed with an eye to scrotal reconstruction (see below).

Management of the injured penis when the wound is circumferential requires complete debridement of all the skin to a level of a few millimetres below the corona. The shaft may then be split-thickness grafted with the seam placed dorsally (b), so that if a contracture occurs along the suture line the corde will be dorsal (and thus functional) rather than ventral. Small defects in the penile skin may be closed primarily, provided they are not circumferential in nature. The grafts are sutured in place and the sutures left long (c) so that they may be used to tie over cotton wadding (d) which is left in place for 5-7 days.

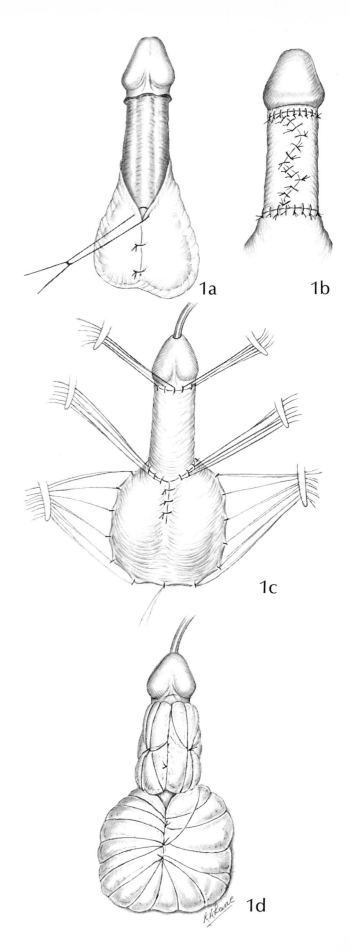

1a

1b

1c

1d

2a & b

Necrotizing gangrene

Necrotizing gangrene requires debridement of all penile skin to within 1–2 mm of the corona, as well as all scrotal and much of the perineal skin. The wound must be left open initially and the testicles and perineum wrapped in dressings. When the infection has been controlled, the testicles are usually found to be partially granulated and have areas of desiccated tissue overlying them. This condition is not amenable to split-thickness grafting, and therefore the preferable procedure is to implant the testes at asymmetrical levels into subcutaneous thigh pockets (a).

Split-thickness graft applied in this situation would require that the wound be left open, and the testicles and their tunics allowed to granulate to the extent that they would accept a graft – a course which requires a 2–3 week period. The testicles may be implanted into the thighs even though portions of the tunics do not appear viable, for when left in this position the tissues surrounding the testicles will become viable and pliable. The perineal defect is covered with a split-thickness graft and the penis grafted as described for degloving injuries.

Reconstruction of the scrotum is accomplished 4–6 weeks later by rotating the superior and lateral-based medial thigh flaps medially and suturing them together in the midline (b). Rounding the ends of the flaps results in a sac-like structure when they are sutured. These flaps are supplied by the external pudendal artery and the medial circumflex femoral artery, as well as by the ilioinguinal and genitofemoral nerve.

This procedure has the advantages of simplicity, superior cosmetic result, maintenance of fertility, maintenance of sensation and early closure of the wound. Patients who have their testes implanted into their thighs invariably complain of pain during ambulation, which disappears when the scrotal flaps are created. In order to maintain fertility, it is important to implant the testes in the thighs in the subdermal tissue with little or no subcutaneous tissue intervening between the skin and testes. This maximizes the chances for maintaining the testicles a degree or two below that of the body core. A cosmetic advantage of such an implantation results from the deposition of haem pigment in the dermis, thus darkening the skin and thereby simulating more closely the colour of the normal scrotum.

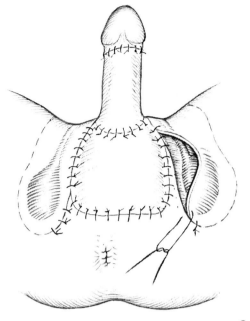

2a

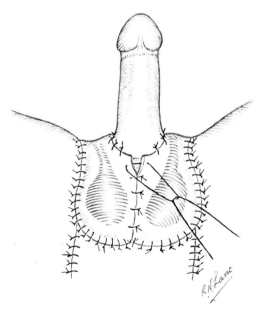

2b

TRAUMATIC INJURIES OF THE FEMALE PERINEUM

The mechanism in female patients who have sustained trauma to the perineum generally involves a straddle-type injury or a direct blow to the perineum. The most common type of lesion is a vulvar haematoma, and this may become massive and quite painful. This is generally treated with icepacks and bedrest initially, followed by hot soaks some 48–72 hours later. On rare occasions the haematoma is so massive that breaks occur in the perineal skin. Under these circumstances, the haematoma should be evacuated. Rarely, packing of the vulvar area may be necessary to control haemorrhage. Vulvar injuries in which there is a loss of tissue are debrided and primary closure gained if possible.

The defects which cannot be primarily closed in the female often do not lend themselves to the application of split-thickness graft, and are better treated by the use either of arterialized pedicle grafts or myocutaneous flaps. They may also be treated by applying wet dressings until the area granulates, at which time a split-thickness graft can be applied.

Commonly associated with vulvar injuries are vaginal lacerations, and these must always be suspected in any patient who sustains trauma to the external genitalia. These injuries can be rather extensive, and can result in massive blood loss leading to hypovolaemic shock. The injury is carefully debrided and sutured with interrupted chromic catgut. The urethra must always be carefully evaluated in patients with this type of injury for it, too, is prone to involvement.

DEEP LACERATION OF THE PERINEUM

Massive trauma to the perineum involving deep lacerations with injury of the rectum or urethra result in a high mortality rate. It is essential in such injuries to form a diverting colostomy. Suprapubic cystotomy should also be performed if urethral integrity is disrupted. These patients are prone to necrotizing fasciitis and unless treated aggressively will not survive their injury. The perineum is debrided, packed and secondarily closed when infection is controlled and haemodynamic stability achieved.

PENILE GANGRENE

Traumatic gangrene of the penis may involve the superficial tissues or the full thickness of the organ, depending upon the mode of damage. The mechanism of injury usually involves placement of a constricting band about the penis, either as a means of maintaining an erection or as a form of child abuse. The objects utilized for this purpose include nuts, pieces of pipe, string, rubber-bands, wire, condoms and hair. The constriction initially impedes venous outflow, causing swelling of the part distal to the constriction and thus increasing subdermal pressure. When this pressure exceeds systolic blood pressure, arterial inflow ceases and gangrene results.

These lesions are treated by removing the constricting device. Hair, string, rubber-bands, wire and condoms can generally be cut. On occasion, it may be difficult to find the offending agent due to the oedema, in which case a vertical incision is made at the junction between normal and oedematous skin. This results in severance of the constricting band. On rare occasions the constricting object may be impossible to cut. Under these circumstances, the skin and areolar tissue distal to the constricting band is removed and the object slid off the penis. The necrotic tissue is debrided and if the debridement results only in loss of the skin of the shaft of the penis, a split-thickness graft may be applied and stented as already described.

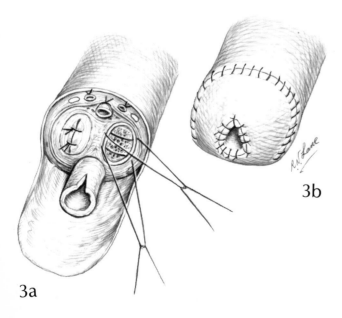

3a

3b

3a & b

However, if the gangrene extends beneath Buck's fascia into the corpora, a partial penectomy is necessary (a). The necrotic distal portion is debrided, a ventral skin flap retained and the corpora closed. The urethra is spatulated and a hole created through the skin flap. The skin flap and urethra are sutured (b).

If the extent of the gangrene is equivocal, the wound may be treated with topical application of mafenide acetate for several days until demarcation is unequivocal, at which time the definite procedure may be accomplished.

AMPUTATION OF THE PENIS

Amputation of the penis with loss of the transected part generally occurs as a result of amputation for malignancy, blast injuries, mechanical trauma, self-inflicted injuries or gunshot wounds. Massive bleeding and shock are common sequelae of such injuries. Under these circumstances, haemostasis should be achieved by compression until the patient can be evaluated.

If the amputated part can be found, the arteries and veins are flushed with a cold, heparinized solution of Ringer's lactate and the part placed in iced Ringer's lactate with streptomycin and penicillin. The dorsalis penis and profunda penis arteries of the stump are identified, cannulated, flushed with heparinized saline and occluded with microvascular clips. A suprapubic cystotomy is performed and a Foley catheter placed *per urethram* through the transected part and into the bladder. This stabilizes the part and aligns the structures. The urethra is then spatulated and sutured in an oblique manner with interrupted 4/0 chromic suture.

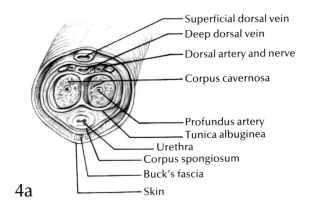

4a

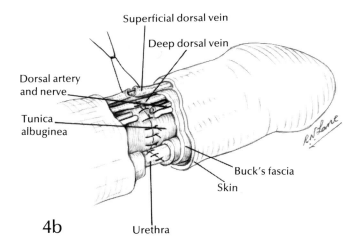

4b

4a & b

Amputation with replantation

The profunda penile arteries are identified and sutured with 9/0 or 10/0 nylon with the aid of a microscope. The tunica albuginea of the corpora are sutured together with interrupted 5/0 Prolene and the deep dorsal vein with 9/0 nylon. Subsequently, the dorsal penile arteries and nerves are sutured with 9/0 nylon, following which the dorsal vein is sutured with 9/0 nylon. The skin is debrided and sutured together.

Commonly, however, the skin distal to the incision line will become oedematous and it may be necessary to remove the distal skin at a later date (as one would with any circumferential injury) and apply split-thickness graft to the wound. Sensation and erectile function return to the penis by about 3 months. Replantations have been successful as much as 18 hours after the injury.

5a–d

Amputation without replantation

The wounds are debrided initially and a perineal urethrostomy performed (a). If the scrotum is intact, a purely non-functional organ may be fashioned by raising a scrotal flap (b), implanting one testicle into the flap, making a tube out of it (c), and suturing the defect in the scrotum at its base (d) in a horizontal manner.

Implantation of the testicle into the appendage is necessary to limit contracture of the flap, for if nothing is implanted it will appear as a small nubbin several months later, thus defeating the purpose of the procedure. The appendage is purely cosmetic and has no functional capabilities. If a functional structure is desired, numerous techniques have been described, which include tubed abdominal pedicle grafts, myocutaneous gracilis flaps and arterialized groin pedicle flaps. In each case, either a rib or a Silastic prosthetic device must be implanted in order to impart function.

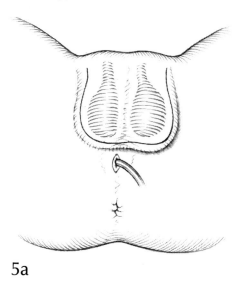

5a

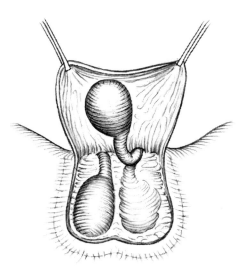

5b

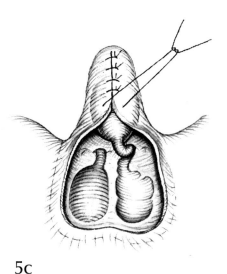

5c

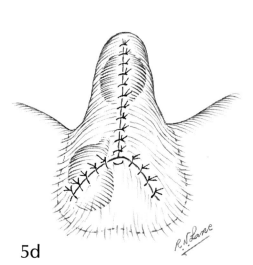

5d

FRACTURE OF THE PENIS

Fracture of the penis occurs when a blow is sustained to the erect penis. During the flaccid state, the corpora is normally 2 mm thick. However, its thickness diminishes to 0.25–0.50 mm during a full erection. A direct blow sustained to the erect penis results in a loud cracking noise, heard at the moment of injury, and a tear which is usually located in the distal two-thirds of the penis. Approximately a third of patients have a concomitant urethral injury. Although non-operative therapy (involving application of icepacks, elevation of the part and injection of enzymatic agents) has been successful, morbidity is reduced and function better preserved if these injuries are explored, lacerations identified and sutured, and the wounds drained. It is, of course, important to prevent erections in the postoperative period, and this may be accomplished by the oral administration of stilboestrol.

TESTICULAR RUPTURE

Blunt scrotal trauma may result in large haematoma formation, which may make it difficult to identify the extent of injury to the testis. Testicular ultrasound is particularly valuable in these circumstances, since a diagnosis of extratesticular haematoma versus rupture of the tunica albuginea may be determined. If the tunica albuginea is ruptured, exploration should be performed. The necrotic and extruded testicular tissue is excised and the tunica albuginea sutured. Two-thirds of patients with rupture of the tunica albuginea treated conservatively can be expected to have an atrophic non-functional testis. On the other hand, early exploration and repair results in an 80 per cent incidence of viable testes.

THE BURNED PERINEUM

Burns of the perineum may either be thermal, chemical or electrical in nature. These injuries are not usually restricted to the perineum, but associated with massive injuries to the rest of the body. Initial therapy depends upon the aetiology of the injury. Thermal injuries may be cooled initially and cold injuries rewarmed. Chemical injuries should be washed thoroughly with water and, if the chemical has been forced into the subcutaneous tissue, this tissue should be debrided immediately. Cutaneous manifestations of electrical injuries often belie the depth of injury below, and exploration of these wounds is necessary as soon as the patient is stabilized to determine the extent of necrosis. Following initial therapy, the wounds are covered with a topical antimicrobial and debrided on a daily basis.

Partial-thickness injuries of the penis and perineum which are superficial will re-epithelialize with management by topical antimicrobial application and the cosmetic and functional result will be quite acceptable.

Deep partial-thickness injuries (deep second-degree) often result in scar and contracture formation. Maturation of the contracture generally takes 4–6 months, and it is at this time that it is released.

Full-thickness injuries require debridement of the eschar on a daily basis and application of topical antimicrobials until a granulating base is obtained which will accept split-thickness graft. On rare occasions, when the thighs are spared from injury, the perineal tissue can be debrided and the testicles implanted into thigh pockets. The shaft of the penis is grafted immediately with split-thickness skin as described above. This accomplishes early closure of the burn wound. The scrotum is reconstructed, as described above, at a later date.

Full-thickness injuries of the ventral aspect of the shaft of the penis will often result in loss of urethral tissue and hypospadias if indwelling Foley catheters are left in place. When this type of injury occurs, it is important to place either a perineal urethrostomy or suprapubic cystostomy. Repair of these injuries can be challenging since, unlike congenital hypospadias, there is an actual loss of distal penile soft tissue. This requires the application of full-thickness and pedicle grafts.

6a–d

CONTRACTURES

Following deep second- or third-degree burn injuries of the perineum, contractures often develop. These are treated 4–6 months post injury. The line of contracture is incised perpendicular to its axis, placing darts at either end of the incision line (a). The resulting extensive defect (b) is covered by a thick split-thickness graft (c) which is subsequently stented in place (d).

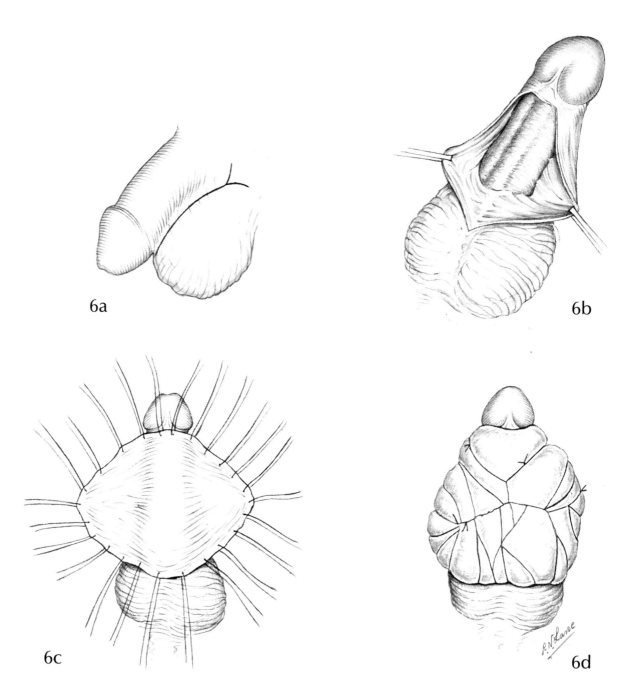

6a

6b

6c

6d

CIRCUMCISION INJURIES

Circumcision injuries are not uncommon and involve damage to the meatus with subsequent meatal stenosis, laceration of the glans and shaft of the penis and denudation of the skin both of the glans and shaft. Meatal injuries, if repaired with fine chromic catgut, generally do not result in long-term complications. Similarly, small lacerations of the glans may be sutured primarily with fine catgut. Loss of skin of the shaft of the penis requires debridement and split-thickness graft application or primary closure, as the defect dictates. Unfortunately, on rare occasions, the glans itself may be partially or completely amputated, in which case the wound must be closed and the urethra spatulated and brought to the skin, much as for a partial penectomy. These patients, unfortunately, suffer from meatal stenosis in the postoperative period.

LYMPHOEDEMA OF THE PENIS AND SCROTUM

Lymphoedema of the penis and scrotum may be due to inflammatory conditions such as tuberculosis, bacterial infections, lymphogranuloma venereum, or parasitic infections; to malignant obstruction; to radiotherapy or to primary aplasia or hypoplasia of the lymphatics. Following lymphatic obstruction, the skin usually becomes thickened and woody and may contain skin tags or warty excrescences. It is prone to secondary bacterial and fungal infection. The part usually becomes asensory and loss of sexual function is invariably the rule. The treatment of this disorder involves complete excision of the skin overlying the penis and scrotum (see *Illustration 1*). Split-thickness graft is applied to the shaft of the penis as described above. The testicles may be implanted into the medial aspects of the thighs if thigh tissue is uninvolved, with reconstruction of the scrotum performed with thigh flaps at a later date. Or they may be sutured together in the midline and split-thickness graft applied. The latter procedure is preferred, since it can be accomplished in one stage.

RADIATION INJURY

Radiation injury is usually a complication of extensive radiotherapy to cutaneous lesions of the perineum. Because of better techniques in radiotherapy, this injury is becoming less common. Initially, the acute injury is manifested by erythema and oedema followed by chronic changes of atrophy of the skin, telangiectasias, hyperpigmentation and excoriation. Generally the lesion is painful and itches, and progresses on occasion to ulceration. If there is no break in the skin, conservative therapy is indicated. However, if ulceration ensues, the area should be excised and pedicle flaps used to close the defects.

HIDRADENITIS SUPPURATIVA

Hidradenitis suppurativa is an infectious process which involves the apocrine glands. The organisms most commonly responsible include *Staphylococcus aureus* and *Aerobacter aerogenes*. The lesion is generally found in adults aged 20–40 years; it is most common in negroes and least common in Orientals. The factors which are thought to contribute to the occurrence of this disease are mechanical irritation, poor hygiene, use of chemical agents, presence of active acne and the use of depilatories. The lesion must be differentiated from perineal abscesses, fistula, tuberculosis, infected sebaceous cysts, lymphadenitis and lymphogranuloma venereum. The incidence of hidradenitis suppurativa is three times greater in women than in men and it may be associated with abnormal steroid metabolism such as is encountered in Cushing's disease. There is a 3 per cent incidence of squamous cell carcinoma in patients who have had active hidradenitis suppurativa for a number of years. X-ray therapy of the groin has been employed but is not ideal, since injury to the testicles is a common complication. The disease is superficial in nature and does not extend beneath the superficial fascia in the thigh or to the level of the tunica vaginalis in the scrotum.

Initially the lesion may be treated with oral antibiotics (tetracycline) and soaks, with incision and drainage of localized abscesses. However, in more extensive cases, it is generally necessary to excise the affected area. In the perineum, this generally involves the suprapubic area as well as the lateral aspect of the scrotum and medial aspect of the thigh, including the groin crease. Skin and subcutaneous tissue are excised to a level of superficial fascia, following which the wound can often be closed primarily. If this is not possible, the immediate application of split-thickness graft (which is stented) provides an acceptable result. If the graft crosses the groin crease it is important not to mesh the split-thickness graft but rather to apply a split-thickness graft which is on the thick side.

Further reading

Flanigan, R. C., Kursh, E. D., McDougal, W. S., Persky, L. Synergistic gangrene of the scrotum and penis secondary to colorectal disease. Journal of Urology 1978; 119: 369–371

McDougal, W. S., Peterson, H. D., Pruitt, B. A. Jr, Persky, L. The thermally injured perineum. Journal of Urology 1979; 121: 320–323

McDougal, W. S., Persky, L Traumatic injuries of the genitourinary system. Baltimore: Willliams and Wilkins, 1981

McDougal, W. S. Scrotal reconstruction of the scrotum using thigh pedicle flaps. Journal of Urology 1983; 129: 757–759

Maull, K. I., Sachatello, C. R., Ernst, C. B. The deep perineal laceration – an injury frequently associated with open pelvic fractures: a need for aggressive surgical management: a report of 12 cases and review of the literature. Journal of Trauma 1977; 17: 685–696

Ovrum, E. Rupture of the penis. Scandinavian Journal of Urology and Nephrology 1978; 12: 83–84

Tamai, S., Nakamura, Y., Motomiya, Y. Microsurgical replantation of a completely amputated penis and scrotum: case report. Plastic and Reconstructive Surgery 1977; 60: 287–291

Vickers, M. A. Jr. Operative management of chronic hidradenitis suppurativa of the scrotum and perineum. Journal of Urology 1975; 114: 414–416

Illustrations by Patrick M. Elliott

Hypospadias

B. S. Crawford FRCS
Consultant Plastic Surgeon, Fulwood Hospital and the Children's Hospital, Sheffield, UK

Introduction

The hypospadiac position of the external meatus on the undersurface of the penis may interfere with normal micturition by making it difficult to direct the stream, and with sexual intercourse because of the associated curvature of the penis (chordee). In mild degrees of the deformity (which are common) and when the opening is on the glans or even at the coronal sulcus, there is seldom any handicap and as a rule an operation is not necessary. In a few cases when the opening is at this level there is meatal stenosis which must be corrected urgently by meatotomy; this procedure can usually be accomplished without accentuating the deformity. On the groove distal to the hypospadiac meatus the opening of a short blind duct usually runs proximally parallel with and dorsal to the urethra. This sinus can be laid open into the lumen of the urethra, thus widening the meatus without moving it proximally[1].

A great many operations have been devised for the correction of hypospadias: most of them can give satisfactory results when carefully performed, but all are subject to complications and are liable to break down if the technique is not meticulous. This is because urethral repair is an exercise in obtaining first intention healing under adverse conditions, namely tissue under tension, oedema, erections, haematomas, friable or scarred tissue, and infection due to moisture and proximity to the anus, all in the face of urine which is evacuated under pressure.

When chordee is slight and the urethral defect less than half the penile length, satisfactory repair can be achieved by a one-stage operation. When chordee is moderate or severe and the urethral defect greater than half the penile length, a two-stage procedure is advisable; the first operation overcorrects the curvature and the second brings the urethral meatus up to or beyond the level of the corona. Attempts to correct these difficult cases in one stage are prone to failure because of the complexity of the defect. It is important to be sure that the chordee has been corrected before proceeding to urethral repair. There are some methods described[2] in which three or more stages are involved, but these are considered to be tedious and unnecessarily taxing for the child and have very few indications. In all operations the aim should be normal micturition with an easily directed stream and normal sexual function without penile curvature. A satisfactory appearance is an important but secondary objective; operations which endeavour to attain perfect normality with the urethra coursing through the glans rather than being placed on its ventral surface risk the creation of a serious stricture.

There are a number of procedures described for the repair of the hypospadiac urethra. One method which has been used extensively is that of Denis Browne. Sommerlad[3] in a follow-up of 24 cases treated by the Denis Browne method, found that over 50 per cent developed a fistula which usually required more than one operation for repair, and in over 50 per cent the meatus was more than 1 cm proximal to the dimple on the glans. Some mistrust this buried strip principle on the grounds that spontaneous healing of the urethral lining leads to scarring which spoils the result. Those who are dissatisfied with their results should change to one or more alternatives of which there are many[4,5]. Each should be studied, because one or more features may be useful in certain circumstances even if the whole method is not adopted. For example, McCormack's[6] method of inserting a full-thickness skin graft to repair what will be the urethral lining is useful in some cases of extreme chordee, and scrotal flaps[2] can be valuable when there is marked shortage of tissue with which to cover the urethra.

In urethral surgery the adverse factors already mentioned must be accepted and avoided by careful technique. The choice of suture material is important – catgut should be avoided for urethral repair in favour of a non-irritant material such as Dexon (polyglycolic acid), nylon or stainless steel wire. Dexon carries the advantage that it does not have to be removed so 'bites' can be close together, resulting in a watertight closure. If leakage is prevented there is no need to divert the urine. Tension must be avoided at all times; in fact, all suture lines must lie loosely because of the danger of erections. Haemostasis is by fine catgut ligatures or bipolar diathermy with the occasional use of a suture ligature. Those who employ conventional diathermy must avoid necrosis by using minimal current and by pressing the penis longitudinally against the abdomen or scrotum when current is applied.

In summary, simple methods should be chosen rather than complicated ones, and those which do not follow the principles of reconstructive surgery should be rejected. Each surgeon will search for methods which he can apply with a high success rate, but he must continue to examine results as objectively as possible and look for improvement. Those who are setting out on this task are advised to gain experience in urology, paediatrics and plastic surgery in order to equip themselves.

Urinary diversion

Many surgeons divert the urine because they believe that urine delays healing. Others do so in order to avoid pain and clot retention. At one time a posterior urethrostomy was popular, but this has been replaced largely by a suprapubic cystotomy which is technically simpler. On the other hand, some surgeons rarely if ever divert the urine. They try to prevent urinary leakage by careful technique and may use a Foley catheter for a few days in moderate and severe cases, or a short Silastic tube passed just beyond the original meatus in mild cases. The use of a caudal block or a dorsal penile nerve block by the anaesthetist and the institution of early micturition before the bladder becomes distended are valuable if diversion is to be avoided.

1

Classification

Mild cases

In these, which are the most common, the meatus opens on the distal half of the penis; chordee is minimal, but occasionally there is an associated anomaly such as meatal stenosis. Patients with a meatus at or distal to the corona are nearly always left alone, but when the meatus opens on the distal half of the penis but proximal to the corona treatment is by a one-stage repair. The prognosis of mild cases (whether operated on or not) is very good in that complications are rare and final function and appearance should be within normal limits.

Moderate cases

The meatus opens on to the proximal half of the penis or scrotum. Chordee is usually severe enough to need correction, and there is a significant incidence of associated anomalies of the urogenital tract. The defect is complex. Consideration must be given to (1) the skin required to cover the ventral surface when the chordee is corrected, (2) the lining layer of the missing portion of the urethra, and (3) the skin required to cover the latter. Owing to the size and complexity of the defect it is wise to repair the defect in two stages. The prognosis is good, but should be somewhat guarded, because fistulae are still a problem and there is always a possibility that other anomalies of the urogenital system are present.

Severe cases

Fortunately these are rare. The meatus is in the perineum, chordee is marked, and many of these patients have cryptorchidism, microphallus, or other anomalies. Each one merits full preoperative investigation, including 17-ketosteroid assay, intravenous pyelography, and sex chromatin studies. There are considerable technical problems in repair, but a satisfactory result should be achieved by using local tissues without having to import from elsewhere, apart from the use of a skin graft to cover the dorsal defect. Boys with microphallus may benefit

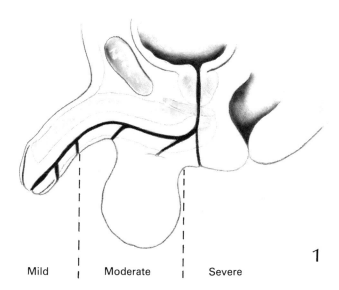

| Mild | Moderate | Severe |

1

from the local application of 5 per cent testosterone acetate cream to increase penile growth[7]. Those who fail to respond may be repaired with scrotum[2], or an abdominal tube pedicle may be introduced after final repair. Cryptorchidism is treated by standard methods; if operation is necessary it can be combined with a stage in urethral repair. The prognosis is guarded. Although a satisfactory repair can be achieved, more operations are required for this group than for the others, and there is always some doubt about fertility.

Age for operation

For psychological reasons it is desirable to secure normal standing micturition before the child goes to school. As it is wise to wait until he is continent, and as there is usually an interval of a year between stages in a two-year repair, chordee correction is carried out at around age 3 years so that treatment may be completed before school age. Severe cases of chordee should be operated earlier as they may need two operations before urethral repair is advisable. One-stage repairs are carried out at age 4 or 5 years.

The operations

One-stage repair

In mild cases (which are very common) a reliable one-stage method should be adopted. Chordee is usually slight and can be corrected at the same time as the urethra is repaired. The success rate should be high[8,9].

THE DORSAL AXIAL FLAP REPAIR (VAN DER MEULEN)

2

Delineation of the lining layer

The buried strip is made as wide as the circumference of the existing urethra (as judged by passing a sound). On the glans, two narrow strips of skin are removed on either side of the midline with scissors to create raw areas which slightly converge, so that the new meatus will be very slightly narrower than the rest of the urethra to avoid spraying. The U-shaped incision which outlines the rest of the strip is continuous with the raw surfaces created on the glans.

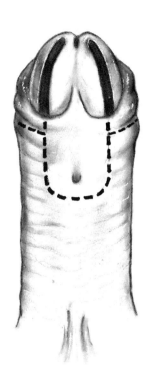

2

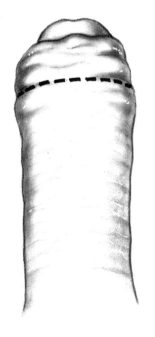

3

3

Incision outlining the covering flap

The penile skin is incised starting at a point 2 mm behind the glans on the edge of the strip. The knife passes laterally in a transverse direction then curves on to the prepuce, following the raphe to the dorsum where it meets the corresponding incision from the opposite side. (The inclusion of skin distal to the raphe carries a risk of necrosis.)

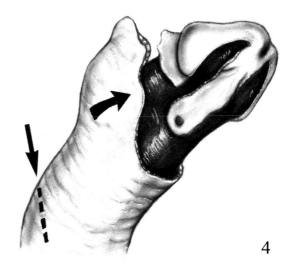

4

4

Raising the flaps

The dorsal penile skin is freely raised as a flap from the deep fascia, preserving the main blood vessels. Tight bands lateral and proximal to the buried strip are divided and a defect is created which helps to correct the chordee. The ventral penile skin is also freed from the deep fascia proximally and laterally until the skin can be completely rotated 180° round the penile shaft with ease. A short 'back-cut' (arrowed) helps the rotation of the dorsal flap to be made with minimal tension, and the base of the flap rotates from the dorsum to the ventral aspect. Haemostasis is ensured.

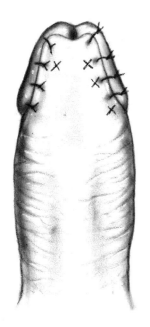

5

5 & 6

Repair

A number of buried sutures (marked X) of 0/0 Dexon are inserted to anchor the dorsal flap ventrally to the glans and penile shaft in order to remove tension from the suture lines, which consist of closely applied interrupted sutures uniting the flap to the raw surfaces of the glans and adjacent penile skin in one layer. The strip, apart from the meatus, is now buried. A catheter is not inserted. The dorsum is repaired using the rotated skin from the front of the penis, together with the preputial remnant. A firm non-encircling dressing holds the penis to the abdominal wall for 24 hours and is then replaced by a light supporting dressing which prevents dangling on to the bedclothes. Early bladder emptying is insisted upon and the child is allowed home in 2–3 days.

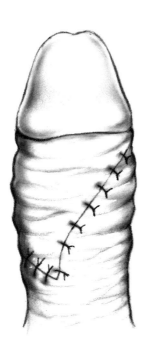

6

7 & 8

CRAWFORD MODIFICATION OF THE ONE-STAGE VAN DER MEULEN REPAIR

This method provides a complete urethral lining which overcomes the objection to the buried strip principle. It also avoids the occasional problem of meatal stenosis[10]. The incisions on the ventral surface of the penis are unchanged but on the dorsum the incisions are carried distal to the preputial pits to reach points 2 mm apart at what will be the ventral lip of the new meatus. The incisions are then carried through the preputial mucosa on either side of the midline to outline a mucosal strip 3 mm wide. The length of the strip corresponds to the extra length of urethra required.

The two triangular mucosal flaps on either side of the preputial strip are raised thinly and based on the glans. They are usually discarded, although part of one may be useful in covering the dorsum. Two strips of skin are also discarded from either side of the prepuce in order to provide anchorage to the glans when the dorsal flap is rotated to the front. The dorsal flap is freed proximally towards the root of the penis in the layer superficial to the deep fascia so that it can be easily rotated to the front. The strip of preputial mucosa is tacked in two or three places to the ventral buried strip in order to fashion a complete urethra. The meatus is made slightly narrower than the urethra, and the buried sutures are inserted to fix the flap and control bleeding from the glans in the usual way. The final appearance is the same as that of the Van der Meulen repair. It is safe to retain tissue distal to the pits provided that the axial vessels are left intact.

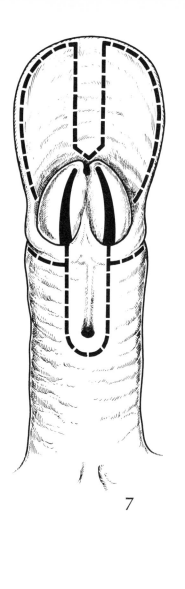

7

8

Two-stage repair

Principles

This method is used when the meatus is proximal to the midshaft of the penis. The curvature is maintained by three factors: (1) the urethra is short, (2) there are multiple fine bands of fibrous tissue running longitudinally from the glans to the region of the meatus in the superficial fascia, and (3) the glans is tilted downwards. The third factor is ignored, but the first two are overcome, indeed overcorrected, by the dissection. In principle, a transverse incision is made just behind the glans (if placed nearer to the scrotum, potentially hair-bearing skin will be introduced into what will be the urethral lining). The incision enables the tight bands on the ventral aspect to be divided. To complete the overcorrection of the chordee, the meatus is freed and retreated towards the perineum;

sometimes a separate incision will be needed to provide access. The prepuce and dorsal skin are now divided to allow the transverse incision to be sutured vertically in the midline. The two halves of the prepuce are now 'parked' on the glans in readiness for urethral repair at the next stage. It will be seen that the objective of the first operation is to make urethral repair safe and effective at the second operation. The siting of the main scar in the midline ensures that all the healing edges (of both the lining layer and the covering flaps) used for urethral repair will be free of scar, and first intention healing will be achieved, provided that tension and other adverse factors are eliminated.

STAGE 1 – CHORDEE CORRECTION

Overcorrection of the chordee is important, particularly in moderate and severe cases, and methods which fail in this regard should be discarded. In principle, the Duplay[11] method is advocated, because the dissection is radical enough to enable all tight bands to be divided. It is useful to 'park' the two halves of the prepuce on the front of the glans for later use in urethral repair[13]. Methods which use up all the available penile and preputial skin to cover the front of the penis are unsatisfactory because nothing is left for urethral repair.

9

Similarly, methods which introduce Z's on to the ventral surface can give good chordee correction but they prejudice a successful urethral repair because of scarring of what will be the buried strip and covering flaps. These scars reduce the healing potential of the skin and may cause strictures and fistulae.

A method should be chosen which overcorrects the chordee, confines the scar to the midline, and avoids introducing hair-bearing skin into what will be the urethra. The operation should rearrange the tissues in such a way that urethral repair will be made easier at the next operation.

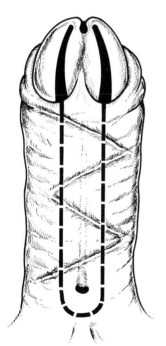

9

10 & 11

The incision

A temporary suture through the tip of the glans helps to steady the part, and bleeding is controlled by finger pressure. The skin on the front of the penis is incised transversely 3 mm behind the glans, from one side of the prepuce to the other. Skin flaps are raised upwards and downwards, giving access to the longitudinal tight bands in the superficial fascia which are divided over the whole width of the penis, to expose a large area of deep fascia. If the deep fascia is accidentally opened, a stitch will control the bleeding. The meatus is freed from its distal attachments (working either from the transverse incision or by a separate V–Y procedure which allows it to move backwards to complete the overcorrection of the chordee). The V–Y is designed to avoid introducing hair-bearing skin into what will be the urethral lining by confining the incision to the hairless strip near the midline.

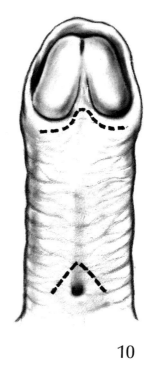

10

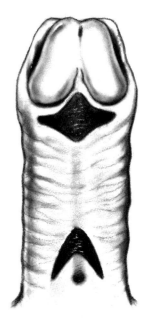

11

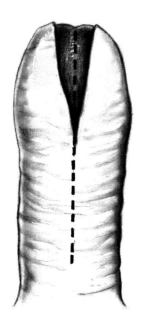

12

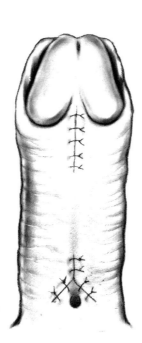

13

12 & 13

Relaxation and suturing

The prepuce is divided dorsally, and the incision is continued for a short distance down the dorsum in the midline until the transverse incision on the ventral aspect can be closed without tension. The dorsal defect is either closed transversely or left to heal spontaneously.

14

'Parking' the prepuce

The opportunity is now taken to unite each half of the prepuce to the glans in readiness for use at the next operation. On each side, full-thickness strips of mucosa and skin 2 mm wide are removed with scissors from the prepuce and glans so they can be sutured together on either side of what will be the new terminal urethra. The choice of suture material is not very important at this stage. A catheter is not inserted.

Dressing

A non-encircling pressure dressing holds the penis to the abdominal wall, leaving the meatus exposed. The dressing is removed in the bath after 48 hours. Early ambulation and discharge home are encouraged.

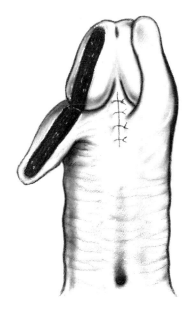

14

Modified Denis Browne method

STAGE II – URETHRAL REPAIR

Conditions that rely on either a suprapubic cystotomy or a perineal urethrostomy impose an unnecessary additional burden on the patient and attendants. Methods that rely on direct advancement under tension are doomed to failure because postoperative oedema will cause sutures to cut out, resulting in leakage of urine and fistula formation. Splitting or tunnelling of the glans is unnecessary and sometimes leads to a late stricture development. A terminal or subterminal meatus can be fashioned by simpler means.

Methods which use very long, narrow, random flaps and those in which a length of prepuce is tubed and applied as a free graft are prone to complications and are better used only in special circumstances.

After chordee correction it is sometimes possible, if the dorsum is unscarred, to repair the urethra using the Van der Meulen method (*see* pp. 550–551). This is generally safer than the modified Denis Browne method because there is less tension on the suture lines. If neither of these methods is feasible the use of scrotum[3] should be considered rather than risk a breakdown.

Proximally, the inclusion of potentially hair-bearing skin in what will be the lining layer of the urethra is avoided by using the moist gutter which is present in the midline. The covering layer is made by advancing skin flaps from the sides of the penis and scrotum and uniting them over the buried strip which is left unsutured. Complete relaxation is obtained by undermining the flaps laterally and proximally and by a dorsal relaxation incision which must be longer than the suture line on the ventral aspect. A watertight repair is ensured by uniting the flaps with two layers of continuous sutures with the 'bites' close together. A catheter is inserted for 2–5 days (depending on the individual case) to make the establishment of micturition easy.

Preliminary operative steps

First, it is important to make sure the prepuce has healed to the glans so there is no risk of a fistula developing along the corona. If a fistula is present, it is excised and repaired at the beginning of the operation. A temporary suture is inserted through the tip of the glans.

15

The incision

The width of the U-shaped buried strip is equal to the circumference of the existing urethra. At the site of the new meatus full-thickness strips are removed to narrow the lumen slightly and create broad surfaces for healing.

Raising the flaps

The flaps which will cover the buried strip are raised as thickly as possible (avoiding opening the deep fascia) and are undermined proximally and laterally until they can be freed from the buried strip.

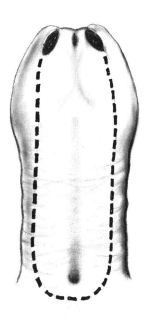

15

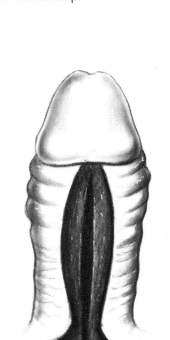

16

16

Relaxation

To avoid tearing the delicate skin by sutures inserted under tension, a generous dorsal slit is made, dividing skin, muscle fibres and veins until the flaps from the sides of the penis will meet loosely in the midline, ventrally, before repair is carried out. To be effective, the relaxation incision must be longer than the ventral suture line. On occasion it will be necessary to make it fork at the pubis. The two extra limbs now run along the junction of scrotum and thigh, dividing the skin until satisfactory relaxation is achieved. The large dorsal defect is skin grafted.

17 & 18

Suture and catheter

A short length of polythene tubing of suitable diameter is passed just beyond the meatus and sutured to the tip of the glans. Alternatively, a 6 or 8 Fr Gibbon catheter is passed into the bladder. The catheter and buried strip are now covered by uniting the flaps in the midline with two layers of continuous 4/0 Dexon. The first suture picks up the subcutaneous tissue, taking care to avoid perforating the skin. The next layer unites the skin edges meticulously. The repair is tested by injecting water along the new urethra; if leakage occurs a few reinforcing sutures are inserted. The dressing is similar to the one already described.

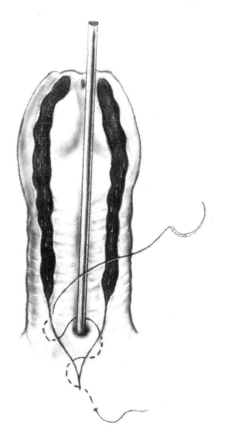

17

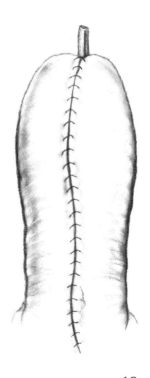

18

Hypospadias cripples

This group of patients comprises those who have had a number of operations but who have failed to make progress[4]. The first duty of the surgeon is to gain the confidence of the patient and his parents who may be demoralized. It should be pointed out that it is seldom possible to repair the deformity in one operation and many patients need multiple procedures. First, the chordee must be overcorrected, hair-bearing skin excised and replaced, and strictures opened and repaired so that recurrence is unlikely. The defects created are repaired using hairless flaps from the dorsum or sides of the penis or preputial remnants; if these sources are no longer available, hairless, free, full-thickness grafts taken from the inner aspect of the upper arm are applied. After at least 6 months the urethra is repaired using the buried strip principle. The lining strip is made on generous lines because it is scarred. It is left unsutured in the interest of safety. Skin cover usually requires the introduction of an unscarred flap from the abdominal wall or thigh.

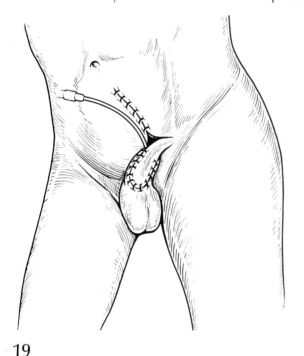

19

Defects of the distal half of the penis

19

These can be repaired using a hypogastric flap[13]. The flap, which contains the superficial epigastric vessels, is usually raised on the left side (to avoid scarring one of the preserves of the general surgeon). It is inset on to a U-shaped defect created on the front of the penis which outlines a generously wide buried strip and includes the original meatus. The U-shaped defect is made by excising a narrow strip of skin and scar. The flap is united to the glans where two triangular raw surfaces are created on either side of the new meatus. A Foley catheter is left in place to make nursing care easier.

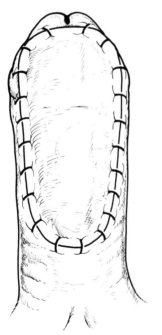

20

20

After 2½ weeks the flap is divided just distal to the level of the new meatus and left to heal spontaneously. The unwanted portion of the flap is discarded or returned to the abdominal wall.

Defects of more than the distal half of the penis

21 & 22

Skin cover can be safely provided using a flap from the superomedial aspect of the thigh[14]. This flap, which contains the medial femoral circumflex vessels, is raised down to the deep fascia. It is inset on to a U-shaped defect created in the same way as the one just described for distal repairs.

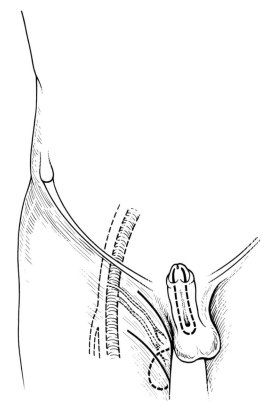

21

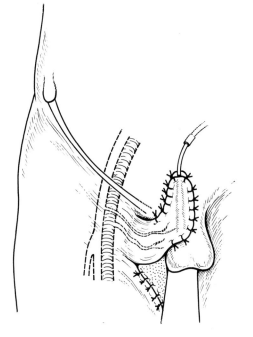

22

23

Proximally, complete closure is not possible so when the flap is divided after 3 weeks a fistula is left. It can be repaired either immediately or some weeks later, using a scrotal flap. Both the hypogastric and adductor flaps are bulky, but they can be thinned by removing unwanted skin and fat after a wait of at least 6 months.

Postoperative care and complications

Oedema is common but is not detrimental. A haematoma, unless it is very small, must be evacuated. Dysuria is avoided by the use of analgesics and baths and the early encouragement of micturition. Fistulae are closed after about 6 months; scarred skin and redundant lining are excised and the buried strip principle applied with full relaxation of covering flaps. The use of a scrotal flap is occasionally of value for large defects. Complete breakdown is rare, but secondary repair is usually successful after an interval of 1 year, using the same principles as before. Occasionally repair is carried out using scrotum when multiple failures have led to scarring and virtual destruction of much of the available skin. Secondary lengthening of the contracted penile dorsum is carried out by scar excision and covering the defect by flaps from the sides of the penis.

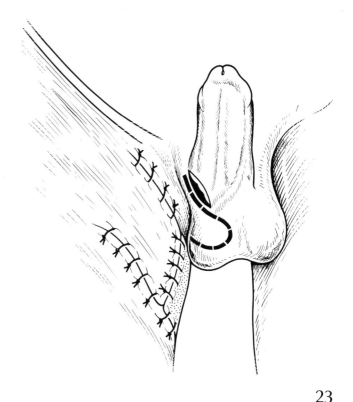

23

References

1. Browne, D. An operation for hypospadias. Lancet 1936; 1:141–143

2. Fraser, K. Hypospadias a Queensland review of 31 major hypospadias repairs using a uniform technique. British Journal of Surgery 1964; 51: 167–178

3. Sommerlad, B. C. British Journal of Plastic Surgery 1975; 28: 324–330

4. Devine, J. C., Horton, C. E. Hypospadias cripples. In: Horton, C. E., ed. Plastic and reconstructive surgery of the genital area. Boston: Little Brown and Co., 1973, 389–392

5. Mustardé, J. C. (ed.) Plastic surgery in infancy and childhood. Philadelphia: W. B. Saunders, 1971

6. McCormack, R. M. Simultaneous chordee repair and urethral reconstruction for hypospadias; experimental and clinical studies. Plastic and Reconstructive Surgery 1954; 13: 257–274

7. Immergut, M., Boldus, R., Yannone, E., Bunge, R., Flocks, R. The local application of testosterone cream to the prepubertal phallus. Journal of Urology 1971; 105: 905–906

8. Van der Meulen, J. C. H. M. Hypospadias Academica, Leyden, 1964

9. Henderson, H. P. One-stage hypospadias repair: a review of 143 cases treated by the van der Meulen technique. British Journal of Plastic Surgery 1981; 34: 144–148

10. Tolhurst, D. E., Gorter, H. A review of 102 cases of hypospadias treated by the van der Meulen procedure. British Journal of Plastic Surgery 1976; 29: 361–367

11. Duplay, S. De l'hypospadias périnéo-scrotal et de sun traitement chirurgical. Archives Generales de Médécine 1874; 1: 513–530, 657–682

12. Yarbrough, W. J., Johnston, J. M. Crawford modification of Denis Browne hypospadias procedure. The Journal of Urology 1977; 117: 782–783

13. McGregor, I. A. Fundamental techniques of plastic surgery: their surgical applications. 5th ed. Edinburgh: E. & S. Livingstone, 1972

14. Hirschowitz, B., Moscona, R., Kaufman, I., Pnini, A. One-stage reconstruction of the scrotum following Fournier's syndrome using a probable arterial flap. Plastic and Reconstructive Surgery 1980; 66: 608

Illustrations by Robert N. Lane

Other techniques of hypospadias repair

W. Scott McDougal MD
Professor and Chairman, Department of Urology,
Vanderbilt University Medical Center Nashville, Tennessee, USA

Introduction

The previous chapter outlines several techniques for hypospadias repair. Two techniques not described which have also gained popularity are the flip-flop flap and the island pedicle flap. It is important that the urologist interested in hypospadias surgery is familiar with many repair techniques so that the most appropriate operation is chosen for each individual.

The flip-flop flap and the island pedicle flap are one-stage procedures. Among their advantages over two-stage operations are that they allow the use of virgin tissue for the creation of both flaps and neourethra, anatomic placement of the meatus at the apex of the glans, and coverage of the penis with unscarred, pliable, non-hair-bearing skin. The goals of any hypospadias repair also include complete chordee release and the creation of a urethra which does not develop a diverticulum, stricture or fistula.

FLIP-FLOP FLAP PROCEDURE

This procedure is used when there is hypospadias and no chordee; a slight modification of this procedure may be employed when the meatus is distal to the midshaft of the penis following release of the chordee.

Procedure

The absence of chordee must be confirmed by an artificial erection, produced by placing a tourniquet at the base of the penis and injecting the corpora cavernosa with saline.

1

A holding suture is placed in the glans. The incision is outlined and infiltrated with 1:100000 adrenaline (epinephrine) and 1 per cent lignocaine (lidocaine) to aid in haemostasis during dissection.

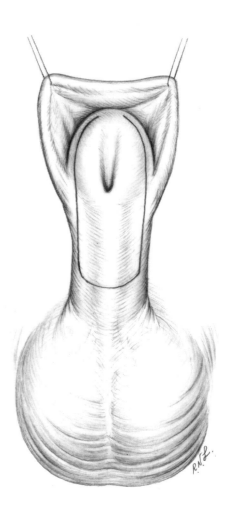

1

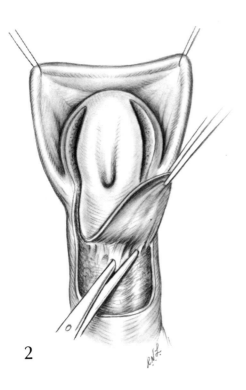

2

2

The proximal portion of the flap is dissected free and rotated distally.

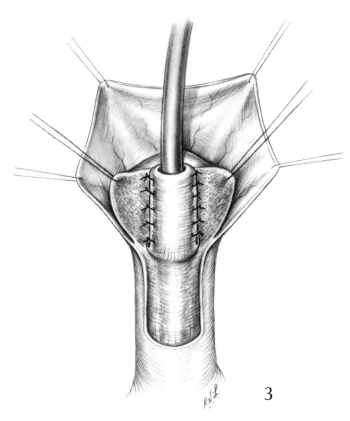

3

A No. 8 or No. 10 feeding tube is placed through the urethra into the bladder. The edges of the flap are sutured together with interrupted 5/0 chromic suture. The foreskin is incised and triangular flaps are raised on the glans.

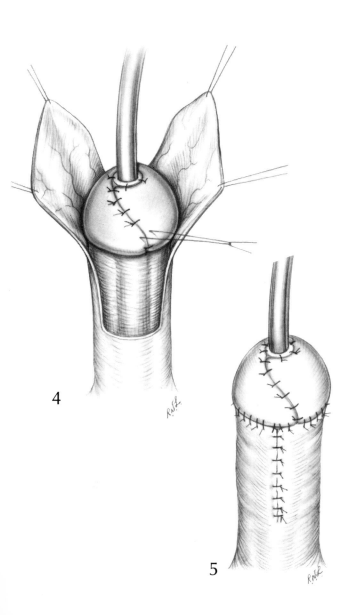

4 & 5

These flaps form a Z-type closure over the glanular urethra. The dorsal foreskin may then be incised around the glans, split, dissected proximally, and sutured ventrally and dorsally to close the skin defect.

MODIFIED PROCEDURE

6

The incision is outlined.

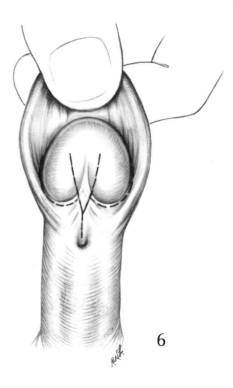

6

7

Notice the creation of triangular flaps on the glans. Following release of chordee the length of urethra is measured and outlined on the proximal portion of the shaft of the penis. The width of the flap is approximately 10–15 mm.

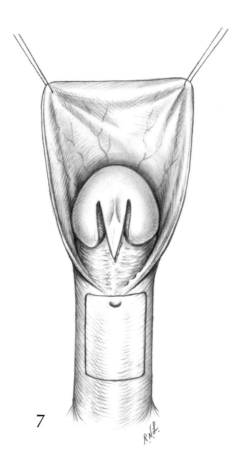

7

8

Using a No. 8 or No. 10 indwelling urethral catheter, the flap is tubed with interrupted 5/0 chromic suture.

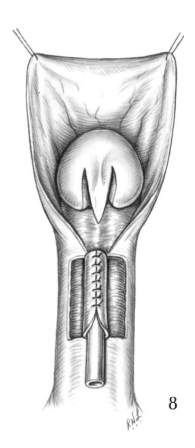

8

9

By flipping the flap distally the suture line is buried, and the distal end is sutured to the triangular flap.

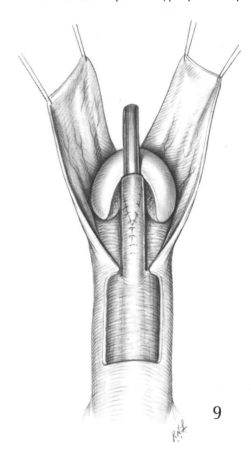

9

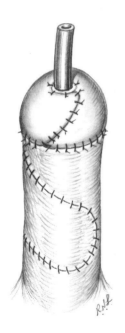

10

10

Using the two lateral triangular flaps, a Z-plasty is formed over the glans, thus bringing the urethral meatus to the tip of the glans. By splitting the dorsal foreskin and rotating it ventrally, the skin defect on the shaft of the penis is covered.

Postoperative care

The wound is dressed by applying Xeroform gauze over the suture lines, followed by light gauze and Elastoplast dressing. The urethral catheter is left indwelling for 10–14 days. Complications of this procedure include strictures (particularly of the glandular urethra) and fistulae. In our experience, the flip-flop flap technique produces fewer complications than the island pedicle technique with only a 5–10 per cent incidence of subsequent surgical procedures.

ISLAND PEDICLE FLAP

This technique allows a one-stage reconstruction in patients whose urethra is located proximal to the midshaft of the penis. Using the island pedicle flap technique a 2–6 cm urethra can be created.

Procedure

11

A holding suture is placed in the dorsal glans, and the subcutaneous tissue is infiltrated with a solution of 1:100000 adrenaline (epinephrine) and 1 per cent lignocaine (lidocaine) to aid in haemostasis. The incision is made around the circumference of the glans and extends vertically from the glans to the meatus on the ventrum of the penis. The chordee is corrected by incising the bands on the ventrum of the penis. Correction of the chordee is confirmed by an artificial erection, and attention can then be given to the creation of the island pedicle.

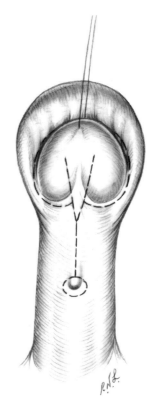

11

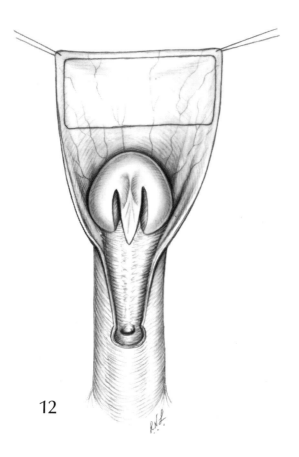

12

12

The proposed site of the island pedicle on the dorsal foreskin is outlined. The length of the flap corresponds to the length of urethra required, and the width is generally 12–15 mm.

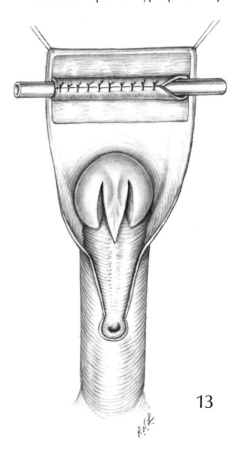

13

A No. 10 red rubber catheter is placed in the island pedicle. The margins of the tube surrounding this catheter are sutured with interrupted 5/0 chromic suture.

13

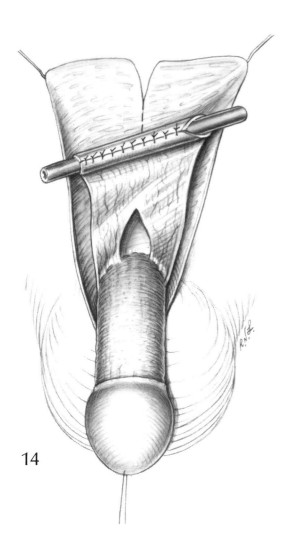

14

14

Following tubing of the island pedicle, the skin of the penis is dissected from Buck's fascia circumferentially. The island pedicle is then carefully dissected and transposed from the dorsum to the ventrum of the penis. For long pedicles a buttonhole in the base of the pedicle may be made, as shown.

15

The proximal portion of the urethra is sutured in an oblique fashion. The distal portion is sutured to the triangle of skin on the glans.

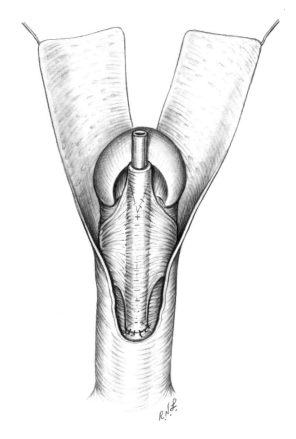

16

The glandular urethra is subsequently covered by a Z-plasty technique. The dorsal foreskin is split, brought around to the ventral aspect of the penis and sutured with 5/0 chromic suture.

A Xeroform dressing is placed over the penile wounds. Soft gauze dressings and Elastoplast support the penis against the abdomen. A No. 8 feeding tube is sutured to the glans and placed in the neourethra. A suprapubic cystotomy is performed for urinary drainage.

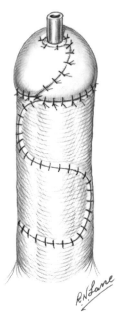

Postoperative care of the urethra

The urethral catheter is left in place for two weeks. After removal of the urethral catheter the suprapubic tube is clamped, allowing one to determine whether complete healing has occurred and whether any fistulae are present. Following establishment of adequate voiding and in the absence of any fistulae, the suprapubic catheter is removed. Using the island pedicle flap technique, excellent results have been obtained, with a secondary procedure being required in about 15–20 per cent of cases. The secondary procedure most commonly involves closure of a small urethral fistulae which usually arises from the proximal suture line.

Further reading

Devine, C. J. Jr., Horton, C. E. Hypospadias repair. Journal of Urology 1977; 118:188–193

Duckett, J. W. The island flap for hypospadias repair. Urologic Clinics of North America 1981; 8:503–511

Illustrations by Rudolf Brammer and Cathy Slatter

Congenital abnormalities of the penis

Herbert B. Eckstein MD, MChir, FRCS
Consultant Paediatric Surgeon, Hospital for Sick Children, Great Ormond Street, London, UK

Introduction

Hypospadias, epispadias and related abnormalities are covered in other sections of this volume and this chapter is limited to some unusual abnormalities of the penis encountered in infancy and childhood.

Micropenis

A very short phallus is a frequent feature of epispadias and exstrophy but the term micropenis is reserved for boys with anatomically normal lower urinary tracts. Penile growth is dependent upon testicular androgen secretion so that bilateral testicular growth failure will result in a small phallus. This situation may arise from pituitary gland lesions – when no gonadotrophic hormone is formed and the testicles remain undeveloped – or from bilateral intrauterine testicular torsion.

The condition causes considerable parental anxiety. The local application of 5 per cent testosterone ointment will usually produce some penile growth, but it is now thought that the effect is from the systemic absorption of testosterone through the skin. Certainly virilization of the mother, produced by her absorbing the hormone through her fingers, is a recognized complication of this treatment. Testosterone injections are therefore a more appropriate form of treatment. Surgery as such has very little to offer in more severe cases, although a sex-change and rearing the infant as a female may be considered[1].

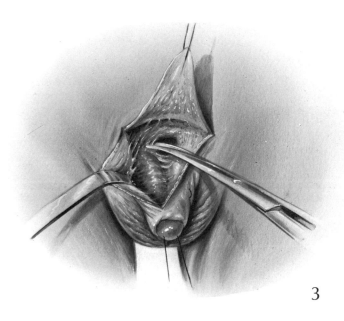

3

1–5

In less severe cases, the length of the phallus can be increased by approximating the widely separated corpora. The corpora are exposed through a V-shaped incision on the dorsal aspect of the penis and are carefully dissected off the pubic arch as far as possible. They are then approximated with interrupted non-absorbable sutures and the skin is finally closed as a Y.

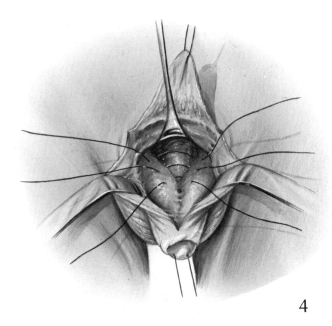

4

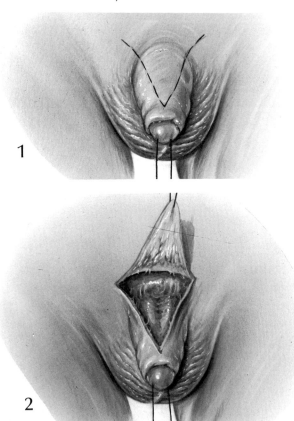

1

2

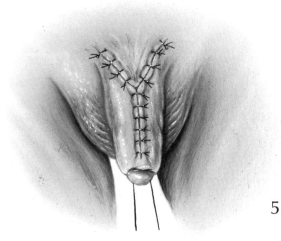

5

Buried penis

In this condition the penis may be virtually invisible or just much too small in relation to the boy's age and size. Palpation will, however, reveal a normal glans and penile shaft which tend to be buried in excessive prepubic fat. It is not surprising that the buried penis is more frequently found in obese little boys than in those of normal weight, and loss of fat on a suitable diet will often produce a satisfactory organ, as will the passage of time. The normal phallus can be demonstrated to the parents by digital pressure applied to the prepubic fat.

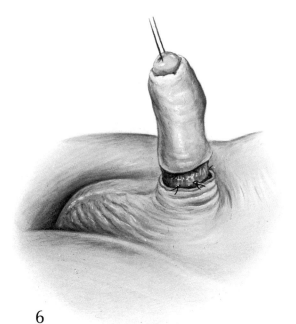

6

6–8

An improvement in the appearance of the penis can be obtained by the following relatively simple procedure[2]. An annular incision is made around the base of the penis (*Illustration 6*), a triangle of skin is excised (*Illustration 7*) and sutures are placed as in *Illustration 8a*. It is important to place the central suture on the dorsal side into the periosteal tissues of the symphysis pubis and the ventral suture through the wall of the corpus spongiosum (*Illustration 8b*).

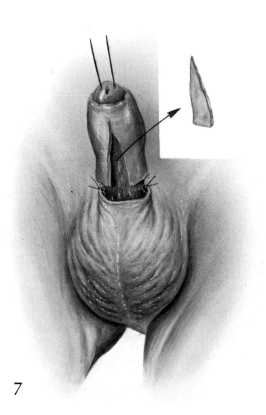

7

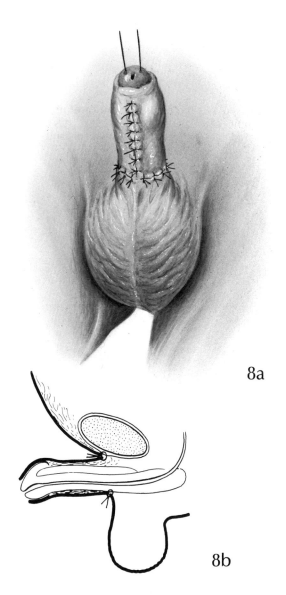

8a

8b

9, 10 & 11

Webbed penis

Sometimes an unusually well developed web of skin between the anterior aspect of the scrotum and the ventral aspect of the penis gives the appearance of a buried penis. This abnormality is easily correctable by a transverse incision into the web which is then sutured longitudinally. Alternatively a Z-plasty can be used.

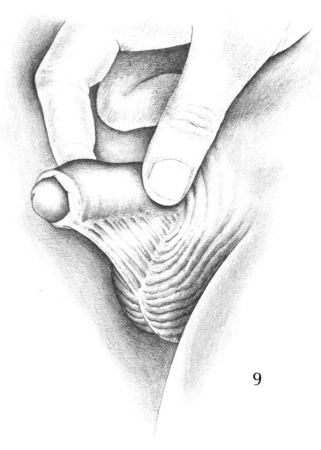

9

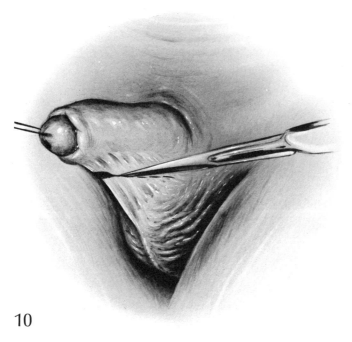

10

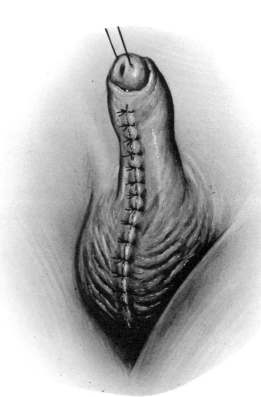

11

Torsion of the penis

Some degree of torsion of the penis is not infrequently encountered in association with hypospadias and can be corrected at the time of the hypospadias repair. Torsion on its own is less common and is almost invariably towards the left. If the angle of torsion reaches 90° surgical correction is indicated.

12 & 13

The operation described by Johnston[2] is simple and effective. A circumferential incision is made near the base of the penis and the skin covering the penile shaft is widely mobilized by blunt dissection. This procedure allows derotation of the glans and urethral orifice and the skin is then sutured so as slightly to over-correct the torsion. Catheter drainage is not needed, but oedema of the foreskin is a common problem.

An alternative technique which avoids this complication has been described[3]. The circular incision is placed at the distal end of the foreskin, as for circumcision, and indeed circumcision can be combined with the derotation procedure. The penile skin is again widely mobilized and resutured (with or without foreskin) so as to over-correct the torsion.

Acknowledgement

Illustrations 1–8 and *10–13* are reproduced from Johnston[2] by courtesy of the Publisher.

References

1. Johnston, J. H. Abnormalities of the penis. In: Williams, D. I., Johnston, J. H., eds. Paediatric urology, 2nd ed. London: Butterworths, 1982: 435–450

2. Johnston, J. H. Other penile abnormalities. In: Eckstein, H. B., Hohenfellner, R., Williams, D. I., eds. Surgical pediatric urology. Stuttgart: Thieme, 1977: 406–413

3. Azmy, A., Eckstein, H. B. Surgical correction of torsion of the penis. British Journal of Urology 1981; 53: 378–379

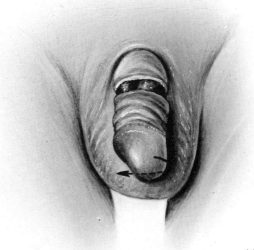

12

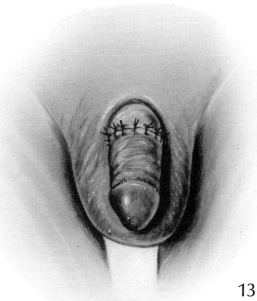

13

Partial and radical penectomy

W. K. Yeates MD, MS, FRCS
Consultant Urologist, Freeman Hospital, Newcastle-upon-Tyne;
Lecturer in Urology, University of Newcastle;
Honorary Senior Lecturer, Institute of Urology, University of London, UK

Introduction

Amputation of the penis is required almost exclusively for cases of carcinoma arising in the preputial sac. The growth may be intraepithelial (carcinoma *in situ*) but is usually papillary, and rather less commonly solid and infiltrating. The papillary variety often forms a large mass with little infiltration either deeply or proximally for a considerable time, but subsequently spreads subcutaneously superficial to Buck's fascia. The infiltrating variety, which may present initially as an ulcer, also extends proximally but tends to invade the corpora cavernosa; the corpus spongiosum is affected only in late cases. All the growths tend to be complicated by infection under the prepuce which has either always been nonretractile or become so as a result of the growth. A dorsal slit may be required to demonstrate the lesion and to obtain a confirmatory biopsy.

Inguinal lymph node enlargement is frequently present, but this is often due to infection. In many cases it subsides after the amputation.

Radiotherapy is usually unsuitable for these growths, particularly because of the severity of the associated infection. It can sometimes be applied with success after a preliminary dorsal slit if the infection resolves rapidly ; it is most suitable for the flat, superficially ulcerating variety.

The choice between a partial and a total amputation depends partly on the superficial extent of the growth and partly on its depth of infiltration. Cases without involvement of the subcutaneous tissues for 2.5 cm distal to the penoscrotal junction may be treated by partial amputation. Proximal extension beyond this point implies that the penile stump after amputation will be so short that a total amputation with or without bilateral orchidectomy is preferable. It should be remembered, however, that coitus is still possible after a partial amputation: unless there is probable involvement of the corpora, these should not be cut shorter than is necessary.

Total amputation of the penis is probably best combined with removal of the scrotum and testes, as this prevents urinary contamination of the scrotum, and incidentally reduces androgen production.

LYMPH NODE DISSECTION

Lymph node dissection should not be carried out at the time of amputation of the penis, partly because it may be unnecessary as the node enlargement is frequently due only to infection, and partly because such infection makes wound breakdown almost certain if excision is carried out at this stage.

Indications

Node dissection is indicated when the enlargement persists for more than 6 weeks after the amputation of the penis and biopsy shows the presence of metastases, or if node enlargement increases after this time. Sometimes only the one node removed for biopsy contains metastases. If the primary growth was well-differentiated, there is a reasonably strong case for confining the dissection to one side, at least initially. Usually, the procedure should include removal of the external iliac group as high as the bifurcation of the common iliac artery. If bilateral dissection is decided upon, it should be carried out in two stages with about a week's interval unless the surgeon is very experienced in the procedure.

Where operability is in doubt, the external iliac nodes should be exposed first. If, as confirmed by frozen section, they are widely involved, it is advisable not to proceed with the inguinal dissection as this will lead to subsequent tumour fungation. Otherwise, it is best to begin with the inguinal dissection and to extend it upwards if the initial dissection has confirmed that the nodes are removable.

The operations

Position of patient

The patient should be operated on in the supine position for partial amputation and in the lithotomy position for total amputation.

PARTIAL AMPUTATION

1a, b & c

The incision may be circular, oblique or fashioned to create a dorsal or ventral skin flap. The latter will be described but the other methods are equally acceptable and may be preferable for growths which are more ventrally situated. The site of the skin section need be no further than 1.5 cm away from the edge of the obvious growth and probably 1 cm is enough. It is easy to remove too great a length of corpora. The correct amount is much easier to assess without using a tourniquet which is quite unnecessary especially before the skin incisions have been made.

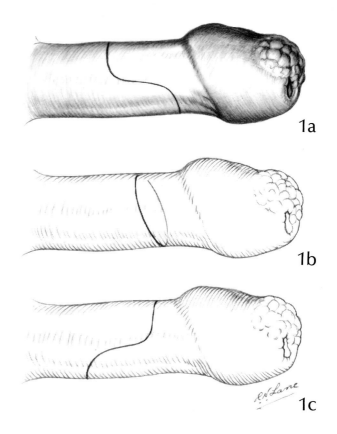

1a

1b

1c

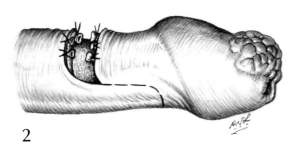

2

2

The skin incision is mapped out with ink or at points with a diathermy needle. The skin is divided with fine scissors; the superficial and then the deep dorsal vessels are isolated, divided and ligated. The site for dividing the corpora cavernosa is selected at the same level as the proximal line of the skin incision and is marked without either retracting the skin or stretching the penis.

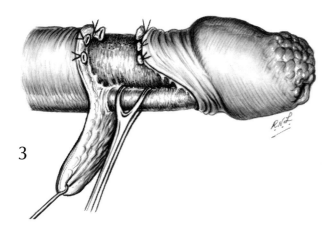

3

3

A tissue forceps is applied to enclose the corpus spongiosum at the level chosen for section of the corpora cavernosa.

4

The corpora cavernosa are compressed either digitally (most conveniently between the assistant's index finger from above and the surgeon's index finger from below) or by applying a rubber tourniquet. The corpora are cut across from above with a knife at the site marked before the application of compression. The dorsum of the corpus spongiosum is closely applied to the central part of the septum but the corpus is protected by the tissue forceps previously applied. The deep arteries in the corpora cavernosa are easily identified by releasing the compression; they are clipped and ligated.

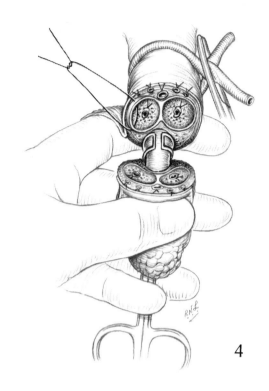

4

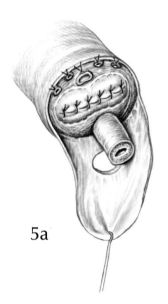

5a

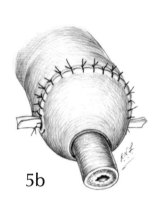

5b

5a & b

The corpus spongiosum is then cut across 1 cm beyond the tissue forceps and dissected free. The corpora are closed by approximating their sheaths either vertically or transversely (in the latter case the sutures pick up the vertical septum). This closure completely controls haemorrhage. The corpus spongiosum with its contained urethra is passed through an adequate stab incision in the flap which is then sutured with fine silk, leaving a small piece of thin rubber drain at either angle.

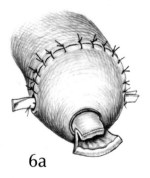

6a

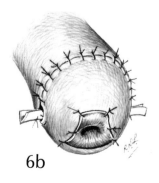

6b

6a & b

The protruding urethra is split dorsolaterally on each side, and the angles created are sutured with catgut to the edge of the stab incision. The larger ventral urethral flap is then sutured at each corner to the outer surface of the skin.

A small (12–16 Fr) balloon catheter is inserted, making sure that the stab incision is large enough to prevent any compression of the protruding urethra.

TOTAL AMPUTATION

7

A vertical midline incision is made in the perineum. The bulbospongiosus muscle is split and the corpus spongiosum is divided about 4 cm from its posterior extremity and then freed for about 2.5 cm. A Foley catheter (size 16–18 Fr) is inserted into the bladder.

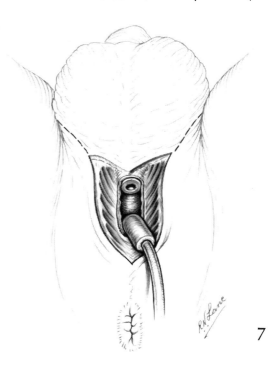

7

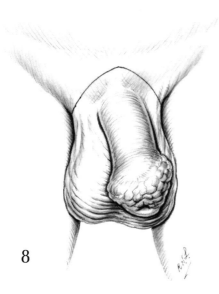

8

8

The penis and base of the scrotum are encircled by a skin incision extending from the prepubic region round each side of the scrotum about 3 cm from its base, joining the midline perineal incision behind.

9

The superficial dorsal and other vessels are divided and ligated. Both spermatic cords are isolated, ligated and divided just below the external inguinal rings.

9

10

The superficial suspensory (fundiform) ligament is divided, followed by progressive incision of the deep suspensory ligament close to the pubis. When the ligament has been completely divided, the deep dorsal vein is isolated, ligated and divided. Slightly more posteriorly, the dorsal arteries are similarly dealt with just after they have perforated the perineal membrane.

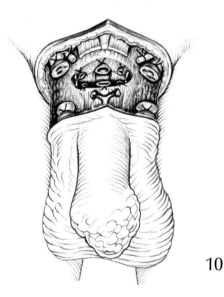

10

11

The ischiocavernosus muscles (omitted from the diagram for clarity) and then the crura of the corpora cavernosa are dissected off the ischiopubic rami. If the total amputation is required because of the extent of superficial spread, the corpora are crushed, divided and ligated about 4 cm from their posterior extremities. If, however, the operation is required because of involvement of the corpora, each crus should be completely removed from the ramus either by a raspatory or diathermy needle. The deep artery of the penis enters the crus about 2 cm from its posterior extremity and may be isolated and clipped before division; it may be necessary to remove the crus and then to under-run the cut end of the vessel as it passes through the perineal membrane. After division of a few remaining attachments to the perineal membrane, the whole mass is removed.

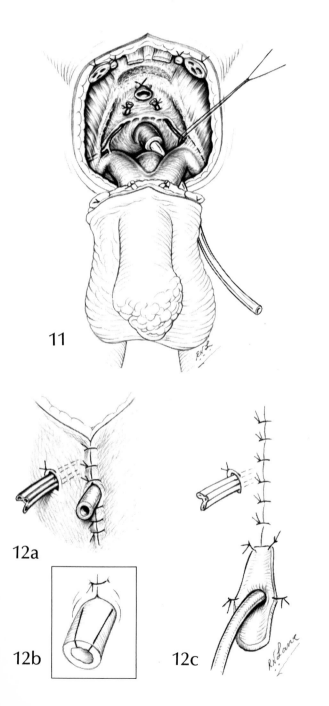

11

12a, b & c

A stab incision is made on one side and a tissue drain inserted (a). The midline incision is closed round the corpus spongiosum, leaving about 2 cm protruding. The corpus is split as in partial amputation into an anterior quarter and a posterior three-quarter segment (b). The angles are sutured with 3/0 chromic catgut to the wound edges and the anterior flap is spreadeagled and sutured to the skin surface. The posterior flap is left free (c).

The skin incision is closed with thick silk sutures; the anterior ones pick up the periosteum of the pubis to tack the skin down to the deeper tissues and so reduce dead space.

Postoperative care

Partial amputation

The drains are removed on the day following operation. The catheter is left in for about 3 days, with the usual precautions to prevent infection being applied during the time of drainage. The skin sutures are removed on the 7th postoperative day.

Total amputation

The tissue drain is removed on about the third day. The catheter is left indwelling for about 5 days.

Complications

Peroperative

With total amputation persistent oozing from the cut ends of the corpus spongiosum occasionally occurs because of persistent erection of the stump. This may require oversewing of the cut surface. Sometimes there is excessive widespread oozing but this is readily controllable by pressure with hot wet mops for a few minutes.

Postoperative

Stenosis of the external urinary meatus may occur following either partial or total amputation, but it is very rare when the above techniques are used. The redundant urethra looks unsightly at first, but when healing is complete the larger segment of the urethral circumference remains as a small protruding rim of pink mucosa, without stenosis (*see Illustration 12c*). If a meatal stricture should develop and require more than occasional dilatation, a small plastic procedure rotating in skin flaps is relatively easily performed.

Further reading

Burton, H. B., Spratt, J. S., Jr, Perez-Mesa, C., Watson, F. R., Leduc, R. J. Carcinoma of the penis. Journal of Urology 1976; 116: 458–461

Catalona, W. J. Role of lymphadenectomy in carcinoma of the penis. Urologic Clinics of North America 1980; 7: 3: 785–792

Droller, M. J. Carcinoma of the penis: An overview. Urologic Clinics of North America 1980; 7: 783–784

Grabstald, H. Controversies concerning lymph node dissection for cancer of the penis. Urologic Clinics of North America 1980; 7: 793–799

Haile, K., Delclos, L. The place of radiation therapy in the treatment of carcinoma of the distal end of the penis. Cancer 1980; 45: 1980–1984

Hoppmann, H. J., Fraiey, E. E. Squamous cell carcinoma of the penis. Journal of Urology 1978; 120: 393–398

Khezri, A. A., Dunn, M., Smith, P. J. B., Mitchell, J. P. Carcinoma of the penis. British Journal of Urology 1978; 50: 275–279

Merrin, C. E. Cancer of the penis. Cancer 1980; 45: 1973–1979

Narayana, A. S., Olney, L. E., Loening, S. A., Weimar, G. W., Culp, D. A. Carcinoma of the penis: analysis of 219 cases. Cancer 1982; 49: 2185–2191

Nelson, R. P., Derrick, F. C., Allen, W. R. Epidermoid carcinoma of the penis. British Journal of Urology 1982; 54: 172–175

Salaverria, J. C., Hope-Stone, H. F., Paris, A. M. I., Molland, E. A., Blandy, J. P. Conservative treatment of carcinoma of the penis. British Journal of Urology 1979; 51: 32–37

Smith, J. A., Jr, Middleton, R. G. The use of fluorescein in radical inguinal lymphadenectomy. Journal of Urology 1979; 122: 754–756

Ilioinguinal lymphadenectomy

W. K. Yeates MD, MS, FRCS
Consultant Urologist, Freeman Hospital, Newcastle-upon-Tyne;
Lecturer in Urology, University of Newcastle;
Honorary Senior Lecturer, Institute of Urology, University of London, UK

Indications

See chapter on 'Partial and radical penectomy', pp. 574–579.

The operation

1

The blood supply to the skin below and lateral to the inguinal lymph nodes is derived mainly from the superficial branches of the femoral artery and vein. These are divided in the course of the dissection, but the deep external pudendal arteries, the long scrotal branches of the internal pudendal and the lateral and terminal branches of the subcostal vessels all communicate to supply and drain this area. Therefore, unless it is necessary to excise skin adherent to the nodes, it is best to plan the incision so that the blood circulation from the medial side is preserved as far as possible (*see* left side of illustration).

If it is necessary to excise an elipse of overlying skin – which is exceptional – a large flap should be planned to rotate downwards either medially or laterally (*see* right side of illustration) to replace any skin which is shown by cyanosis to have a defective circulation at the end of the operation.

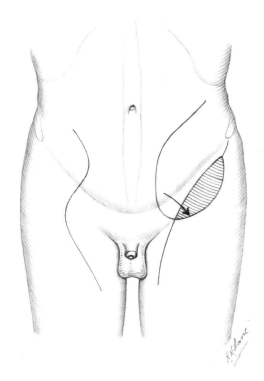

1

2

Skin flaps about 5 mm thick are raised to just beyond the boundaries of the femoral triangle. The external oblique aponeurosis is exposed about 2 cm above the inguinal ligament and the overlying fat is dissected downwards until the inguinal ligament and the spermatic cord emerging from the external inguinal ring are seen.

The deep fascia over the sartorius is incised from just below the anterior superior iliac spine to about the apex of the femoral triangle. The muscle fibres of the adductor longus are similarly exposed medially. The long saphenous vein is divided superficially to where these two incisions will intersect.

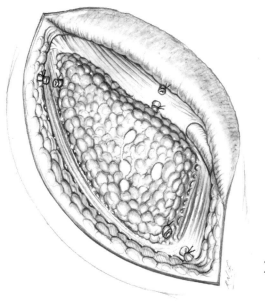

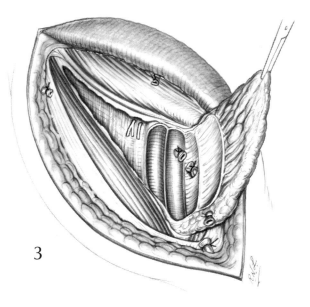

3

The deep fascia medial to the sartorius is then elevated by easy sharp dissection from the fascia overlying the psoas. This fascia also covers the deep branch of the femoral nerve which is not seen. The superficial branches of the femoral nerve are divided as they cross the plane between the fascias.

The anterolateral aspect of the femoral artery is felt and the femoral sheath is opened. The incision in the sheath and its adventitial continuation lower down is extended distally as far as the apex of the triangle. The sheath is easily elevated from the artery by dividing the former just below its attachment to the inguinal ligament. The septum between the artery and the vein is incised from above downwards. Further medial elevation of the femoral sheath readily displays the saphenofemoral junction. The saphenous vein is ligated and divided at the junction.

4

The lower angle and medial part of the delineated mass is dissected upwards and laterally, exposing the lateral part of the adductor longus and the medial part of the pectineus. Only the contiguous pectineal fascia and the medial wall of the femoral sheath and the contents of the femoral canal now remain undisturbed. The dissection can be terminated at this stage by dividing these remaining attachments and removing the contents of the femoral canal with the main mass.

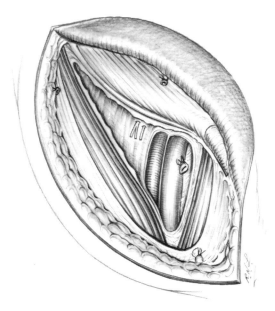

5

When, however, the external iliac group is also to be removed (as is usual), the contents of the femoral canal are left until the final stage of the dissection. The inguinal canal is opened and the spermatic cord is mobilized and elevated. The posterior wall of the inguinal canal is incised and the incision continued upwards and laterally towards McBurney's point. The deep epigastric vessels are ligated and divided.

The peritoneum is elevated upwards and medially until the bifurcation of the common iliac artery is seen. The sheath of the external iliac vessels is incised transversely and then longitudinally along the outer margin of the external iliac artery. The sheath and its associated lymph nodes, particularly those lying along the medial side of the femoral vein, are stripped downwards to the inguinal ligament. Sometimes this ligament can be elevated easily so the continuity of the external iliac and inguinal lymph nodes is clearly demonstrated. If not, the inguinal ligament is divided by incising the pectineal part medially and dividing the ligament itself at its attachment to the pubic tubercle. The whole mass is then removed.

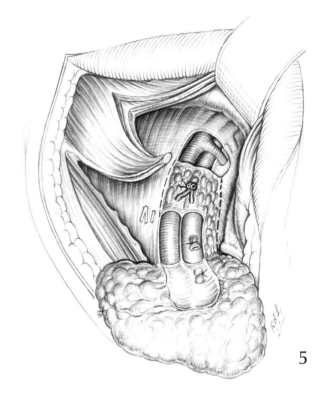

5

6

The wound is reconstructed in layers, the inguinal ligament and conjoined tendon being sutured to the pectineal ligament with chromic catgut. A tension-relieving incision into the lower part of the rectus sheath helps this approximation.

The femoral vessels are protected by dividing the sartorius muscle near its origin, mobilizing it and suturing the free cut end to the inguinal ligament by a few interrupted catgut sutures. This provides a covering for the vessels should the overlying skin slough.

A tissue drain (preferably of the suction type) is passed through a short stab incision below and lateral to the main incision. The wound is closed with interrupted silk sutures.

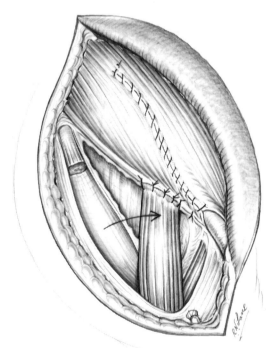

6

Postoperative care

The dressing is kept firmly applied with a spica bandage, and this is reapplied each time the dressing is changed. Drainage is maintained as long as there is much fluid discharge which is usually a few days.

Sometimes there is sloughing of the skin over an area of about 2 cm². After separation of the slough, healing occurs by secondary intention. Occasionally the sloughing is more extensive and it is subsequently necessary to graft the granulating surface.

A moderate amount of oedema may persist in the upper half of the thigh for weeks or months, but it very rarely involves the lower leg. In fact in such circumstances one should suspect that there is lymphatic involvement beyond the field of operation.

Further reading

See list at end of previous chapter.

Illustrations by Robert N. Lane

Operations for priapism

John P. Blandy   MA, DM, MCh, FRCS
Professor of Urology, The London Hospital Medical College;
Consultant Urologist, St Peter's Hospital, London, UK

Introduction

Priapism is usually a surgical emergency. With the possible exception of priapism in sickle cell disease, where exchange transfusion is recommended rather than operation[1], in most instances the sooner the blood in the distended corpora cavernosa is shunted into the flaccid glans penis or corpus spongiosum the better. There are exceptional cases where surgical shunting may not be feasible for one reason or another, and the alternative technique of blocking off the pudendal artery with autologous clot may be considered[2,3]. Ganglion-blocking agents do not work: anticoagulant therapy is usually ineffective (since the blood in a priapism does not coagulate – a fact well known to John Hunter). In practice the surgeon confronted with a priapism should proceed in steps, for not every case will respond to each technique, and it is prudent to progress from the least traumatic to the more difficult, step by step.

The operations

WATERHOUSE'S AND WINTER'S PROCEDURES

1a & b

It is easily confirmed, by simple palpation of the penis in a priapism, that the knobs of the erected corpora cavernosa protrude well up under and into the flaccid glans penis. In Waterhouse's manoeuvre a sharp knife is used to cut through the glans and the fascia covering the obstructed, bulging part of the corpora.

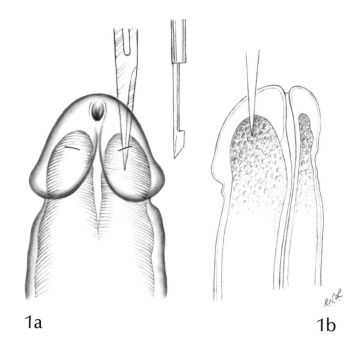

1a   1b

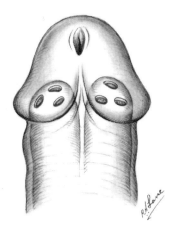

2

2

In Winter's procedure the same operation is done, only using a Trucut biopsy needle to remove a circle of the fascia in the hope of keeping the communication open between the tense and distended corpora cavernosa and the flaccid glans and its adjacent corpus spongiosum.

In the writer's experience Waterhouse's manoeuvre is the easiest and quickest, but does not always work. Similarly, cutting out a core with the Winter technique sometimes works, but not always, and not for long enough in the majority of cases. And so one progresses to the next step – namely, a corporocorporal anastomosis

CORPOROCORPORAL ANASTOMOSIS

3

This is a quick and easy operation. A short midline incision is made over the shaft of the penis at any convenient site. Dissection is done in the plane between the corpus spongiosum and the hard distended corpus cavernosum.

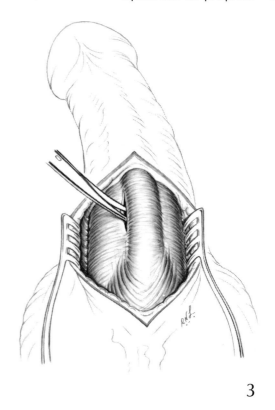

3

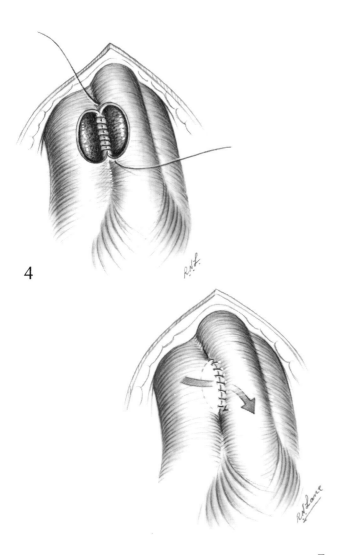

4

5

4 & 5

A generous window, about 1 cm × 1 cm, is cut away from the fascia covering the spongy tissue of each corpus. The sludge from the corpus cavernosum is irrigated using heparinized saline until bright 'arterial' blood appears and the erected penis is emptied out by firm pressure. The fascial edges of each window are anastomosed using very fine non-absorbable suture material, e.g. 5/0 Tevdek or 7/0 Prolene.

Even this operation is not always successful. In the event that the priapism has returned in the morning, the next procedure is to make an anastomosis between the saphenous vein and the corpus cavernosum.

SAPHENOCORPORAL ANASTOMOSIS

The saphenofemoral junction is exposed through a short incision like that used for the Trendelenburg operation for varicose veins.

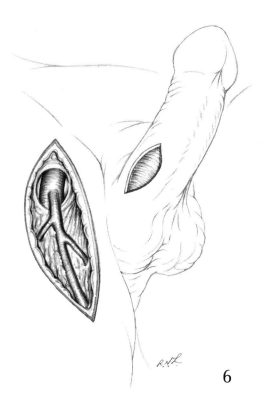

6

7

The saphenous vein is dissected out for 10 cm, each of its tributaries being carefully ligated. The vein is distended with heparinized saline, while one makes sure that any fascial bands on its adventitia are not obstructing the lumen.

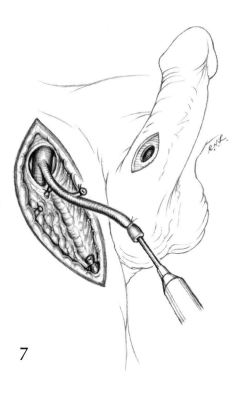

7

8

A tunnel is made under the fat between the fossa ovalis, where the saphenous vein enters the femoral vein, and the root of the penis. There, through a separate incision, Buck's fascia is exposed, window cut away and the end of the vein anastomosed to the fascial edge with 5/0 Tevdek or 7/0 Prolene. The penis is irrigated thoroughly with heparinized saline to eliminate the accumulation of thick sludge.

The immediate effect of this procedure is to allow the penis to collapse. Late effects are not so satisfactory. Often the penis remains somewhat thickened and semirigid. Fibrosis occurs in the septa of the corpus cavernosum, and the normal erectile system may never function properly again. Usually the bypass becomes blocked off within a week, but rarely (as may be shown by a cavernosogram) it is patent and may have to be tied off to allow normal erection to return.

Because the results of any operation for priapism cannot be guaranteed, the patient should be warned of the possibility of future impotence.

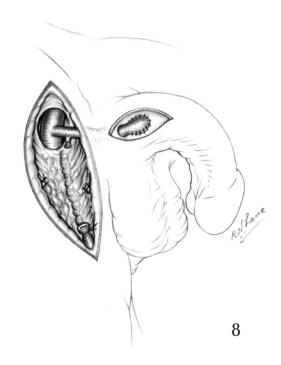

8

References

1. Baron, M., Leiter, E, The management of priapism in sickle cell anemia. Journal of Urology 1978; 119: 610

2. Winter, C. C. Cure of idiopathic priapism: new procedure for creating fistula between glans, penis and corpora cavernosa. Urology 1976; 8: 389–391

3. Crummy, A. B., Ishizuka, J., Madsen, P. O. Post-traumatic priapism: successful treatment with autologous clot embolisation. American Journal of Radiology 1979; 133: 329–330

Further Reading

Carter, R. G., Thomas, C. E., Tomskey, G. C. Cavernospongiosum shunts in the treatment of priapism. Urology 1976; 7: 292–295

Eadie, D. G. A., Brock, T. P. Corpus-saphenous bypass in the treatment of priapism. British Journal of Surgery 1970; 57: 172–174

Hinman, F. Priapism: reasons for failure of therapy. Journal of Urology 1960; 83: 420–428

Wear, J. B. Jr, Crummy, A. B., Munsen, B. O. A new approach to the treatment of priapism. Journal of Urology 1977; 117: 252–254

Circumcision, meatotomy and meatoplasty

John P. Blandy   MA, DM, MCh, FRCS
Professor of Urology, The London Hospital Medical College;
Consultant Urologist, St Peter's Hospital, London, UK

Circumcision

Indications

Circumcision of newborn babies is a religious rite, not a surgical emergency, but there are very rare instances where the foreskin is provided with a true pinhole meatus and a circumcision may justifiably be performed in order to overcome obstruction. Later on in childhood recurrent balanitis, the development of a secondary meatal stenosis, or an inability to wash behind the foreskin are real indications for circumcision, and it is possible to make a good case for routine circumcision of children who are likely to be brought up in parts of the world where soap and water are rare commodities. Such a policy would prevent the large numbers of penile carcinomas seen in contemporary Africa.

A general anaesthetic is necessary, except perhaps in the newborn. For this reason it is preferable to postpone circumcision if possible until the child is about 3 years of age.

1, 2 & 3

Whatever technique is followed, the first step in circumcision is to make sure that the foreskin has been thoroughly separated from the glans penis. It is still a common error to see boys in whom the corona glandis has been left covered, and smegma has been retained under it. First a probe separates the foreskin from the glans. The foreskin is then stretched and pulled down, any adhesions between its mucosa and the glans being gently broken with a moist dissecting swab until the coronal sulcus is quite clean.

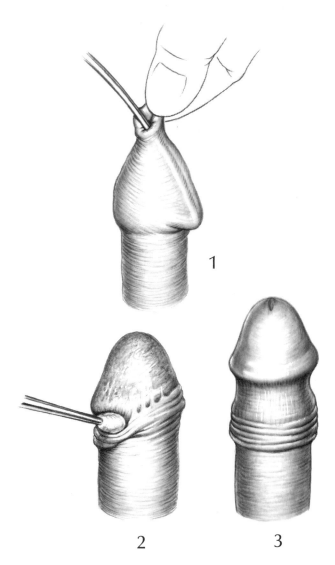

1

2   3

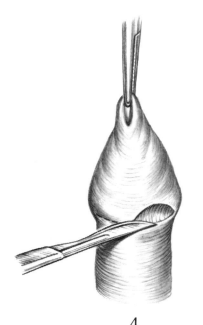

4   5

4 & 5

It is very difficult to cut a clean edge with scissors, and preferable to incise the skin and mucosa with a knife. The foreskin is pulled back over the glans, and allowed to lie in a natural position. This will allow the surgeon to choose the right position for the incision through the foreskin, which should coincide with the corona glandis. The knife is carried through skin only, and on the ventral surface of the penis may take the direction shown in order to liberate a frenum which is short.

6–11

The foreskin is now pulled back and, again using a knife, an incision is made some 3 mm away from the coronal sulcus through epidermis and into the underlying areolar tissue. The surplus foreskin is removed with scissors. Small vessels are meticulously caught and ligated with 4/0 catgut. Particular attention is paid to the artery in the frenum which must be carefully ligated. The skin edges are approximated with 5/0 interrupted catgut sutures.

No dressing is necessary. To prevent bedclothes from adhering to the suture line, it may be lightly smeared with sterile Vaseline. Haemostatic dressings should be unnecessary and may give rise to severe skin reactions, even amounting to necrosis.

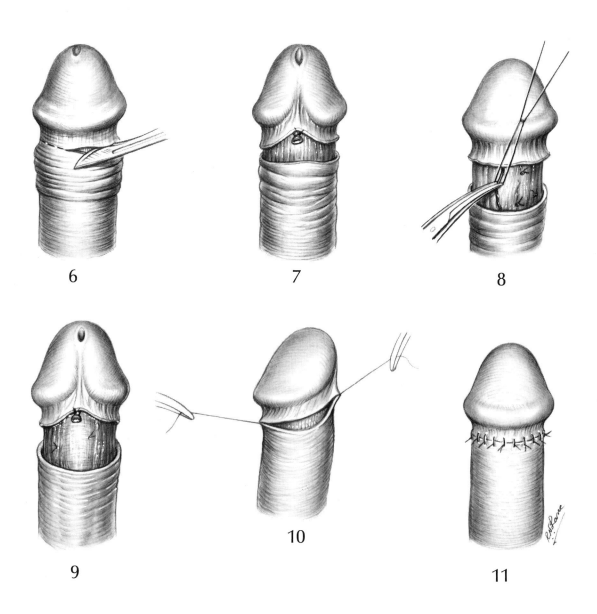

6   7   8

9   10   11

Aftercare

A child may be allowed home at the end of the day of the operation. The mother may bathe it in the usual way and should be instructed to dry the part gently, but not to apply any dressing. Adults will probably need to remain in a little longer in order to become accustomed to the sensitivity of the exposed glans. In those adult patients in whom the two layers of the foreskin have become particularly adherent, and in whom sharp dissection has been necessary in order to remove the foreskin, one must allow a considerable period of time for the glans to epithelialize. It is never necessary to apply skin grafts, for the new glandular skin will completely regenerate in time and give an almost normal appearance.

PLASTIBELL TECHNIQUE

12, 13 & 14

The Hollister Plastibell, and similar devices, are of interest to surgeons obliged to perform circumcision on neonates. The principle is simple: a plastic device is pushed into the cleft between glans penis and foreskin and a ligature (supplied sterile with the device) is tied tightly around the lip of the 'bell'. Surplus foreskin is cut off with scissors and the handle of the plastic bell snapped off. It is essential that the child is examined at intervals until the plastic device has been recovered. The surplus skin separates with a clean line of demarcation, leaving a fine, neat scar. Complications are rare.

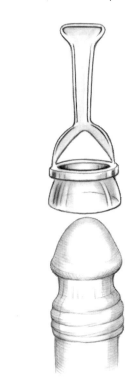

12

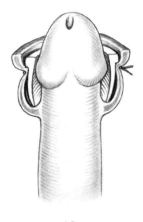

13

14

Meatotomy

Meatotomy may by itself result in a permanent cure of a meatus narrowed as a result of the trauma of urethral instrumentation. But in most adults it is followed by restenosis, and a meatoplasty is a more certain way of dealing with the problem.

15, 16 & 17

If meatotomy is performed, it should be carried right down into the normal urethra, forming a more generous incision than the circumstances may seem to warrant. However, unless a large incision is made, restenosis is inevitable. A few sutures may be inserted to achieve haemostasis, and the apical suture should attempt to approximate urethral mucosa to skin.

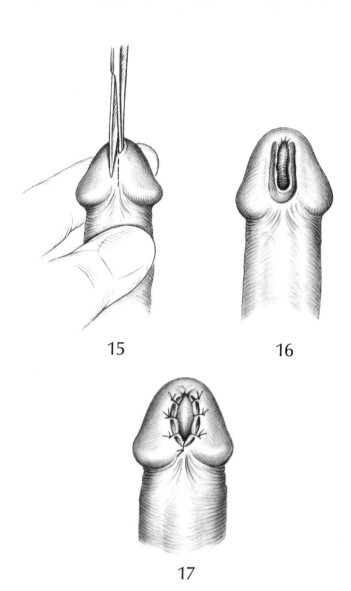

15

16

17

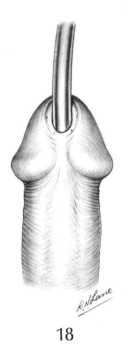

18

18

Following meatotomy a patient should be provided with a suitable bougie and advised to pass it at increasing intervals until the risk of restenosis has passed.

Meatoplasty

A more sure way to overcome meatal and submeatal stenosis, as seen after surgical trauma and in cases of balanitis xerotica obliterans, is to insert a ∩-shaped flap of skin into the opened-up urethral meatus.

19–24

A curved ∩-shaped flap is made of the skin on the ventral surface of the penis and this is allowed to drop back. A very generous incision is now made along the ventral midline of the meatus, care being taken that the incision enters healthy urethra and unscarred corpus spongiosum. In many cases of balanitis xerotica obliterans the hard scar tissue extends proximally for 2–3 cm and it is easy to make this incision too short. The ∩-shaped flap of skin is now tucked into the defect. Using 5/0 plain catgut with a double-ended needle, the skin is sewn in position with fine, even bites, making sure that the skin is approximated neatly to the mucosal surface of the urethra. Where the urethra is very scarred at its distal centimetre, the edges should be loosely brought together so that the end-result is like a congenital glandular hypospadias.

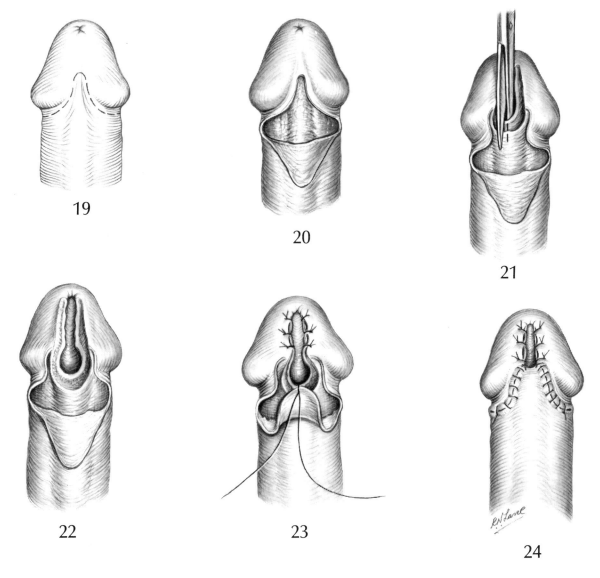

Instrumentation is avoided during the period of follow-up. The author has seen one recurrence in 32 cases – in a patient with balanitis xerotica in whom the original incision was probably not carried far enough proximally, or else the condition recurred. One tiresome complication is mentioned by these patients, namely that on voiding the stream sprays. With a little manipulation and side-to-side compression of the glans, this disability is usually overcome.

Surgical treatment of Peyronie's disease

Robert A. Roth MD
Department of Urology, Lahey Clinic Medical Center, Burlington, Massachusetts, USA

Introduction

1

Peyronie's disease is the presence of an inelastic plaque of fibrous tissue involving the tunica albuginea of the corpus cavernosum of the penis. These plaques may cause penile curvature toward the plaque even in the flaccid state and occasionally pain. The deformity is greatly accentuated in erection. Extensive fibrosis distal to the plaque may impair full erection. Corrective surgery is indicated for persistent pain, penile deformity sufficient to preclude coitus, or erectile impotence.

Two types of procedure currently used are plaque excision and overlay graft, and placement of intracorporeal penile prosthesis with or without plaque incision.

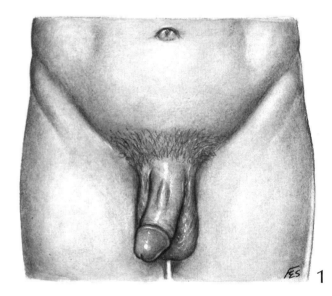

1

The operation

The patient is placed in the supine position. A Foley catheter is passed into the bladder through the urethra for identification of the urethra and for traction. A complete circumferential incision is made 1 cm proximal to the corona of the glans, cutting through the subcutaneous tissue to expose Buck's fascia. The shaft is denuded by pulling the skin down to the base of the penis. The plaque can then be palpated as an indurated area, usually in the dorsal midline position. It may, however, occur in other areas.

2

To simulate an erection under anesthesia, a 6 mm Penrose drain is placed as a tourniquet at the base of the penis, and saline solution is injected via a butterfly needle into one corpus cavernosum[1]. Both corpora will fill through cross-connections and the extent of the deformity can be observed.

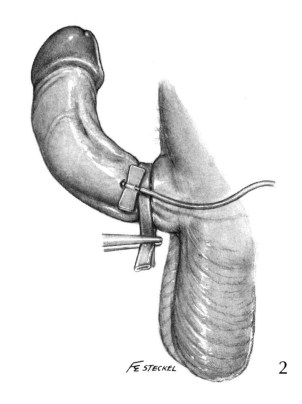
2

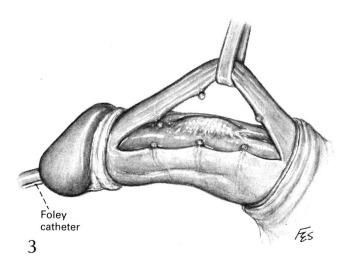
Foley catheter
3

3

The plaque is midline dorsal. Buck's fascia is incised and small bleeding vessels are controlled. The dorsal neuro-vascular bundle is carefully dissected off the plaque and retracted in an atraumatic fashion with a tape. Damage to the nerve may cause a sensory deficit to the distal penis.

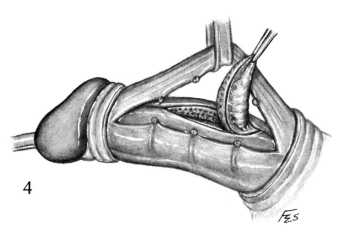
4

4

The plaque is delineated with a marking pen and sharply and completely excised until the normal spongy tissue of the corpus cavernosum is exposed in all areas. In an extensive lesion, the location of the urethra is always confirmed by palpating the urethral catheter to avoid inadvertent damage to this structure. A tourniquet is not necessary, as manual compression suffices to control bleeding.

5

Anatomical relation of penis and plaque is shown in cross-section. The neurovascular bundle is above the plaque. Plaque is often ill-defined and involves not only the tunica albuginea but also extends superficially into the corpus cavernosum.

Overlay grafts are used to cover the defect, to control bleeding and to provide support for subsequent erection. Various types of materials have been used for this purpose including fascia, skin grafts and artificial fabrics. At present there is no clear correct choice of material. We have noted favourable experience with both tunica vaginalis[2,3] and dermal graft[4] for overlay grafts.

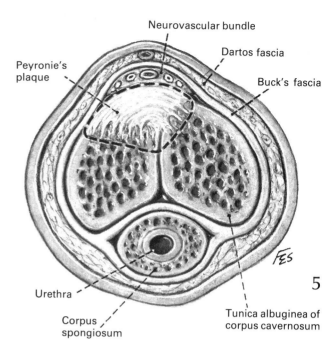

6

The technique of overlay grafts varies only in procurement of graft material. Tunica vaginalis is obtained by making a scrotal incision over either testis. The testis and its enveloping tunics are delivered into the incision. A generous section of tunica is outlined over the testis (not epididymis).

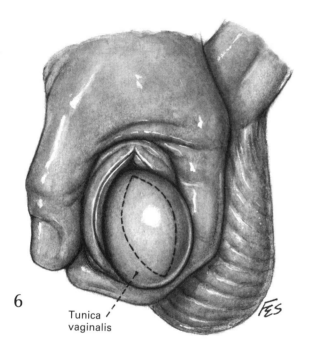

7

A patch of the tunica vaginalis is generously excised to expose the testis. The graft is kept between sponges moistened with saline solution until it is sewn in place. The glistening parietal surface is sewn into the defect toward the spongy tissue with a running 4/0 absorbable suture. The scrotum is closed in the usual way.

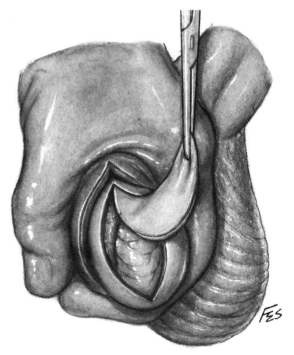

8

The suturing technique for placement of the overlay graft is the same regardless of the material used. The graft is sewn into place with several absorbable running sutures closely placed for haemostasis. The graft is trimmed to size as the suture line is being completed but is cut slightly generously.

An artifical erection is again produced to ascertain the degree of correction and to be sure it is fluid-tight. If a significant deformity is still present, a Nesbit[5] tuck is made on the tunica albuginea of the opposite side. The penile skin is reapproximated with absorbable sutures. A light pressure dressing is kept in place for 48 hours and is removed when the Foley catheter is removed.

Dermal graft is obtained by using a dermatome to remove 0.3 mm (0.012 inch) thickness of epidermis and excising the underlying dermis generously with a knife. The fat is trimmed from underneath the dermal graft, and the graft is sewn into place with running sutures.

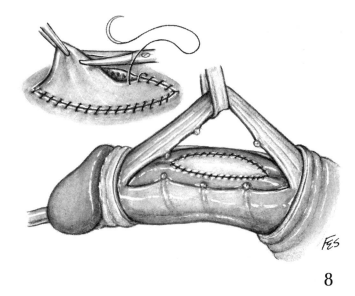

8

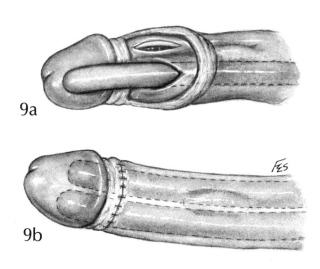

9a

9b

9a & b

Insertion of a penile prosthesis should be considered for the patient who has concomitant erectile impotence or extensive disease[6]. The rigid type of prosthesis (Small-Carrion, Finney or Jonas) is preferable. In some instances, placement of the rigid rod will give sufficient straightening without incision of plaque. For moderate curvature, insertion of the prosthesis will correct the deformity alone. The patient's own tumescence will add to penile length and girth. Insertion is accomplished by the surgeon's preferred method. The technique shown is that described by Jonas.

10

When the penile plaque is extensive and insertion of the prosthesis does not provide sufficient correction, the plaque should be incised transversely down to the rod. Tension from the rod tends to pull the incision open and thus correct the deformity. Electrocutting through the plaque works well and will not cut inadvertently into the prosthesis.

An overlay graft is not necessary unless significant haemorrhage has occurred. The skin is replaced back over the shaft and sutured into place and treated as in the overlay grafting technique. Whenever prosthetic materials are used, systemic prophylactic antibiotics are used before and after operation until the Foley catheter is removed. A modest circumferential pressure dressing is applied and the Foley catheter is removed in 24–48 hours.

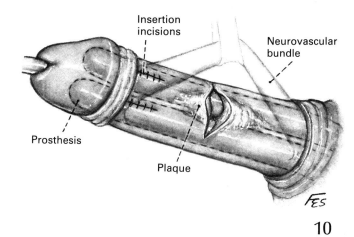

10

References

1. Gittes, R. F., McLaughlin, A. P., III. Injection technique to induce penile erection. Urology 1974; 4: 473–474

2. Das, S. Peyronie's disease: excision and autografting with tunica vaginalis. Journal of Urology 1980; 124: 818–819

3. Amin, M., Broghamer, W. L. Jr, Harty, J. I., Long, R. Jr. Autogenous tunica vaginalis graft for Peyronie's disease: an experimental study and its clinical application. Journal of Urology 1980; 124: 815–817

4. Horton, C. E., Devine, C. J. Jr. Peyronie's disease. Plastic and Reconstructive Surgery 1973; 52: 503–510

5. Nesbit, R. M. Congenital curvature of the phallus: report of three cases with description of corrective operation. Journal of Urology 1965; 93: 230–232

6. Raz, S., Dekernion, J. B., Kaufman, J. J. Surgical treatment of Peyronie's disease: a new approach. Journal of Urology 1977; 117: 598–601

Illustrations by Nancy Heim

Penile prostheses

Drogo K. Montague, MD, FACS
Head, Section of Urodynamics and Prosthetic Surgery,
Department of Urology, Cleveland Clinic Foundation, Cleveland, Ohio, USA

Introduction

Considerable progress has been made since the first description of implantation of a prosthesis for treatment of erectile impotence[1]. Early penile prostheses were single, rigid, midline devices usually implanted beneath Buck's fascia in the shaft of the penis. These devices did not extend into the perineum and consequently cosmetic and functional results were generally disappointing. Primarily because of this, early prostheses failed to gain widespread recognition and use.

With the introduction of paired, intracorporal prostheses, the modern age of penile prosthetic surgery began. The Small-Carrion prosthesis was the first of the paired semirigid prostheses[2]. Later the Finney[3] and Jonas[4] semirigid rod prostheses became available. The Scott-Bradley-Timm inflatable penile prosthesis[5] was introduced at the same time as the Small-Carrion prosthesis. Since its introduction, numerous modifications have been made both in the inflatable prosthetic device and in techniques for its implantation. This has led to a steadily decreasing incidence of mechanical and surgical complications.

The principal advantage of a semirigid rod penile prosthesis is its simplicity. Compared to the inflatable prosthesis, the costs of the prosthesis and the surgical procedure are lower and there is less chance of subsequent mechanical malfunction. The disadvantage of the semirigid prosthesis is that the cosmetic appearance of the erection is less realistic than with the inflatable penile prosthesis and the patient maintains a constant state of artificial erection. The Finney prosthesis is 'hinged' to allow the prosthesis to be bent downwards for micturition and to be raised to an upward position for coitus. The Jonas prosthesis has a silver alloy wire down the middle of each of the rods. With this prosthesis, the penis can be bent into a downward position and can also be brought into an upward position for coitus. The Jonas prosthesis maintains these positions better than either the Small-Carrion or Finney prostheses.

All candidates for a penile prosthesis should have an opportunity to choose between the inflatable penile prosthesis and one of the semirigid rod prostheses. An objective description of the relative advantages and disadvantages of each prosthesis should be given so the patient can make an intelligent decision about which prosthesis is best for him.

The inflatable penile prosthesis

1

The inflatable penile prosthesis consists of a fluid reservoir implanted in the retropubic space, a pump with both an inflation and deflation mechanism implanted beneath the fascia of the scrotum, and two penile cylinders implanted in the corpora cavernosa. The various parts of the prosthesis are connected by tubing which has been trimmed to appropriate length. Tubing connections are made over stainless steel connectors to form one continuous hydraulic system. Sterile saline can be used for the hydraulic fluid. If the surgeon wishes the prosthesis to be radiographically visible, he can use an intravenous contrast agent.

With the inflatable penile prosthesis, the penis remains in a flaccid state. When the patient wishes to have coitus he compresses the inflation bulb. This forces fluid into the penile cylinders while the inflation bulb refills by drawing fluid out of the reservoir. This is repeated until the patient has an erection which he finds most satisfactory for coitus. The man with an inflatable penile prosthesis can not only control when he has an erection but he can also control the size and firmness of the erection within certain limits. Although the glans penis does not erect with any prosthesis, the inflatable prosthesis gives the shaft of the penis more girth and thus a more natural appearance than it has when semirigid rods are implanted.

When coitus is completed, the deflation button can be depressed through the scrotal skin. The fluid, which is under pressure in the penile cylinders, returns to the reservoir and the penis resumes a flaccid postion.

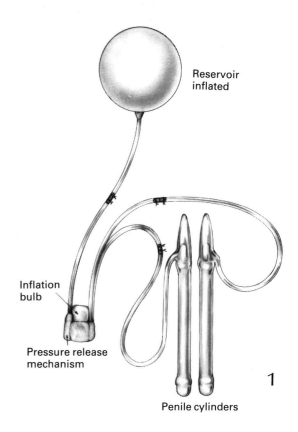

Reservoir inflated

Inflation bulb

Pressure release mechanism

Penile cylinders

1

The operation

Following the induction of general or spinal anaesthesia, a broad-spectrum bactericidal antibiotic is administered intravenously. This is continued for 48 hours postoperatively. The patient is placed in the lithotomy position; the lower abdomen and genital area are shaved, and a 15 min scrub is performed. An adhering plastic drape is placed across the perineum just anterior to the anus to exclude the anus from the surgical field. The remainder of the field is then draped in the usual fashion.

2

The location of the incision is outlined. Also shown in outline are the underlying corporal bodies. The incision is approximately 2–3 cm in length, and it lies along the median raphe at the base of the penis. Care must be taken not to place the incision too far distally on the shaft of the penis. An 18 Fr silastic Foley catheter is inserted and left indwelling throughout the procedure.

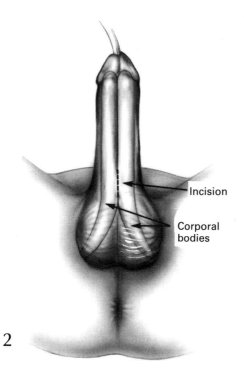

Incision

Corporal bodies

2

3

The Scott ring retractor is used to maintain exposure. A piece of polyethylene tubing is placed just above the break in the retractor and this tubing runs behind the penis. An elastic skin hook stay is placed dorsally in the meatus of the penis. The penis is then stretched in a cephalad direction, and the stay is placed through a slot at the 12 o'clock position of the ring. It is the combination of this meatal stay exerting cephalad traction and the polyethylene tubing that keeps the retractor in place. The remaining skin hook stays are then used to expose one of the corpora lateral to the urethra.

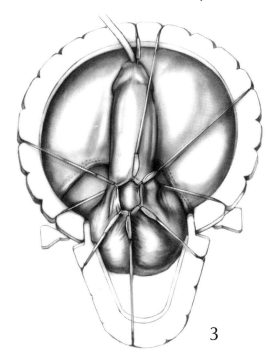

3

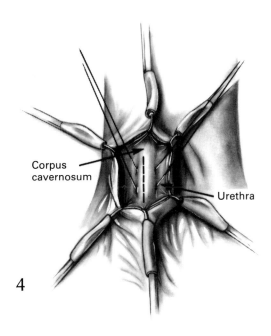

4

4

The location of the urethra can be determined initially by palpation of the catheter and later by direct vision. The scrotal fascia is opened just lateral to the urethra; in this case, the right corpus cavernosum is being exposed. After the scrotal fascia has been opened to expose the corpus carvernosum, Buck's fascia is also opened longitudinally just lateral to the urethra. The hook elastic stays are then placed so they retract both Buck's fascia and the skin. The medial stays will retract the urethra out of the operative field. The corporotomy, which is 2 cm in length, is outlined. 3/0 Prolene sutures are placed through the tunica albuginea on either side of the proposed incision.

5

The tunica albuginea is sharply incised between the stay sutures. The thickness of the tunica albuginea and the appearance of the underlying erectile tissue should be noted. Next 2/0 Prolene sutures are placed full thickness through the tunica albuginea as shown and the original 3/0 Prolene sutures are removed. Bleeding from the erectile tissue is usually minimal; however, if it is excessive, temporary upward traction on the stay sutures will reduce it.

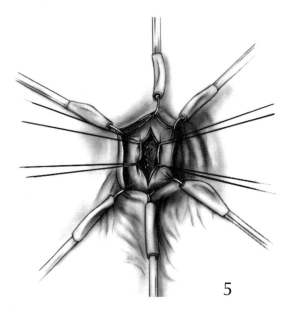

5

6

The proximal portion of the corpus cavernosum (or crus) is dilated, beginning with a number 8 and proceeding through a number 12 dilator. Care must be taken to ensure that dilatation proceeds all the way down to the insertion of the crus on the ischial tuberosity.

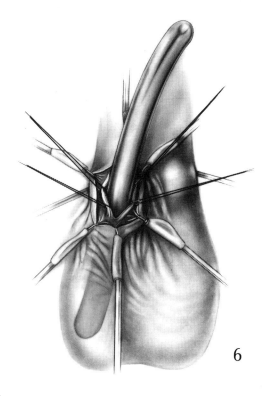

6

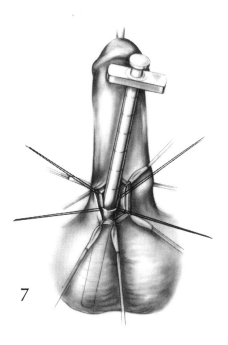

7

7

The Furlow instrument is inserted down to the ischial tuberosity to obtain a measurement. The measurement is made from the end of the crus to the caudalmost extent of the corporotomy.

8

The Scott cylinder inserter is used for distal dilatation, measurement and cylinder insertion. The tip of the instrument is introduced beneath the tunica albuginea of the ventrolateral aspect of the corpus cavernosum (away from the urethra) and passed to the end of the corpus cavernosum which should lie beneath the midportion of the glans penis. The surgeon's index finger is used to palpate the tip of the instrument through the glans penis. Once the instrument is in its proper position, and the penis is on full stretch, a measurement can be taken directly from the instrument. This measurement is taken from the most cephalad extent of the corporotomy.

The distal measurement used to select a penile cylinder of appropriate size should correspond to the inflatable portion of the penile cylinder. The solid rear tip portion of the cylinder, which is 4 cm long, can be lengthened by the use of rear tip extenders to match the proximal measurement. The paired cylinders are then filled with 50 per cent Hypaque diluted with 3 parts sterile water. The remaining portions of the prosthesis are also filled with 12.5 per cent Hypaque. After the reservoir is filled with solution and all the air is evacuated, the reservoir is emptied again ready for implantation.

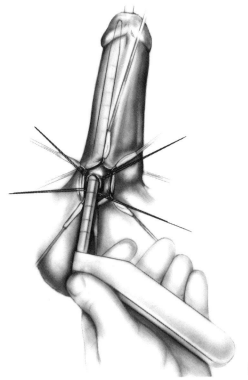

8

9

The penile cylinder has a thread running through the tip of the cylinder, and both ends of this are threaded through a 5 cm Keith straight needle. This needle is embedded in the tip of the plastic wedge that is provided with the Scott inserter, and the wedge is introduced into the inserter as shown. The handle on the inserter should be opposite the rear tab on the wedge. As the wedge is inserted, the corpus cavernosum is dilated to the size of a number 13 Hegar dilator while the needle is carried through the corpus cavernosum and emerges through the glans penis. The Keith needle should then be grasped with a haemostat and pulled through. When the sutures come through the skin on the glans penis, they are grasped with the haemostat. Next the wedge is removed and finally the Scott inserter is removed.

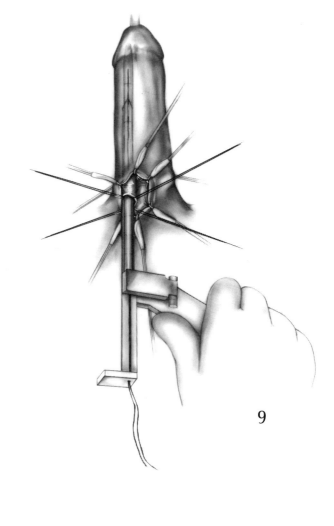

9

10 & 11

The suture through the tip of the penis is used to guide the cylinder into the distal half of the corpus cavernosum. The proximal corporal measurement determines the number and size of rear tip extenders. The solid rear portion of the penile cylinders are 4 cm in length. Rear tip extenders are available in 1, 2 and 3 cm sizes. These rear tip extenders can be combined by stacking them.

10

11

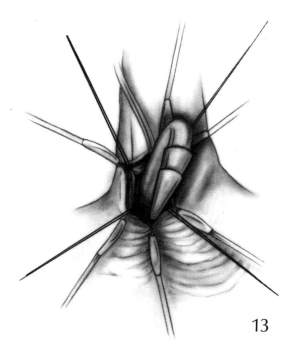

12

12 & 13

Two rear tip extenders are shown being applied to the cylinder. This should be done so that when the cylinder is inserted down the crus of the penis (*Illustration 13*), it will reach the ischial tuberosity, providing a snug fit.

13

14

The tubing from the cylinder should exit directly from the posterior-most aspect of the corporotomy. The closure is begun by placing a 2/0 Prolene suture immediately in front of the tubing, closing the tunica albuginea snugly around it and taking care not to kink or compress the tubing. This suture is tied and left long. The remainder of the corporotomy, beginning at the cephalad portion, is closed with a 2/0 Prolene horizontal mattress suture. It is finally tied to the suture which was previously placed in front of the cylinder tubing.

14

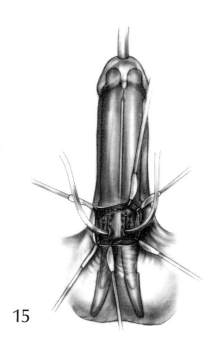

15

15

This procedure is repeated on the opposite side.

16

A subdartos pouch is made to create a pocket between the dartos fascia and the tunica vaginalis. By convention this is usually done on the right side.

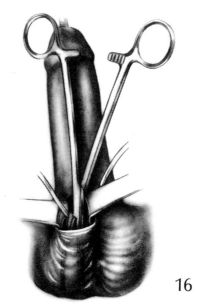

16

17

The pump is placed in this pouch so that the deflation button is located inferiorly and anteriorly. The pump (inset) consists of two parts. On top is the compressible bulb which pumps fluid into the cylinders. The lower portion of the pump houses the tubing. One tube leads to each of the two penile cylinders from one end of the housing; at the opposite end a single tube goes to the reservoir. The end of the reservoir tubing is cut obliquely, the ends of the cylinder tubings perpendicularly. The deflation button, located on the outside of the housing at the reservoir end, allows the fluid to drain from the cylinders.

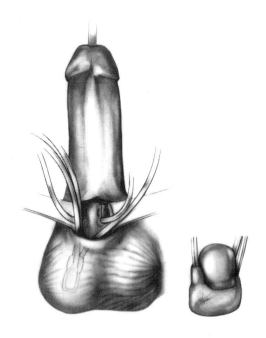

18

Once the pump is in place, the tube leading to the left cylinder is inserted through the medial wall of the pouch by a tubing passer. This serves to fix the pump in the scrotum so it cannot ride up or rotate unduly.

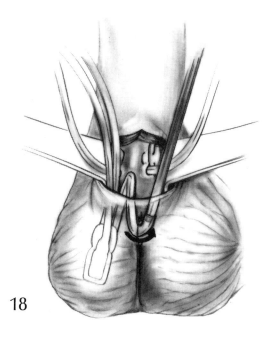

19

The tube rubber-shod clamps are applied to the left cylinder tube and to the tube leading from the left penile cylinder. Blood is washed off the tubing with an antibiotic solution and the tubing is cut to length. Connection is made over a straight stainless steel connector; this connection is secured with double 3/0 Prolene ties.

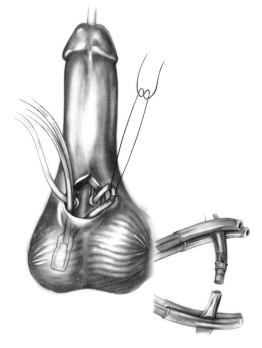

20

The connection to the right cylinder is made in similar fashion except that there is no need to bring the tube from the pump through any scrotal tissue.

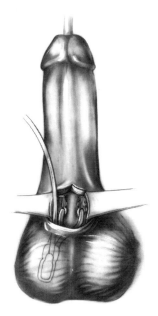

20

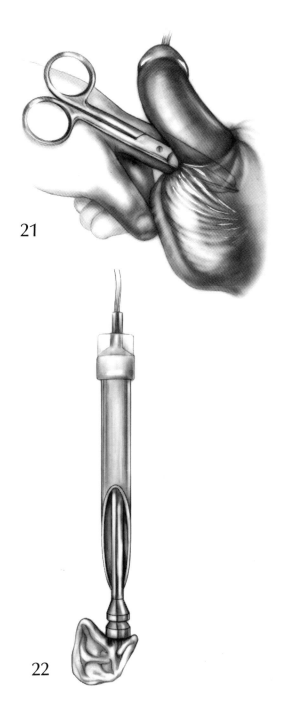

21

21

Prior to insertion of the reservoir, the bladder is completely drained by removing the plug on the Foley catheter. The surgeon's index finger is placed through the incision and into the right external ring. Metzenbaum scissors are inserted along the medial aspect of the ring and the fascia in the floor of the ring is perforated. The index finger can then be introduced into the retropubic space. It should be possible to feel clearly the back wall of the symphysis pubis and the empty bladder.

22

The Scott reservoir inserter has a small, hollow plunger which fits inside a larger, outer cylinder. The tubing from the empty reservoir is fed through the inner part and is pulled down until the reservoir bell sits in the ball-shaped cup of the plunger. The plunger is then fitted into the outer cylinder as shown and is drawn back until the folded, empty reservoir is inside the oblique opening of the cylinder.

22

23

The empty reservoir is then inserted. The surgeon's finger is left in the fascial defect and the inserter is introduced alongside the finger. As the inserter dilates the fascial opening the finger is gradually withdrawn. The plunger of the reservoir introducer is released and depressed to introduce the reservoir into the retropubic space. The outer portion of the reservoir introducer is removed and 30 ml of 12.5 per cent Hypaque solution is injected into the reservoir. The plunger is also removed and the surgeon checks to make sure that the tubing bell exits directly from the fascial defect. If it does not, the partially filled reservoir can easily be rotated. Once this is accomplished, an additional 35 ml of 12.5 per cent Hypaque solution is injected into the reservoir so that it contains a total of 65 ml of 12.5 per cent Hypaque solution.

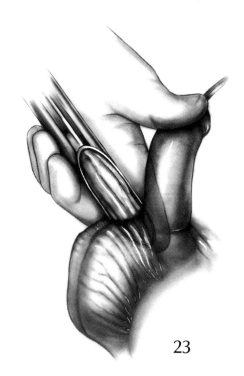

23

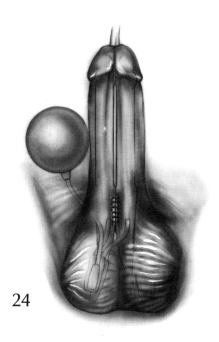

24

24

The reservoir is connected to the reservoir tubing from the pump over a straight stainless steel connector. The prosthesis is then inflated and the symmetry of the erection is observed. Both cylinder tips should be well seated in the distal corpora under the glans penis to give it good support. The prosthesis is deflated, and the procedure is repeated several times.

After antibacterial solution irrigation the wound is closed in two layers. Running absorbable sutures are used for a subcuticular closure.

SEMIRIGID ROD PROSTHESES

Various surgical incisions can be used for implantation of the semi-rigid rod prostheses. Among those more commonly used are the perineal incision, the penoscrotal incision, a subcoronal incision, and a longitudinal incision on the dorsal shaft of the penis. The author prefers the penoscrotal incision and uses the same preoperative preparation as outlined for the inflatable penile prosthesis. Again the patient is placed in the lithotomy position and prepped and draped as described above. The incision is located in the same area and exposure is maintained with the Scott ring retractor. A catheter is placed in position at the start of the procedure to allow ready identification of the urethra.

The operation

25

After one corpus cavernosum is exposed, a longitudinal corporotomy is made between stay sutures. This incision should be approximately 50 per cent longer than the inflatable prosthesis corporotomy to allow for insertion of the more rigid rod prosthesis.

Dilatation proximally down the crus of the penis proceeds from a number 8 through a number 12 Hegar dilator, and the proximal measurement is made as for the inflatable penile prosthesis.

The distal dilatation proceeds with the Scott dilating instrument as described above, except that the wedge is inserted without the needle. After measurements and dilatation proximally and distally, a paired prosthesis is selected. The measurements are added up and then 1 or 2 cm are allowed for the length of the corporotomy, which is approximately 3 cm. With experience, the surgeon will be able to judge how much should be allowed for the corporotomy. If one size is tried initially and does not fit, then it should be removed and the next larger or smaller size should be tried.

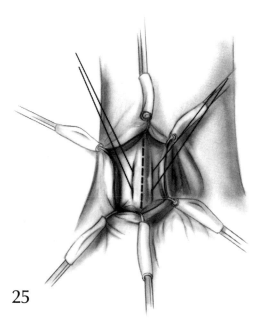

25

26

After the penile prosthesis has been selected, the distal end is inserted up to the glans penis.

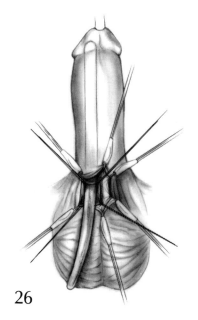

26

27

The proximal end is twisted in order to introduce it into the proximal portion of the corpus cavernosum. Pressure can then be put on the tail of the prosthesis so that it lies in the same direction as the course of the crus of the penis.

28

Once the prosthesis is in place, palpation distally should reveal that the tip of the prosthesis is out in the distal corpus cavernosum and gives good support to the glans penis. The corporotomy is closed with a running 2/0 Prolene suture. The procedure is repeated on the opposite side. The incision is closed in two layers (*see above*) and, once again, throughout the procedure the wound is irrigated with antibacterial solution.

Postoperative care

The postoperative care is the same for both the inflatable and the semirigid rod penile prostheses. The urethral catheter is removed on the first morning following surgery and ambulation is begun. It has been our practice to discharge patients on the morning of the 3rd postoperative day.

For patients with a semirigid rod prosthesis, if it is a Jonas the prosthesis is placed in a dependent position by the surgeon prior to the patient's discharge. At the first postoperative visit 4–6 weeks later, the patient is instructed how to position the prosthesis in both the dependent position and the upward coital position. If the patient is pain-free or nearly pain-free, he is instructed to begin coitus. He and his partner are advised to use lubricating jelly at least for the first few episodes of coitus to insure adequate lubrication. If the female partner is anxious with the first coitus, there may not be sufficient natural lubrication; this is particularly true in the oestrogen-deficient, postmenopausal female partner.

Patients with the inflatable penile prosthesis are not instructed on inflation and deflation of the prosthesis until the first postoperative visit 4–6 weeks after surgery. At this time, they are usually pain-free, or nearly so, and instruction is easy. Because the sheath that formed around the cylinders has not yet been stretched, there is considerable pain for the first few inflations. However, this rapidly subsides. The patient is instructed to inflate and deflate the prosthesis twice daily for at least a month for practice. He is instructed to begin coitus when he is pain free with inflation. Once again, the initial use of artificial lubricants is recommended.

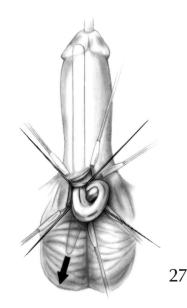

27

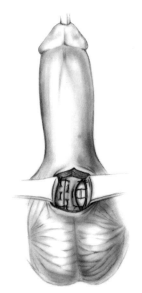

28

References

1. Goodwin, W. E., Scott, W. W. Phalloplasty. Journal of Urology 1952; 68: 903–908

2. Small, M. P., Carrion, H. M., Gordon, J. A. Small-Carrion penile prosthesis. A new implant for management of impotence. Urology 1975; 5: 479–486

3. Finney, R. P. New hinged silicone penile implant. Journal of Urology 1977; 118: 585–587

4. Jonas, U., Gunther, H. J. Silicone-silver penile prosthesis: description, operative approach, and results. Journal of Urology 1980; 123: 865–867

5. Scott, F. B., Bradley, W. E., Timm, G. W. Management of erectile impotence: Use of implantable inflatable prosthesis. Urology 1973; 2: 80–82

Illustrations by Nancy Heim

Prostheses for urinary incontinence

Drogo K. Montague MD, FACS
Head, Section of Urodynamics and Prosthetic Surgery, Department of Urology,
Cleveland Clinic Foundation, Cleveland, Ohio, USA

Introduction

Severe urinary incontinence constitutes one of urology's greatest challenges. Most women with stress urinary incontinence can be treated with surgical procedures which do not involve the use of prosthetic devices. However, some women with severe urinary incontinence may have so little sphincter function that restoration of continence with surgical procedures utilizing their own tissues is impossible. Furthermore, the male with post-prostatectomy urinary incontinence invariably requires implantation of a prosthetic device. The incontinence associated with selected forms of neurogenic bladder can also be managed by implantation of an artificial sphincter. Before an artificial sphincter can be considered, patients with these disorders should be able to completely empty their bladder, and they should be able to store reasonable volumes of urine under low pressure.

Preoperative preparation

The patient must have sterile urine prior to the implantation procedure. On the day before the procedure the patient takes two baths, scrubbing with a surgical scrub solution from the nipples to the knees for 20 min. When the patient is called to the operating room, a broad-spectrum, systemic bactericidal antibiotic is given. After the induction of either general or spinal anaesthesia the operative field is shaved and then a 15 min scrub is administered.

Artificial urinary sphincters

1

The AS 791 consists of a sphincter cuff which is implanted around the bulbous urethra. There is also a capsule-shaped deflation bulb which is implanted subcutaneously in one side of the scrotum. The balloon, which serves both as a reservoir and as a pressure measuring device, is implanted in the retropubic space. Tubing from each silicone rubber portion of the prosthesis is trimmed to appropriate lengths and attached to a stainless steel assembly which contains valvular mechanisms and a delayed fill resistor.

With this device, the cuff stays full of fluid except during micturition. When the patient wishes to void, he repeatedly squeezes and releases the deflation bulb through the skin of the scrotum. Each time the bulb is squeezed, the fluid inside it returns to the balloon-reservoir. When the bulb is released it fills, taking fluid out of the cuff. When the cuff is empty, the bulb stays collapsed. Generally, it takes between two and three squeezes to empty a urethral cuff. The patient voids after deflating the cuff. The balloon pressure remains constant whether the cuff is inflated or not. For a urethral cuff the balloon pressure is usually 50–60 cmH$_2$O (various pressure range balloons are available to be used at the judgement of the surgeon). As soon as the cuff is empty, flow begins from the balloon back into the cuff. A delayed fill resistor in the stainless steel assembly slows the return of fluid to the cuff so that the patient has adequate time to void. Fluid will flow from the balloon back into the cuff until the pressure in the balloon and the cuff are equal; this takes approximately 2 min. Once this has taken place, the pressure in the cuff will be between 50 and 60 cmH$_2$O. This is enough to produce passive continence; however, it is not so great as to impede blood flow into the tissues under the cuff.

When the patient performs a stress manoeuvre (such as coughing, sneezing or lifting), the pressure forces transmitted to the bladder are also conducted to the elastic balloon. Consequently, with this system pressure in the balloon increases transiently during these physical activities and stress incontinence is prevented.

2

The AS 792 is the artificial sphincter designed for implantation around the bladder neck. In the male, either the bladder neck or the bulbous urethra can be chosen for cuff implantation. Obviously in the female only the bladder neck can be used. The only difference between the AS 791 and the AS 792 is that with the AS 791 the port for the connection of cuff tubing is on the same side as the pump port, whereas in the AS 792 the cuff port is on the same side of the stainless steel assembly as the balloon port. This facilitates connections of tubing to the stainless steel assembly. Otherwise, the AS 791 and AS 792 stainless steel assemblies can be used interchangeably.

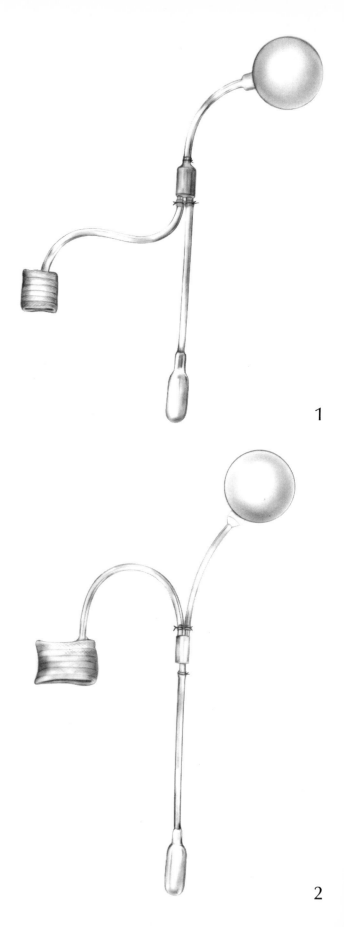

1

2

Implantation of AS 791

The patient is placed in the lithotomy position and, after suitable preparation, an adhering plastic drape is placed to cover the anus and exclude it from the operative field. The remaining operative field is then draped. A urethral catheter is inserted to facilitate identification of the urethra throughout the procedure.

3

A longitudinal incision is made in the perineum over the bulbous urethra.

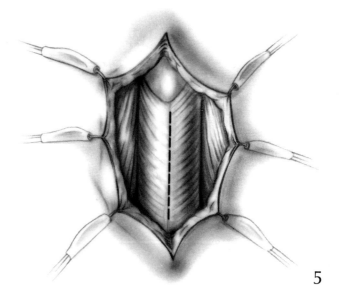

3

4

The bulbous urethra is exposed through this incision. The Scott ring retractor can be used for exposure as shown, or any type of self-retaining retractor may be used.

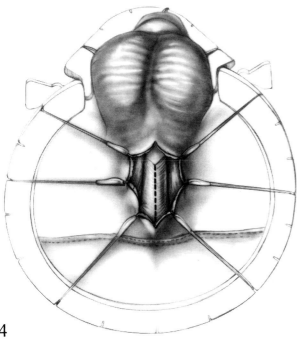

4

5

This close-up shows the bulbocavernosus muscles; the dotted line indicates where they can be separated in the midline.

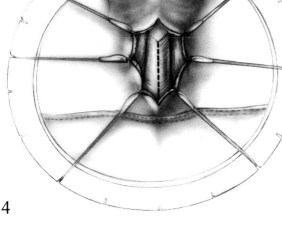

5

6

Once the bulbocavernosus muscles are separated, they are reflected laterally to expose the underlying bulbous urethra.

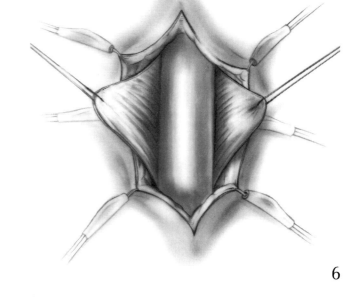

6

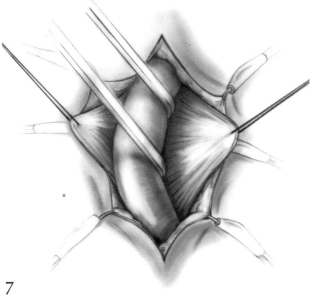

7

7

The urethra is mobilized utilizing sharp and blunt dissection under direct vision. This is not usually difficult, except at the 12 o'clock position where the urethra is adherent to the underlying intracrural septum. Great care must be taken at this position to avoid urethral injury.

8

Once the dissection is completed, a clamp can be placed around the urethra.

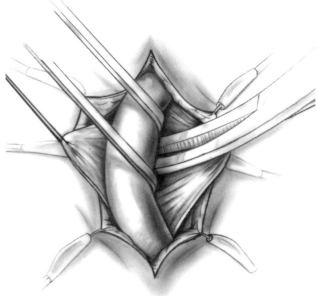

8

9

Umbilical tape is brought around the urethra and used to measure the circumference of the urethra. After it is cut, it can be removed and laid along the centimetre ruler to obtain a direct circumference measurement.

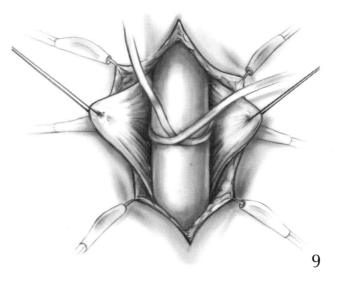

9

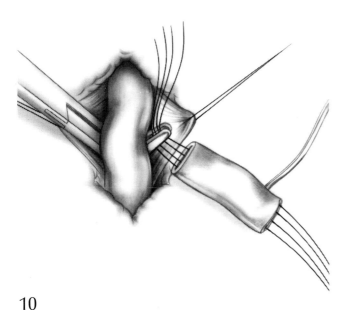

10

10

A cuff of suitable length is selected. Usually a 4.5 or 5.0 cm cuff will be suitable for the bulbous urethra. A 12.5 per cent Hypaque solution is prepared by diluting 25 per cent Hypaque solution with one part of sterile water. The cuff and other portions of the prosthesis are then filled with this fluid. Once the cuff and balloon are filled with solution and all the air is displaced from them, the solution is removed: the cuff and balloon are implanted. The cuff is then drawn around the urethra.

11

The ends of the cuff are brought and held together by tying the four sutures which are imbedded in the back of the cuff.

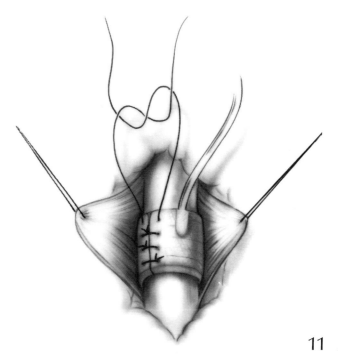

11

12

While the surgeon is implanting the urethral cuff, an assistant makes a transverse incision immediately above the symphysis pubis and carries this down to the anterior rectus fascia. The tubing for the cuff is passed through the bulbocavernosus muscle; it is then passed lateral to the base of the penis to emerge between Scarpa's fascia and the anterior rectus fascia in the suprapubic incision. After the tubing has been passed up into the suprapubic incision, the bulbocavernosus muscles are approximated over the cuff with interrupted sutures of 4/0 chromic catgut. The scrotal fascia is closed with catgut and the skin is approximated with running subcuticular absorbable suture.

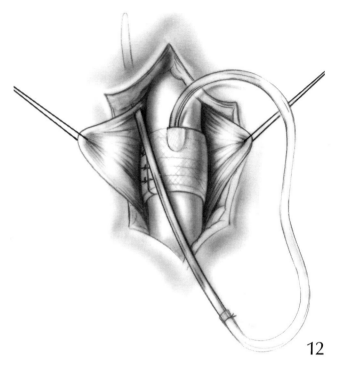

12

13

This shows the suprapubic incision with the cuff tubing entering the incision deep to Scarpa's fascia and superficial to the anterior rectus fascia. The anterior rectus fascia has now been incised transversely.

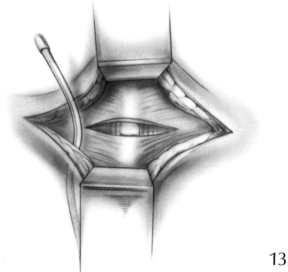

13

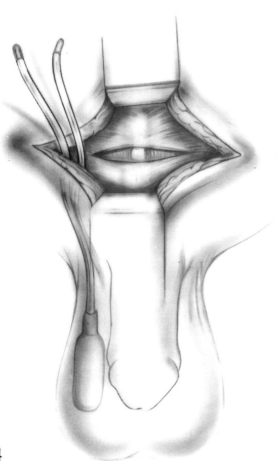

14

14

Through the suprapubic incision, a passageway deep to Scarpa's fascia is made into the right hemiscrotum. A blunt clamp is used to do this. The deflation bulb is inserted as low in the scrotum as possible.

15

The rectus muscles are separated in the midline and the retropubic space is entered. The empty balloon is placed on top of the bladder in the retropubic space. The tubing from the balloon is brought through the right rectus muscle and through the superior leaf of the anterior rectus fascia with a tubing passer. Once the balloon is in place, exactly 18 ml of 12.5 per cent Hypaque solution are added to the balloon.

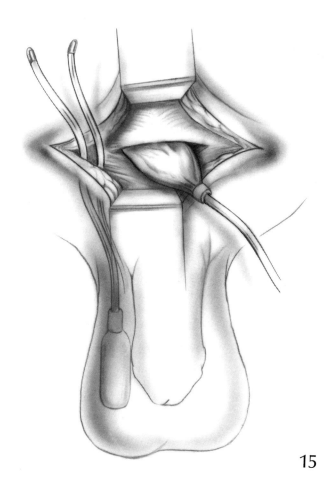

15

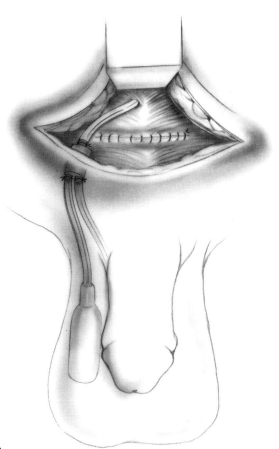

16

16

The AS 791 stainless steel assembly is placed in position. The balloon port is marked on the stainless steel assembly with a B; the cuff and pump ports are marked with C and P respectively. Rubber-shod clamps are placed on the tubing to prevent fluid escape from the system. The tubes are cut to appropriate lengths and then connected to their respective ports on the stainless steel assembly. Each connection is secured with a double 3/0 Prolene tie. The anterior rectus fascia is closed, followed by closure of Scarpa's fascia over the tubing and stainless steel assembly. The remaining wound layers are closed.

Implantation of the AS 792

The AS 792 assembly is selected when a vesical neck cuff is to be implanted electively in the man or of necessity in the female. The female patient is placed in the supine position, and the thighs are abducted so the external genitalia and vagina can be prepared and included in the operative field. A urethral catheter is inserted so the urethra can be readily identified during the dissection.

17

A transverse suprapubic incision is made and the anterior rectus muscles are mobilized and detached. The bladder neck and urethra are exposed.

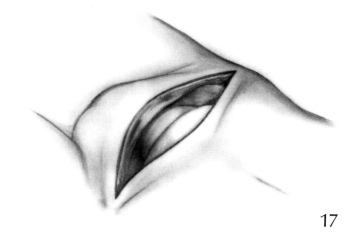

17

18

With downward traction on the catheter, the inflated balloon of the Foley catheter can be palpated at the bladder neck. It is at the bladder neck that the dissection around the urethra begins. Great care must be taken to ensure that the underlying vagina is not entered. An assistant can place his hand in the vagina during the procedure to help identify this structure if necessary. Once the bladder neck and proximal urethra have been mobilized, an umbilical tape is brought around them.

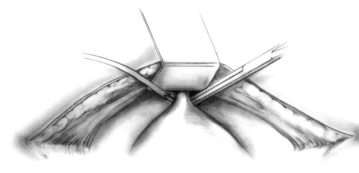

18

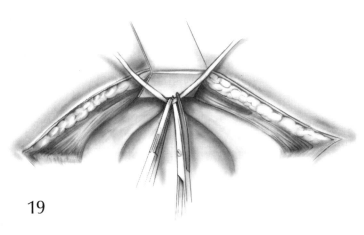

19

19

The ends of the tape are brought together, cut and removed.

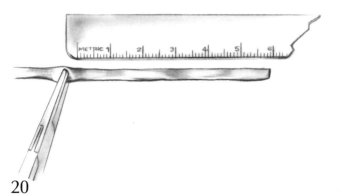

20

20

The tape is measured against a centimetre ruler to determine the circumference of the bladder neck.

21

A cuff of suitable length is selected, filled with 12.5 per cent Hypaque solution to displace the air, and then emptied. It is inserted into the cuff passer supplied by the manufacturer of the prosthesis.

22

A right-angle clamp is placed around the bladder neck and used to guide the cuff passer into place. Once the cuff passer has passed posteriorly around the bladder neck, it can be removed: this will leave the cuff in place.

23

The ends of the cuff are brought together and tied, utilizing the four sutures which are imbedded in the back of the cuff.

24

The cuff is rotated so the cuff tubing lies in the midline.

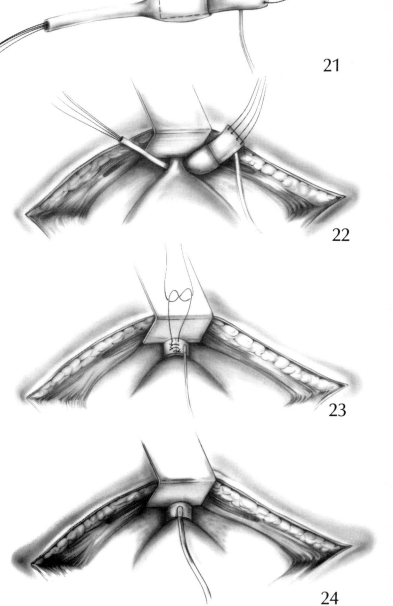

21

22

23

24

Once this is done, the cuff tubing is brought through the anterior rectus fascia with the tubing passer. The deflation bulb is placed subcutaneously in either the right or left labium majus. Once again, passageway down into either labium is made just beneath Scarpa's fascia.

After the cuff is in place, a balloon of appropriate pressure range is selected. This range is determined both by the patient's usual blood pressure and by the blood supply and thickness of the tissue under the cuff. A 70–80 cmH$_2$O pressure balloon is often selected.

The balloon is filled with exactly 18 ml of 12.5 per cent Hypaque and connected temporarily to the cuff by joining cuff and balloon tubings together over a stainless steel connector. The rubber-shod clamps are removed, the balloon is allowed to pressurize the cuff and the cuff

tubing is clamped. The balloon is disconnected, emptied, and refilled with exactly 16 ml of 12.5 per cent Hypaque. The balloon is placed in the space of Retzius and the balloon tubing is brought out through the rectus fascia.

The cuff, pump and balloon tubing should be placed so they can be connected to the AS 792 stainless steel assembly in the area of one of the external inguinal rings. Once again, rubber-shod clamps on the tubes prevent leakage of fluid while the tubes are cut to appropriate length and connected to their respective ports on the stainless steel AS 792 assembly. Each tubing connection is secured with a double 3/0 Prolene tie.

The rectus fascia is closed, Scarpa's fascia is closed over the tubing and assembly, and the remaining portions of the incision are closed in layers.

Postoperative care

The urethral catheter is removed on the first postoperative day after deflating the cuff. The patient is instructed on the use of the device.

Delayed activation of the AS 791 or AS 792

The AS 791 and AS 792 are semi-automatic devices. Deflation of the cuff is achieved with the deflation bulb; the cuff, however, automatically reinflates with either device. This is an obvious advantage for patient convenience. A disadvantage of both these prostheses is that the cuff cannot be left in the open position.

If the urethral or bladder neck tissues are injured during dissection, healing may not take place and cuff erosion into the urinary tract may occur. If the cuff is implanted in an empty state and left deflated, there is a greater chance of primary healing. Consequently, many surgeons prefer to use a delayed activation technique. With the first surgical procedure, the empty cuff is placed around the bulbous urethra or bladder neck and the deflation bulb and balloons are placed in their normal locations. The tubing from the cuff and the pump are connected to each other over a straight stainless steel connector and an implantable plug is placed in the tubing from the balloon. The wound is closed and the patient, after recovering from the procedure, is discharged from the hospital. The patient is readmitted 6 weeks later for the activation procedure. After cystoscopy to confirm that cuff erosion has not occurred, the suprapubic incision is opened, the stainless steel assembly put into place and the tubes trimmed to appropriate lengths and connected to their respective ports on the stainless steel assembly. Many implanting surgeons feel that this delayed activation technique decreases the risk of cuff erosion.

References

1. Scott, F. B., Bradley, W. E., Timm, G. W. Treatment of urinary incontinence by implantable prosthetic sphincter. Urology 1973; 1: 252–259

2. Montague, D. K. The Scott-Bradley-Timm artificial urinary sphincters. Journal of Urology 1981; 125: 796–798

Illustrations by Patrick M. Elliott

Genitourinary abnormalities associated with imperforate anus

Evan J. Kass MD
Associate Professor of Urology and Child Health and Development,
George Washington University School of Medicine and Health Sciences;
Attending Pediatric Urologist, Children's Hospital National Medical Center, Washington, DC, USA

General considerations

Children with imperforate anus commonly have unsuspected anomalies of the urinary tract. Therefore every child with this condition must have an excretory urogram and a voiding cystourethrogram performed early in the newborn period. The most common urological abnormalities encountered include renal agenesis, hydronephrosis, vesicoureteral reflux and neuropathic bladder. The management of these conditions proceeds along standard lines.

1

A fistulous communication between the terminal colon and urethra is typically found in males with supralevator types of imperforate anus. This fistula is an integral part of the anomaly and should be excised at the same time that the rectal pull-through procedure is performed by the paediatric surgeon. The urologist may be called upon to assist in the management of postsurgical complications related to this fistula.

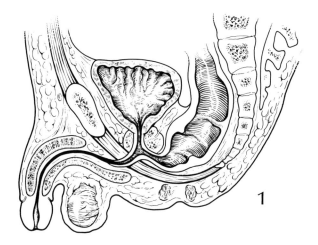

1

2

If, at the time of the original surgery, the fistula is transected too close to the urethra so that the urethral lumen is narrowed upon closure, a urethral stricture may result. Rarely, the urethra itself may be mistaken for the fistula and transected, leaving the original fistula in place.

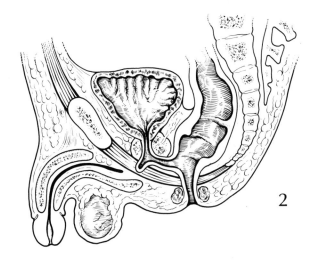

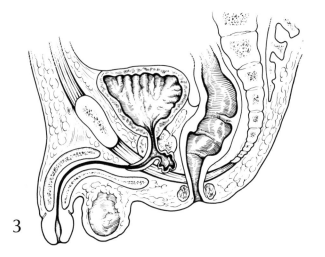

3

Alternatively, too much fistula may be left, creating a urethral diverticulum which can predispose to urinary infection and/or calculus formation within the diverticulum itself. A metal sound passed through the urethra at the time the fistula is transected will simplify the pull-through procedure and help obviate these complications.

4

The original fistula may be missed completely at the time of the original surgery and pulled down along with the rectal segment. Symptoms associated with this complication include passage of urine *per rectum* or of faeces and air *per urethram*. This complication was more common when the pull-through procedure was performed exclusively using the perineal approach, but has been seen only occasionally since a combined abdominal/perineal approach has become popular. The presence of a persistent fistula can be confirmed best radiographically with a voiding cystourethrogram or barium enema. The fistula itself may be difficult to visualize, but contrast material is often seen to pass from the urinary tract into the rectum. If such transport of contrast media occurs, then one can assume that a fistula is present even if the actual fistulous tract itself cannot be identified radiographically.

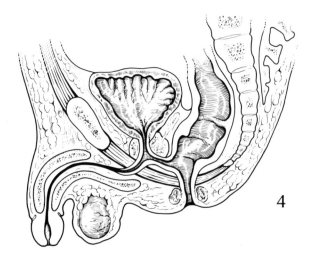

Preoperative

The bowel is prepared with a mechanical cleansing and an antimicrobial agent for 2 or 3 days prior to operation.

Anaesthesia

General anaesthesia administered through a small intra-tracheal tube is the most satisfactory. A small plastic cannula should be inserted into a vein in the operating theatre and left in place for the administration of fluids.

The operation

The perineal approach is satisfactory when a low-lying diverticulum or fistula is found to be present. The patient is placed in the exaggerated lithotomy position. Cystoscopy is performed at this time, to confirm that the urethra is entirely normal, and an attempt is made to pass a ureteral catheter endoscopically through the urethra into the rectum. Left in place, this catheter can greatly simplify the surgical procedure.

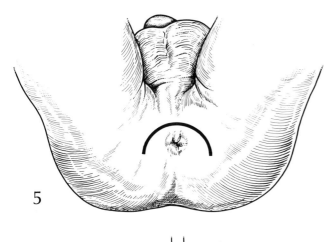

5

An elliptical incision is made in the perineum and a plane of dissection created close to the rectum to reduce the potential for urethral injury. A finger placed in the rectum periodically during the dissection is most helpful in this regard. If a small rent is made in the bowel it can usually be closed with two layers of 3/0 or 4/0 chromic catgut sutures. A larger injury will usually require temporary colostomy diversion, but proximal intestinal diversion is not routinely employed unless such an injury occurs.

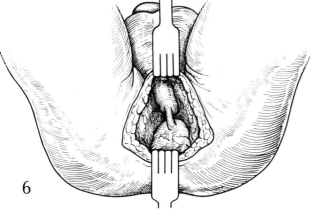

6

Once the fistula or diverticulum is identified it is very important to delineate the urethra prior to transection. A metal sound passed per urethrum will greatly simplify this process and help define its anatomical limits.

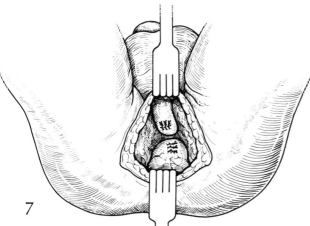

7

In excising the fistula, just enough tissue is left so that when the defect is subsequently closed the urethra is not narrowed and no diverticulum is created. The urethra is closed in a single layer of 4/0 chromic catgut or polyglycolic acid sutures, and the bowel is closed in two layers of 3/0 or 4/0 sutures.

8

The interposition of well vascularized tissues between the urethra and rectum will minimize any potential for recurrent fistula formation.

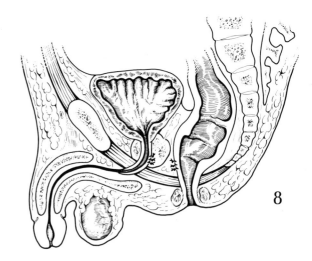

8

9

The skin is closed with interrupted sutures of 4/0 chromic or polyglycolic acid suture. A drain is not routinely employed, but an indwelling silicone-coated Foley catheter is always left in place for 7–10 days postoperatively. Prior to removal of the catheter it is helpful to have a voiding cystourethrogram to ensure that the suture line is intact and no leakage present. If any leakage is documented, then the catheter is left in place for an additional week and the study repeated.

When the fistula or diverticulum is located particularly high in the pelvis, or the surgical exposure through a perineal incision alone might be too limited, a combined abdominoperineal or transsacral approach may have to be performed in conjunction with a paediatric surgeon.

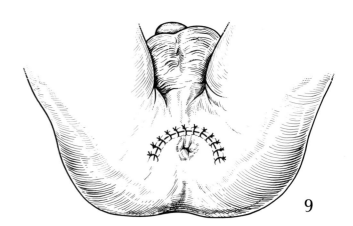

9

Further reading

Belman, A. B. Imperforate anus and cloacal exstrophy. In: Kelalis, P. P., King, L. R., Belman, A. B., eds. Clinical pediatric urology, Vol. 2. Philadelphia: W. B. Saunders Co., 1976: 600–614

DeVries, P. A. Complications of surgery for congenital anomalies of the anorectum. In: DeVries, P. A., Shapiro, S. R., eds. Complications of pediatric surgery. New York: John Wiley and Sons, 1982: 233–262

Lewis, L. G. Repair of recto-urethral fistulas. Journal of Urology 1947; 57: 1173-1183

Thomas, G. G., Molenaar, J. C. The management of a fistula between the rectum and the lower urinary tract. Journal of Pediatric Surgery 1979; 14: 65–73

Williams, D. I., Grant, J. Urological complications of imperforate anus. British Journal of Urology 1969; 41: 660–665

Illustrations by Robert N. Lane

Operations for incontinence of urine in the female

Stuart L. Stanton FRCS, MRCOG
Senior Lecturer in Obstetrics and Gynaecology, St George's Hospital Medical School, London;
Consultant Obstetrician and Gynaecologist, St Helier Hospital, Carshalton, Surrey, UK

Introduction

The surgical procedures discussed here are for the correction of stress incontinence due to urethral sphincter incompetence (genuine stress incontinence) in the female. Incontinence due to detrusor instability is less successfully managed by surgery and should, in the first instance, be treated medically.

There are several factors responsible for incompetence of the urethral sphincter mechanism. Among these are: loss of urethral contractility or resistance; descent of the bladder neck outside the abdominal zone of pressure; loss of hermetic sealing by the urothelium; and absence of posterior support to the proximal urethra during physical effort. These factors may operate singly or in combination.

1

To be continent, the urethral pressure should exceed the bladder pressure at rest; this produces a positive urethral closure pressure. The bladder neck is normally situated within the abdominal zone of pressure and any rise in abdominal pressure is usually transmitted to the bladder and the proximal urethra, thus preserving the pressure gradient. Disturbance of this equilibrium resulting in incontinence can occur in two ways: either the bladder neck descends and no longer receives transmission of intraabdominal pressure or the urethral contractility/resistance is decreased (e.g. following repeated bladder neck surgery).

The importance of the posterior urethrovesical angle is no longer credible, relying as it does on morphology rather than physiology.

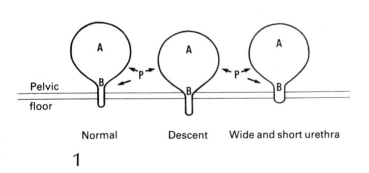

Normal   Descent   Wide and short urethra

1

Preoperative preparation

All patients should have a midstream urine for culture and sensitivity and any urinary tract infection should be treated before surgery. While not every patient needs urodynamic investigations, these are indicated in the following situations: when symptomatology is multiple and complex; following one failed procedure to establish continence; and when procedures are known to produce voiding difficulties (e.g. sling operations), or when there are symptoms of voiding difficulty. Cystoscopy is indicated when intravesical pathology is suspected.

While detrusor instability is not an absolute contraindication to corrective surgery for stress incontinence, these cases should initially be treated medically. If these measures fail to control stress incontinence, bladder neck surgery can be undertaken, providing the patient is cautioned that success is less likely when stress incontinence is due to detrusor instability rather than urethral sphincter incompetence alone. It is important to emphasize that frequency and urge incontinence may not necessarily be corrected. Occasionally these symptoms may be made worse.

Neither are voiding difficulties an absolute contraindication to bladder neck surgery, but these must be considered individually. In some cases an Otis urethro-tomy, carried out beforehand, will improve the flow rate.

Notwithstanding the patient's history, it is mandatory that urinary loss should be demonstrated preoperatively, either on physical examination or by investigation.

As subsequent vaginal deliveries are likely to prejudice the surgical care, the patient should be warned about this and advised that either she should have completed her family or that further children should be delivered by Caesarean section.

Choice of procedure

There is controversy over whether the conventional anterior repair is preferable and as effective as a suprapubic procedure, such as a Marshall-Marchetti-Krantz or colposuspension operation, for correction of primary urethral sphincter incompetence. For the latter with anterior vaginal wall relaxation, either the anterior repair or a colposuspension would be appropriate. For recurrent incontinence or primary incontinence with minimal anterior vaginal wall descent, a suprapubic procedure appears preferable.

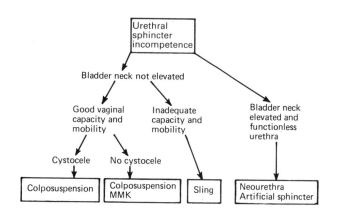

2

2

The choice of suprapubic procedure is made according to the anatomical position of the bladder neck. If the bladder neck is not elevated, a colposuspension, Marshall-Marchetti-Krantz (MMK) or sling procedure is appropriate and the indications will be discussed under those procedures. If the bladder neck is elevated, incontinence is likely to be due to a decrease in the urethral resistance which may be confirmed by a reduced urethral closure pressure at rest. This will be treated appropriately by a neourethra or an artificial sphincter.

It is frequently suggested that there is an improved chance of cure of incontinence if a hysterectomy is performed at the same time as a continence procedure. The author does not know of any data to support this and only performs a hysterectomy when uterine pathology is present.

Postoperative care

The great majority of these procedures induce temporary acute retention of urine and require postoperative catheter drainage. It is more sterile and easier for the patient to commence this in the operating theatre. Opinion is divided on the benefits of suprapubic and urethral catheter drainage. Urinary tract infection appears to be less using a suprapubic catheter[1], and this is certainly a more comfortable method for patients. In addition the patient is able to commence voiding while a suprapubic catheter is in place, allowing its removal when voiding has become normal.

The author's choice is always to use a suprapubic catheter such as the Bonanno catheter. The bladder should be filled before the catheter is inserted and it is left to drain freely for the first 24–48 hours after operation, depending on the patient's condition. The catheter is then clamped in the morning and released either 8 hours later or earlier if pain and retention develop. A residual urine is performed by lying the patient on one side and draining the suprapubic catheter for 15–30 min. An accurate fluid input and output chart is maintained and when the residual is less than 100 ml (and provided the patient has been voiding 100–200 ml during the day), the catheter is clamped overnight. The patient is woken once or twice during the night to void and the residual checked in the morning. If neither retenton nor incontinence has developed the catheter may be removed. The track heals within 24 hours.

All patients may be mobilized in the normal manner, commencing on the first postoperative day. When the operation involves repositioning of tissues (e.g. anterior repair, Marshall-Marchetti-Krantz, colposuspension or sling), avoidance of heavy lifting is advised. Ideally this should be forever, but this is not practical, especially in young women who wish to continue athletic activity, in which case heavy lifting should be avoided for 2 months.

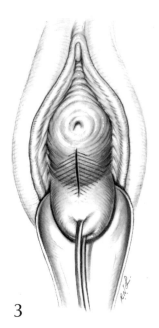

3

The procedures

ANTERIOR REPAIR (COLPORRHAPHY)

Numerous eponyms are associated with this procedure. Almost a century ago, Donald in Manchester[2] described a combination of operations to narrow the anterior and posterior vaginal walls with amputation of the cervix, a procedure later written up by Fothergill[3]. This was renamed the Manchester repair by Shaw in 1933. That the bladder neck is crucial to the mechanism of incontinence was recognized by Kelly[4], who described coaptation of bladder neck tissue by sutures placed from side to side, across the bladder neck region. This is now the basis of the anterior repair. Further modifications were described by Pacey[5], who performed extensive lateral dissection to enable him to coapt pubocervical fascia and pubococcygeus muscle in the midline, beneath the bladder.

The aim of this procedure is to elevate the bladder neck. There is no objective evidence to suggest that the anterior repair produces outflow obstruction as part of its mechanism of continence[6].

Preoperative preparation

No special preparations are necessary, apart from the administration of metronidazole suppositories, 500 mg twice a day for 24 hours preceding the operation, as prophylaxis against anaerobic infection.

Anaesthesia and position of patient

The patient is given a general anaesthetic with relaxation, or an epidural or spinal anaesthetic, and placed in the lithotomy position. The perineum is prepared and draped in a sterile manner.

Technique

The bladder is catheterized to make reduction of the cystocele easier. A solution containing adrenaline 1:200 000 is injected into the midline of the anterior vaginal wall and into the tissues around the bladder base for haemostasis and to delineate tissue spaces prior to dissection.

3

A Sims or Auvard vaginal speculum is inserted into the vagina, to depress the posterior wall. A vertical midline incision is made in the anterior vaginal wall, starting 0.5 cm below the external urethral meatus and extending downwards over the maximum prominence of the cystocele. Using a scalpel or scissors, with blunt dissection, the anterior vaginal wall flaps are separated laterally from the underlying bladder and held apart by small Kochers forceps, and dissection continued until the bladder base, bladder neck and proximal urethra are exposed. The pubocervical fascia will be found laterally, attached to the undersurface of the anterior vaginal wall flap. Some bleeding will occur and this can be arrested by diathermy. Venous oozing may be left; it will cease on closing the wound.

4

A bladder neck or Kelly suture of No. 1 polyglycolic acid suture (Vicryl or Dexon) is inserted into the paraurethral tissue at the level of the bladder neck and tied, and a further suture inserted just lateral to this and tied. These elevate the bladder neck,

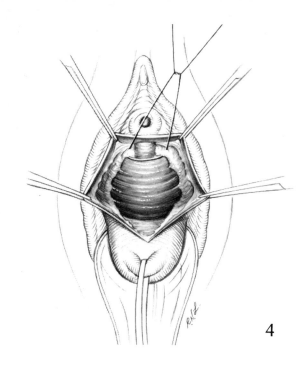

4

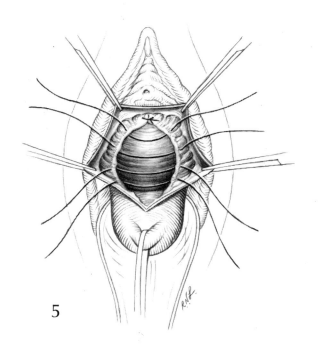

5

5

Starting at the base of the bladder, three or four sutures of the same material are inserted into the lateral margins of the pubocervical fascia and are left untied.

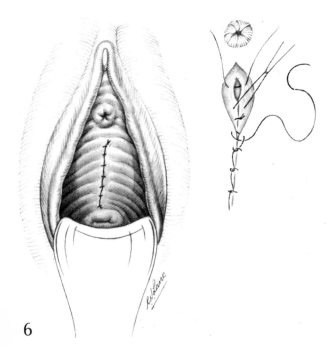

6

6

Surplus vaginal skin is now excised from both flaps and a continuous locking suture of No. 0 polyglycolic acid suture is used to close the anterior vaginal wall, beginning at the lower end of the midline incision. The locking suture provides haemostasis and prevents shortening of the anterior vaginal wall. As suturing proceeds, the underlying pubocervical sutures are tied in order.

Complications

The major complications are trauma to the urethra and bladder and haemorrhage. The former occurs through inability to find and remain within the correct plane of dissection. This is more likely to occur when there has been previous surgery to the bladder neck. In this situation, a urethral diverticulum may be opened; two-layer closure without tension, using a fine polyglycolic acid suture and catheter drainage, are necessary. Haemorrhage may result from trauma to the perivesical veins. This may be managed by a combination of diathermy, oversuturing and prompt closure.

Results

Most results in the literature are inferior to those for suprapubic surgery. Nevertheless, a careful technique and selection of patients may produce a satisfactory cure rate. Subjective results of between 40 per cent cure[7] and 96 per cent cure[8] are found.

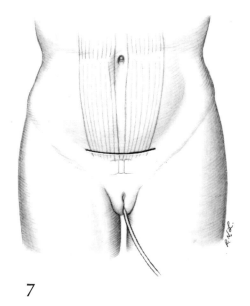

7

THE MARSHALL-MARCHETTI-KRANTZ OPERATION

This was described by its authors in 1949[9] and its main modification has been a reduction in the number of sutures. The principle, in common with other suprapubic procedures, is elevation of the bladder neck.

Preoperative preparation

No special preoperative preparations are necessary.

Anaesthesia and position of patient

A general anaesthetic with relaxation is used and the patient placed in the lithotomy position with head-down tilt. Both the abdomen and the perineal areas are cleaned and draped so that the operator has access to the vagina, to aid dissection. A transurethral resection drape (3M type 1071) is used, with the condom inserted into the vagina, to provide a sterile field and to avoid glove changing. A 16 Fr Foley catheter on open drainage is passed to empty the bladder and to delineate the urethra and bladder neck. The operator stands on the patient's left.

Technique

7

A low Pfannenstiel incision is made. The rectus sheath is incised transversely and upper and lower flaps are dissected off the underlying rectus muscles, which are separated in the midline.

8 & 9

A Denis Browne ring retractor will give an excellent exposure. The space of Retzius is entered and the bladder and urethra are dissected off the posterior aspect of the symphysis pubis. It is best to start in the midline and dissect laterally. Caution should be exercised if a previous suprapubic operation has been performed, as it is easy to enter the bladder accidentally. Any bleeding from perivesical veins may be arrested by diathermy.

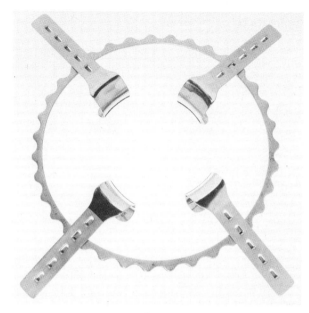

8

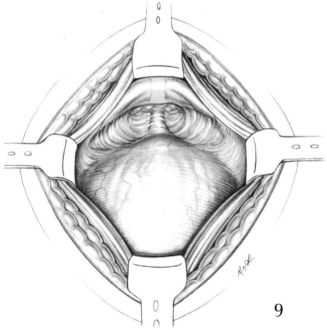

9

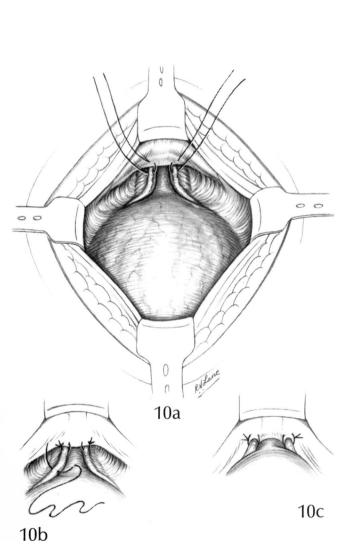

10a

10b

10c

10a, b & c

With the surgeon's left forefinger in the vagina to elevate the anterior vaginal wall, the right hand is used to dissect the paraurethral tissues free at the level of the bladder neck, so that a polyglycolic acid suture is placed either side of the bladder neck, into the paravaginal tissue. If non-absorbable material is used, care must be taken to avoid penetrating the bladder or urethra, as a calculus may be formed. Further distal sutures may be inserted either side of the bladder neck. These are then inserted in order into the periosteum or perichondrium of the posterior aspect of the symphysis pubis.

11

The assistant elevates the anterior vaginal wall and the sutures are tied, starting with the most distal one first. The wound is closed in layers and a Redivac drain is left in the space of Retzius. The bladder is filled via the Foley catheter, which is withdrawn once a suprapubic catheter has been inserted.

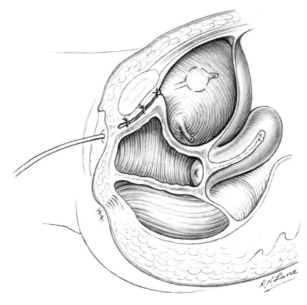

11

Complications

Trauma to the bladder can occur on entry to the space of Retzius. This is treated by a one or two layer closure using an absorbable suture and an indwelling urethral catheter for 5–7 days. Antibiotic or chemotherapeutic cover is given. Osteitis pubis is a late complication in about 5 per cent of cases. This is treated by antibiotic chemotherapy and drainage if any abscess occurs.

Postoperative care

Routine mobilization and care of a suprapubic catheter are carried out. The Redivac is removed on the second postoperative day.

Results

Most papers quote a subjective improvement rate exceeding 90 per cent for patients where this has been a primary procedure[8, 10]. Where recurrent incontinence has been treated, the improvement rate is expected to be lower.

COLPOSUSPENSION

Burch described this procedure in 1961, when he used it to correct stress incontinence and cystocele in a series of 53 patients. Elevation of the bladder neck and anterior vaginal wall is achieved by suturing the paravaginal fascia of each lateral vaginal fornix to the corresponding ileopectineal (Cooper's) ligament.

Preoperative preparation

No special preparations are necessary.

Anaesthesia and position of patient

The patient is anaesthetized and positioned in the same way as for the Marshall-Marchetti-Krantz operation, except that the author prefers the horizontal lithotomy position, with no head-down tilt. The bladder is catheterized with a 16 Fr Foley catheter and allowed to drain freely. The operator stands on the patient's left.

Technique

12

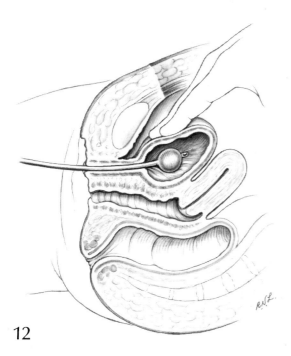

12

A low Pfannenstiel incision is made and the space of Retzius entered as described previously.

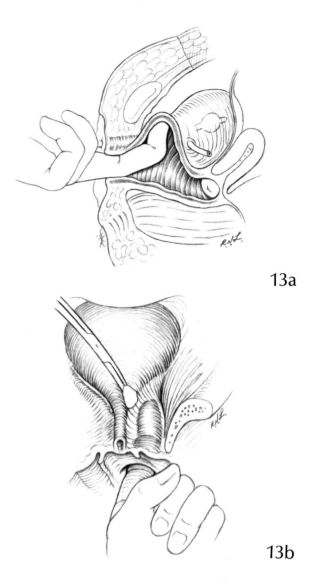

13a

13b

13a & b

The left forefinger is inserted into a lateral vaginal fornix, which the surgeon elevates. With the right hand, the surgeon cautiously begins to sweep the bladder base and neck off the paravaginal fascia, using a sponge, forceps or a small swab on a curved Roberts forceps. The fascia appears as white tissue and is of variable thickness. Caution should be exercised in the elderly as this is readily torn. Perivesical veins may be traumatized and haemostasis is achieved by diathermy at this stage. The dissection continues until the surgeon is able to approximate the lateral fornix to the corresponding ileopectineal ligament.

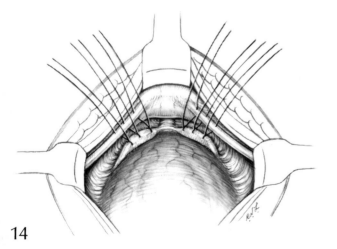

14

14

The author inserts three pairs of No. 1 polyglycolic acid suture on each side, placing one suture at the bladder neck; the subsequent two are placed progressively more cephalad. An 18–20 cm Finochetti needle holder (with an angled jaw) is most useful. The sutures are tied on the fascia to provide haemostasis and to prevent the suture sliding when it is tied onto the ileopectineal ligament. It does not matter if a full thickness of vaginal wall is penetrated by the suture providing an absorbable material is used. Retraction of the previous suture by the assistant eases the insertion of the next suture.

The author finds it easier to remain on the left-hand side of the patient for the entire operation, using his left hand to insert the appropriate sutures into the left ileopectineal ligament.

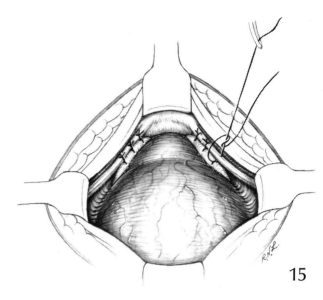

15

15 & 16

Once all sutures have been inserted into the ileopectineal ligaments and haemostasis obtained, the sutures are tied, starting at the most distal suture and tying alternate sides. There is no need for the assistant to elevate the anterior vaginal wall as this is achieved by pulling taut that suture which passes through the ileopectineal ligament and tying the other limb of the suture around this.

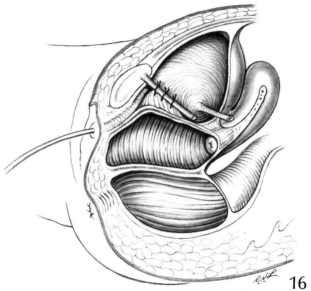

16

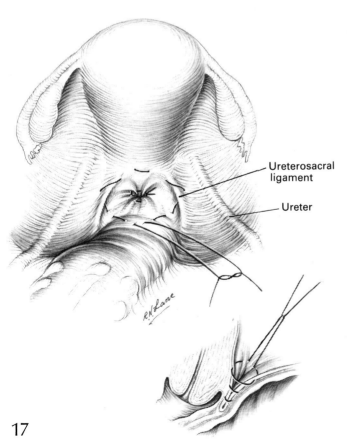

Ureterosacral ligament

Ureter

17

If an enterocele is present, it should be repaired from within the peritoneal cavity as it is likely to become more prominent after a colposuspension operation. A Moschowitz procedure, whereby the pouch of Douglas is closed by successive purse-string sutures of No. 1 linen inserted into the pouch of Douglas peritoneum, passing through the uterosacral ligaments is employed. Care should be taken to avoid the ureters.

A Redivac drain is inserted into the cave of Retzius and the wound closed. A suprapubic catheter is inserted as previously described.

17

Complications

Trauma to the bladder and the urethra can occur during dissection and should be repaired using a one- or two-layer closure technique. Haemorrhage from perivesical veins is a frequent occurrence and can be minimized by cautious dissection, diathermy and over-sewing. If these do not suffice, venous haemorrhage will cease once the fascial sutures are tied and the lateral fornices are elevated. Failure to dissect the ureterovesical junction clear from the fascia may result in ureteric ligation. Prompt detection and removal of the ligature (occasionally achieved at endoscopy) may suffice, but usually ureteric reimplantation is required. If the para-vaginal fascia is torn it should be closed and the operation continued. Prophylactic intravenous metronidazole may be given.

Sometimes it is impossible to approximate the lateral fornix to the corresponding ileopectineal ligament. Providing there is elevation, some lack of distal approx-imation is acceptable, but, in gross cases, the procedure should be abandoned and a sling operation performed, or a unilateral hitch to the ileopectineal ligament attempted. In the author's opinion, the obturator fascia is rarely strong enough to support these sutures.

Postoperative care

Routine mobilization and care of the Redivac drain and suprapubic catheter are as previously described.

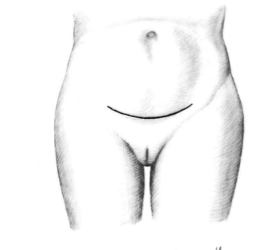
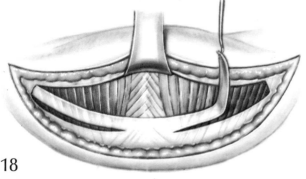

18

Results

Burch[11] reported on results with 143 patients, followed for varying intervals up to and beyond 5 years. He found a 93 per cent subjective cure rate of stress incontinence and a 2.8 per cent recurrence of cystocele.

The author followed up a group of 60 patients (out of a total series of 370 patients) for 5 years and found a subjective cure rate of 87 per cent and an 83 per cent objective cure rate over 1 year, decreasing to a 72 per cent objective cure rate over 5 years[13]. For cystocele, there was a 7.7 per cent recurrence rate over 5 years.

SLING PROCEDURES

Sling procedures have been in use for 70 years and are classified according to whether organic or inorganic tissue is used for the sling. Of the former, the Aldridge procedure[14], described in 1942, is well established and widely used. The Morgan[15] sling technique makes use of inorganic tissue, mainly polypropylene mesh (Marlex), and will be described as an alternative method.

Slings produce elevation of the bladder neck and often partial outflow obstruction. Organic tissue is without foreign-body reaction and is obtained from the rectus sheath or fascia lata. It is inconsistent in strength. Inorganic tissue is of consistent strength, but, if it becomes infected, it has to be removed. The choice remains that of the individual surgeon.

Preoperative preparation

No special preparation is necessary

Anaesthesia and position of patient

No special preparation is necessary, and the patient is anaesthetized and positioned as for the colposuspension operation.

Aldridge procedure

18

A low Pfannenstiel incision is made and the rectus sheath opened 2 cm above the symphysis. The upper flap is dissected off the midline raphe and retracted. A second transverse incision is made through the rectus sheath 1.5 cm below the first, leaving a central 3 cm island intact. The incisions create two strips of rectus fascia attached centrally.

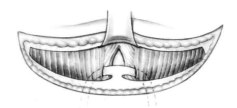

19

A short transverse incision is made through the anterior vaginal wall at the level of the bladder neck, and this is then exposed. A curved haemostat, inserted through the vaginal incision, is passed retropubically in an upward direction along the lateral side of the bladder neck, to emerge behind the symphysis. One end of the rectus flap is grasped and pulled down alongside the bladder neck. This is repeated on the other side. The slings are crossed below the bladder neck and sutured under slight tension. The vaginal and abdominal wounds are closed and a suprapubic catheter is inserted.

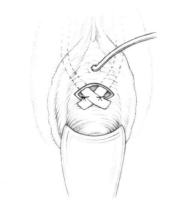

19

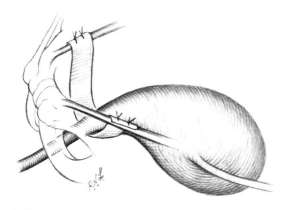

20

Morgan procedure

Although Morgan describes a combined vaginal and abdominal approach, the sling can be inserted via an abdominal route only. This is advantageous when using inorganic tissue as it lowers the risk of sling infection. The retropubic space is entered via a low Pfannenstiel incision and the bladder and urethra freed from the posterior aspect of the symphysis pubis.

20

If a vaginal incision is made, the bladder neck is exposed as described in the Aldridge technique, and a 1–2 cm wide sling of polypropylene is passed into the space of Retzius on either side of the bladder neck, so that the sling supports the bladder neck as a hammock. It is secured to the bladder neck by No. 1 polyglycolic acid sutures. The two ends of the sling are retrieved in the abdominal field and secured under slight tension to the corresponding ileopectineal ligament by similar sutures.

21 & 22

If the abdominal route alone is chosen, a tunnel is created under the bladder neck by scissors and blunt dissection. The sling is passed through and secured to each ileopectineal ligament. Caution is necessary to avoid trauma to the perivesical plexus of veins and to the bladder and urethra during dissection from the underlying vaginal wall. A Redivac drain is left in the retropubic space and a suprapubic catheter is inserted.

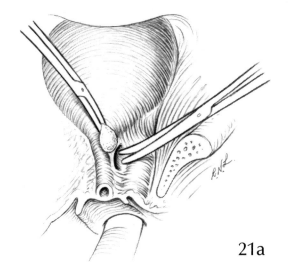

21a

Complications

Operative complications include haemorrhage, trauma to the bladder and urethra during separation from the symphysis and during tunnelling under the bladder neck. Postoperative complications include delayed spontaneous voiding with persistent retention and erosion of the sling through the urethra. Difficulty in voiding or retention may require release or removal of the sling. Erosion should be treated by sling removal (if it is inorganic).

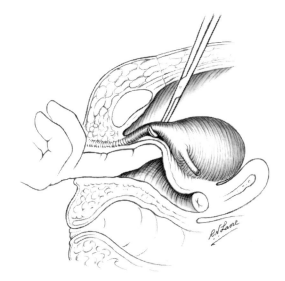

Postoperative care

This is the same as for the colposuspension, except that delayed voiding is more common.

21b

Results

Morgan and Farrow[16] found that 118 out of 127 patients (93 per cent) were cured of stress incontinence on subjective assessment.

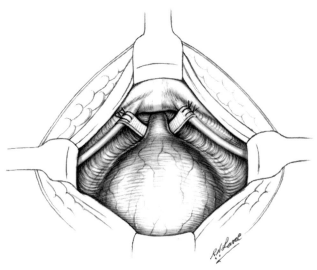

NEOURETHRA

The technique of replacement of the urethra by a tube constructed from the anterior bladder wall was described by Tanagho and Smith in 1972[17] and again by Tanagho[18] 8 years later. The anterior bladder wall adjacent to the internal urethral meatus has a large proportion of transverse fibres. A tube constructed from this area is likely to have abundant circularly orientated fibres and should be able to impart some sphincteric function to this tubular segment. The operation is appropriate for cases where urethral function and resistance are markedly reduced, where previous continence surgery has been attempted and failed, and in epispadias where it may be used as a primary procedure.

Preoperative preparation

An intravenous urogram is necessary to exclude any abnormality of the upper urinary tract, such as an ectopic ureter, but otherwise no special preparation is necessary.

Anaesthesia and position of patient

As for a colposuspension operation.

Technique

23

The bladder and proximal urethra are approached via a low Pfannenstiel incision. The bladder is severed from the urethra at the bladder neck level.

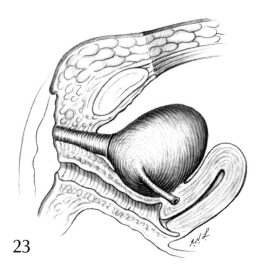

23

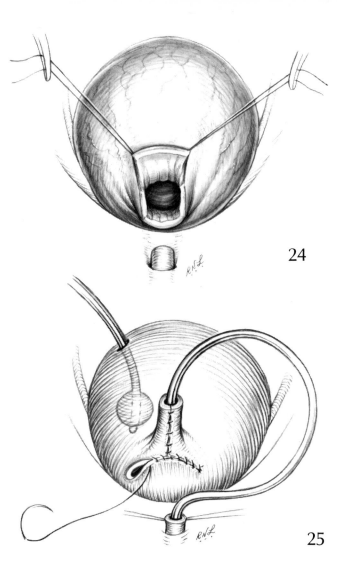

24

24 & 25

An anterior bladder flap measuring 2.5 by 2.5 cm is raised with its base attached to the bladder wall. This is furled around a 12–14 Fr Nelaton or non-retaining catheter and closed in one layer with a continuous locking 3/0 polyglycolic acid suture. At this stage a suprapubic catheter (14 Fr) is inserted. The remainder of the bladder is closed

25

26

A neourethra, approximately 2.5 cm in length, is now formed and is anastomosed to the proximal end of the divided urethra, using a single layer of interrupted 3/0 polyglycolic acid sutures. The urethral catheter is left in place as a stent and to drain the bladder. A retropubic Redivac drain is inserted and the wound closed.

The stent may be removed on the 7th day and the suprapubic catheter clamped and removed when voiding is satisfactorily established.

Complications

If any urinary leakage occurs, the catheters should be left in for an additional week and then reviewed. Stricture at the site of the anastomosis may occur 2–3 months after the operation and this may be treated by urethral dilatation or cautious anterior urethrotomy.

Results

The author has operated on 7 patients, each of whom had between 2 and 5 previous operations to cure incontinence (mean 3.6). Two patients were cured, 3 improved and 2 remained wet.

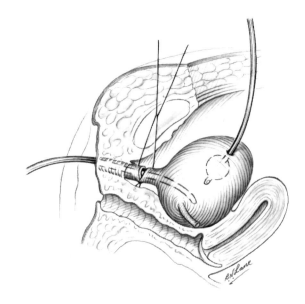

26

ARTIFICIAL URINARY SPHINCTER

The artificial urinary sphincter was introduced by Scott, Bradley and Timm in 1973[19] to control incontinence in the male and female and to allow voiding to continue via an intact lower urinary tract. The sphincter has undergone several modifications and is now available as a bladder neck sphincter (AS792) for the female and male, and as a bulbous urethral sphincter (AS791) for the male.

27

The sphincter consists of a silicone rubber occlusive cuff placed around the bladder neck, a reservoir or balloon situated in the abdominal cavity, a stainless steel control assembly comprising a delay fluid resistor, a pump placed in the left labium majus and interconnecting silicone fluid-filled tubing. The device mimics the urethral sphincter by the opening and closing action of the occlusive cuff, obtained by transfer of fluid from the reservoir and activated at will by digital control of the deflation pump.

This procedure is performed following failed bladder neck operations to correct urethral sphincter incompetence. In addition, it is indicated to correct incontinence due to: detrusor instability which has failed to respond to medical or surgical treatment; myelomeningocele or other neurological disease; epispadias or exstrophy. Absence of lower urinary tract obstruction is important.

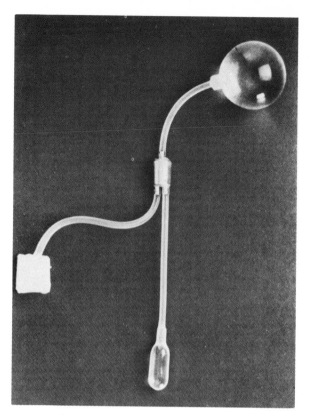

27

Preoperative preparation

Urodynamic studies should confirm urinary leakage and the absence of lower urinary tract obstruction. Strict asepsis is required. The urine should be sterile for at least 48 hours prior to surgery. Antibiotic cover may be given for 24 hours prior to and continuing for 7–10 days after surgery. On the day preceding surgery, the abdomen and perineum should be scrubbed using either hexachlorophane or iodoform.

Anaesthesia and position of patient

The patient has a routine anaesthetic with relaxation and is placed in the horizontal lithotomy position. The abdomen and perineum are scrubbed for 15 min with Betadine and then draped. A 16 Fr Foley catheter is inserted.

Technique

28

A low Pfannenstiel incision is performed and the bladder neck and proximal urethra displayed. The bladder neck is cautiously dissected off the paravaginal fascia as for the abdominal approach for the sling procedure. The size of the cuff is judged by using a cuff sizer, marked in centimetres, which is placed around the bladder neck. The reservoir is chosen according to required cuff pressure (usually 50–60 cm H_2O in the female) and is filled with 18 ml of isotonic 25 per cent Hypaque; 2 ml of this is used to prime the cuff. The reservoir is placed abdominally, and its tubing, together with that of the cuff, is led via the inguinal canal into the left inguinal space. A deep pocket is created by blunt dissection in the left labium majus to hold the pump, which has been filled beforehand with the same solution.

All three parts are now carefully attached to the respective parts of the control assembly using 3/0 Prolene which has been flushed beforehand to exclude air.

If either the bladder or urethra has been traumatized, or if the blood supply is compromised or the tissue appears in any way to be devitalized, primary deactivation is performed to avoid cuff erosion. All the parts of the prosthesis are inserted but the cuff and the control assembly are not connected. Instead the cuff is left deflated and its tubing temporarily sealed. The control assembly is flushed through and the reservoir and the pump are both filled with Hypaque and connected. Secondary activation is carried out under a local or general anaesthetic, 6–10 weeks following surgery.

After haemostasis has been ensured, the wound is closed without a retropubic drain or a suprapubic catheter, to avoid risk of infection. The urethral catheter is left in place.

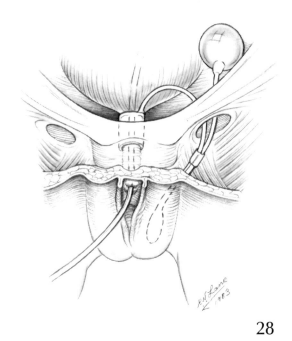

28

Complications

The prosthesis may be complicated by cuff erosion, infection or mechanical failure. The first two will require removal of part or all of the prosthesis. Mechanical failure includes kinking of the tubes, leakage of Hypaque and failure of individual parts. Failure is most common in the cuff, followed by the balloon, then the pump and control assembly. The overall survival rate of the parts is 77 per cent at 30 months. This may be managed by surgical exploration and review or renewal of the part concerned.

Postoperative care

29

A pelvic X-ray is taken at 48 hours to show the device *in situ*. Beginning on the 3rd day, depending on tenderness, the patient is instructed to deflate the pump twice a day. When this can be achieved without discomfort (usually about the 6th or 7th day), the catheter may be removed. The patient should be cautioned that urinary infection, haematuria, incontinence or other malfunction of the sphincter should be reported back promptly to the surgeon. She will carry a card with her name, the name of the surgeon and the hospital where the sphincter was implanted. There is a diagram of the sphincter and simple instructions in what to do and what not to do should catheterization be required.

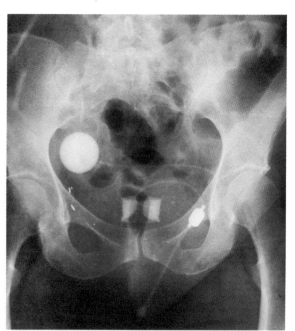

29

Results

Furlow[20] reported overall results for male and female patients: 43 out of 47 patients (91 per cent) achieved continence with a follow-up of 6–30 months. Hald (personal communication, 1982) achieved 74 per cent continence and 12 per cent improvement in a series of 69 male and female patients. American Medical Systems[21] published life-table analyses of 486 patients who had been followed up for 27 months and showed a 77 per cent cure rate.

References

1. Anderson, J. T., Fisher-Rasmussen, W., Molsted Pedersen, L., Nielsen, N. C. Suprapubic bladder drainage reduces rates of urinary infection and of impaired voiding ability after colposuspension/vaginal repair. A randomised trial. Proceedings of 12th Annual Meeting. International Continence Society Leiden, 1982: 96–98

2. Shaw, W. F. Plastic vaginal surgery. In: Kerr, J. M., Johnston, R. W., Phillips, M. H., eds. Historical review of British obstetrics and gynecology, 1800–1950. Edinburgh: Livingstone, 1954: 370–381

3. Fothergill, W. E. On the pathology and the operative treatment of displacements of the pelvic viscera. Journal of Obstetrics and Gynaecology of the British Empire 1908; 13: 410–419

4. Kelly, H. A. Incontinence of urine in women. Urologic and Cutaneous Review 1913; 17: 291–293

5. Pacey, K. The pathology and repair of genital prolapse. Journal of Obstetrics and Gynaecology of the British Empire 1949; 56: 1–15

6. Stanton, S. L., Hilton, P., Norton, C., Cardozo, L. Clinical and urodynamic effects of anterior colporrhaphy and vaginal hysterectomy for prolapse with and without incontinence. British Journal of Obstetrics and Gynaecology 1982; 89: 459–463

7. Low, J. A. The management of anatomic urinary incontinence by vaginal repair. American Journal of Obstetrics and Gynecology 1967; 97: 308–315

8. Green, T. Urinary stress incontinence: differential diagnosis, pathophysiology and management. American Journal of Obstetrics and Gynecology 1975; 122: 368–400

9. Marshall, V. F., Marchetti, A. A., Krantz, K. E. The correction of stress incontinence by simple vesicourethral suspension. Surgery, Gynecology and Obstetrics 1949; 88: 509–518

10. Parnell, J. P., Marshall, V. F., Vaughan, E. D. Primary management of urinary stress incontinence by the Marshall Marchetti Krantz vesicourethropexy. Journal of Urology 1982; 127: 679–682

11. Burch, J. C. Urethrovaginal fixation to Cooper's ligament for correction of stress incontinence, cystocele and prolapse. American Journal of Obstetrics and Gynecology 1961; 81: 281–290

12. Burch, J. C. Cooper's ligament urethrovesical suspension for stress incontinence. American Journal of Obstetrics and Gynecology 1968; 100: 764–774

13. Stanton, S. L., Hertogs, K., Cox, C., HIlton, P., Cardozo, L. Colposuspension operation for genuine stress incontinence: a five-year study. Proceedings 12th Annual Meeting International Continence Society. Leiden, 1982: 94–96

14. Aldridge, A. H. Transplantation of fascia for the relief of urinary stress incontinence. American Journal of Obstetrics and Gynecology 1942; 44: 398–411

15. Morgan, J. E. A sling operation using Marlex polypropylene mesh for treatment of recurrent stress incontinence. American Journal of Obstetrics and Gynecology 1970; 106: 369–377

16. Morgan, J. E., Farrow, G. A. Recurrent stress urinary incontinence in the female. British Journal of Urology 1977; 49: 37–42

17. Tanagho, E., Smith, D. R. Clinical evaluation of a surgical technique for the correction of complete urinary incontinence. Journal of Urology 1972; 107: 402–411

18. Tanagho, E. Neourethra: rationale, surgical technique and indications. In: Stanton, S. L. and Tanagho, E. eds., Surgery of female incontinence. Heidelberg: Springer-Verlag, 1980: 111–117

19. Scott, F. B., Bradley, W. E., Timm, C. W. Treatment of urinary incontinence by an implantable prosthetic sphincter. Urology 1973; 1: 252–259

20. Furlow, W. Implantation of a new semi-automatic artificial genitourinary sphincter: experience with primary activation and de-activation in 47 patients. Journal of Urology 1981; 126: 741–744

21. American Medical Systems (1982). House files

Illustrations by Bayard H. Colyear III

Endoscopic suspension of the vesical neck for correction of urinary stress incontinence in the female

Linda M. Dairiki Shortliffe MD
Assistant Professor of Surgery (Urology), Division of Urology,
Stanford University School of Medicine, Stanford, California;
Chief, Urology Section, Veterans Administration Medical Center, Palo Alto, California, USA

Thomas A. Stamey MD
Professor of Surgery (Urology), Chairman, Division of Urology,
Stanford University School of Medicine, Stanford, California, USA

Introduction

Endoscopic suspension of the vesical neck was first described in 1973[1]. It has several advantages over open retropubic urethrovesical suspensions like the Marshall-Marchetti-Krantz procedure[2]. The incision is superficial; the bladder and bladder neck are not dissected; and the suspending sutures of heavy monofilament nylon are buttressed vaginally with a 1 cm tube of knitted Dacron. More important, the cystoscope is used to ensure placement of the nylon sutures exactly at the vesical neck without penetration of the bladder wall. Our operation is still performed as originally described in 1973[1]. It has proved to be a highly successful procedure for the correction of stress urinary incontinence in the female, especially useful in those patients who have had unsuccessful retropubic operations, and in those whose incontinence is complicated by obesity, pelvic trauma or pelvic irradiation.

Preoperative

Patient evaluation

Symptoms of stress incontinence may be divided into three grades: Grade 1, leakage associated with severe stress alone (coughing, laughing, sneezing); Grade 2, leakage with minimal activity such as walking; and Grade 3, total incontinence. When considering urinary leakage associated with stress, it is important to recognize those patients who describe additional loss of urine after sensing the urge to urinate (urgency incontinence) and those who have suprapubic pain associated with a full bladder; they do not have simple stress urinary incontinence. In our experience, patients with an urgency component to their stress incontinence have not shown bladder instability and usually have been cured by endoscopic suspension of the bladder neck[3], but patients who describe loss of urine *only* after sensing the urge to urinate may have a neuropathic, unstable bladder. Patients who have suprapubic pain associated with a full bladder may have interstitial cystitis. As a result, patients with these two symptoms may need further evaluation.

The actual demonstration of stress-induced incontinence is the most important part of the evaluation, and this must be demonstrated during the physical examination. When the patient has a strong desire to urinate, and feels she has a full bladder, she is asked to void in the bathroom in her normal sitting position. A measuring pan is placed under the toilet seat to measure the voided volume. This volume is recorded and the patient immediately catheterized with a 14 Fr urethral catheter to measure the residual urine in the bladder. A residual volume of greater than 10 per cent of the voided bladder volume may indicate a neuropathic, noncontractile bladder which may not empty spontaneously after surgical suspension of the vesical neck, and may need further preoperative evaluation. After the residual volume is recorded, the bladder is filled slowly via the urethral catheter attached to the empty barrel of a 50 ml catheter tip syringe. By holding the catheter and attached syringe barrel vertically, the bladder is filled with water by gravity flow. When the patient states she is comfortably full, usually at some volume less than the amount voided, the volume of fluid in the bladder is recorded. Any sudden rises in the water column observed during the bladder filling phase should be noted because these are signs of spontaneous uninhibited bladder contractions which may need further evaluation. With the bladder comfortably full, the patient – still in the lithotomy position – is asked to cough. If the patient has demonstrable leakage coincident with the cough, the examination for surgically curable, urinary incontinence is complete. If no leakage occurs, the head of the table is tilted up to 45° and again the patient is observed for evidence of urethral incontinence when she coughs. Finally, if the patient does not demonstrate leakage in this position she is asked to stand and cough with her legs apart. Leakage in this position must be almost coincident with the cough in order to avoid mistaking a cough-induced spontaneous bladder contraction for a sign of stress incontinence. A cough-induced bladder contraction will lag 5-15 s after the cough.

Before conclusion of the examination, the patient should be inspected for a rectocele and cystocele. Significant rectoceles can be corrected at the time of surgery, and small to moderate cystoceles will be corrected automatically with suspension of the vesical neck tissues; larger cystoceles which protrude through the vaginal outlet on straining require deepening of the vaginal incision and appropriate repair. The patient should have a bimanual pelvic examination at this time and Pap smear if needed. Perineal sensation to check S2, S3 and S4 pelvic nerves can be tested, but we have never found this useful. On completion of this examination, the patient is given 24 hours of an antimicrobial agent, such as nitrofurantoin, or trimethoprim-sulphamethoxazole, to prevent a urinary tract infection caused by catheterization.

Urethrocystoscopy, cystometrograms and lateral chain cystograms are not routinely used for evaluation. These may be included in the evaluation if the patient has unusual symptoms, a pathological urinary sediment, signs of a neuropathic bladder, or has had multiple previous surgeries for correction of incontinence.

Preoperative management

The evening before surgery the patient undergoes routine preoperative preparations including soap-suds enemas, povidone-iodine douche and perineal and suprapubic shaving and scrubbing. Urinalysis and urine culture are obtained, but blood is not usually cross-matched for this procedure. Any known urine infections should have been treated prior to the patient entering the hospital. Usually a parenteral dose of an aminoglycoside (tobramycin or gentamicin 80 mg) is given the evening before surgery to try to ensure that the patient's urine will be sterile at the time of surgery in case a urinary infection is present. A second parenteral dose of aminoglycoside is given the following morning an hour before surgery. This dose is used to produce a tissue level of antimicrobial during the surgery to reduce the risk of postoperative wound infection.

Anaesthesia

The patient should be given the form of anaesthetic best suited to her general health. However, most of the time this procedure can be performed under a spinal block with a sensory level of anaesthesia to at least T10. Anaesthesia should be planned to last at least 90–120 min.

The operation

1

The operation is performed with the patient in the modified lithotomy position. The knees are bent and elevated laterally while the lower abdomen is kept flat. The patient's buttocks must be placed far enough below the edge of the table for the weighted posterior vaginal retractor to be used.

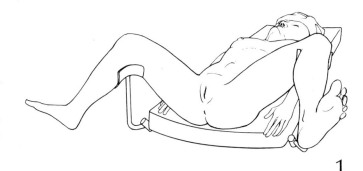

1

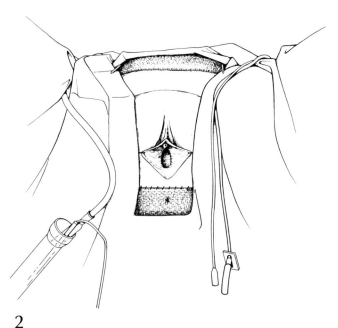

2

2

After careful shaving and scrubbing of the entire perineum, vagina and suprapubic area, a cloth drape attached to a sticky plastic drape is sutured across the perineum to exclude the anus from the surgical field. Both labia minora are sutured laterally to expose the vaginal introitus. The legs and abdomen are draped, but the pubis and 4–5 cm of the suprapubic area and perineum are kept within the operative field. It is convenient to drape the fibreoptic cord of the cystoscope and water tubing over one of the patient's legs and the suction tubing and electrocautery over the other.

3

Two symmetrical transverse 2–3 cm skin incisions are made on both sides of the midline just above the point at which the upper edge of the symphysis pubis can be palpated. A clamp is used to spread the subcutaneous tissue below these incisions to the level of the rectus fascia and a dry gauze sponge is packed into each incision while the vaginal portion of the operation is in progress. The urethral length is measured by inserting a urethral catheter into the bladder and inflating the balloon; the catheter balloon is placed at the internal vesical neck without traction while the urethral meatus is marked on the catheter with a haemostat. When the catheter is withdrawn, the balloon is reinflated so that the urethral length, from balloon to haemostat, can be measured.

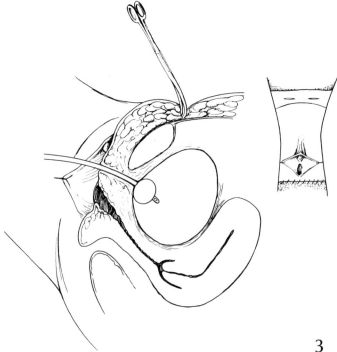

3

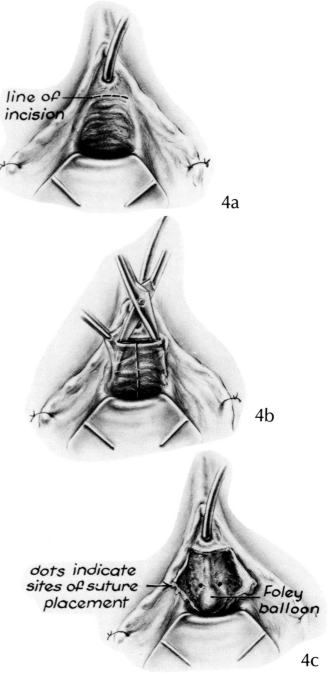

4a

4b

dots indicate
sites of suture
placement

Foley
balloon

4c

(*Reproduced from Stamey[1]*)

4a, b & c

The surgeon is now ready to start the vaginal portion of the operation. The catheter is reinserted into the bladder and the balloon inflated with 10 ml of air. The weighted posterior vaginal retractor is placed. The vaginal mucosal incision will be made underlying the urethra in the shape of a 'T'. If the urethral length is short (2.5 cm or less) the transverse portion of the 'T' incision should be started near the urethral meatus. If the urethra is longer, this incision may be made deeper in the vagina. This transverse incision may be started sharply with the scalpel in the vaginal mucosa and should be 2–2.5 cm. The anterior vaginal tissue can be separated from the urethra by gently spreading the blunt, curved scissors in the plane between these tissues. Keeping the scissor tips pointing downwards and parallel to the floor will prevent the scissors from inadvertently entering the bladder or urethra. The scissors should not be used to spread the tissues vertically alongside the vesical neck because this weakens the pubocervical fascia which forms part of the suspending support. The vertical portion of the 'T' incision (*b*) is made in the vaginal mucosa which has already been separated from the urethra. When the tip of the index finger can be placed at the bladder neck on each side of the catheter, the vaginal incision is complete (*c*).

5

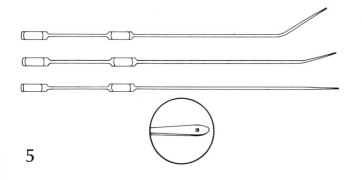

5

The Stamey long, blunt steel needles are specially designed for this procedure*. The straight needle is used in the majority of cases. A needle with the tip angled at 15° or 30° is often useful when the patient has had earlier open retropubic surgery for urinary incontinence and it is necessary to stay close to the undersurface of the pubis to avoid entry into the bladder.

* These needles are available from the Pilling Company, Delaware Drive, Fort Washington, PA 19034, USA

6a & b

After the weighted retractor is removed, both hands are used to insert the Stamey needle into the medial edge of one of the suprapubic incisions and through the rectus fascia just at the upper edge of the symphysis pubis.

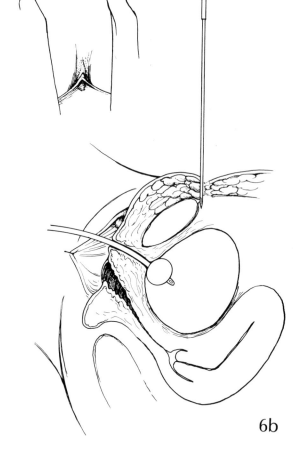

6a

6b

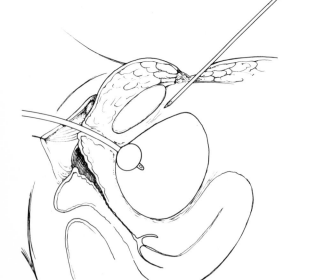

7

7

The superior edge of the symphysis can be probed with the tip of the needle to find the undersurface of the symphysis, and the needle is passed about 1–2 cm parallel to the posterior surface of the symphysis pubis. Both hands are used to guide the tip of the needle to this point in the operation.

8

The left (non-dominant) index finger is placed in the vaginal incision at the ipsilateral bladder neck, while the right (dominant) hand is used to move the needle into position onto the tip of this finger. Sometimes a vertical bouncing motion of the needle in the retropubic space (without advancing the needle) is helpful in locating the point of the needle over the left index finger. The needle is then guided alongside the vesical neck, through the endopelvic and pubocervical fascia, into the periurethral tissues adjacent to the bladder neck, as judged by the surgeon's left (nondominant) index finger which is in the vaginal incision. During this manoeuvre the urethral catheter is held without tension in the palm of the left hand so the catheter balloon can be palpated as it marks the position of the bladder neck. It is important to avoid pulling on the urethral catheter; this will telescope the urethra and cause the surgeon to misjudge the position of the vesical neck.

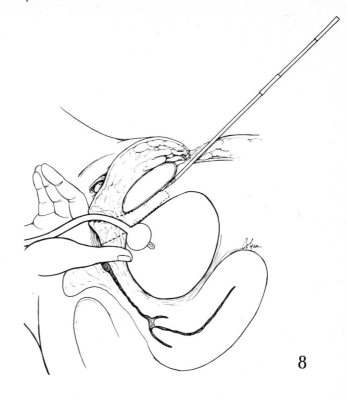

8

9

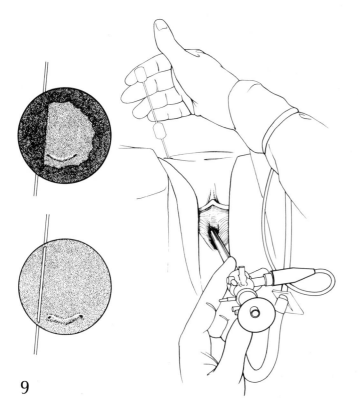

9

The right angle (70° or 110° lens) cystoscope is then inserted into the urethra to view the position of the needle in relation to the vesical neck. If the needle is in the correct position it will indent the ipsilateral vesical neck when moved slowly from right to left suprapubically. The dome and ipsilateral bladder wall are also examined to ensure that the needle did not pass through the bladder. The course of the needle outside the bladder can be determined by pushing the entire needle medially; this causes an indentation or fold inside the bladder. If the needle has been passed intramurally rather than outside the bladder muscle, the same identation or fold can be seen without pushing the needle medially; in such cases, especially when the fold is seen at volumes less than 250 ml, the needle should be removed and passed more laterally. Should the needle pass into the bladder, or if its position is incorrect, it is removed and repassed. It is important that the posterior weighted retractor is removed for this portion of the procedure so the tissues are not distorted by posterior pressure. When the surgeon is satisfied with the needle placement, a No. 2 monofilament nylon suture is threaded through the eye of the needle which protrudes into the vaginal incision. One end of the suture is pinched in a Mayo clamp and the other end follows the needle as it is withdrawn suprapubically. Once the needle is removed the suture end extending through the suprapubic incision is clamped as well. The nylon suture now has one end within the suprapubic incision and the other in the vagina.

10

A second needle pass is made 1 cm lateral to the first in the manner previously described. While this pass is being made, the nylon suture may be placed on tension to help direct the needle. The position of this needle, once passed, should be checked cystoscopically. Before the vaginal end of the nylon suture is threaded through the eye of the needle, a 1 cm length of 5 mm diameter Dacron graft is placed over the nylon to buttress the periurethral tissues from the vagina. The nylon is threaded into the eye of the needle which is withdrawn suprapubically. The periurethral tissues on one side of the urethra have now been suspended exactly at the vesical neck. The same procedure is repeated on the opposite side of the bladder neck.

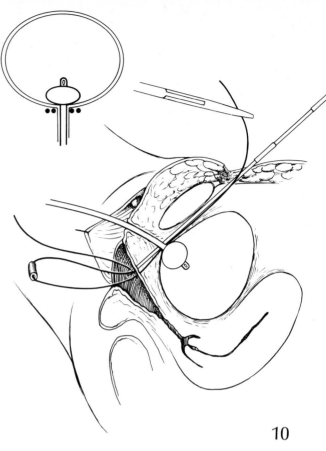

10

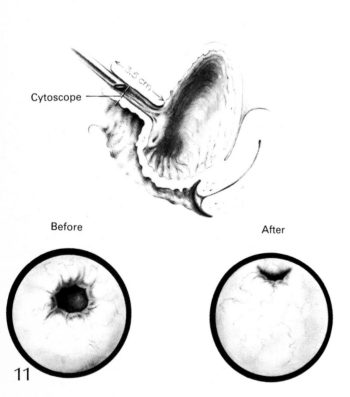

Cytoscope

Before

After

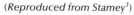

11

11

The foreoblique (30° or 150°) lens is now placed in the urethra to evaluate closure of the bladder neck when either of the nylon suspending sutures is pulled upward.

(Reproduced from Stamey[1])

12

Functional closure of the vesical neck can be observed when the cystoscope is removed and the bladder has been filled with 300–500 ml of irrigating solution. If the cystoscope is gently depressed as it is removed (to remove the suspending tension of the Dacron tubes), gross leakage of fluid from the urethral meatus will usually occur. This stream should be stopped promptly and easily with gentle upwards traction on either or both suspending nylon sutures. In the occasional difficult case with severe periurethral scarring, unusual suture placements can cause the vesical neck to close functionally when an individual suture is suspended, but paradoxically cause the vesical neck to open when *both* periurethral sutures are suspended simultaneously. In such instances, the suspending sutures must be replaced to avoid paradoxical opening of the vesical neck; or, one side can be removed and the operation concluded with a single, unilateral suspension of the vesical neck. When placement of the two sutures is satisfactory, the vaginal incision is irrigated with an aminoglycoside solution (usually 80 mg of tobramycin or gentamicin in 200–300 ml sterile water) and closed with a continuous 3/0 chromic suture. Both pieces of Dacron graft should be buried well beneath this suture line. It is important to close the vaginal incision before tying the suprapubic nylon sutures because elevation of the bladder neck and periurethral tissues which accompanies suspension makes the incision difficult to reach afterwards. A dry vaginal pack is left in position overnight.

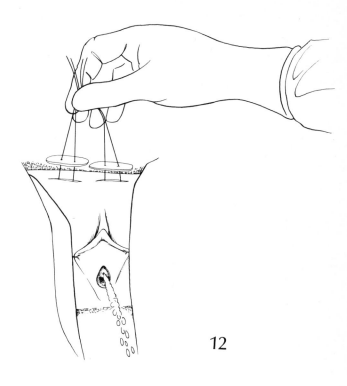

12

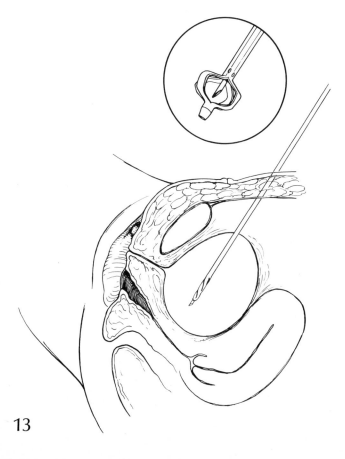

13

While the bladder is still full, a percutaneous polyethylene 14 Fr suprapubic Malecot (Stamey suprapubic catheter) or other percutaneous catheter may be placed. Position of the bladder can be confirmed by aspirating bladder fluid with a 21 gauge spinal needle. A 3–4 mm cutaneous stab incision is made 3–4 cm above the suprapubic incision. The polyethylene catheter with its obturator locked in position is then passed into the bladder with the needle entering the skin at a 30° angle above the vertical. The obturator is removed and the catheter is taped into position at the completion of the procedure. If the patient has had low abdominal surgery and there is concern of low-lying bowel, or if there is difficulty placing a catheter which drains easily, or if the patient is so obese that her pannus interferes with the suprapubic tube, a 16 Fr urethral catheter may be left in place at the end of the procedure.

13

14

Before the two suprapubic suspending sutures are tied, both suprapubic incisions are irrigated with aminoglycoside solution and the weighted vaginal retractor must be removed. The bladder is emptied with the cystoscope sheath. The two suprapubic suspending sutures are gently pulled upwards until there is no slack in the loops. Occasionally it will be necessary to press a finger onto the rectus fascia to ensure that extra slack is removed. The tension is then released and the sutures are both tied without tension so the knot lies flat on the rectus fascia. At least 5–6 throws are placed on the knot. Skin and subcutaneous tissue are closed in one layer with several interrupted vertical mattress sutures of 3/0 nylon. If the rectus fascia is shredded and weak from previous surgery or lax musculature, two flat silicone bolsters may be made and placed on the sutures so the knot is tied over the bolsters[4].

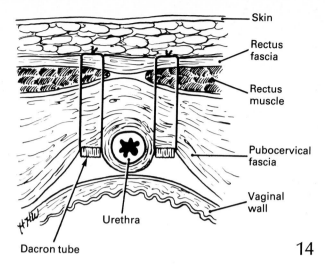

14

(Reproduced from Stamey[1])

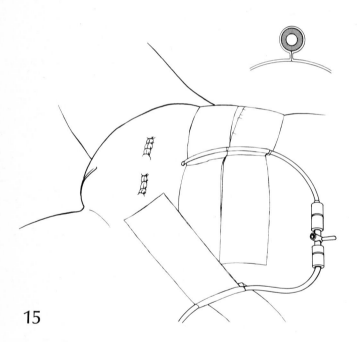

15

15

The suprapubic tube is then taped onto the abdomen using waterproof adhesive tape with benzoin placed on the catheter and abdomen prior to adhesion. It is important to make a mesentery of the tape extending from the catheter to the abdomen, so the catheter is not dislodged when the patient moves. In addition, the taping should start from the point where the tube exits from the abdomen. No gauze needs to be placed around the base of the catheter. A dry gauze dressing may be placed over the two suprapubic incisions.

Postoperative management

Parenteral aminoglycoside prophylaxis is usually continued for 24 hours after surgery. The vaginal pack is removed the morning following surgery and the patient may use a perineal pad for any further vaginal bleeding or discharge. Since most patients have minimal postoperative discomfort, they are able to start voiding trials 2 or 3 days after surgery. At that time the patient can be taught how to control the stopcock or clamp which regulates the drainage through her suprapubic catheter. For the voiding trials the stopcock is closed and the patient is told to increase her fluid intake. When she feels her bladder is very full, and she has a strong urge to urinate, she should void into a measuring pan placed beneath the toilet seat. Whether or not she is able to void, she should return to her bed and open the stopcock for 5 or 10 minutes to empty her bladder. The time, the volume of urine voided into the measuring pan, even if it is zero, and the residual volume drained through the suprapubic tube should be recorded on a chart near the patient's bedside. Usually the patient can be taught to perform these simple manoeuvres herself and to record these volumes at least 3 or 4 times a day.

When the patient is consistently able to void 75 per cent of her total bladder volume the suprapubic catheter may be removed. If she is unable to void this volume 5 or 6 days postoperatively, the patient can be discharged with the catheter in place and told to continue recording the results of her voiding trials at home. She can then be re-evaluated during outpatient visits.

If the patient has a urethral catheter left in postoperatively, she can be instructed to perform intermittent self-catheterization. Catheterizations may be stopped when residuals are 25 per cent or less of the total bladder volumes. Antimicrobial agents are not used as long as the suprapubic catheter is in place or while the patient is on intermittent catheterization. Once catheterization ceases, or the suprapubic catheter is removed, the patient is treated for several days with a broad-spectrum oral antimicrobial agent to sterilize the urine.

When the patient returns to the office after the suprapubic catheter has been removed, or intermittent catheterization has been discontinued, and all antimicrobial agents have been stopped for 2 weeks or more, the postvoid residual urine should be measured by catheterization and a portion of the specimen should be cultured. Prophylactic antimicrobial agents should then be administered for 24 hours to prevent a catheter induced infection of the bladder.

Discussion

The surgical results of this procedure have been reported earlier[1,3,4]. Using this method of elevation of the bladder neck, 91 per cent of 203 consecutive patients followed for at least 6 months (47 of those followed for more than 4 years) were cured of stress urinary incontinence. Of these 203 patients, 188 had undergone previous surgical attempts to correct stress urinary incontinence, so the majority did not have simple Grade 1 stress incontinence[4]. In fact, 41 had total urinary incontinence, holding no more than 30 ml in their bladder when standing, and 32 of these were cured by this operation[4]. The presence or absence of a uterus did not affect the success of this procedure. The median period of postoperative suprapubic drainage in these 203 patients was 7 days, although the range was from 1 to 120 days.

The complications of this operation have been few[4]. One patient had erosion of one nylon suture into the bladder 7 years after surgery. This suture was cut endoscopically and the patient has remained continent with only one intact suture. Another patient, a diabetic who was found to have a small periurethral abscess intraoperatively, developed postoperative *Staphylococcus aureus* suprapubic and vaginal wound infections which necessitated removal of the sutures and Dacron bolsters. In two patients the anterior vaginal incisions failed to heal completely, resulting in an exposed Dacron tube. In each case the exposed tube and suture were removed and the patient remained continent with the remaining suture. The occasional patient who has had persistent postoperative suprapubic pain from a nylon suture has had the offending suprapubic suture removed under local anesthetic with relief of discomfort and continuing continence with the remaining suture. Finally, there was one death from a cardiopulmonary event on the 4th postoperative day.

This method of elevating the urethrovesical neck using two permanent heavy nylon sutures bolstered by a Dacron graft has proved to be a successful means of correcting stress urinary incontinence and even total urinary incontinence in females. The use of the cystoscope to guide placement of the nylon sutures at the vesical neck ensures exact placement and the Dacron buttress greatly strengthens the suspension in a manner that cannot be accomplished in open retropubic urethropexies. This technique is less invasive and causes less postoperative discomfort than many other operations currently used to correct incontinence. It may be used in women who have undergone other procedures unsuccessfully and may be combined with abdominal or vaginal procedures being performed for other purposes with good results. Furthermore, obese women are no more difficult to operate on than thin women. Endoscopic suspension of the vesical neck is the ideal operation for the difficult surgical pelvis complicated by multiple surgery, previous trauma with pelvic fractures, or prior irradiation for carcinoma. Since it has been so successful in surgically difficult cases, it is an excellent choice for the routine case.

References

1. Stamey, T. A. Endoscopic suspension of the vesical neck for urinary incontinence. Surgery, Gynecology and Obstetrics 1973; 136: 547–554

2. Marshall, V. F., Marchetti, A. A., Krantz, K. E. The correction of stress incontinence by simple vesicourethral suspension. Surgery, Gynecology and Obstetrics 1949; 88: 509–518

3. Stamey, T. A., Schaeffer, A. J., Condy, M. Clinical and roentgenographic evaluation of endoscopic suspension of the vesical neck for urinary incontinence. Surgery, Gynecology and Obstetrics 1975; 140: 355–360

4. Stamey, T. A. Endoscopic suspension of the vesical neck for urinary incontinence in females: report on 203 consecutive patients. Annals of Surgery 1980; 192: 465–471

Illustrations by Geoff Lyth

Surgical management of urinary bilharziasis

Mahmoud M. Badr MCh, FRCS, FACS, FICS
Professor of Urology, Cairo University, Egypt

Introduction

Urinary bilharziasis (schistosomiasis) constitutes a group of diseases caused by the haematobium species of parasite which infests the venous system in man. The veins which drain the urinary organs are the most heavily affected, especially the vesicoprostatic plexuses. Pathological changes occur when the parasite (adult coupled worms) reaches the smallest venules and the female starts to lay its eggs. Only the final 'fixed pathological states' which are irreversible are of concern to surgeons. It may be useful to list the various pathological manifestations of urinary bilharziasis. These are set out as a chronological chain in the table below.

Chain of pathological manifestations of urinary bilharziasis

Structural changes

I. *Initial lesion*
    Mural mesenchymal response is granuloma formation: 'bilharzioma' (ovideposition, foreign body cellular reaction, granulomatosis, fibrosis)

II. *Subsequent lesions*
    A. Mucosal reactions
       1. Non-specific
          (a) Hyperaemia
          (b) Elevations (nodules, plateau)
       2. Specific
          (a) Atrophic lesions (sandy patches, ulcers, etc.)
          (b) Hypertrophic lesions (generalized, localized)
    B. Mesenchymal reactions
       Granulomatosis and fibrosis of:
       1. Muscular layer
       2. Adventitial layer

III. *Final states*
    A. Favourable 'healing'
    B. Development of 'fixed pathological states'
       1. Mucosal
          (a) Atrophic (chronic ulceration)
          (b) Hypertrophic (enclosures, leucoplakia, polyps)
       2. Mesenchymal (fibrotic contractures)
          (a) Localized (stricture)
          (b) Generalized (organ contracture)
    C. Complications
       1. Secondary microbial infection
       2. Back pressure effects
       3. Calculosis
       4. Fistulization
       5. Renal failure
       6. Malignant transformation

Functional changes

I. Renal insufficiency
    Relating to:
    A. Excretory functions (altered body fluid balance, uraemia and/or metabolic disorders)
    B. Endocrine functions (systemic hypertension and possibly haematopoietic changes)

II. Conductive system alterations
    A. Neuromuscular
    B. Obstructive
    C. Atonic

Operations for epithelial lesions of the bladder

CHRONIC VESICAL ULCERATIONS

Ulcers suspected clinically and confirmed by cystoscopy are of three types: superficial, deep and stellate or fissure ulcers. The main causes of their development and chronicity are submucous ovum deposition at various stages of disintegration (calcific plaque) and dense extended fibrosis.

1, 2 & 3

The logical management of these ulcers is surgical excision by partial cystectomy. The extent of tissue removal is shown. It includes the ulcer with its bordering pathological mucosa, the ulcer base with the calcific plaque and the surrounding fibrosis in the underlying muscle and adventitial layers, especially in the case of deep and stellate or fissure ulcers.

Meticulous haemostasis is essential to prevent intramural haematoma following excision. Closure of the wound should be in three layers, two mural and one inverting mucosal suture. The bladder is closed around a suprapubic tube which is kept *in situ* for 7–10 days. Endoscopic or open electrocauterization has proved ineffective because of deep fibrosis and will leave a persistent ulcer.

Associated pathological complications are common. Bladder neck obstruction is often found; it should be suspected preoperatively from the symptoms and confirmed at cystoscopy. Calculi and secondary infection are also common. Stones should be removed and the bladder neck obstruction corrected at the time of surgery. The infection can then be controlled by chemotherapy.

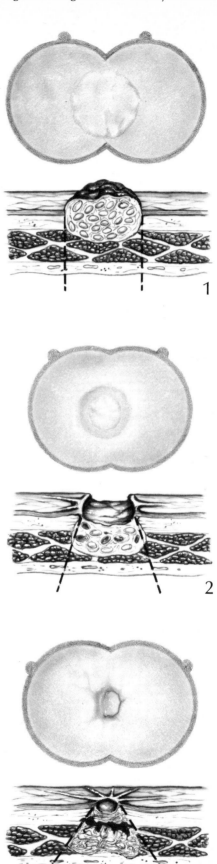

BILHARZIAL POLYP

Polyps correspond to papillomas in non-bilharzial lesions, although they are not considered neoplastic or precancerous. They are more common in active bilharziasis and may disappear under medical treatment or slough away, leading to ulceration which may heal or become chronic and require excision. In chronic bilharziasis, polyps are rare, but they may occur anywhere in the bladder.

4

The usual gross pattern and pathological state of the underlying vesical wall is shown. The neighbouring ureteric orifice may be stenosed. The logical treatment is surgical excision with correction of the associated ureteric disorder. The extent of the incision is illustrated. It should include the polyp mass with bordering pathological mucosa, the ova-stuffed submucosa and superficial muscle layer but it should not extend to partial cystectomy as the lesion is mucosal and hypertrophic rather than cancerous. Again, endoscopic treatment followed by fulguration is not effective.

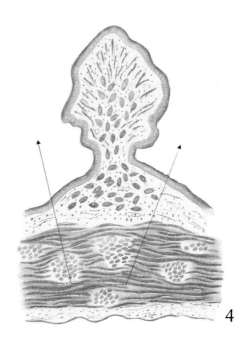

4

GROSS LEUCOPLAKIA

Leucoplakia is the most important localized mucosal lesion. These patches are considered to be precancerous. They may be flat or occasionally verrucous in form. Histological studies show a variety of lesions: squamous metaplasia, carcinoma *in situ* or infiltrating carcinoma.

Treatment consists of excision of the patches together with the submucosa and at least the superficial half of the muscle layer. The author advises full-thickness partial cystectomy.

VESICAL CARCINOMA

Vesical carcinoma is a common complication of bilharziasis. It is found 4–5 times more frequently than spontaneous carcinoma the general Egyptian population and hence constitutes a national problem.

The patient is, as a rule, relatively young (30–50 years of age) and pursuing an active, usually agricultural life. This often implies a low socioeconomic background and sometimes poor nutritional state. Late consultation and diagnosis are inevitable in these circumstances.

The bladder is totally involved in bilharziasis with multiple precancerous stigmata and intramural fibrosis. The urine is heavily infected and its outlet is invariably contracted. The tumours rarely involve the trigone. They are often multiple with largely intraluminal spread. Lymph node metastasis is late and distant metastases are rare. Squamous carcinoma based on pre-existing squamous metaplasia is the most common pathological finding in carcinoma cases.

Treatment is inevitably cystoprostatectomy and the diversion preferred is a ureterosigmoidostomy. Fortunately the upper urinary tract is usually well preserved. When hydronephrosis is present an ileal conduit must be used; occasionally, in advanced cases with uraemia, an emergency cutaneous ureterostomy is the only procedure possible. Total cystectomy and diversion can usually be performed in one stage. The cystectomy can be a simpler procedure than the radical operation described in the chapter on 'Simple and radical cystectomy' (*see* pp. 348–354) because of the low incidence of lymph node metastasis. Except in the case of vault carcinoma, this can be conducted extraperitoneally.

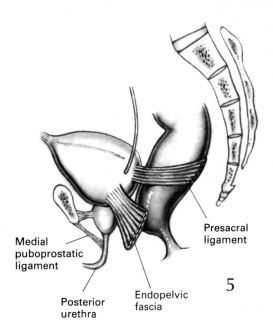

5

Cystectomy

5 & 6

The anatomical basis of the operation is shown.

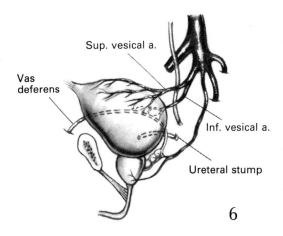

6

7–10

Author's 10-step technique

First the bladder is freed in the posterior midline. Then the posterolateral structures are sectioned in turn: the superior vesical and vesicodeferential vessels, the vas deferens and the ureters. Finally the apex of the prostate is mobilized; the presacral ligament, the inferior vesical vessels, the endopelvic fascia and the medial puboprostatic ligament are severed; and the urethra is transfixed.

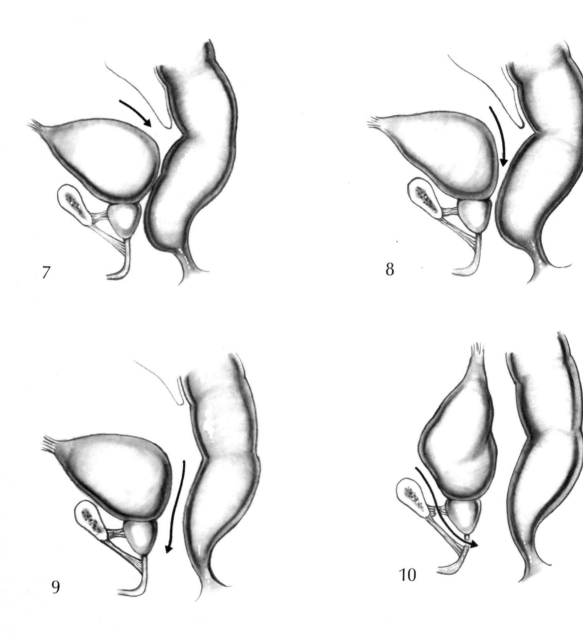

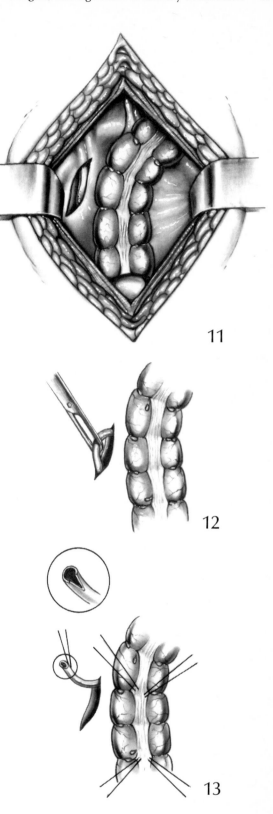

Ureterosigmoidoscopy

The technique preferred by the author is shown.

11, 12 & 13

The ureter is identified, mobilized and cut obliquely.

14, 15 & 16

An incision is made in the taenea, the submucosa freed and a small rent made in the mucosa at the distal end of the incision.

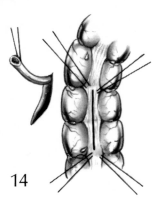

14

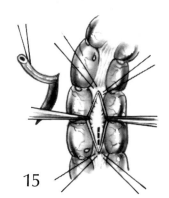

15

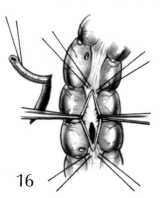

16

17, 18 & 19

Using absorbable fine chromic catgut suture, the ureter is anastomosed to the enteric mucosa-submucosa. The taenea is closed over the ureter.

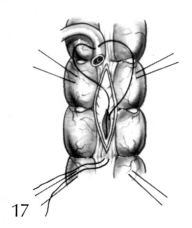

17

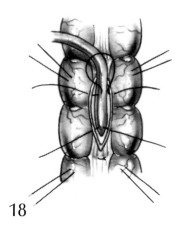

18

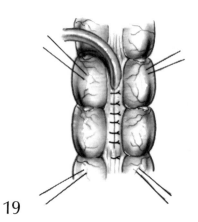

19

20, 21 & 22

The anastomosis is retroperitonealized.

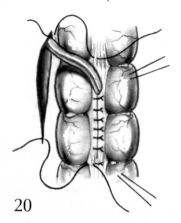

20

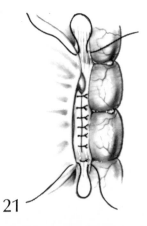

21

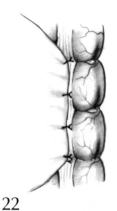

22

Operations for mesenchymal lesions

BLADDER NECK OBSTRUCTION

In bilharziasis, bladder neck obstruction results from alteration of the opening mechanism of the bladder neck at the time of micturition. This change is due to replacement of the subtrigonal plate by granulomatosis and fibrosis in response to massive ovum deposition. According to the degree and extent of the resulting fibrosis, the disease is graded by clinical, radiological, endoscopic and operative criteria into three stages.

23

Stage 1

The mucosa is congested and hypertrophic. The subtrigonal plate exhibits ovum deposition, fibroblastic reaction and granulomatosis. At this stage a stricture is in the process of forming and this has to be treated by repeated dilatation, and ironing out the posterior lip of the bladder as the dilator is withdrawn.

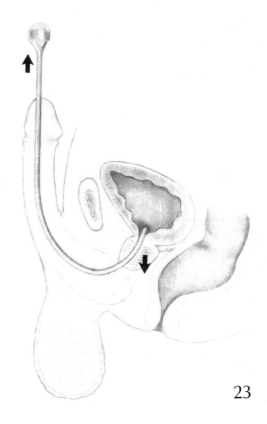

23

24

Stage 2

The mucosa is anaemic, the muscle partly atrophied with more fibrosis around disintegrating ova. At this stage there is a formed stricture with maximal posterior fibrosis, extending laterally to a variable extent. It is treated by wedge excision of the posterior lip of the vesical outlet, with or without lateral sphincterotomy, depending upon the tightness and resilience of the stricture. The operation may be done endoscopically or through an open suprapubic cystotomy if concomitant disease demands open forms of surgery. Midinterureteric bar incision or partial excision is carried out when a shortened or hypertrophied ureteric ridge causes ureteric orifices to be approximated with ureteral angulation.

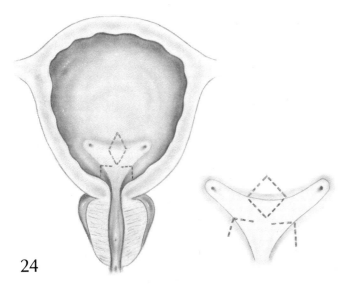

24

25

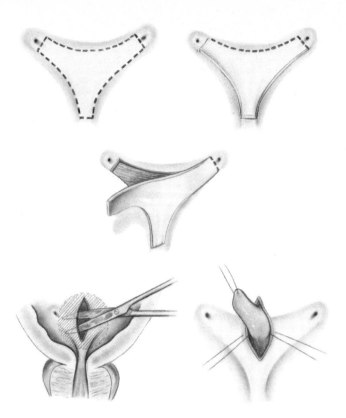

Stage 3

The mucosa is atrophic and partially shed, the muscle is replaced by fibrous tissue and the trigonal plate replaced by a calcified plaque. This formed stricture and trigonal atrophy is treated by trigonectomy, i.e. excision of the inactive fibrosed trigone and underlying subtrigonal plate. In the occasional case where the trigone is intact, subtrigonal plate excision is indicated, preserving the superficial layer. The principle of the latter operation, introduced by the author, is to obviate the hazards of the trigonectomy, i.e. retrograde ejaculation with attendant sterility.

CONTRACTED BLADDER

On rare occasions there is an exaggerated reactive fibrosis to ovum deposition resulting in a contracted bladder. This condition is characterized by marked reduction in capacity, sometimes as low at 50 ml or less, leading to intractable frequency and nocturia – not unlike the late stages of tuberculous cystitis. The pathological changes involve well marked perivesical fibrolipomatosis, fibrous replacement of the detrusor muscle, mucosal atrophy and ulceration and bladder neck obstruction. The lower ureter, however, is often spared and the upper urinary tract is therefore often preserved.

The logical treatment is surgical and involves some form of cystoplasty. Most of the known procedures described in the chapter on 'Cystoplasty' (see pp. 335–344) have been applied to bilharzial cases but certain peculiarities must be noted. In selecting a case for surgery the possibility of fibrotic hepatolienal or pulmonary lesions must be assessed, since they will lead to a poor general outlook. The technique of the operation involves a decortication, removing the surrounding fibrolipomatous tissue. The anastomotic stoma between the bladder vault and the intestine must be as wide as possible. It should be intraperitoneal and sutured with three separate layers. The correction of associated bladder neck obstruction is essential. In advanced cases with bilateral ureteric stricture, urinary diversion by ureterosigmoidostomy or ileal conduit is indicated.

STRICTURES OF THE URETER

26

Strictures of the ureter are common in urinary bilharziasis, second only to vesical lesions and often found in association with them. In accordance with the general rule governing the distribution and intensity of the bilharzial lesions (i.e. development in the rich venous plexus) ureteric strictures develop at two main sites. These are, in order of frequency: the lower pelvic ureter, either juxtavesical or intramural; and the lumbar ureter affecting the junction between the upper and middle third. These strictures occur more often on the left side where there is a venous pool formed by ureteric, testicular, mesenteric and retroperitoneal veins.

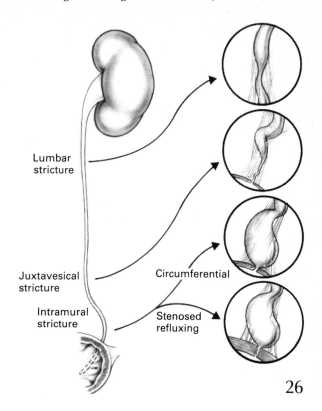

26

The usual indications for surgery are the onset of secondary bacterial infection, urinary calculi and back pressure with progressive deterioration of renal function. However, earlier cases may well be recognized from dilatation of the ureter with good preservation of renal function, and there may be associated bilharzial lesions requiring surgical intervention.

The operations to be performed are similar to those applied to non-bilharzial cases. Occasionally in short, localized lumbar strictures a meticulous ureterolysis will suffice. This can be supplemented by a simple plastic procedure on the wall of the ureter, but more often the stenosed segment must be excised and continuity restored. In the lumbar region this can be done by spatulation of the ends and direct anastomosis. At the lower end reimplantation of the ureter will be required.

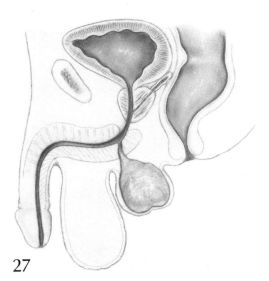

27

EXTERNAL FISTULAE IN RELATION TO THE URETHRA

27

The pathological process starts as periurethral cellulitis around bilharzial granulations developing in the roof of the bulbous urethra. Unless vigorously treated with both antibilharzial and antimicrobial therapy the cellulitis progresses to the formation of abscess which may be incised surgically or rupture spontaneously. At this stage medical treatment may well lead to closure of the wound. More often, however, a fistulating mass develops – the result of chronic urinary extravasation from the breach in the urethral wall into capacious perineal cavities which are secondarily infected. The mass is fibrolipomatous, surrounding a bizarrely branching and partly epithelialized track. The urethra is usually strictured and surgical correction aims chiefly at removing the fistulous mass.

28

The plan of treatment should include incision of the abscesses, medical treatment of the bilharzia and secondary infection, suprapubic cystotomy and fistulectomy. The mass is removed through a wide perineal exposure in order to ensure complete excision of the mass without retraction but with preservation of the perineal vessels, nerves and muscles.

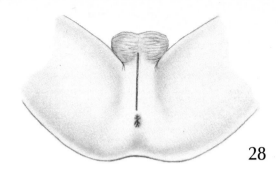

28

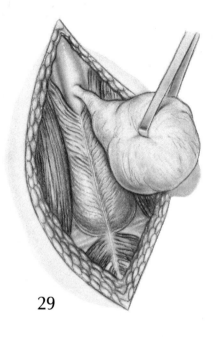

29

29

The mass is usually flask-shaped, tapering towards its point of origin in the urethra.

30

The urethra is usually preserved. A catheter is introduced up to but not through the internal urinary meatus and kept in place for 5 days so that urine will not trickle alongside the catheter and contaminate the wound. The perineal wound is closed in two fascial layers and the skin closed around two drainage tubes which remain in place for 3–5 days. A few urethral dilatations are advised after removal of the catheter to prevent postoperative stricture.

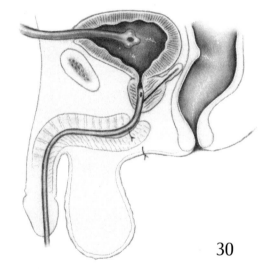

30

Further reading

Badr, M., Zaher, F. Ileocystoplasty in the treatment of bilharzial contracted bladder. Journal of the Egyptian Medical Association 1959; 42: 33–47

Badr, M., Zaher, M., Fawzy, R. Further experience with bilharzial bladder-neck obstruction. Journal of the Egyptian Medical Association 1958; 41: 624

Dimmette, R. M., Sayegh, E. S., Sproat, H. F. Chronic ulcers of the bladder, associated with schistosomiasis. Surgery, Gynecology and Obstetrics 1955; 101: 721–731

Ibrahim, A. Bilharziasus of the ureter. Lancet 1923; 2: 1183

Sayegh, E. S. Late complications of urinary bilharziasis. Journal of Urology 1950; 63: 353–371

Smith, J. H., Kelada, A. S., Khalil, A. Schistosomal ulceration of the urinary bladder. American Journal of Tropical Medicine and Hygiene 1977; 26: 89–95

Orchidectomy

J. E. A. Wickham   MS, BSc, FRCS
Director of the Academic Unit, Institute of Urology, University of London;
Senior Consultant Urological Surgeon, St Bartholomew's Hospital, London;
Consultant Surgeon, St Peter's Hospital Group, London, UK

Preoperative

UNILATERAL ORCHIDECTOMY

Indications

Orchidectomy, or the removal of one testicle, is performed for unilateral testicular disease. The indications for operation are as follows.

1. In testicular maldescent, when orchidopexy is not possible owing to lack of cord length or where a maldeveloped testicular remnant is not worthy of salvage.
2. For trauma in crush injuries when complete testicular disruption may necessitate the removal of the non-viable organ.
3. For torsion. Where failure to relieve torsion has resulted in total testicular infarction, it may be necessary to remove the destroyed organ.
4. For infection. On rare occasions in uncontrolled acute pyogenic or tuberculous infection, testicular destruction with scrotal ulceration may occur and orchidectomy is required to secure healing.
5. For malignant disease. A tumour arising in the body of the testis is by far the most common indication for orchidectomy.
6. In conjunction with hernial repair. In fat elderly men, with large inguinal hernias, it may occasionally be necessary to perform orchidectomy in order to secure a sound repair by obliteration of the inguinal canal.

Preoperative preparation

In all cases of orchidectomy the patient should be reassured that the removal of one testicle will in no way affect potency or fertility.

In cases of malignant disease of the testicle, a preoperative chest X-ray should be performed.

BILATERAL ORCHIDECTOMY – CASTRATION BY THE SUBCAPSULAR METHOD

Indications

Bilateral orchidectomy is indicated for the endocrine control of prostatic malignant disease. This treatment is based upon the demonstration that the activity of the prostatic malignant process is subject to the hormonal influence of the testicular androgens. Elimination of the latter by castration or its suppression by oestrogen therapy provides a simple method for the control of the malignant disease. The psychological effect of castration may be considerable but this can be mitigated to some extent by the performance of a subcapsular as opposed to a bilateral radical orchidectomy for, by the performance of subcapsular orchidectomy, some semblance of the original organ may be maintained.

Anaesthesia

A general anaesthetic should be administered.

Position of patient

The patient should be lying on his back with his legs slightly abducted.

The operations

SIMPLE ORCHIDECTOMY

When removing the testicle it is customary to tie the spermatic cord at the level of the internal inguinal ring.

1

The incision

The skin incision, which is made 1.25 cm above and parallel to the inguinal ligament, is 5 cm long and extends from just above the pubic tubercle to the mid-inguinal point. Fat, superficial and deep fascia are divided in this line to expose the aponeurosis of the external oblique muscle and the external inguinal ring.

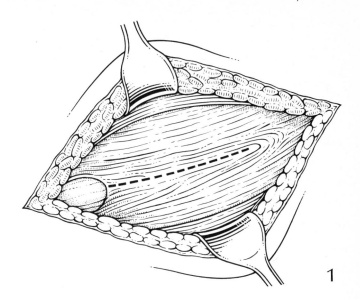

2

Exposure of spermatic cord

The aponeurosis is now divided in the line of its fibres from the apex of the external ring to the level of the internal ring, exposing the underlying spermatic cord; the cord is then mobilized.

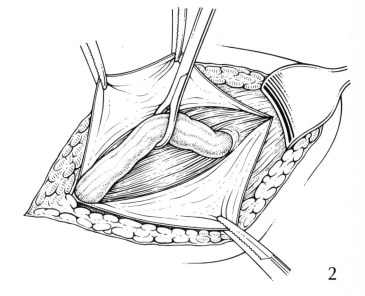

3

Ligation of cord

At the internal ring the testicular veins join to form two or three well defined vessels. These are identified, dissected free and ligated flush with the muscles at the internal ring. The vas is next identified, clamped and divided, and finally the remaining portion of the cord containing the testicular artery and the artery of the vas is ligated and divided. It is considered important to proceed in this order when dealing with malignant disease of the testicle in order to minimize venous embolization of malignant cells prior to manipulation of the tumour.

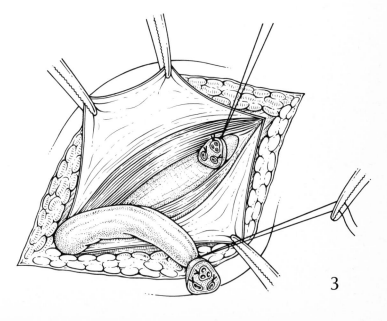

4

Delivery of testis

The distal portion of the cord is now mobilized from its bed and gentle traction is exerted to deliver the testis from the scrotum into the lower margin of the wound. Attachments of the external spermatic fascia and the cremaster muscle to the scrotal wall and surrounding tissues are gently separated by blunt dissection until the gubernacular attachment of the lower pole of the testis to the scrotal wall is reached. This fibrous attachment is then divided between haemostats and the testis removed.

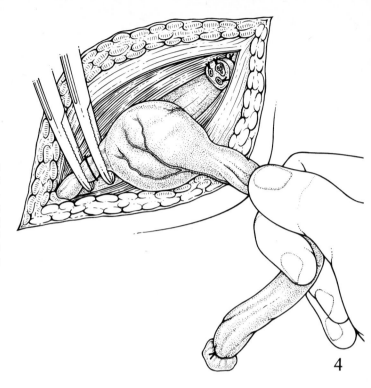

4

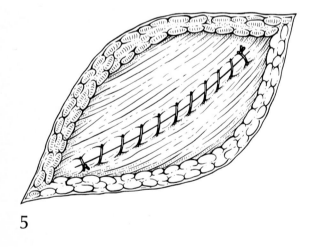

5

5

Closure

After careful haemostasis the external oblique aponeurosis is reapproximated with a continuous 1/0 chromic catgut suture, obliterating the external inguinal ring. A few interrupted 3/0 catgut sutures may be used to reunite the superficial fascia in the obese patient. Skin closure is then effected with interrupted 3/0 silk sutures. Drainage of the wound is not necessary.

Postoperative care

On rare occasions a small haematoma may form in the scrotal cavity but this should be avoided by careful haemostasis. At the conclusion of the operation the empty scrotal sac may be compressed against the thigh by a firmly applied length of 3 inch Elastoplast strapping.

SUBCAPSULAR ORCHIDECTOMY

6

The incision

The scrotum is elevated and a longitudinal incision is made through the stretched skin and dartos muscle to expose both testes.

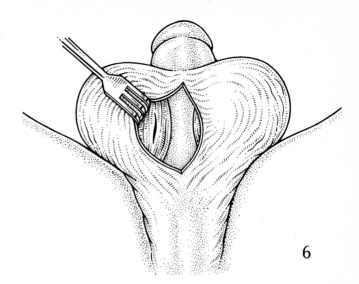

7

Evagination of testes

Each testis is evaginated from the scrotum together with its coverings. The tunica vaginalis is incised vertically and the testicle and epididymis exposed.

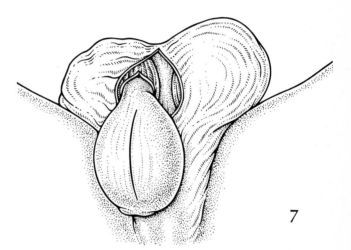

8

Incision of tunica albuginea

The visceral tunica is incised vertically over the globe of the testis.

9

Removal of testicular substance

The testicular tissue is separated from the inner surface of the tunica albuginea by blunt and sharp dissection. Careful haemostasis is required in the region of the rete testis at the upper pole.

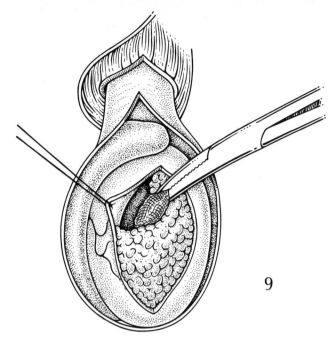

9

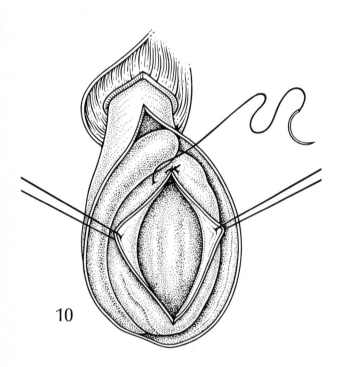

10

10

Closure of tunica

When all visible testicular tissue has been removed the tunica is closed with a continuous 3/0 plain catgut suture and the testicle is replaced in its scrotal coverings.

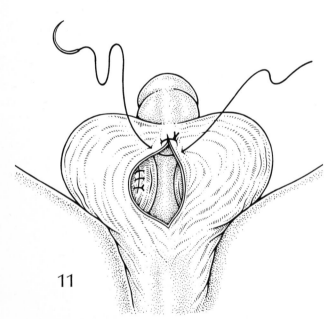

11

11

Closure of scrotum

The scrotum is closed in two layers with a continuous vertical 3/0 chromic catgut suture to the dartos layer and interrupted 3/0 nylon or Dexon sutures to the transverse skin incision. There is no need to drain the scrotum.

Note: After a few weeks the residual cavity in the tunica albuginea, which becomes filled with blood clot, organizes to form a palpable nodule similar in size to a small testis.

Testicular prostheses

Should a better simulation of the testicular body be required it is possible to insert a Silastic prosthesis into the tunica albuginea at the time of operation. These prostheses are commercially available from the Dow Corning Co.

Illustrations by Robert N. Lane

Epididymectomy

J. E. A. Wickham MS, FRCS
Director of the Academic Unit, Institute of Urology, University of London;
Senior Consultant Urological Surgeon, St Bartholomew's Hospital, London;
Consultant Surgeon, St Peter's Hospital Group, London, UK

Preoperative

Indications

There are only two principal indications for this operation which is rarely performed:

1. For degenerative cystic disease of the epididymis, where the caput epididymis may be replaced by numerous small, tense and occasionaly painful cysts.
2. For the removal of a fungating tuberculous infection of the epididymis. This is now a rare occurrence and most tuberculous disease of the epididymis, even if ulcerated, will heal on antituberculous therapy.

Preoperative preparation

It is important that these patients should be warned before operation that complete orchidectomy may perhaps be necessary at exploration.

Anaesthesia

A general anaesthetic should be given.

Position of patient

The patient should be placed lying on the back with the legs slightly abducted.

The operation

1

The incision

If a sinus or ulcer is present in the skin of the scrotum the incision is planned to encircle the involved area, leaving a clear margin of normal skin. If the skin is uninvolved a posterior incision should be made with the scrotum elevated. If tuberculous disease involves the whole of the spermatic cord it is desirable to remove this up to the level of the internal inguinal ring and a second inguinal incision is required for this. If disease is localized to the epididymis a scrotal incision will suffice.

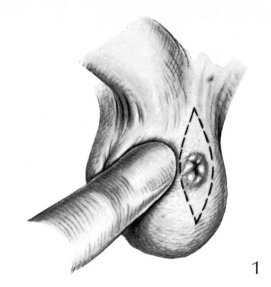

1

2

Opening the tunica vaginalis

The skin around any sinus is mobilized and the testicle is delivered from the scrotum with its coverings. The tunica vaginalis is opened and the testicle and epididymis exposed.

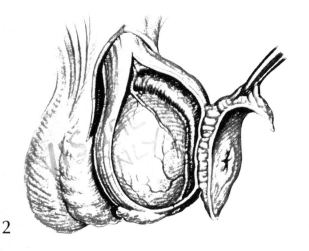

2

3

Excision of epididymis

With sharp dissection in the cleft between the epididymis and the body of the testicle the whole epididymis is mobilized from the inferior testicular pole upwards. At the upper pole of the testicle the vasa efferentia are divided and at the apex of the epididymis a small branch of the testicular artery should be identified and ligated. Care should be taken to avoid the main branch of the artery supplying the testis. The diseased epididymis may now be removed.

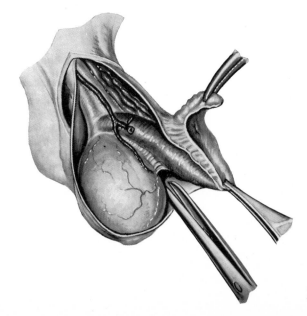

3

4

Removal of diseased cord

If tuberculous disease extends into the cord, an inguinal incision should be made as for orchidectomy and the cord exposed. The cord is divided at the internal ring and the distal portion mobilized down into the scrotum. With slight traction on the separated epididymis and vas the whole of the vas and cord may be pulled down from the scrotal incision.

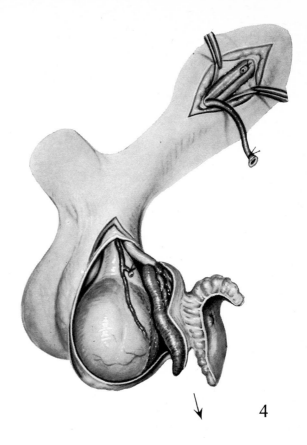

4

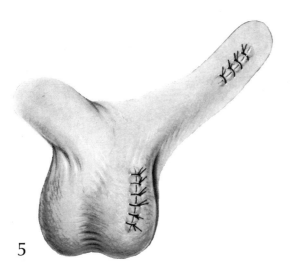

5

5

Replacement of testis

The testis is replaced in the scrotum without suturing the tunica vaginalis, and the scrotal skin is closed with one layer of interrupted 3/0 chromic catgut sutures to the dartos layer, and interrupted 3/0 silk sutures to the scrotal skin. No drainage is required. If an inguinal incision has been necessary it is closed in the manner described for orchidectomy.

Illustrations by Philip Wilson

Operation for testicular torsion

J. E. A. Wickham MS, BSc, FRCS
Director of the Academic Unit, Institute of Urology, University of London;
Senior Consultant Urological Surgeon, St Bartholomew's Hospital, London;
Consultant Surgeon, St Peter's Hospital Group, London, UK

Introduction

Torsion of the testis or its appendages most commonly occurs in the child or young adolescent. Previous attacks of scrotal pain may have occurred. The definitive attack occurs suddenly, frequently following physical exertion such as riding a bicycle. The scrotum becomes rapidly swollen and exquisitely painful, particularly on palpation, so that it is normally impossible to define the various parts of the scrotal contents with any certainty.

Torsion must be differentiated from the following.

Acute epididymo-orchitis. This develops much less acutely than a torsion. The scrotum, although swollen, is usually reddened and it may be possible to distinguish a normal body of testis from a swollen and tender epididymis. There may also be a history of urinary tract or urethral infection.

Mumps Orchitis. This may simulate a torsion very closely, although the onset of symptoms is usually less acute.

Testicular tumour. Also gives rise to a tender scrotal mass, but again the length of history will normally distinguish a tumour from a torsion.

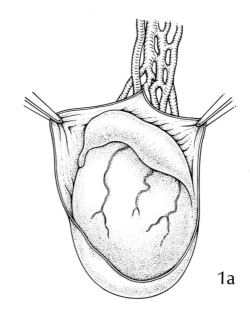

1a

1a & b

Torsion occurs because an abnormal unobliterated prolongation of the tunica vaginalis completely invests the
epididymis and distal spermatic cord. (a) shows the
normal anatomy and (b) shows abnormal anatomy with
torsion potential. In (b) the testis is in effect suspended in
the scrotum from a stalk and is free to rotate within the
tunica vaginalis. Rotation of the testis twists the spermatic
cord, obstructs the contained blood vessels and produces
testicular ischaemia with ultimate necrosis.

Torsion is one of the few urological emergencies. There
is no place for manipulative management and the
treatment is urgent surgical exploration which must be
undertaken within 3–4 hours if the testicle is to be saved
from ischaemic necrosis.

Preoperative preparation

A Ryle's tube should be passed to empty the stomach
before anaesthesia. A general anaesthetic should be used,
and the patient should be placed supine on the operating
table.

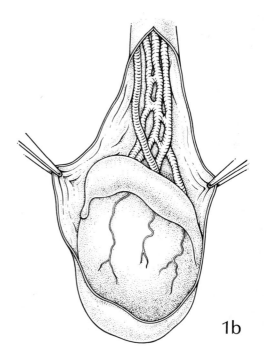

1b

The operation

The testicle is delivered from the scrotum by an anterolateral incision. The skin, dartos fascia and tunica vaginalis are all incised in this line.

2

The testicle, frequently surrounded by a secondary hydrocele containing serosanguinous fluid, is delivered gently from the tunica. The epididymis is usually distended and haemorrhagic and the globe of the testis is swollen and cyanotic. The torsion is visualized as the cord comes into view when the direction of twist is usually quite obvious. This is untwisted until the cord lies normally.

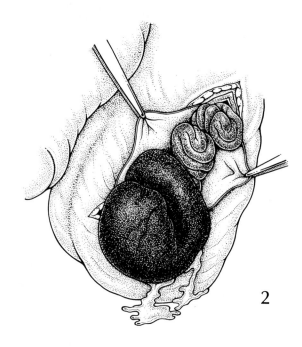

2

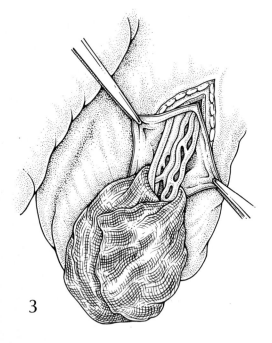

3

3

Conservation or removal of the testicle

The untwisted testicle is wrapped in moist warm swabs for 5–10 minutes and its colour carefully observed. If vascular perfusion has been re-established, with a return to normal, or near normal, colour, the testis is conserved. If the testis is obviously black and necrotic, or the circulation is not re-established on untwisting, then the testicle should be removed. It is better to err on the side of conservation if in doubt. A torted testicle may partially recover and, although small, may function hormonally if not spermatogenically.

4

Removal of the testicle

The cord should be divided between clamps and ligated with a transfixion ligating stitch of 2/0 chromic catgut.

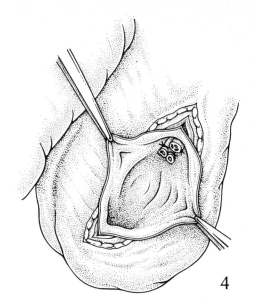

4

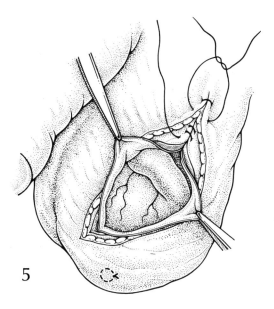

5

5

Replacement of the testicle

If the testicle is replaced, a small 'tack' suture of 2/0 catgut should be used to attach the lower pole of the testis to the inside of the scrotal cavity to prevent recurrence. The wound is closed with continuous 3/0 chromic catgut suture to the tunica vaginalis and dartos layer, and interrupted sutures of 3/0 chromic catgut or Dexon to the skin.

Fixation of contralateral testicle

The abnormal condition of the tunica vaginalis giving rise to torsion usually occurs bilaterally. Therefore, when the twisted testicle has been dealt with, the contralateral testis should be explored and similarly secured in the scrotum with a 'tack' suture of 2/0 chromic catgut passed between the lower pole of the testis and the tunica vaginalis. This manoeuvre is even more strongly indicated if orchidectomy has been performed for the torsion.

Illustrations by Barbara Hyams

Hydrocele, spermatocele and orchiopexy

Peter H. Lord, MChir, FRCS
Consultant Surgeon, Wycombe General Hospital, High Wycombe, Buckinghamshire, UK

Introduction

The clinical differentiation between hydrocele and spermatocele can be difficult and even after care and thought a mistake can be made. Fortunately, even when an incorrect diagnosis is made, the appropriate procedure of the two to be described can be selected without difficulty once the operation has begun.

The operations

HYDROCELE

The operation for hydrocele described in this chapter consists of plication of the tunica vaginalis in order to obliterate the hydrocele space. The testis is returned to the scrotum without its tunica vaginalis covering. The procedure differs from many others in that the hydrocele is not delivered out of the scrotum. If the surgeon begins an operation for hydrocele by making an incision and delivering the complete hydrocele out of the scrotum there is inevitably bleeding from the scrotal areolar tissue which has to be dissected off the hydrocele. The blood vessels retract into the areolar tissue and it is difficult to avoid a haematoma. Occasionally this results in a large haematoma, giving rise to appreciable morbidity. The plication procedure, however, is an almost bloodless one.

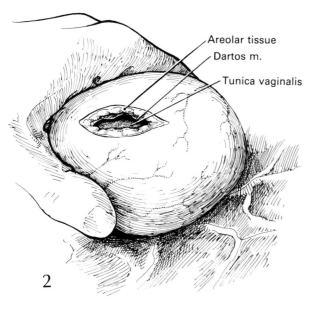

1

After the usual skin preparation and towelling, the surgeon (if right-handed) stands on the patient's right and grasps the hydrocele in the left hand in such a way as to stretch the skin, particularly at the point where the incision is to be made. The 4 cm incision should be made on the far side of the hydrocele from the testis.

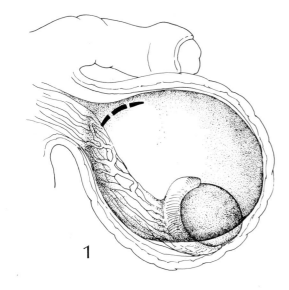

Areolar tissue
Dartos m.
Tunica vaginalis

2

Maintaining the skin on tension, the incision is made through the skin, areolar tissue and dartos muscle down as far as but without opening the tunica vaginalis. As the incision deepens, the knife can be replaced by blunt scissors to avoid premature opening of the hydrocele.

3a, b & c

If the tension on the skin has been well maintained by the left hand there should be minimal oozing from the cut edges and further bleeding is prevented by applying Allis forceps in the manner shown. Each Allis forceps is applied by slipping one blade under the cut edge, picking up all the divided tissue, closing the forceps and turning it over. Three Allis forceps on each side should control bleeding completely.

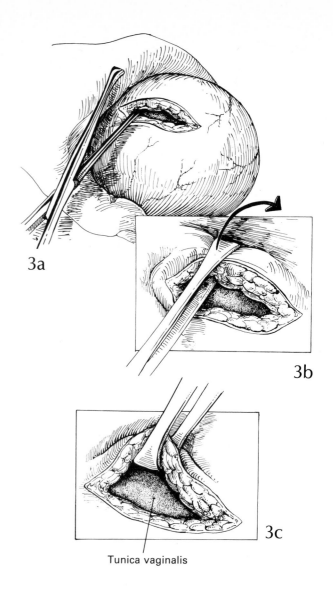

3a

3b

3c

Tunica vaginalis

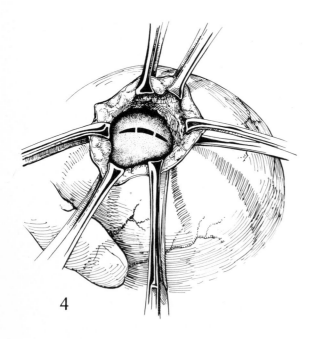

4

4

With the forceps in place, the tension on the skin from the left hand can now be released.

Cut edge of tunica vaginalis

Sucker

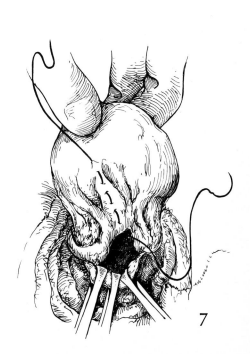

5

5

The tunica vaginalis is incised and the fluid in the hydrocele drawn off with the sucker.

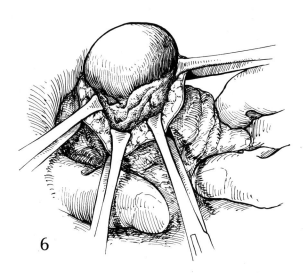

6

6

The testis is now raised clear of the scrotum. As it is lifted up, the tunica vaginalis is turned inside out, to hang down like a curtain from the testis to the cut edge of the scrotum.

7

This curtain of modified peritoneum must now be gathered by plication suture so that it forms a narrow ruff around the mediastinum testis thus obliterating the cavity occupied by the hydrocele. This is done by picking up the cut edge of the tunica vaginalis and, taking small bites at 1 cm intervals, forming a gathering stitch to run from the cut edge towards the testis.

7

8

This stitching is repeated at intervals all round the tunica, requiring eight to ten sutures in all. Each suture is tied as it is inserted.

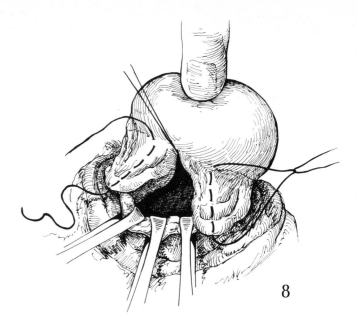

8

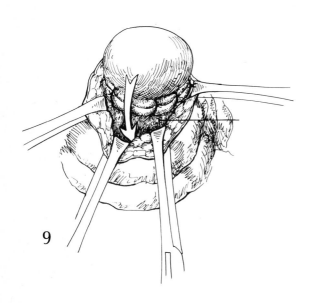

9

9

The tunica vaginalis and hydrocele having been obliterated, the testis is then returned to the scrotum. As there is no actual cavity within the scrotum waiting to receive it, the testis has to be eased back gently. The areolar tissue of the scrotum has to stretch to accommodate the testis, which it does without tearing and, therefore, without risk of haematoma formation.

10

A Lane's tissue forceps is applied to each end of the incision, which can then be put on the stretch, and full-thickness interrupted Dexon sutures are inserted, thus maintaining the haemostatic function of the Allis forceps which are removed in pairs as the stitches are placed.

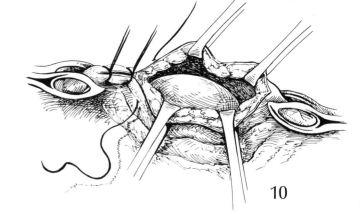

10

SPERMATOCELE

11

The operation for spermatocele should also be bloodless. A spermatocele or epididymal cyst starts as a tiny swelling in the head of the epididymis. Gradually it enlarges, bringing its own blood supply from the epididymal head, and pushes aside the areolar tissue of the scrotum to make a space for itself. Unless there is an infection or the cyst has been aspirated with a needle, there is no reason why scrotal blood vessels should enter the wall of this simple benign cyst. It follows, therefore, that there must be a completely bloodless plane between the cyst and the surrounding areolar tissue. The object of this operation is to use this plane to remove the cyst without risk of scrotal haematoma.

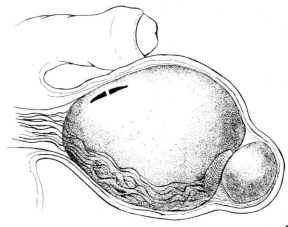

11

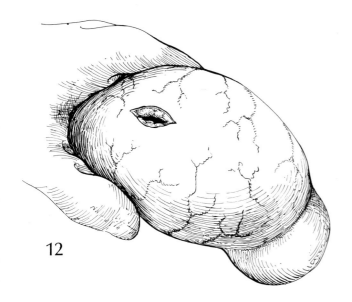

12

12

The surgeon stands to the right of the patient and takes the cyst in the left hand, placing the skin on tension. The incision can be quite small (say 2 cm) and is made over the cyst as far removed as possible from the testis.

13

Allis forceps are applied to each side of the incision and turned over to secure haemastosis of the scrotal coverings. Using curved artery forceps for blunt dissection, the areolar tissue is pushed aside until the bluish appearance of the wall of the cyst is visible. The cyst wall is grasped and some of the contained fluid allowed to escape.

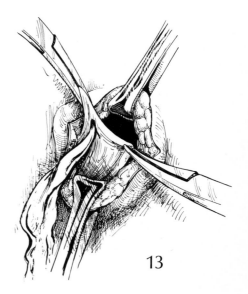

13

14

Gentle traction on the cyst wall should allow it to come through the scrotal incision and the plane of cleavage between it and the areolar tissue should be found easily. About ⅔ of the cyst fluid is allowed to escape, after which a Duval forceps is applied to the hole in the cyst wall so as to retain the remaining fluid as a guide to identifying the cyst during the rest of dissection.

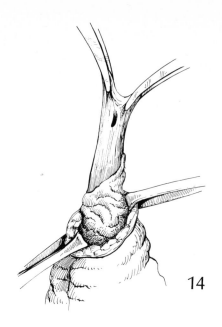

14

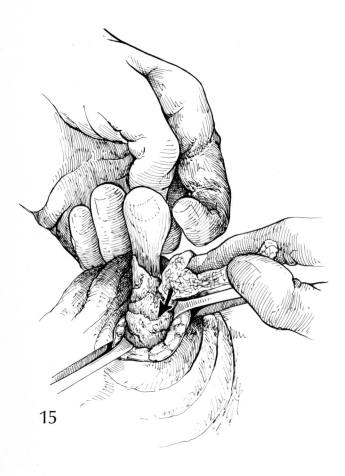

15

15

As the cyst is gently teased out of the scrotum the areolar tissue can be stripped off it by wiping with a swab.

16

Alternatively, fine-toothed forceps can be used to pick away the areolar tissue until the whole cyst is exteriorized and the head of the epididymis from which it arises is pulled out into the wound.

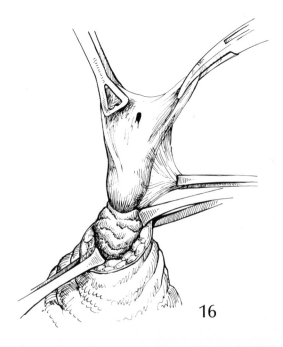

16

17

The small blood vessels which arise from the head of the epididymis and run over the wall of the cyst must be controlled either by diathermy or by ligation with 3/0 Dexon.

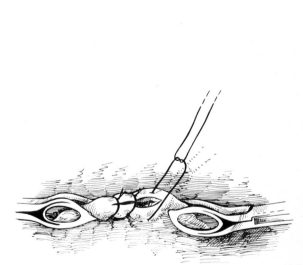

17

18

Now the cyst can be separated from the head of the epididymis. Often smaller cysts are also present and these should be dealt with in a similar way.

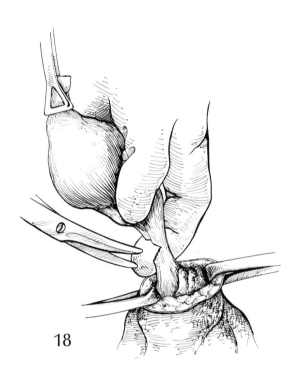

18

19

Lane's tissue forceps are applied to each end of the short scrotal incision, which is closed with interrupted Dexon suture.

Postoperative care

Postoperative care after either hydrorelectomy or spermatorelectomy includes a dry dressing applied to the wound and the scrotum supported in a suspensory bandage. The patient is allowed to shower after 24 hours and either the Dexon sutures can be left to hydrolyse or they can be removed, whichever is more convenient. Both procedures are suitable for day-case management.

19

ORCHIOPEXY

The indications for orchiopexy are still controversial. At one extreme are surgeons who recommend that any testicle not in the scrotum should be brought down by 2 years of age. At the other extreme are surgeons who believe that the majority of undescended testes will descend spontaneously and that few of those which fail to descend are worth saving.

If the testes are in the scrotum at birth, although they may retract and not be seen again for many years, they will return to the scrotum by puberty. Surgical intervention is not indicated. Likewise, the testis that can be pushed into the scrotum in a small boy will almost certainly descend spontaneously as he matures.

Whereas unilateral maldescent is not a desperate problem (since there is presumably a normal testicle on the other side), bilateral cryptorchidism causes considerable anxiety to surgeon and the child's parents alike. Most surgeons believe that at least one testis should be brought down to the scrotum before the age of 5 years. It may be that testes which come down easily and stay down satisfactorily are those which would have descended spontaneously.

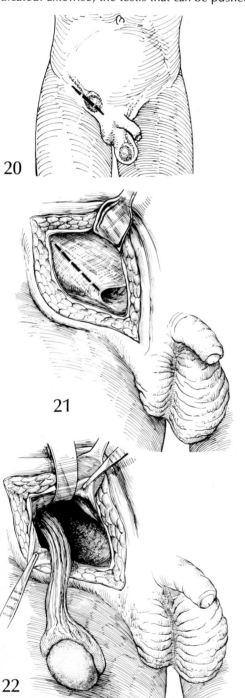

20

In true cryptorchidism the testis lies within the inguinal canal or more cephalad. The majority of patients undergoing surgery have a testis which lies in the superficial inguinal pouch or superficial to the external oblique muscle (ectopic testis).

21

The operation requires a generous inguinal incision for good access, and the external oblique should be split along the direction of its fibres, starting at the external ring.

22

The testis, its coverings and the cord should be dissected free from all attachments with the aim of getting as much length of cord as possible to allow the testis to come down into the scrotum. It is not normally necessary to divide the inferior epigastric vessels, which lie just medial to the internal ring, though it is alleged that this gives more length.

23

A finger pushed down inside the somewhat underdeveloped scrotum helps to create space for the testis, but it sometimes proves difficult to guide it to the bottom of the scrotum. To facilitate its passage, a Killian's nasal speculum is passed into the scrotum and opened. A blunt silver probe is passed down between the blades of the speculum and pushed through the scrotal skin. The probe carries a monofilament nylon suture which penetrates the loose coverings of the testis, avoiding damage to the body itself. The suture pulls the testis into the scrotum, although care must be taken to avoid any twisting of the cord.

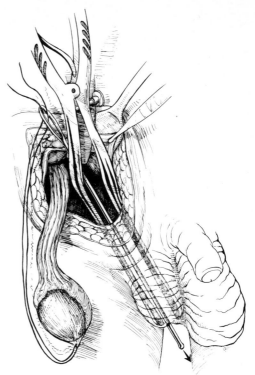

23

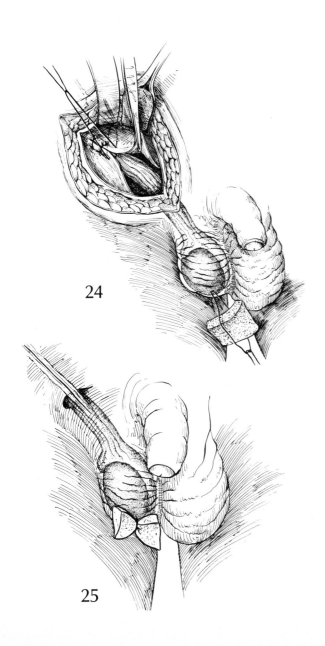

24

24 & 25

The external oblique is closed with interrupted Dexon sutures and the skin incision is closed in the usual manner.

There are three methods of fixing the testicle to remain in the scrotum. The simplest is to tie the nylon suture used to pull down the testicle over a pad of sterile plastic foam or a sterile cotton dental roll.

25

26

Alternatively, the suture can also be tied is such a way as to include a rubber band which is attached under tension to the opposite thigh (just above the knee). If this method is used, the child tends to stand and sit with the opposite thigh flexed at the hip, but during sleep the rubber band tightens, helping to pull down the testis.

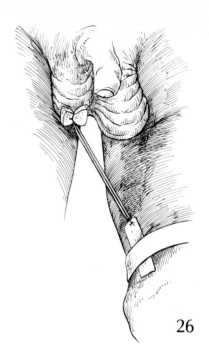

26

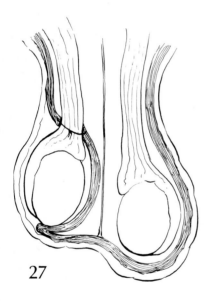

27

27

A third way of fixing the testis in the scrotum is to create a pocket between the scrotal skin and the dartos muscle. The scrotal skin is incised, the space between skin and dartos opened up with scissors and the testis pulled through the dartos into the pocket. The scrotal skin is then closed with interrupted Dexon sutures.

Postoperative care

Where there is an external suture over a pad the suture is removed on the 11th postoperative day.

Illustrations by Ronald J. Ervin

Vasectomy

David C. Saypol MD
Resident, Department of Urology,
University of Virginia School of Medicine, Charlottesville, Virginia, USA

Stuart S. Howards MD
Professor of Urology and Associate Professor of Physiology,
University of Virginia School of Medicine, Charlottesville, Virginia, USA

Preoperative

Indications

Vasectomy is the most common method of permanent male sterilization with a success rate of nearly 100 per cent. In conjunction with transurethral resection of the prostate, vasectomy will reduce the incidence of postoperative epididymiditis by about 60 per cent. In rare cases it is indicated as a treatment for recurrent epididymiditis.

The individual who requests a vasectomy should be psychologically stable and have complete understanding of the potential risks and complications described below. Decisions regarding such a procedure in a single man, childless married man, or men whose wives are unaware of the intended procedure are best left to the individual physician and patient.

The surgical technique should achieve lasting sterilization without compromising the possibility of reversal at a later date. Nevertheless, certain measures, reviewed below, can be taken to enhance the success of future vasovasostomy should this be necessary.

Preoperative preparation

A thorough discussion of vasectomy is essential, making certain that the patient is aware of the following:

1. The operation is intended to be irreversible.
2. Unprotected intercourse is safe only after the ejaculate is free of sperm.
3. Ejaculate volume may decrease but this should not alter sexual pleasure.
4. Recanalization may occur in approximately 0.5 per cent of cases[1].
5. Preliminary studies in vasectomized monkeys showed possible increases in the development of atherosclerosis although this has not been shown in humans[2].
6. Vasovasostomy and sperm banks are available should they be needed.
7. Alternative forms of birth control are available.

The patient's scrotum should be shaved and treated with antiseptic solution.

Anaesthesia

Lignocaine (lidocaine) 1 per cent infiltrated in the area of the incision provides adequate anaesthesia. We have found injection of 0.25 per cent bupivacaine injected in the area of the cord useful in preventing the abdominal pain associated with traction on the vas and helpful in eliminating postoperative pain for 24–48 hours.

The operation

1

Bupivacaine 0.25 per cent is infiltrated to achieve a cord block. Gentle caudal traction on the testis facilitates palpation of the vas by the other hand. The vas is secured between the thumb and two forefingers at a high level in the spermatic cord. Lignocaine (lidocaine) 1 per cent is infiltrated subcutaneously over the vas and extended into perivasal tissue. A 1–2 cm vertical skin incision is made over the vas.

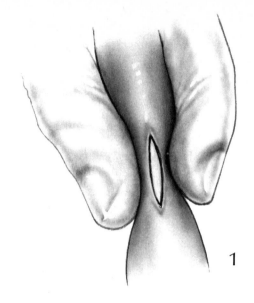

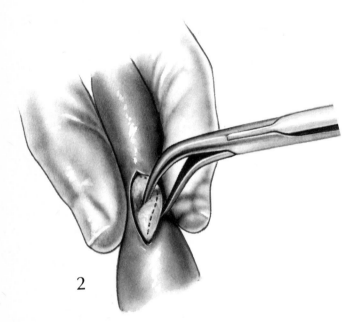

2

The vas and surrounding fascia are grasped with a towel clamp, making certain that the teeth of the instrument are placed around and not through the vas.

3

With traction on the towel clamp a second 5–10 mm vertical incision is made over the vas and carried through surrounding vasal fascia and vessels, thus freeing the vas from supportive tissue.

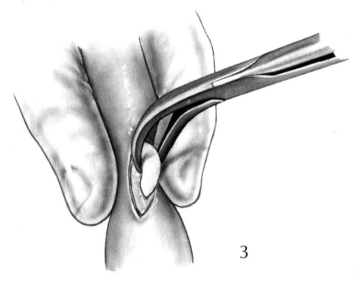

4

Following exposure of a 2–3 cm portion of vas, a straight haemostat is used to grasp the mid portion of the vas.

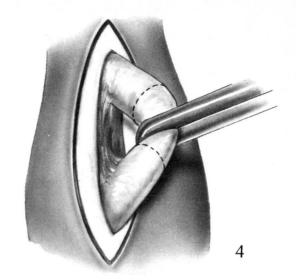

4

5

A 3/0 silk tie or ligature is tied around the distal end (testis side being proximal) and the vas is incised 2–3 mm distal to the clamp.

5

6

The distal end is dropped and the perivasal fascia is approximated over this area with a running 4/0 chromic suture, thus providing a fascial barrier to the proximal vas.

The proximal vas is incised 2–3 mm proximal to the haemostat and the lumen is fulgurated with an electrocautery. The 7–8 mm section of excised vas is sent for pathological confirmation.

The proximal vas is returned to the scrotum without approximation of overlying fascia and the skin is closed with an interrupted 3/0 catgut suture. The wound is dressed with collodion. The remaining side is treated in a similar manner.

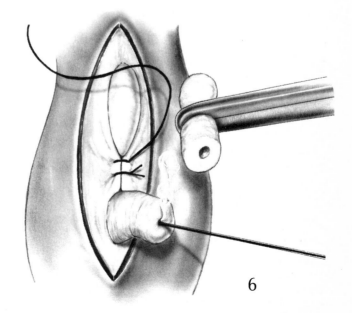

6

Postoperative care

A scrotal support is worn for 4–7 days. Patients should continue preoperative contraceptive methods for about 4 weeks and at least 8–10 ejaculations. A semen specimen should then be submitted to confirm azoospermia.

Results

Spontaneous reanastomosis of the divided vas is reported to occur in less than 1 per cent of cases[3]. However, closure of the fascial sheath over the distal end and fulguration of the vasal lumina was associated with no recanalization in over 1500 cases[4]. Operative failures occur in about 3 per cent[3] of vasectomies and are due to failure to identify a duplicated vas, ligation and division of the same vas twice, or merely mistaken ligation of a vas-like structure – an error which is discovered when pathological diagnosis is returned.

Sperm granulomas, which are usually asymptomatic, occur in 20–35 per cent of patients. They may be more common in individuals who have undergone ligation of the proximal end. When electrocoagulation is substituted for this step, the incidence is reduced. The recurrence of sperm-agglutinating or -immobilizing antibodies does occur in some men, but the significance and long-term effects await further study.

References

1. Esho, J. O., Ireland, G. W., Cass, A. S. Recanalization following vasectomy. Urology 1974; 3: 211–214

2. Clarkson, T. B., Alexander, N. J. Long term vasectomy: effect on the occurrence and extent of atherosclerosis in rhesus monkeys. Journal of Clinical Investigation. 1980; 65: 15–25

3. Schmidt, S. S. Complications of vas surgery. In: Sciarra, J. J., Markland, C., Speidel, J. J., eds. Control of male fertility. New York, London: Harper & Row, 1975: 78–88

4. Schmidt, S. S. Vasectomy should not fail. Contemporary Surgery. 1974; 4: 13–17

Illustrations by Ronald J. Ervin

Varicocele repair

David C. Saypol MD
Resident, Department of Urology,
University of Virginia School of Medicine, Charlottesville, Virginia, USA

Stuart S. Howards MD
Professor of Urology and Associate Professor of Physiology,
University of Virginia School of Medicine, Charlottesville, Virginia, USA

Preoperative

Indications

Surgical repair of varicoceles in certain infertile men appears to augment sperm motility, increase the total count and result in improved fertility in selected couples. Recent evidence suggests that varicoceles impair spermatogenesis by causing haemodynamic changes that result in increased capillary flow and bilateral temperature elevation[1].

Ligation of the internal spermatic vein is indicated in the rare painful varicocele and in an infertile man with varicocele who is oligospermic (less than 20 million/ml) and has poor semen quality. The patient should have no endocrinological abnormalities and his wife should undergo pertinent gynaecological evaluation[2]. The repair of so-called subclinical varicoceles is of uncertain benefit at this time.

Preoperative preparation

The lower abdomen is shaved and treated with antiseptic solution. Positioning of the patient in a slight reverse Trendelenberg position aids the identification of the spermatic veins.

Anaesthesia

Either general or epidural anaesthesia is used.

The operation

1

A short transverse incision is made 2–3 finger breadths medial and 1–2 finger breadths inferior to the antero-superior iliac spine.

The external oblique aponeurosis is incised in the direction of its fibres and the underlying internal oblique muscle is identified.

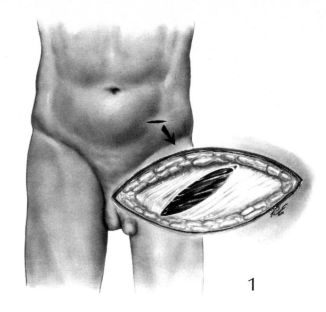

1

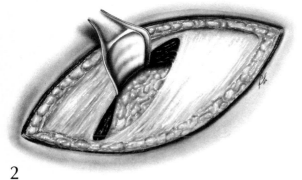

2

2

A phrenic retractor is placed over the inferior edge of the internal oblique and retracted superomedially. The area near the internal ring is then seen.

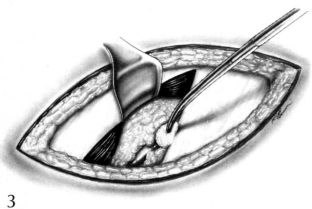

3

3

The retroperitoneal space is gently dissected with a Kittner dissector. The major branch of the internal spermatic vein is identified and dissected proximally as far as the wound will allow, about 5–8 cm.

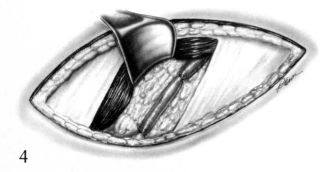

4

4

Ligatures of 2/0 silk are placed distally and proximally and a small section of vein is removed. No special effort is made to identify the testicular artery.

5

Blunt dissection lateral or medial to the ligated branch often reveals a second smaller branch of the testicular vein which is ligated similarly. The vas deferens is easily identified slightly medial and caudal to this second branch. A careful search is then made for additional venous branches.

The external oblique aponeurosis is closed with interrupted 3/0 silk sutures and the skin closed with an absorbable running subcuticular suture.

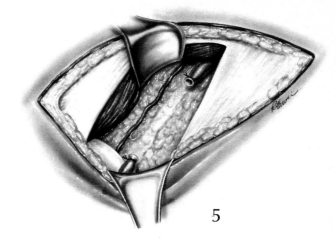

5

Postoperative care

The patient is discharged from hospital the day after surgery and is instructed to avoid strenuous activity for about 3 weeks. A semen analysis is done 3 months after surgery.

Results

The largest series of infertile men undergoing ligation of the internal spermatic veins is that of Dubin and Amelar[3]. Of 986 surgically treated patients there were pregnancies in 53 per cent of couples and 70 per cent of the men had improved semen quality. Other series report pregnancies in 20–55 per cent of previously childless couples after vein ligation[2].

The Ivanissevich[4] and the Palomo[5] procedures are commonly used alternatives to our method but offer no specific advantage. The high ligation herein described is simple, safe, associated with minimal postoperative discomfort and yields a success rate comparable to the more popular procedures. We feel it has the advantages of being high enough to avoid multiple venous collaterals and low enough to be a very simple procedure.

References

1. Saypol, D. C., Howards, S. S., Turner, T. T., Miller, E. D., Jr. Influence of surgically induced varicocele on testicular blood flow, temperature, and histology in adult rats and dogs. Journal of Clinical Investigation 1981; 68: 39–45

2. Saypol, D. C. Varicocele. Journal of Andrology 1981; 2: 61–71

3. Dubin, L., Amelar, R. D. Varicocelectomy. 986 cases in a twelve year study. Urology 1977; 10: 446–449

4. Ivanissevich, O. Left varicocele due to reflux, experience with 4470 operative cases in 42 years. Journal of the International College of Surgeons 1960; 34: 742–755

5. Palomo, A. Radical cure of varicocele by a new technique: preliminary report. Journal of Urology 1949; 61: 604–607

Illustrations by Ronald J. Ervin

Testicular biopsy

David C. Saypol MD
Resident, Department of Urology,
University of Virginia School of Medicine, Charlottesville, Virginia, USA

Stuart S. Howards MD
Professor of Urology and Associate Professor of Physiology,
University of Virginia School of Medicine, Charlottesville, Virginia, USA

Preoperative

Indications

Biopsy of the testis is performed to complete the evaluation of certain infertile men and to rule out testicular relapse in childhood leukaemia[1]. The availability of accurate assays for male gonadotropic hormone and androgen has made testicular biopsy in most infertile men unnecessary. Biopsy is, however, imperative in azoospermic men with normal-sized testes to differentiate ductal obstruction from primary spermatogenic failure[2]. The incidence of leukaemic infiltrates in the testis is sufficiently high to warrant such identification prior to instituting additional chemotherapy.

Preoperative preparation

The scrotum should be shaved and treated with antiseptic solution.

Anaesthesia

Either general or local anaesthesia can be used. Lignocaine (lidocaine) 1 per cent infiltrated in the area of the incision is adequate. We have found the addition of 0.25 per cent bupivacaine injected in the area of the cord useful in preventing the abdominal pain often associated with incision of the tunica albuginea and helpful in eliminating postoperative pain for 24–48 hours.

The operation

1

The testis should be held firmly on its posterior aspect to allow the scrotal skin on the anterior surface to stretch tightly in the area of incision. This forces the epididymis to remain posterior and allows the scrotal skin to part without the need for retraction. A 1–2 cm vertical skin incision is made.

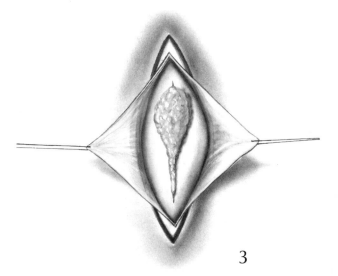

2

The incision is carried down to the tunica vaginalis which is incised with efflux of several drops of clear fluid. It is helpful to place two 4/0 chromic stay sutures in the tunica vaginalis for retraction and to aid closure.

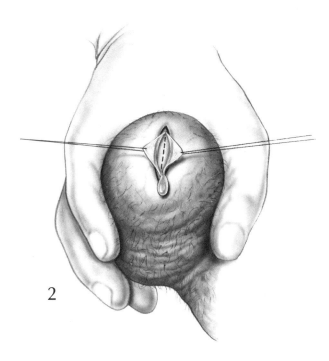

3

Making certain that the underlying tissue is testis and not epididymis, a 3–4 mm incision is made in the tunica albuginea. The pressure on the posterior aspect of the testis is increased slightly and testicular parenchyma will protrude beyond the tunica albuginea.

4

The biopsy is taken with a sharp knife or razor blade by shaving the bulging tissue using a no-touch technique. The specimen is immediately placed in Bouin's, Zenker's or a similar fixative without being handled by a forceps or gauze. Formalin should be avoided as it distorts the germinal epithelium. However, if the pathologist is not familiar with special fixatives, it may be better to use formalin. The tunica albuginea, tunica vaginalis and skin are closed in three separate layers of running 4/0 catgut.

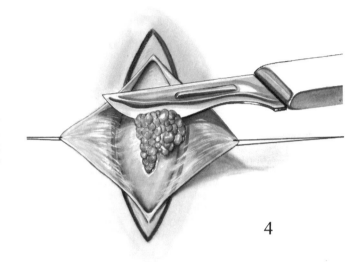

4

Postoperative care

The patient should wear a scrotal support for 3–5 days.

Results

The morbidity associated with testis biopsy is minimal. Rowley, O'Keefe and Heller[3] have demonstrated a significant drop in sperm count following testicular biopsy in normal volunteers, although this deficit resolves spontaneously within 4–5 months. The suggestion that this temporary suppression of spermatogenesis is secondary to sperm antibodies is probably unfounded. In fact, Ansbacher and Gangai[4] found no sperm antibodies up to 14 days following testicular biopsy in oligospermic men.

Testicular biopsy is safe and in spite of the findings of Rowley it is useful in reaching a definite diagnosis in selective infertile men.

References

1. Kim, T. H., Lui, V. K-S., Woodruff, R. D., Ragab, A. H. Testicular biopsy prior to termination of leukemic therapy. Journal of Pediatrics 1979; 94: 95–96

2. Sherins, R. J., Howards, S. S. Male infertility. In: Harrison, J. H., Gittes, R. F., Perlmutter, A. D., Stamey, T. A., Walsh, P. C., eds. Campbell's urology, Vol. 1, 4th ed. Philadelphia, London: W. B. Saunders, 1978: 739–740

3. Rowley, M. J., O'Keefe, K. B., Heller, C. G. Decreases in sperm concentration due to testicular biopsy procedure in man. Journal of Urology 1969; 101: 347–349

4. Ansbacher, R., Gangai, M. P. Testicular biopsy: sperm antibodies. Fertility and Sterility 1975; 26: 1239–1242

Vasography

David C. Saypol MD
Resident, Department of Urology,
University of Virginia School of Medicine, Charlottesville, Virginia, USA

Stuart S. Howards MD
Professor of Urology and Associate Professor of Physiology,
University of Virginia School of Medicine, Charlottesville, Virginia, USA

Preoperative

Indications

Radiographic evaluation of the vas deferens and seminal vesicles is imperative in azoospermic males with normal spermatogenesis. Only after definitive localization of the site of obstruction can reparative surgery be undertaken. In addition, vasography may aid in the identification of distal Wolffian duct structures in patients without ambiguous genitalia. Contrast medium can be injected either directly into the vas or in a retrograde fashion via the ejaculatory ducts although the latter method is often technically difficult[1].

Preoperative preparation

The scrotum should be shaved and treated with an antiseptic solution.

Anaesthesia

Local lignocaine (Xylocaine) 1 per cent provides adequate anaesthesia.

The operation

1

A small transverse scrotal incision is made over the area of the midcord, and the vas is surgically exposed. A spaghetti loop is placed around the vas for traction.

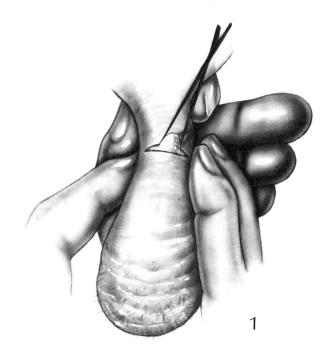

1

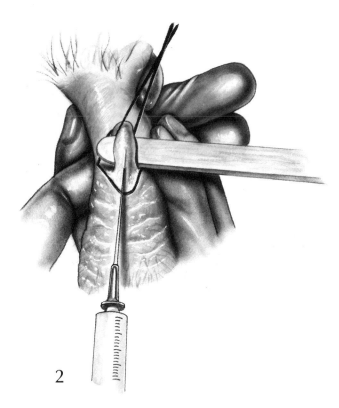

2

2

The vas is placed on a flat tongue depressor and a 23 or 25 gauge needle is inserted into the vas, pointing cephalad. Contrast material used for intravenous urography is diluted with 2 parts sterile saline and 2.5 ml of the mixture are injected.

3

Supine and sometimes oblique radiographs are obtained; the latter are useful for demonstrating the ejaculatory ducts which otherwise might be obscured by contrast medium within the proximal urethra.

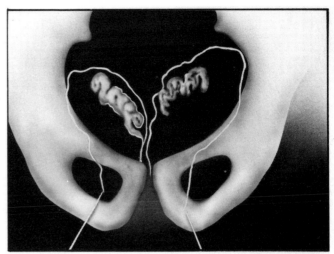

3

4

The needle is removed and, if indicated, reinserted pointing caudad while 0.5 ml of contrast is injected to demonstrate the convoluted vas and epididymis.

The skin is closed with chromic sutures.

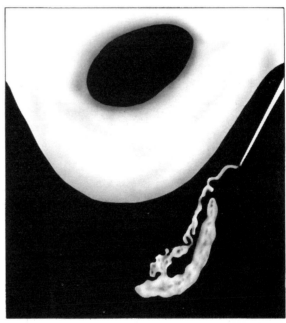

4

Postoperative care

A scrotal support is worn for 1–2 days.

Results

During vasovasostomy, the patency of the distal vas can be ascertained by injecting methylene blue and noting the coloured efflux from a urethral catheter. This method, however, yields no information about the seminal vesicles and epididymis and should not be used elsewhere.

We have found it unnecessary to make a transverse vasotomy and have had no difficulty inserting a needle into the lumen without such an incision. Using modern contrast agents and the technique described above, there has been no stricture formation or other complications.

Reference

1. Sherins, R. J., Howards, S. S. Male infertility. In: Harrison, J. H., Gittes, R. F., Perlmutter, A. D., Stamey, T. A., Walsh, P. C., eds. Cambell's urology, Vol. 1, 4th ed. Philadelphia, London: W. B. Saunders, 1978: 738–739

Illustrations by Ronald J. Ervin

Vasovasostomy

David C. Saypol MD
Resident, Department of Urology,
University of Virginia School of Medicine, Charlottesville, Virginia, USA

Stuart S. Howards MD
Professor of Urology and Associate Professor of Physiology,
University of Virginia School of Medicine, Charlottesville, Virginia, USA

Preoperative

Indications

Except in rare cases of ductal obstruction, vasovasostomy is indicated primarily in men who have undergone either voluntary or iatrogenic vasectomy. The number of men requesting vasectomy reversal has increased steadily over the past few years. Changing attitudes regarding family size and remarriage account for the increased numbers of vasovasostomies performed. The surgical technique which is most effective in restoring vasal patency and fertility is probably one that is performed using optical magnification, although equal pregnancy rates using macroscopic and microscopic techniques are reported[1]. We feel that formal two-layer microscopic closure offers no specific advantage over the modified technique herein described[2]. Our technique considerably shortens operating room time and the resultant anastomosis is strong, watertight and yields a patency rate equal to the two-layer method.

Preoperative preparation

The acquisition of appropriate equipment for microscopic surgery is the most important aspect of preparation for this operation. The following equipment is required: (1) a zoom operating microscope with foot controls; (2) microsurgical instruments including a needle-holder, scissors, two straight-toothed forceps, two straight-smooth forceps and a polished J-shaped jewellers forcep; (3) a vas deferens clamp; (4) Ethicon 10/0 Ethilon suture (1711G) on a GS-16 needle and 8/0 monofilament suture; (5) an operating table which allows the surgeon to sit comfortably; (6) bipolar microdiathermy; and (7) a small syringe with a fine blunt needle for irrigation. The patient's scrotum should be shaved and treated with antiseptic solution prior to surgery.

Anaesthesia

Either general or continuous epidural anaesthesia is used with the choice ultimately left to the patient and anaesthesiologist. With appropriate sedation and the use of lignocaine (lidocaine) 1 per cent locally, surgery can be performed on an outpatient basis in selected situations.

The operation

1

The patient is placed on the operating room table in the supine position. A vertical incision avoiding the base of the penis is made in the scrotum, and the testis, epididymis and proximal vas deferens are delivered through the incision. The site of previous vasectomy is identified by palpation of the scarred ends of the vas.

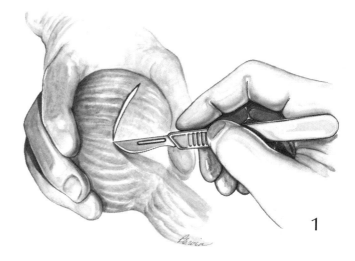

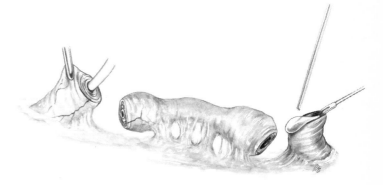

2

The vas deferens is isolated proximal and distal to the scarred areas. Small elastic 'spaghetti' tapes are passed around the vas deferens both proximal and distal to the scarred site of the previous vasectomy. The tapes are used as retractors during the dissection of the vas.

3

The surgeon's hands should rest on a platform of towels to stabilize them during the microvascular phases of the procedure. With the scarred area placed on the knife handle, the proximal end of the vas is then cut back until fluid is seen. The fluid is collected by capillary action into a small pipette placed directly on a microscopic slide, and viewed under the microscope; a better prognosis is associated with the presence of spermatozoa. The distal end of the vas is resected until normal lumen and a well vascularized wall is seen. The distal lumen is very gently dilated with the jeweller's forceps. The patency of the distal segment may be confirmed quickly and easily by passing a 4/0 nylon or Prolene suture into the lumen. Bleeding is carefully controlled with bipolar microdiathermy. Devascularization of the vas has not been a problem.

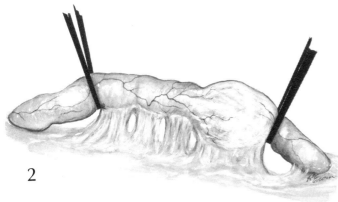

4

The two ends of the vas are then placed in a vas deferens approximator clip. If the outer diameter of the vas deferens is small, it is useful to place a sterile piece of rubber tubing over one arm of the clip. A thin sterile piece of blue plastic material is then placed under the two ends of the vas. This provides an excellent visual background, and puncture of this plastic material with a fine needle allows blood and irrigation solution to drain adequately.

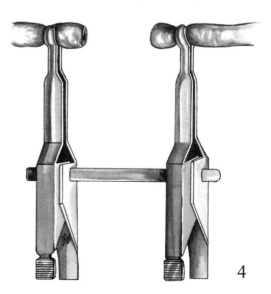

4

5

A 10/0 suture is passed through the entire thickness of the vas deferens, puncturing the serosa of the proximal segment, its mucosa, the mucosa of the distal end and finally the distal serosa. The suture is then tied.

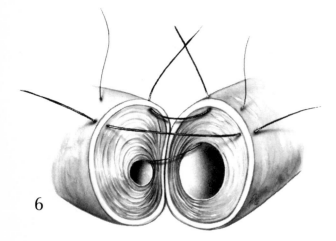

5

6

6

Two 8/0 sutures are placed on either side of the 10/0 suture, but do not enter the lumen.

7

Three more 10/0 luminal stitches are placed in each of the remaining three quadrants and reinforced on either side with one or two 8/0 nonluminal sutures.

The posterior quadrant suture can be placed by rotating the vas deferens approximator clip 180°. If the anastomosis is made to the proximal convoluted vas deferens or to the epididymal tube itself, it is often easier to use six to eight through-and-through luminal sutures in a single layer. The testis and epididymis are returned to the scrotum, and the dartos muscle and skin are closed in layers using absorbable sutures.

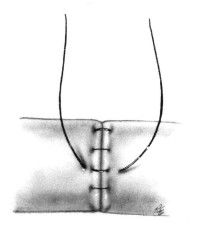

7

Postoperative care

Patients are discharged from hospital the day after operation. They are able to return to work within a few days but are advised to wear a scrotal support for about 2 weeks. Heavy lifting and intercourse should also be avoided for approximately 2 weeks. Aspirin or paracetamol (Tylenol) is a sufficient analgesic. Three months postoperatively the semen analysis often reveals a good sperm count with poor motility. After 6 months, the count usually is stable or slightly improved and motility is significantly improved.

Results

More than 90 per cent of patients in whom spermatozoa were present in the fluid obtained from the distal vas deferens at operation will have spermatozoa in their postoperative ejaculate. The subsequent pregnancy rate is approximately 40–71 per cent[3]. The reasons for the discrepancy between incidence of patency and fertility are unknown. Possible factors include testicular malfunction secondary to the previous vasectomy, abnormal epididymal function, delayed transport of spermatozoa, immunological abnormalities and female infertility. It does seem evident that the fertility rate following vasovasostomy slowly decreases as the interval between vasectomy and reanastomosis increases.

The surgical procedure of choice has not yet been established, but results do support the contention that the experience of the surgeon is more important than the technique used. Thomas *et al.*[4] have investigated the effect of surgical technique on the results of vasovasostomy in dogs and found that excellent patency could be achieved with both the unstented microscopic and the non-microscopic technique. However, more sperm leakage occurred after non-microscopic techniques. In addition, there was no significant difference between the success rates of the one-layer and two-layer microscopic anastomoses. Lee and McLoughlin[1] found that 17 out of 37 (46 per cent) patients who underwent macroscopic vasovasostomy and 14 out of 26 (54 per cent) patients who underwent microscopic vasovasostomy became fathers[1]. The results obtained from both groups were not statistically different.

The modified surgical technique for microscopic single-layer closure described here is less tedious and more cost-effective than the formal two-layer anastomosis. By placing through-and-through sutures in the first row, 2 hours of operating room time are saved. According to our laboratory studies and clinical results, these modifications do not compromise the results of surgery.

References

1. Lee, L., McLoughlin, M. G. Vasovasostomy: a comparison of macroscopic and microscopic techniques at one institution. Fertility and Sterility 1980; 33: 54–55

2. Sharlip, I. D. Vasovasostomy: comparison of two microsurgical techniques. Urology 1981; 17: 347–352

3. Silber, S. J. Vasectomy and its microsurgical reversal. Urologic Clinics of North America 1978; 5: 573–584

4. Thomas, A. J., Pontes, J. E., Buddhdev, H., Pierce, J. M. Vasovasostomy: evaluation of four surgical techniques. Fertility and Sterility 1979; 32: 324–328

Illustrations by Ronald J. Ervin

Vasoepididymostomy

David C. Saypol MD
Resident, Department of Urology,
University of Virginia School of Medicine, Charlottesville, Virginia, USA

Stuart S. Howards MD
Professor of Urology and Associate Professor of Physiology,
University of Virginia School of Medicine, Charlottesville, Virginia, USA

Preoperative

Indications

Epididymal obstruction is likely to be the cause of azoospermia in a man whose testicular biopsy demonstrates normal spermatogenesis, and who has seminal fluid which is positive for fructose, and normal vasograms. Most commonly these patients will have postinflammatory obstructive lesions or a congenital blockage.

The classic procedure used to perform vasoepididymostomy is macroscopic and involves an incision into the body of the epididymis transecting multiple lumina. A longitudinal incision is made in the vas which is sewn side-to-side with the epididymal tunica. The success of the procedure is dependent upon formation of a sperm fistula between these two structures.

Microscopic anastomosis of the vas deferens to a single epididymal tubule is conceptually the ideal procedure[1]. Although this new technique has not proved to yield more pregnancies than the macroscopic method, it certainly is more physiological. The equipment and general techniques necessary for microscopic surgery are described in the chapter on 'Vasovasostomy' (see pp. 700–703).

Preoperative preparations

The patient should have two to three semen analyses demonstrating azoospermia, a positive fructose and histological proof of normal spermatogenesis. The biopsy can be performed as a preliminary procedure or at the time of scrotal exploration and sent for frozen section. A vasogram must be obtained but most often is done in the operating room at the start of the vasoepididymal procedure. The scrotum is shaved and treated with antiseptic solution.

Anaesthesia

General or continuous epidural anaesthesia can be used.

The operation

1

The patient is placed on the operating table in the supine position. A vertical incision is made in the hemiscrotum and carried through the parietal layer of tunica vaginalis. The testis, epididymis and vas are delivered out of the scrotal compartment.

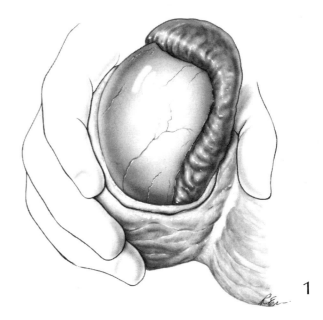

1

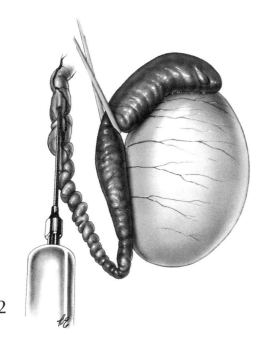

2

2

Visual inspection of the epididymis will often reveal a dilated epididymal tubule. In the absence of an obviously dilated tubule, the microscope is used at low magnification to localize tubular dilatation.

Following identification of the site of probable obstruction, the epididymis is dissected distally, freeing it from the testis. An elastic loop is placed around this portion of the epididymis. To be certain that no vasal obstruction is present, the vas is dissected free just distal to the convoluted portion and a vasogram is performed.

3

After confirming vasal patency, the vas is divided distal to the convoluted area. The epididymis is transected immediately distal to the site of presumed obstruction. If no obvious site of obstruction is identified, an arbitrarily chosen distal location is transected. Each of the incised tubules is examined for egress of luminal fluid which when seen, is sampled with a capillary tube and examined microscopically for the presence of sperm. In the absence of sperm, we have found it useful to remove a 5 mm transverse section of the epididymis on the distal side of the transection and examine this tissue microscopically[2]. If sperm are not evident, the epididymis needs to be transected more proximally. The presence of sperm confirms transection proximal to the site of obstruction.

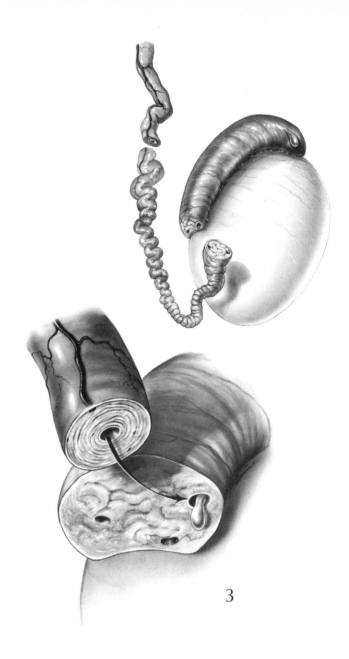

3

4

The tubule from which fluid is effluxing is best identified by applying pressure to the proximal epididymis, swabbing the transected epididymal surface and microscopically observing the cut surface.

This tubule is anastomosed to the vas using the vas approximating clamp. Three to five 10/0 nylon sutures are passed through the individual epididymal tubule and the vas.

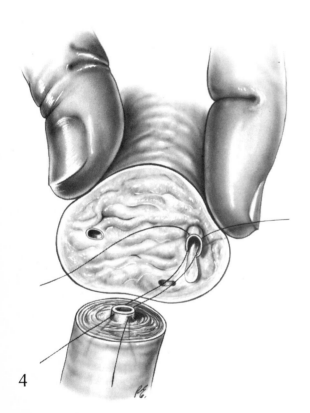

4

5

Six to 10 8/0 nylon sutures are used to approximate the seromuscular layer of the vas to the tunica of the epididymis. A 5/0 chromic seromuscular suture is placed in the vas just distal to the anastomosis and this portion of vas is pexed to the adjacent tunica albuginea, thus preventing postoperative tension on the anastomosis. The testis is returned to the scrotum which is closed in separate layers using chromic sutures.

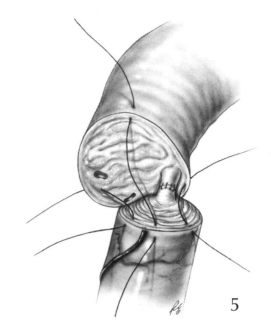

5

Postoperative care

A scrotal support is worn for 6–8 weeks and sexual activity is avoided for 2–3 weeks. Semen analysis is obtained 3 months after surgery.

Results

Using the classic side-to-side vasoepididymostomy, Amelar, Dubin and Walsh[3] reported sperm in the ejaculate of 50 per cent of patients with postinflammatory obstruction but pregnancies in only 20 per cent. Silber[1], whose technique we use with minor modification, reported sperm in the ejaculate in 12 out of 14 patients. Follow-up in his report and our own experiences is too short to evaluate pregnancies, although 1 out of 5 patients followed for greater than 1.5 years has reported a pregnancy[4].

While convincing data are insufficient at this time regarding the advantages of microscopic vasoepididymostomy, we feel the direct tubular anastomosis is physiologically and anatomically the preferred procedure.

References

1. Silber, S. J. Microscopic vasoepididymostomy: specific microanastomosis to the epididymal tubule. Fertility and Sterility 1978; 30: 565–571

2. Turner, T. T., Howards, S. S. Microscopic vaso-epididymostomy: examination of epididymal lumen content for presence of spermatozoa. Fertility and Sterility 1981; 36: 533–534

3. Amelar, R. D., Dubin, L., Walsh, P. C. Male infertility. Philadelphia, London: W. B. Saunders, 1977

4. Silber, S. J. Vasoepididymostomy to the head of the epididymis: recovery of normal spermatozoal motility. Fertility and Sterility 1980; 34: 149–153

Illustrations by Rudolf Brammer and Cathy Slatter

Intersex – the surgery of the external genitalia in girls

Herbert B. Eckstein   MD, MChir, FRCS
Consultant Paediatric Surgeon, Hospital for Sick Children, Great Ormond Street, London, UK

Introduction

While clitoral hypertrophy, vulval or introital stenosis and vaginal atresia tend to occur together and are usually related to an endocrine abnormality (of which the adrenogenital syndrome is the commonest), these abnormalities can occur in isolation and without any known cause. It should, however, be remembered that the maternal ingestion of androgens (used in the treatment of threatened abortion) may be an aetiological factor.

The surgical treatment of clitoral hypertrophy will therefore be dealt with, together with vaginal reconstruction, under the heading of 'Adrenogenital syndrome'.

VULVAL (INTROITAL) STENOSIS

This condition is not infrequently seen as an isolated abnormality but it is essential to exclude any endocrine disease before embarking on surgical treatment. Early correction (well before school age) is advocated so as to reduce possible emotional disturbances which may otherwise follow surgery.

1

In the less severe form, a posterior Y-V plasty will widen the vaginal introitus adequately. The lower third of the vagina is incised posteriorly in the midline and the incision is continued as a V in the perineum.

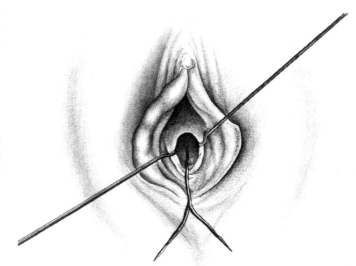

1

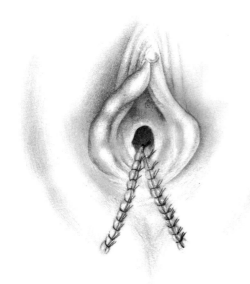

2

The V-shaped flap is fully mobilized and is advanced into the vagina where it is held with interrupted sutures. A vaginal pack reduces postoperative bleeding and the bladder is catheterized for a few days to keep the perineum dry.

2

3

In the more severe form of stenosis, a posterolateral flap allows for a greater area of pedicled skin to be transposed. On the whole, this procedure is preferred. The lower third of the vagina is incised posterolaterally (a left-sided incision is easier to suture for the right-handed surgeon) and the incision is carried into the perineum as shown so as to produce a large flap with a posterior based pedicle.

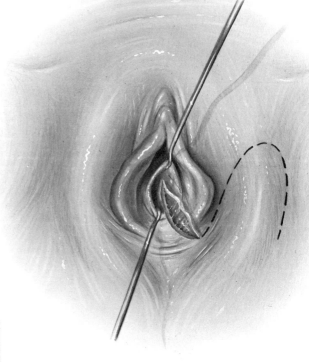

3

4

The pedicle is rotated into the vagina and its apex is fixed to the deepest part of the incision.

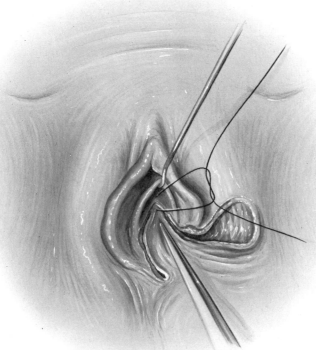

4

5

The procedure is completed using interrupted absorbable sutures.

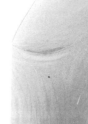

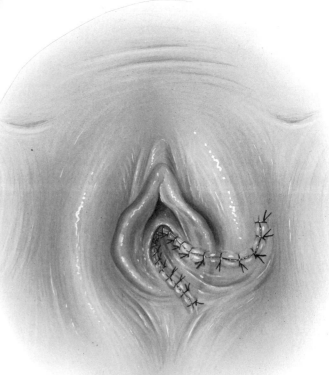

ADRENOGENITAL SYNDROME

In adrenogenital syndrome (AGS) there is an enzyme defect which prevents the full elaboration of hydrocortisone. A serious electrolyte disturbance may result and there is an excessive output of ACTH by the pituitary gland. In female infants this disturbance will lead to masculinization with clitoral hypertrophy and there may or may not be an associated and life-threatening salt-losing syndrome. In any event, all patients with AGS require a careful endocrine study before surgery is contemplated and hydrocortisone may have to be given for the rest of the patient's life. Menstruation develops normally and pregnancy is possible.

Before discussing the management of AGS it is helpful to consider the available techniques for dealing surgically with the enlarged clitoris. The following options exist: clitoridectomy; clitoral recession; and partial clitoridectomy or clitoroplasty. The surgical exposure of the clitoris and of the crura is the same in all three techniques.

Clitoridectomy is technically simple: the crura are ligated and divided and the complete clitoris is excised or amputated. While this technique was popular in the past, there is no doubt that it leads to a loss of libido and gives rise to considerable emotional problems at the time of sexual maturity. The technique should, therefore, no longer be used.

Clitoral recession was introduced to avoid the loss of libido following clitoridectomy. The corpora are exposed and mobilized as for clitoridectomy but are not divided. Instead they are plicated in a concertina fashion with a series of mattress sutures through the tough fibrous covering so that the clitoris is effectively shortened[1,2]. While the procedure preserves clitoral sensation it gives rise to considerable discomfort and even pain during sexual activity and erection and for this reason can no longer be recommended.

Partial clitoridectomy as described below reduces the bulk of the erectile tissue while at the same time preserving clitoral sensation. Careful preservation of the blood and nerve supply is, however, essential[3].

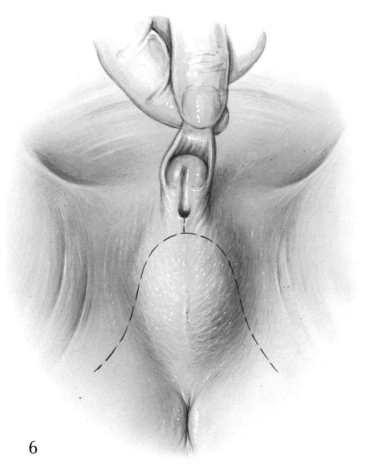

Partial clitoridectomy

The operation is performed in the lithotomy position with the head end of the operating table tilted down. It is essential to have blood crossmatched as serious bleeding may be encountered.

6

An inverted U-shaped incision is made in the perineum which is extended in the midline to the urethral orifice; note sagittal extension to urethral opening.

6

7

A full-thickness flap is raised, the urethral tissue is defined and a self-retaining retractor is inserted.

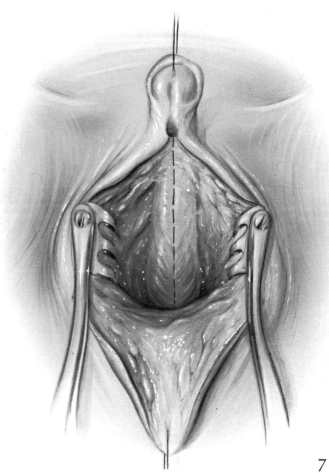

7

8

The urethra is then incised in the midline from the external meatus backwards, using a pair of straight scissors, until the vaginal orifice comes into view.

It is convenient to insert a Foley type of balloon catheter into the bladder at this stage and a second balloon catheter can be inserted into the vagina so as to allow the vaginal opening to be pulled downwards towards the operator once the balloon has been inflated.

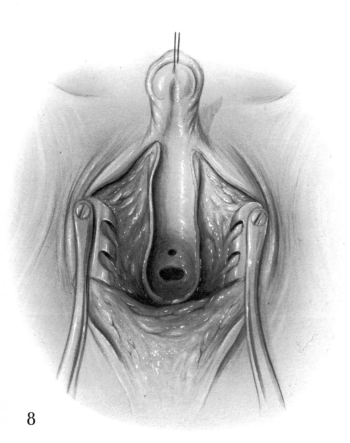

8

9

The apex of the skin flap is then carefully sutured to the vaginal margin and to the posterior edge of the urethral strip. The vaginal balloon catheter can now be removed. The skin incisions are then carried forwards and are joined by curved incision around the dorsal part of the clitoris.

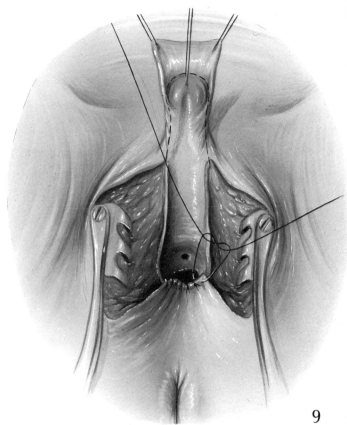

9

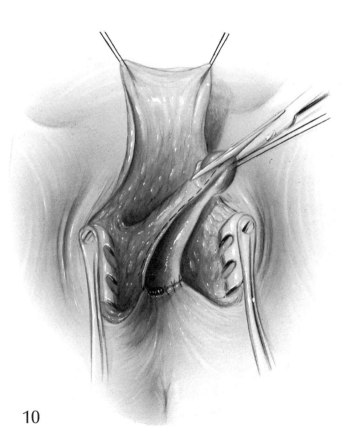

10

10

The foreskin of the clitoris is then opened up so as to produce a large area of skin with a proximal blood supply. An incision is made across the glans clitoris so that the ventral portion (to be preserved) consists of one-third of the organ, while the dorsal two-thirds, attached to the corpora, are ultimately resected.

11

The corpora are carefully dissected out and the blood supply to the glans which lies between the two corpora is carefully preserved and is left attached to the urethral strip.

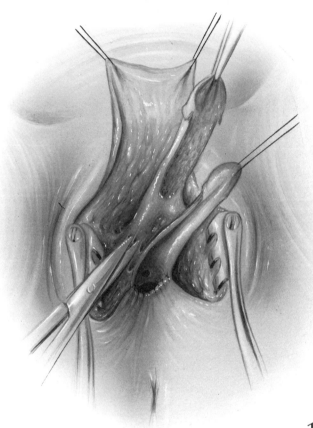

11

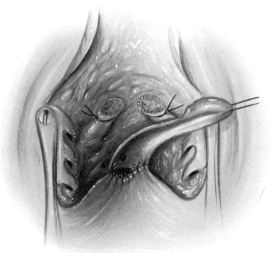

12

12

It is essential to dissect out the crura well proximal to their junction so that the right and left crura can be transfixed, ligated and divided separately. The phallus is excised.

13

The urethral strip and ventral portion of the glans are anchored to the fibrous tissue under the pubic arch at the appropriate level and the preputial skin is split longitudinally so as to form two rectangular skin flaps. The apex of this incision should encircle the glans.

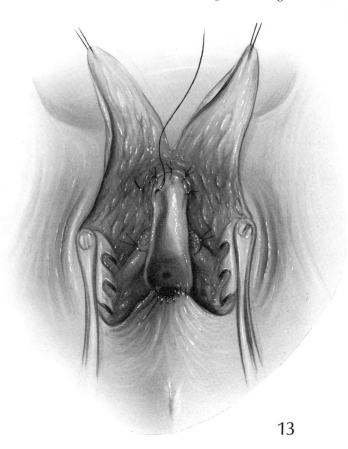

13

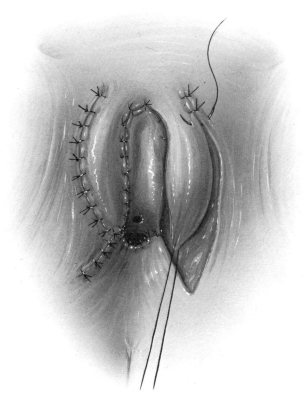

14

14

The preputial flaps are now sutured into position to form the new labia minora and the skin defect is completely closed.

A pressure dressing is applied to ensure haemostasis and catheter drainage is maintained to keep the suture lines dry.

Further surgery to the vaginal orifice should not be required in the majority of patients.

Acknowledgement

Illustrations 3–14 have been reproduced from Williams[3] by courtesy of the Publishers.

References

1. Hendren, W. H., Donahoe, P. K. Correction of congenital abnormalities of the vagina and perineum. Journal of Paediatric Surgery 1980; 15: 751–763

2. Randolph, J., Hung, W., Rathley, M. C. Clitoroplasty for females born with ambiguous genitalia: a long-term study of 37 patients. Journal of Paediatric Surgery 1981; 16: 882–887

3. Williams, D. I. Adrenogenital syndrome. In: Eckstein, H. B., Hohenfellner, R., Williams, D. I., eds. Surgical pediatric urology. Stuttgart: Thieme, 1977: 437–440

Illustrations by Gary M. James, A. E. Cottrell, Michael J. Courtney and T. R. Tarrant

Urethroscopy and cystoscopy

J. P. Mitchell CBE, TD, MS, FRCS, FRCS(Ed)
Honorary Professor of Surgery (Urology), University of Bristol, UK

Preoperative

Indications

Cystourethroscopy provides a means of inspecting the bladder wall, bladder neck and urethra. Any endoscopic surgery or open operation on the bladder or urethra should always be preceded by a preliminary cystourethroscopy, preferably under the same anaesthetic.

Contraindications

It is inadvisable to carry out a cystoscopy in the presence of acute urethritis, acute prostatitis, or epididymitis without appropriate antibiotic cover, as this may result in local or even systemic spread of infection.

Preparation of instruments

A supply of sterile water is essential. This can be provided either from sterile bottles or from a closed sterile piped water system. It is an advantage if this is distilled water, so the surgeon is free to use the diathermy if necessary. In addition, a nonelectrolytic isotonic solution should be available for use during transurethral prostatic resections. The water should be delivered to a reservoir which can be varied in height in relation to the patient's bladder, so that the exact pressure of water delivery to the endoscope is controlled.

The pressure should normally not exceed 60 cmH$_2$O. In order to achieve this the distance from the middle of the delivery bag to the symphysis pubis should not exceed 60 cm. The tubing from the reservoir to the cystoscope should contain some form of non-return valve so that when the patient coughs or strains none of the bladder content refluxes into the reservoir, thereby contaminating it for subsequent patients on the same operating list. The water should be delivered at approximately body temperature.

The telescope itself should be checked before sterilization to ensure that the lighting is intact and the view is optically clear. Any blurring or distortion of the field or a crescentic loss on one or both sides indicates that the telescope is damaged.

The instrument should be disinfected by immersion in a solution of chlorhexidine (Hibitane 1:200 in 70 per cent spirit) or gluteraldehyde (Cidex), or by exposure to a disinfecting vapour such as ethylene oxide, or by some form of heat pasteurization. Bactericidal fluid or vapour is dependent for effective disinfection on thorough contact with the entire instrument. Many modern endoscopes can be boiled and a few can be passed through a limited autoclave procedure. The safest method of disinfecting endoscopes is by pasteurization, either in water at 80 °C or in a low-pressure (half an atmosphere) autoclave, where steam is delivered at 73 °C. The latter method gives the most efficient penetration for disinfection and is suitable for all types of urological endoscopes.

The instrument is stored in a sterile pack, ready for immediate use. This avoids delay when special endoscopes are required at short notice.

1

Types of cystoscope

Two types of urological endoscope are in common use: the end-viewing urethroscope (0° angle of view) and the right-angled cystoscope (usually 70° angle of view). These endoscopes are combined in the cystourethroscope sheath by changing from the 0° to the 70° telescope. The direct vision urethroscope is useful for inspecting the length of the urethra as well as the bladder neck but will give only a tangential view of that part of the bladder wall near the internal urinary meatus; however, it provides a good view of the posterior wall of the bladder and can be used for inspecting the interior of a diverticulum

The cystoscope with a 70° telescope can view all parts of the bladder wall, as well as the proximal prostatic urethra down to the verumontanum. The optical system is constructed in such a way that the operator can view objects as close as 3 mm and as far as 5–6 cm from the objective lens of the telescope.

The size of the cystourethroscope sheath need not be more than 18 Fr for a simple inspection endoscopy. For the passage of a ureteric catheter a 22 Fr sheath may be necessary. Smaller sizes of endoscope down to 8 Fr are available for use in infants and children. In a newborn male an external urethrotomy via the bulbous urethra may be necessary to introduce the 8 Fr instrument.

Additional telescopes are constructed for viewing at 30° for operative endoscopy or for viewing at 120° on occasions when the anterior wall of the bladder is in a slightly retroverted position to the bladder neck.

Illumination

Most urological endoscopes today depend for illumination on light transmitted via glass fibre cables. These convey the light by total internal reflection from an external source of illumination. This equipment provides a constant, reliable light, but there are two major disadvantages: first, the fibre cables are likely to be fractured by any acute flexion, thus reducing the amount of light transmitted; and, second, the pillar on the telescope to which the cable is fixed cannot be rotated, which tends to limit the freedom of movement of the endoscope.

The junction points between the light source and the cable and between the cable and the telescope light pillar should match, as the size of the port of entry and exit must be equal.

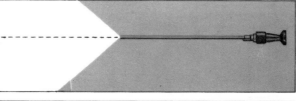
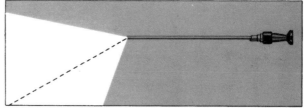
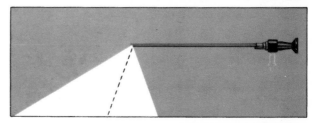
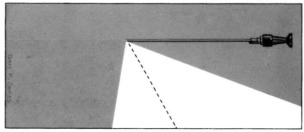

1

2

Preparation of patient

The patient should be placed in a forward lithotomy position with the thighs flexed to 45°. Flexion of the thighs more than 45° makes it more difficult to pass the endoscope as greater pressure on the suspensory ligament of the penis is needed to straighten the urethra. Moreover, in elderly patients, extended lithotomy is likely to result in a painful back following examination, presumably from disturbance of any lumbar osteoarthritis.

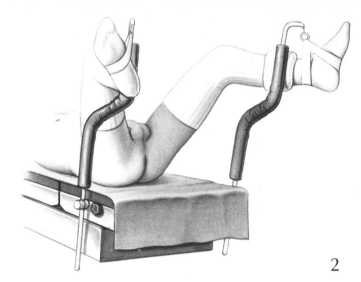

2

Anaesthesia

General anaesthesia is preferable for most males, children and younger females, while the majority of married females will tolerate the examination under a local anaesthetic only. The local anaesthetic can be given as for catheterization (i.e. lignocaine and chlorhexidine in methyloxycellulose jelly. It should be appreciated, however, that this is liable to create optical difficulties when viewing the urethra, and the jelly has to be washed ahead of the objective lens of the telescope with a good strong flow of irrigating fluid. The lignocaine and chlorhexidine should be avoided if any disease is suspected in the urethra itself, or if any specimen of urine is required for culture from the bladder, as the chlorhexidine will inhibit the culture.

The urethral antiseptic should also be given immediately after the endoscopy has been completed and before any further endoscopic procedure, such as transurethral resection.

Surgical diathermy

A diathermy plate should be applied to the patient, either under the buttocks or around the thigh in preparation for possible diathermy coagulation. The patient should be draped and sterile precautions taken, as for any surgical procedure. The penis should be wrapped in a sterile swab so that only the external meatus remains uncovered after the towelling has been completed.

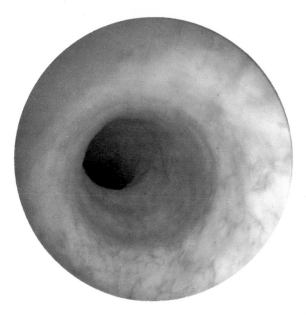

Normal anterior urethra
Illustration 4 from page 719

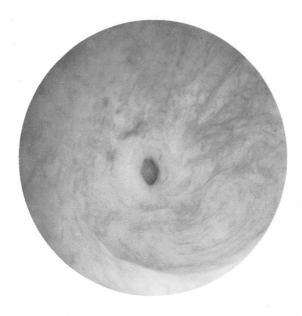

Stricture
Illustration 8 from p. 720

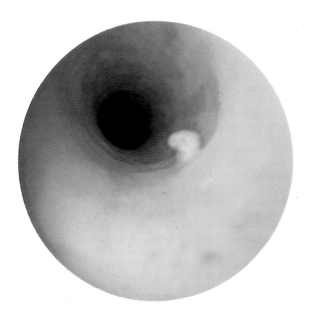

Neoplasm
Illustration 9 from p. 720

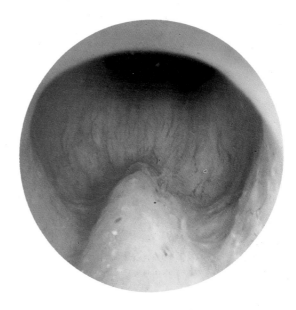

Verumontanum and prostatic urethra
Illustration 11 from p. 721

The operation

URETHROSCOPY

If the patient is under general anaesthesia, the panendoscope should be lubricated with chlorhexidine in 0.5 per cent glycerine, to avoid any possible contamination of the urethra from organisms in the region of the external meatus. This solution also acts as a suitable water-soluble lubricant for the endoscope. Although liquid paraffin is the best urethral lubricant, it is not recommended for endoscopy: globules of oil may interfere with the optical system of the telescope and may remain on the urethral wall. This will damage any part of a latex catheter such as the self-retaining balloon which may rupture, as latex is soluble in liquid paraffin.

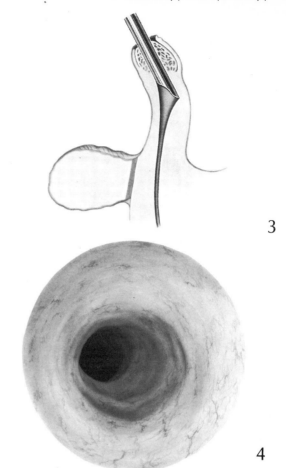

3

3, 4 & 5

In the male the urethroscope should be passed before any other urethral instrument, in order to inspect the virgin urethra. If a 0° telescope is not available, a 30° one may be used, but it should be remembered that the view is fore-oblique. Therefore, the beak of the instrument is directed 30° away from the line of view and is likely to impale the mucosal lining of the urethra on the opposite wall. The penis should be drawn upwards so that the instrument slides down the distal urethra to the triangular ligament.

4

Normal
This illustration may also be seen in the colour plate section facing p. 718

6

Difficulty may be encountered if the beak of the instrument fails to follow the right-angled change of direction through the triangular ligament (the urogenital diaphragm) and becomes lodged in the depression at the posterior end of the bulbous urethra. This, however, will be obvious when using the 0° (direct vision) telescope and can be smoothed out if the penis is drawn well upwards. As soon as the beak of the instrument has negotiated the triangular ligament, the shaft of the cystoscope is depressed between the patient's thighs in order to guide the beak of the instrument through the prostatic urethra and over the neck of the bladder.

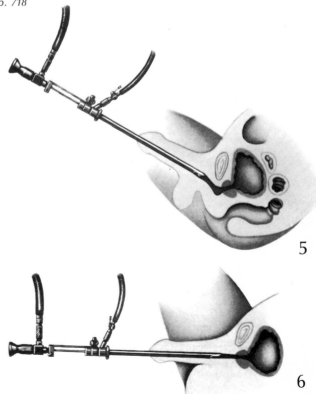

5

6

7

A deep dip (depression of the eyepiece) of the instrument may be required to negotiate an enlarged middle lobe of prostate or an occasional ridge at the bladder neck as in 'prostatism sans prostate'. As the instrument is passed slowly along the urethra, a gentle but very slight oscillatory movement in and out of the urethra will discourage any artificial fold of the mucosa being lifted by the beak of the instrument. Again, with a direct vision telescope this should be obvious before any damage is done to the mucosa.

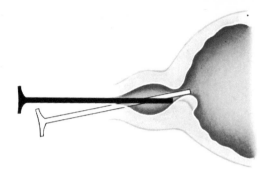

7

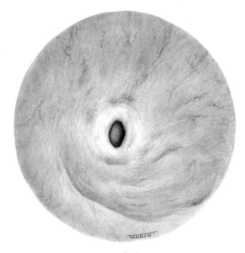

8

8

The urethra is inspected for possible stricture, causing stenosis of the lumen, which may further obstruct the passage of the instrument along the urethra. The face of the stricture can be examined in detail and, if necessary, the sheath of the endoscope can be changed in order to dilate or cut the stricture. This may be performed either under direct vision or by the use of blind urethral dilators. The length of the stricture can then be estimated by further endoscopy.

Stricture
This illustration may also be seen in the colour plate section facing p. 718

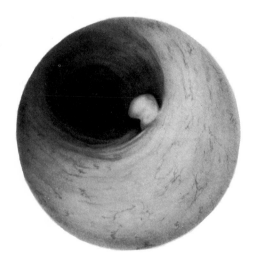

9

9

Urethroscopy may be helpful in the examination of a false passage, made by previous instrumentation of the urethra. Occasionally neoplasms may be seen as primary growths of the urethra or secondary seedlings from a transitional cell carcinoma of the urothelium in the more proximal urinary tract.

Neoplasm
This illustration may also be seen in the colour plate section facing p. 718

CYSTOSCOPY

10 & 11

After passage of the cystourethroscope using the 0° telescope under direct vision, the bladder and prostatic urethra are inspected with the 70° telescope. The trigone, bladder neck and both ureteric orifices are identified, and the instrument is withdrawn slowly through the prostatic urethra to observe the lobes of the prostate gland and verumontanum. Although the two latter features have been inspected already by urethroscopy with the direct vision telescope, a further perspective is obtained by the 70° telescope. The short focal distance of the 70° telescope makes this near vision in the prostatic urethra possible in nearly all male patients.

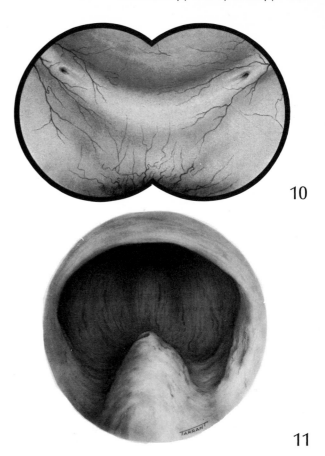

10

11

Verumontanum and prostatic urethra
This illustration may also be seen in the colour plate section facing p. 718

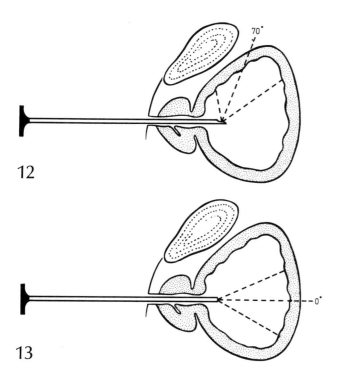

12

13

12 & 13

The instrument is moved slowly forward into the bladder, which is inspected systematically from the neck to the mid-posterior wall. Oscillation of the instrument in and out is repeated with each few degrees of rotation, first from the midline posteriorly (6 o'clock), rotating the instrument anticlockwise to the right by a few degrees at a time, until the whole of the right half of the bladder up to the vault (12 o'clock) has been inspected. The same movement is then repeated on the left side of the bladder. Finally, it is essential to make sure that the central point of the posterior wall has been thoroughly inspected, as this point is likely to be a blind spot for most right-angled telescopes. If there is any doubt about the inspection of this area of the bladder, the operator is advised to reintroduce the direct vision (0°) telescope, which may also be necessary for viewing the interior of a diverticulum.

14

A 120° telescope will give an excellent view of the anterior wall of the bladder, which may otherwise be slightly out of view with the conventional 70° telescope.

The ureteric orifices are inspected and any difference in size, shape or position is noted. The efflux from each side is observed, although if the patient is under general anaesthetic and on restricted fluids there may be a long delay before any efflux is seen. Indigo carmine (5 ml) may be given intravenously to demonstrate the efflux by a colour change of the urine.

Occasionally the ureteric orifice is stenosed and the underlying intramural ureter may balloon with each efflux. A ureterocele is a permanently distended intramural part of ureter which bulges into the bladder.

Finally, the effects of distension of the bladder on the appearance of the ureteric orifices are noted. It is necessary to see whether the orifice remains closed as the bladder reaches full distension. An orifice that opens with distension of the bladder suggests the probability of vesicoureteric reflux.

The effects of previous surgery may be seen, such as stenosis from surrounding scar, or a rigid patent orifice which can also result from diathermy scarring. A rigid patent orifice, from whatever cause, is likely to result in vesicoureteric reflux, and a micturating cystourethrogram should be performed at a later stage.

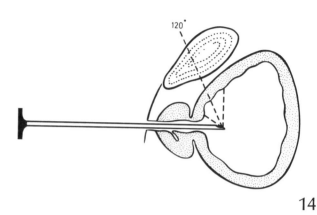

14

15

The bladder wall should be inspected for any localized lesions, such as a hyperaemic patch, a proliferative area of bullous cystitis, a neoplasm, or an ulcer of either infective or neoplastic origin. The degree of trabeculation and sacculation or diverticulum formation should be noted as an estimate of mechanical obstruction or neurological abnormality. Some trabeculation, limited to the posterior wall of the bladder, is physiologically within normal limits and may be increased in the 'unstable' bladder, though in this condition the trabeculation will not extend over the entire bladder wall and will not be associated with any saccules. If the water used for irrigating the bladder is well below body temperature, the mucosa of the bladder wall may contract into rugae, imitating the appearance of trabeculation; hence the water supply should always be as near to body temperature as possible. The capacity of the bladder should be estimated and recorded. Calculi in the bladder will usually have been noted previously on X-ray.

Generalized lesions of the bladder wall, such as cystitis, will appear as either infection of the blood vessels or a 'fuzziness' of definition due to oedema which gives the impression that the bladder wall is slightly out of focus. Sometimes in severe acute cystitis the whole of the bladder wall will appear haemorrhagic. Occasionally the lesion of cystitis may be localized at the base of the bladder; this is the case in patients who have been bedridden for some time and have accumulated a sump of pus at the bladder base, while they pass the supernatant clear urine.

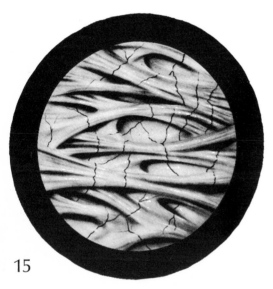

15

Trabeculation

16

The thickness of the bladder neck should be estimated cystoscopically and palpated with a finger per rectum against the cystoscope. The length of the prostatic urethra can be measured by sliding the instrument in and out from the bladder neck to the verumontanum and gauging the extent of this movement against a fixed point externally.

Finally, if any localized lesion is seen in the bladder, a biopsy should be taken.

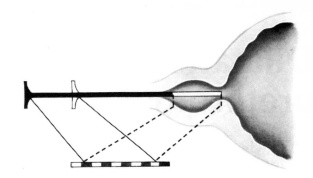

16

Postoperative care and complications

The most essential part of the technique of endoscopy of the urethra or the bladder is to maintain accurate orientation. It may be difficult to reorientate oneself once the drill of a systematic inspection is abandoned.

Complications that may be encountered at the time of cystoscopy are: stricture of the urethra which may prevent the passage of the instrument and require dilatation before the endoscope can be passed into the bladder (this, however, would have been noted in the preliminary urethroscopy); the limited capacity of the bladder itself, which can make inspection difficult as the bladder wall cannot be distended sufficiently to obtain a satisfactory view. The prostate may be so enlarged that the length of the conventional cystoscope may not be sufficient to reach the bladder.

Bleeding may be so profuse from a lesion from within the bladder, or at the neck of the bladder, that the view is obliterated despite repeated washings. Neoplasms may be large and extensively fronded, making it difficult to view the normal bladder wall.

The patient should be advised to drink copiously following the inspection (i.e. about 2.8 litres (5 pints) of fluid in the succeeding 24 hours). The passage of dilute urine will be less uncomfortable than the passage of concentrated urine over the urethral mucosa. There may be some relief from leaving a small quantity of water in the bladder at the end of the cystoscopy so that the patient can satisfy his inevitable urge to micturate when he recovers from the anaesthetic.

Illustrations by Michael Courtney

Dilatation and endoscopic urethrotomy for urethral stricture

J. P. Mitchell   CBE, TD, MS, FRCS, FRCS(Ed)
Honorary Professor of Surgery (Urology), University of Bristol, UK

Introduction

The number of patients requiring regular urethral dilatations has decreased markedly in the past 25 years. This reduction has been due to a combination of factors, the most important of which are the successful treatment of gonococcal urethritis, the improvement in the technique of urethroplasty, the development of smaller endoscopic instruments, such as the 24 Fr resectoscope, and the use of inert materials for indwelling urethral catheters. In addition to these factors, the improved management of ruptured urethra has reduced the number and severity of post-traumatic strictures. A factor which has improved the time interval between dilatation of urethral strictures is the removal of the formalin oven, which was used for sterilizing or, more correctly, disinfecting urethral dilators. After this process, despite careful rinsing, a thin film of aldehyde remained on the surface of the instruments and this was transferred onto the surface of the stricture with the next dilatation, thus aggravating the fibrosis. All urethral dilators can now be sterilized either by autoclave, ethylene oxide gas or soaking in a disinfectant.

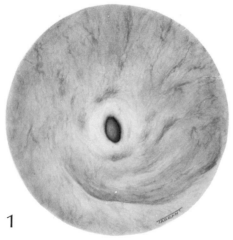

1

Stricture

1

If a stricture of the urethra is encountered at urethral endoscopy, it will probably be too stenosed to allow the further passage of the endoscope until dilatation has been performed. This can be carried out either under direct vision or using one form of urethral dilator. This is an operation which should never be relegated to inexperienced staff as a false passage will severely aggravate what may at first be a simple stricture easily treated by occasional dilatation. A rigid stricture may require urethrotomy which, again, can be performed under direct vision, or blindly with the aid of a urethrotome.

Instruments required

2

Endoscopic dilators For dilating under direct vision, an endoscope fitted with an appropriate dilating beak will be required for use with the 0° telescope. The dilating beak may be a rigid probe or a flexible filiform attachment which can be screwed to the tip of the endoscope sheath.

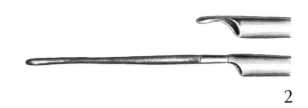

2

3

Solid dilators For blind dilatation, metal or plastic dilators may be used. Of the rigid metal dilators, Clutton's sounds appear to be popular with most urologists, as the angle is the most convenient for manipulating the curvature of the male urethra. Alternatively, plastic bougies may be preferred. These are available either as filiforms with followers that screw on to the end of the filiforms, or as graduated sizes of dilating bougies.

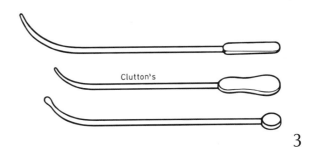

Clutton's

3

4 & 5

The endoscopic urethrotome For endoscopic urethrotomy, either the rigid urethrotome with a blade in the beak of the sheath, or a retractable urethrotome with the blade mounted on a carrier may be used, so that the cutting edge can be withdrawn completely within the sheath. Each will require a 0° direct vision telescope.

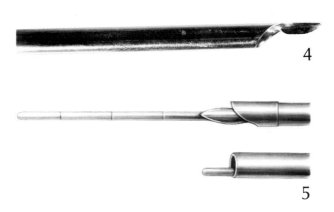

4

5

Preparation

The preparation for urethral dilatation is the same as for any urethral instrumentation. The position and the towel draping of the patient should be as for cystourethroscopy. General anaesthesia is probably advisable for the first dilatation, when the extent of the stricture has yet to be explored. Any subsequent dilatation can usually be carried out under local anaesthesia (lignocaine 2 per cent in methyloxycellulose jelly, with chlorhexidine 0.05 per cent added).

Sterilization of endoscopes and dilators

As for sterilization of cystourethroscopes, the most satisfactory method is by low-pressure steam with formaldehyde.

The operation

Dilatation by direct vision

The face of the stricture is approached with the beak of the panendoscope or the flexible filiform tip. This is threaded gently through the minute orifice of the stricture, under the direct vision of the 0° telescope. Repeated withdrawal of the dilating beak will ensure that it is maintaining the correct channel of the stricture, as each time the tip of the beak is inserted into the orifice of the stricture it disappears temporarily from view. Most strictures are less than 1 cm long and very shortly the healthy urethra beyond comes into view.

6

The shaft of the dilating endoscope will probably be only 17 Fr in size. After dilating the stricture with the beak of the endoscope up to 17 Fr, further dilatation can be achieved by using a sheath which is 17 Fr at the tip and 24 Fr at the eyepiece end.

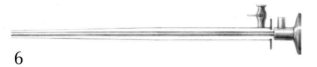

6

Alternatively, a filiform guide can be passed under visual control. If a urethroscope with a large operating channel is available (24 Fr), the optimum method of dilatation with a filiform is to pass the bougie down the endoscope under direct vision with the 0° telescope. A large size endoscope will be necessary as the screw thread on the filiform has to be drawn down the lumen of the endoscope. The orifice of the stricture face can be seen and the filiform directed into it. Once the filiform has been passed through the stricture the endoscope is withdrawn, leaving the filiform *in situ*.

With the filiform *in situ* and its tip in the bladder, follower dilators are screwed onto the end of the filiform. Before advancing the filiform follower through the stricture, it is advisable to ensure that the screw thread is gripping satisfactorily and is completely closed. A gentle pull should be made on the two ends of the thread to ensure that the joint is secure. Progressively larger followers are passed until the stricture is adequately dilated.

Urethrotomy by direct vision

7

If the stricture is very rigid and the beak of the dilating endoscope makes little impression without the use of excessive force, it is advisable to use the direct vision urethrotome. The stricture face is cut gently and a little at a time until the whole stricture has been divided on its ventral aspect. The urethrotome knife should not be turned into the 12 o'clock position for fear of damaging the corpora cavernosa. In the hands of a skilled endoscopist it should be possible to negotiate all strictures under direct vision.

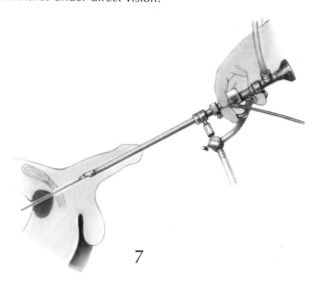

7

Either the rigid or the retractable urethrotome can be used in conjunction with a fine ureteric catheter, passed through the stricture under direct vision, to act as a guide for the direction in which the urethrotome knife should cut, particularly when used for longer strictures.

Following endoscopic urethrotomy, a soft silicone catheter should be inserted into the bladder to reduce the risk of intramural extravasation of urine into the interstices of the wall of the urethra, thus increasing the postoperative fibrosis and recurrence of stricture, as well as increasing the risk of bacteraemia.

8a & b

Passing the catheter after endoscopic urethrotomy

Passage of the catheter can be aided by the use of the catheter guide passed with the urethrotome and lying over its sheath. This guide is a split tube of only ⅝ of a circle, and the guide can therefore be slid over the catheter after its self-retaining balloon has been inflated.

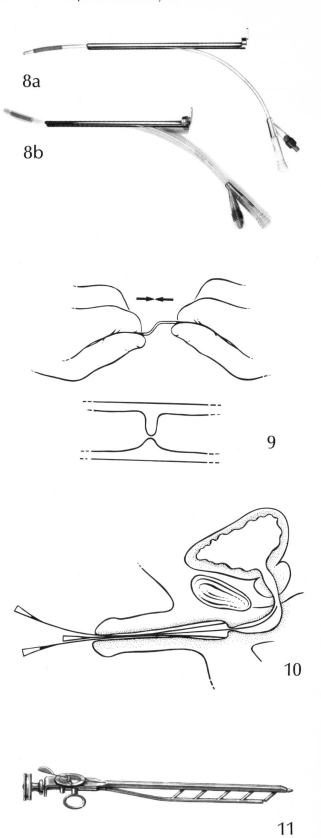

8a

8b

9

It may help to shape the tip of the filiform into a dog-leg to give some rotational control.

Once the filiform is in the bladder and the operator is certain it has not buckled or coiled up in the distal urethra the followers of increasing size are screwed on in turn and passed through the stricture.

10

Multiple filiform bougies may be passed together at the same time until one passes the stricture (the 'faggot' method). Although this is popular in all textbooks, in practice it is not as effective as the descriptions would have us believe.

9

Blind urethrotomy

11

Urethrotomy is best carried out by means of the viewing urethrotome, but this does require the special skill of endoscopy. Blind urethrotomy can be carried out by the use of the Otis urethrotome. This can be attached to a filiform bougie, and used in the form of a follower. After passing the Otis urethrotome the blade is extruded to a given distance and counterpressure is applied by opening the opposing bar. The knife blade is then slid down the full length of the urethra as the instrument is withdrawn. The knife edge of the urethrotome should always be directed ventrally and never towards the corpora cavernosa, otherwise any penetration of the corpora can result in severe chordee. It is essential that the operator is familiar with the use of this instrument as severe bleeding can occur from the corpus spongiosum. In fact, the author believes that there would appear to be no place for this instrument when the surgeon has mastered the technique of urethral endoscopy, as urethrotomy under visual control is safer, more effective and much less likely to be followed by severe urethral bleeding or subsequent chordee deformity.

10

11

Postoperative care and complications

Dilatation of a urethral stricture is probably one of the most difficult operations in urology to perform successfully on all occasions. There is no justification for delegating this procedure to a junior member of staff. The more experienced the surgeon performing the dilatations, the less frequently will dilatation of a stricture be required.

Haemorrhage

Bleeding following urethral dilatation usually indicates that the stretching has been excessive, that too much force has been used, or, worse still, that a false passage has been made. The patient should be encouraged to drink copiously and pass water frequently. If the bleeding is heavy and persistent it may be necessary to insert a catheter.

False passage

Any complete breach of the full thickness of the urethra demands urinary diversion by a suprapubic cystotomy for 4 or 5 days until the false passage has healed. A breach of the mucosa only will heal of its own accord, but, in due course may aggravate the urethral stricture.

Bacteraemia

Many patients with urethral stricture have urinary tract infection. Whether the organisms are present in the urine, or merely come to light when the fibrous tissue of the stricture is split, or cut, is a moot point. The fact remains that many patients, after urethral dilatation, will suffer from a bacteraemia. A positive blood culture can often be obtained within 5 min of a urethral dilatation.

Instillation of chlorhexidine with the local anaesthetic will be adequate prophylaxis in the majority of patients. Occasionally patients may be encountered who still show symptoms of bacteraemia despite this prophylactic precaution. If this occurs, for subsequent dilatations, in addition to the chlorhexidine instilled beforehand, 5 ml of chlorhexidine in glycerine or in methyloxycellulose jelly should be instilled immediately after the dilatation of the urethra. After the final dilator has been passed, a catheter can be introduced and 50 ml of 1:5000 chlorhexidine can be instilled into the bladder so that the first passage of urine over the split stricture bed will be sterile. Finally, coverage by an appropriate antibiotic for 24 hours before and 48 hours after dilatation is advisable.

Calculi

Stones associated with a stricture are usually an indication of past if not present infection. The stricture may preclude the use of the lithotrite and suprapubic lithotomy is advisable.

All the complications, in particular haemorrhage and bacteraemia, can also follow endoscopic urethrotomy. However, they should be considerably reduced by urinary diversion via an indwelling urethral catheter.

Indications for urethroplasty

When the interval between dilatation of the urethral stricture can no longer be extended, and the patient has stabilized to a pattern of dilatation at regular intervals, then the possibility of urethroplasty should be discussed. If the dilatation becomes increasingly difficult with each successive instrumentation, then urethroplasty should be considered.

Further reading

Mitchell, J. P. The endoscopic surgery of urethral stricture: urethrotomy. In: Mitchell, J. P. Endoscopic operative urology. Bristol: John Wright, 1981: 176–195

Ravasini, G. Die kontrollierte Urethroskopische Elektrotomic für die Behandlung der Harnröhrenstricturen. Urologia 1957; 24: 229–231

Sachse, H. Zur behandlung der Harnröhrenstriktur: Die transurethrale Schlitzug unter Sicht mit scharfem Schnitt. Fortschritte der Medizin: 1974; 92: 12–15

Smith, P. J., Dunn, M., Dounis, A. Sachse optical urethrotome in management of urethral stricture in the male. Journal of the Royal Society of Medicine 1978; 71: 596–599

Transurethral biopsy of the bladder and diathermy destruction of bladder neoplasms

J. P. Mitchell   CBE, TD, MS, FRCS, FRCS(Ed)
Honorary Professor of Surgery (Urology), University of Bristol, UK

BIOPSY OF THE BLADDER

Preoperative

Indications

A biopsy should be obtained in all neoplasms or suspected neoplasms of the bladder, since the mode of treatment and prognosis will depend on the depth of invasion and histology. Also, further biopsies should be taken from tumour recurrences, especially when they appear to have changed macroscopically. If tumours are multiple and differ in appearance, it is advisable to take biopsies of each.

Any unexplained appearance of the bladder mucosa should also be biopsied. Occasionally, a suspected diagnosis of 'carcinoma *in situ*' of the bladder mucosa demands quadrant biopsy (one bite in each quadrant of the bladder), even though the mucosa may appear normal on endoscopy.

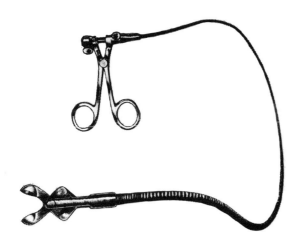

1

Contraindications

There should be scarcely any contraindications to the biopsy of the bladder wall, but a brief delay may be justified while infection is controlled. Biopsy taken from the bladder wall when there is urinary infection present can result in bacteraemia unless antibiotic coverage is provided.

The minute anterior urethra of an infant precludes the introduction of any biopsy instrument, but a perineal urethrotomy via the wider bulbous urethra will usually allow the passage of the smallest sheath of the infant's resectoscope (8–10 Fr), though the indications for a biopsy in an infant are rare. A child's urethra will admit the 14–16 Fr resectoscope and an adult urethra, even with a stricture, can be dilated to 24 Fr for the standard resectoscope sheath without any harm.

Orientation and endoscopic assessment in a small capacity bladder may be difficult, but this should not prevent the taking of a biopsy.

Extreme care must be taken in the female bladder, as the wall can be very thin. Certain disease processes, such as tuberculosis of the bladder or refractory ulcerative cystitis (Hunner's ulcer), can reduce the thickness of the bladder wall. Even so, if histological evidence is required, there should be no hesitation in attempting to take a biopsy of any bladder lesion.

Instruments

1

The essential feature of any biopsy forceps is that the bite of tissue taken should be large enough to provide a representative histological section. The biopsy forceps designed to pass down the operating channel of a conventional-sized cystoscope are too small to obtain a substantial bite of a proliferative tumour, but are ideal for taking a minute piece of mucosa of the bladder when, for example, carcinoma *in situ* is suspected.

2

Alternatively, the rigid 'cold cup' biopsy forceps can be used with greater accuracy, both in aiming at the target site and in the volume of tissue removed. There are two types, with blades either above or below the telescope. Neither of these minute biopsy forceps can be relied upon to cut cleanly and, in most instances, the small bite of mucosa is in fact avulsed.

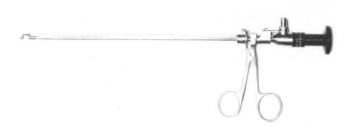

2

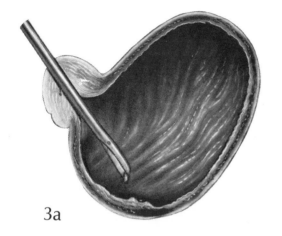

3a

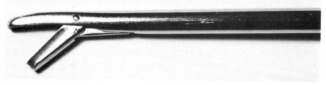

3b

3a & b

Lowsley forceps have the disadvantage that no view can be obtained until the blades of the instrument are separated as the telescope is passed down the interior of the instrument.

The jaws of these biopsy forceps should be checked before use to ensure that the blades are overlapping when they cut, as the fulcrum can wear so that the blades only meet, in which case the tissue biopsy will be avulsed rather than cut cleanly.

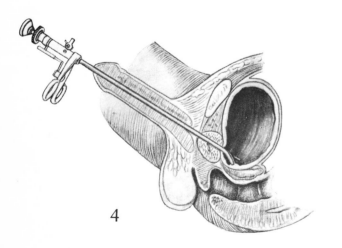

4

4

Young's and Riches' forceps give the operator a better view of the tissue to be biopsied, but their calibre is as large as the smallest sheath of the adult resectoscope. A 24 Fr sheath, which is available for most resectoscopes, is probably the most suitable for taking a biopsy and has the advantage that any bleeding point from the biopsy site can be controlled by diathermy coagulation.

The operation

5 & 6

Biopsy by Lowsley's or Riches' forceps

The instrument is passed in the same manner as a cystoscope, but it is advisable to leave the water tap running so that there is a flow through the instrument, preventing debris or blood clot from obscuring the view. After locating the lesion, as large a biopsy as possible is then taken from its margin.

Biopsy by diathermy resectoscope

See description in chapter on 'Transurethral biopsy of the bladder and diathermy destruction of bladder neoplasms', pp. 729–738.

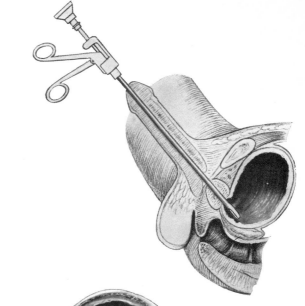

5

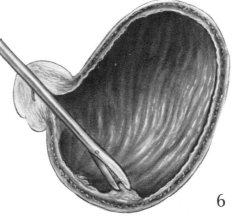

6

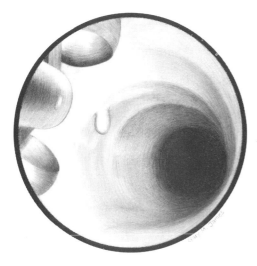

7

7

Biopsy by cold cup biopsy forceps

The object is to remove a representative sample of mucosa, approximately 1 mm in diameter. At the same operation random biopsies of the bladder mucosa can be taken in each of its quadrants. Each biopsy site should be inspected for bleeding and any persistent oozing of blood should be touched with the diathermy electrode.

DIATHERMY DESTRUCTION OF BLADDER NEOPLASMS

Preoperative

Indications

An adequate biopsy should always be obtained of any new bladder tumour, or of any recurrence with altered appearance, before it is destroyed by diathermy.

When there is no macroscopic evidence on cystoscopy of infiltration of the bladder wall, a tumour should be treated by diathermy destruction. Small neoplasms, i.e. less than 1 cm in diameter, will probably have been destroyed *in toto* by the biopsy, but if there is any residual tumour remaining this can be destroyed by cystofulguration. This method is not suitable for larger neoplasms as the core of the fulgurated mass may still remain viable. For tumours up to 5 cm in diameter, transurethral resection is preferable, as this gives total destruction of the proliferative parts of the tumour and fulguration of its base into the bladder wall.

Any bladder neoplasm which is palpable bimanually as an area of induration, or seems to be tethered to the lateral wall of the pelvis (T3 or T4, UICC), although not curable, is operable by the transurethral route. However, only the intravesical, peripheral part of the tumour can be resected. The residual tumour, beyond the limits of the resection, is then treated by high-voltage therapy.

Contraindications

Any tumour larger than 5 cm in diameter will probably be difficult to resect transurethrally as the view will be obscured by the extent of waving tumour fronds. Such tumours can be reduced in size by Helmstein's intravesical pressure therapy. A large balloon catheter is introduced into the bladder and distended to a pressure just above the patient's diastolic blood pressure. This causes necrosis of a large part of the tumour, which can then be approached easily by transurethral resection 3 weeks later.

Tumour in a diverticulum should be removed by diverticulectomy. Gross prostatic hypertrophy is often a contraindication to a transurethral resection of a coexistent bladder tumour, as the adenoma may obstruct access to the part of the bladder wall bearing the tumour. This will almost certainly precipitate an attack of acute retention. This is therefore better treated by an open transvesical prostatectomy with open diathermy destruction of the bladder tumour. A small adenoma of prostate or a bladder neck obstruction is not a contraindication to transurethral resection of a bladder tumour as both the adenoma and the bladder neoplasm can be resected under the same anaesthetic without any increased risk[1] of seedling implant.

Preparation and position of patient

The patient should be shaved and otherwise prepared as for cystoscopy. A previous intravenous pyelogram should always be performed to exclude any similar neoplasm in the upper urinary tract. A haemoglobin estimation is advisable if there has been recent heavy haematuria.

Anaesthesia

Although small neoplasms of the bladder wall can be destroyed when the patient is under a local anaesthetic, this method of anaesthesia is inadequate for tumours in the region of the trigone, which is much more sensitive than the rest of the bladder wall. Single tumours larger than 1 cm in diameter, or multiple tumours, demand a general anaesthetic or epidural anaesthesia with good relaxation.

Tumours on the lateral wall of the bladder may have their base situated in the proximity of the obturator nerve, and troublesome adductor spasms may embarrass the operator if the anaesthetic does not include an efficient relaxant.

Instruments required

For cystodiathermy a series of three different sizes of cystodiathermy blunt electrodes are advisable, graduated from 4 Fr to the largest size which the 22 Fr cystoscope will accept via its operating channel.

8

For transurethral resection there is a variety of electric resectoscopes available (*see* chapter on 'Transurethral prostatectomy', pp. 739–743), but all of these operate on the same principle: a loop of wire, activated by short-wave diathermy current, is withdrawn into the operating sheath of the resectoscope.

The sheath of the resectoscope should not be more than 26 Fr and preferably 24 Fr. For resection of bladder tumours the loop should be of fine wire alloy which does not fragment with short-wave diathermy current.

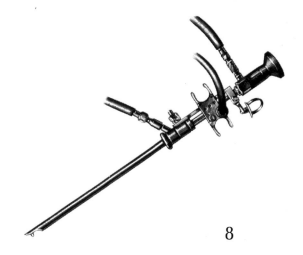

8

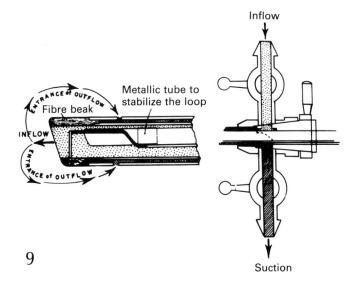

Inflow

Metallic tube to
stabilize the loop

ENTRANCE of OUTFLOW

Fibre beak

INFLOW

ENTRANCE of OUTFLOW

Suction

9

9

The continuous flow resectoscope has proved to be a great advance in the management of bladder tumours: it keeps the bladder at a constant volume so that the tumour does not recede out of view and out of reach as the bladder distends.

10

All resectoscopes should be designed so they can be used just as comfortably in the anterior part of the bladder as on the posterior wall (fully rotatable). This is difficult to achieve with the fixed pillar of the telescope which transmits the fibre illumination. A laterally fixed pillar (i.e. 90° from the vertical) will allow access to each side of the bladder without the light pillar impacting against the patient's thigh in the endoscopy position of the bladder.

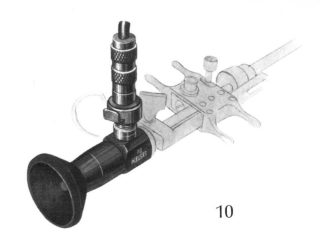

10

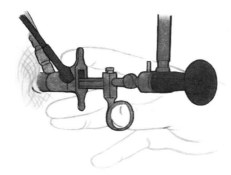

11a

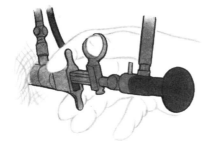

11b

11a & b

Alternatively, completely free rotation can be achieved using a direct vision telescope (0° angle of view) with no beak on the sheath of the resectosope. However, a 0° telescope has limited view and access to the anterior wall of the bladder close to the bladder neck.

In surgical diathermy for transurethral resection the machine must provide a high-frequency sine wave output for cutting under water, and this type of current can only be produced either by a valve oscillating or a transistorized generator. The spark-gap diathermy will give excellent coagulation but is unsatisfactory for cutting under water.

The operation

12 & 13

Cystofulguration

This should be performed only after adequate biopsy of the tumour has been obtained. With the blunt electrode of suitable size passed via the cystoscope, the tip is placed in contact with the tumour. Activation of the diathermy current at the appropriate setting will produce white coagulation of the tumour surface. If the strength of the current is increased, fulguration will occur with some black charring. This, however, does not produce better tumour destruction or haemostasis than simple white coagulation.

Transurethral resection of the tumour

The 24 and 26 Fr resectoscope sheath is either passed under direct vision using a 0° angle telescope, or it may be passed blindly with the aid of the Timberlake obturator, which gives a conveniently angled beak to the instrument. Once in the bladder the 0° telescope is removed and replaced by the 30° telescope. The tumour can be viewed with the water flowing but, as the tumour is lying on the bladder wall, it appears to recede while the bladder distends. Allowance must be made during resection for the movement of the target. In this respect, removal of a bladder tumour is considerably more difficult than resection of the prostate or bladder neck, which do not move as the bladder distends. The continuous flow resectoscope obviates this difficulty.

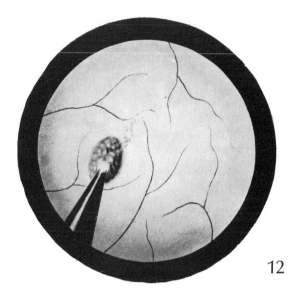

12

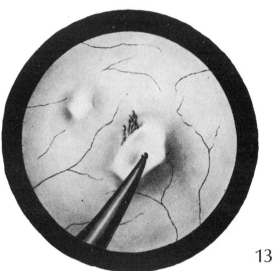

13

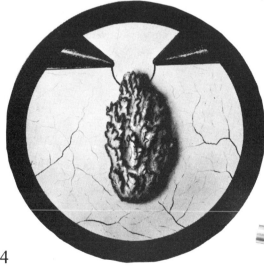

14

14 & 15

The resection begins at the part of the tumour farthest away from the telescope, and the cuts are always made towards the operator. The objective should be to cut into the muscle of the bladder wall so that shallow infiltration of the muscle layer will be destroyed.

15

16

It is worth noting that when the bladder is empty the bladder wall may be folded. Consequently there is a risk that the loop may cut across one of the folds and perforate the wall of the bladder.

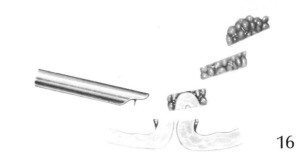

16

17a & b

Difficulty of access may be experienced in resecting tumours of the anterior wall of the bladder, particularly when these are near the bladder neck. Suprapubic pressure applied with the left hand helps to bring the target area into range.

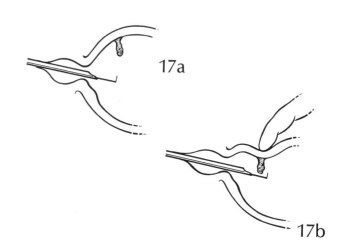

17a

17b

18

When the entire tumour has been resected so that the bladder wall appears flat, the base of the tumour, which should be well down into muscle, is coagulated with the button electrode. Firstly this produces complete haemostasis, and secondly, it destroys any tumour cells which remain on the surface or may have infiltrated deeper into the muscle layer.

Evacuation of bladder tumour cuttings

The Ellick evacuator filled with fluid is then attached to the end of the resectoscope sheath and the cuttings are aspirated. The resectoscope is removed and a bimanual examination is performed while the patient is still anaesthetized, in order to confirm that there is no induration in the tumour area. The bladder is then drained by an indwelling catheter. During transurethral resection of a bladder tumour, every effort must made to cut through the submucosal layer and into the muscle layer, which will leave the bladder wall thin. A catheter should be left indwelling.

With simple cystodiathermy fulguration or transurethral resection of a well pedunculated tumour, the catheter can usually be removed after 24–48 hours, when the drainage is clear of blood.

18

Postoperative complications

Perforation of the bladder wall

19a & b

In a successful biopsy, an attempt is made to take a piece of the bladder wall, as well as the margin of the lesion, with the result that the thickness of the bladder wall at this site may be considerably reduced.

After destruction of a bladder neoplasm, perforation of the bladder wall may be noticed at the time of operation as a hole appearing in the bladder wall with a dark cobweb area beyond. It may also become apparent, when the pieces of tumour are evacuated with the Ellick evacuator, that an incomplete bladder return is obtained. If the perforation has been missed during the operation, it will soon be obvious as the patient recovers from the anaesthetic. The pulse rate rises, the abdomen appears rigid and the patient's general condition deteriorates due to absorption of extravasated fluid which may result in significant electrolytic disturbances.

Perforation, however, may be delayed and occur 2–7 days after operation, in which case it is due to delayed breakdown of a necrotic area from the diathermy destruction (fulguration). The treatment required is immediate drainage of the retropubic area. A suprapubic catheter in the bladder is rarely necessary unless the perforation is extensive. It is usually sufficient to insert a drain into the retropubic space with an indwelling urethral catheter in the bladder.

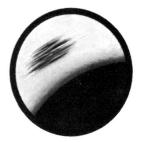

19a

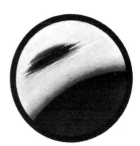

19b

Spasm from stimulation of the obturator nerve

Considerable inconvenience at operation sometimes arises from stimulation of the obturator nerve, which lies along the lateral wall of the distended bladder at 3 and 9 o'clock. If a tumour appears to be situated in this area of the bladder wall, a violent adductor spasm is liable to occur when the diathermy electrode reaches the sensitive area. This spasm can be so violent that it has been known to result in perforation of the bladder by the electrode. Anaesthesia using an effective muscle relaxant is helpful.

Also, cutting slowly with diathermy, using repeated brief touches on the footswitch, reduces the violence of the adductor contractions. Infiltration with 1.5 per cent glycine, using a long spinal needle, into the perivesical tissue just beneath the point on the lateral wall of the bladder where the tumour is situated, may give relief from the troublesome adductor spasm. Saline should not be used for this infiltration as it will continue to conduct the activating current.

Haemorrhage

After transurethral resection of a bladder neoplasm, and even after a simple biopsy, the site may bleed profusely. The loop of the resectoscope is changed for a coagulating button, and the bleeding points fulgurated until the fluid return is clear.

20 a–d

Extreme care must be taken during the postoperative period to ensure free drainage of the bladder. Any obstruction, resulting in distension of the bladder wall, will stretch the coagulated vessels and renewed bleeding will occur. A closed drainage system should be employed, preferably with the capability of performing irrigations.

If there is blood or pus in the bladder, irrigation may be advisable. An irrigation apparatus may be connected to the bladder catheter by means of a Y-junction. If the bulb of a Higginson's syringe is incorporated in the lower limb (outflow) of the Y-junction, forced irrigation and suction can be applied to the bladder in order to clear any clot or bolus of mucus. The rubber bulb of the Higginson's is emptied into the drainage bag. By changing the position of the clamps it is then refilled from the irrigation bottle. With both limbs clamped beyond the bulb, forced irrigation and suction can be applied directly to the bladder.

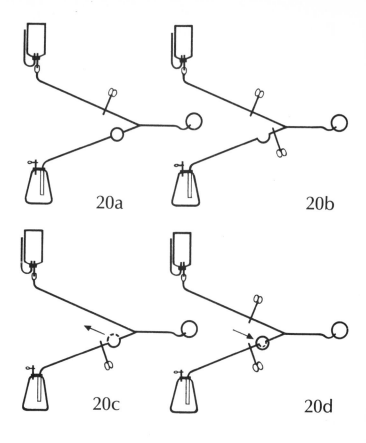

20a   20b
20c   20d

Further reading

Blandy, J. P. Transurethral resection. London: Pitman Medical, 1971

Cifuentes Delatte, L. Cirurgia urologica endoscopica. 2nd ed. Madrid: Editorial Paz Montalvo SA, 1980

Greene, L. F., Segura, J. W., eds. Transurethral surgery. Philadelphia: W. B. Sanders Co., 1979

Iglesias, J. J., Sporer, A., Gellman, A. C. *et al.* New Iglesias resectoscope with continuous irrigation. Journal of Urology 1975; 114: 929–933

Miller, A., Mitchell, J. P., Brown, N. J. The Bristol Bladder Tumour Registry. British Journal of Urology 1969; 41: Suppl. 1

Mitchell, J. P. Endoscopic operative urology. Bristol: John Wright, 1981

Morera, J. Reseccion transuretral. Buenos Aires: Lopez Libreros Editores, 1977

Reuter, H. J. Atlas of urologic endoscopic surgery. English ed. Philadelphia: W. B. Saunders, 1982

Transurethral prostatectomy*

Herbert Brendler MD
Professor, Department of Urology, The Mount Sinai Medical Center, New York, USA

Preoperative

Indications

In the past, the transurethral route, as opposed to one or another of the open operations, i.e. retropubic, suprapubic (transvesical) or perineal, has, except in a few specialized centres, usually been reserved for glands estimated to be 40 g or less. The present trend, however, is in favour of transurethral resection for glands of virtually any size, so that at least 60–70 per cent of all prostatectomies in the United States are now being performed by this technique. Occasionally, very large glands may require two sittings for completion. Under certain circumstances the transurethral operation may be difficult, even impossible, for example in patients with severe arthritis involving the hip joints which interferes with abduction. Strictures of the anterior urethra do not ordinarily constitute a contraindication because they can be bypassed via a temporary perineal urethrotomy.

Equipment

Instruments

These should always be in perfect repair, and replacements and spare parts must be available. Sheaths include sizes No. 24, 26 and 28 Fr. The type of working element is optional, e.g. Stern-McCarthy, Iglesias, Nesbit, Baumrucker, Storz, etc. Since the cutting wire loops are subject to breakage they should be checked before use. Loops may also need to be adjusted to ensure proper shearing action when drawn back into the sheath. Telescopes include the foreoblique, right angle (either as part of the resectoscope or a separate cystoscope), retrograde and forward-vision (Vest) lenses. Illumination may be by electric bulb or the fibreoptic system. A complete set of sounds should be available, as well as filiforms and followers. Manual irrigators such as the Ellick evacuator and the Toomey piston syringe are essential, with stiff, large-calibre rubber tubing and tight adaptor connections.

Electrosurgical unit

This provides cutting and coagulation currents. The unit should be checked and adjusted periodically.

Irrigating fluids

Non-haemolyzing solutions, such as 1.1 per cent glycine, are generally used, although some urologists still prefer sterile water because of better visibility.

Table

Leg supports should be arranged to permit adequate manoeuvrability for the resectionist. A commodious drainage tray is essential.

Anaesthesia

Spinal anaesthesia is preferred as it permits early detection of abdominal pain and rigidity in the event of perforation and extravasation.

Preoperative management

In cases of impaired renal function, or ureteric reflux, a preliminary suprapubic cystostomy may have to be performed. In addition to protecting the kidneys, this considerably shortens and simplifies subsequent transurethral prostatectomy by allowing continuous run-off of irrigating medium.

The value of prophylactic antibiotic therapy is uncertain. Many urologists prefer to withhold antibacterials unless they are indicated.

An ample supply of matched whole blood should be immediately available.

* This chapter has been reprinted from the 3rd edition

The operation

1

Inspection of prostatic urethra at the level of the verumontanum shows hypertrophied lateral lobes.

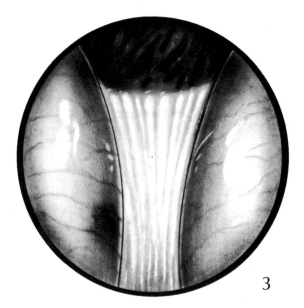

2

The resectoscope has now been advanced proximally, permitting the enlarged middle lobe to come into view.

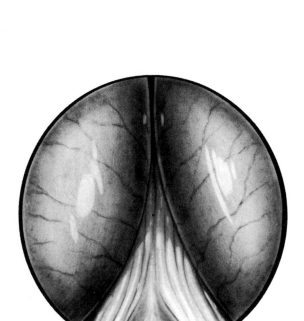

3

As the instrument enters the bladder, the enlarged lateral lobes separate further. Note the vertical markings on the elevated middle lobe – the so-called 'waterfall' appearance.

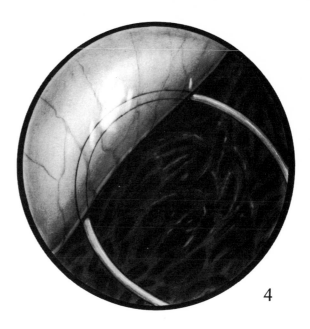

4

4

The bladder neck is resected first. Operation commences on the roof, or anterior aspect, at 11 o'clock and is carried around counter-clockwise until the right side of the bladder neck has been cleared.

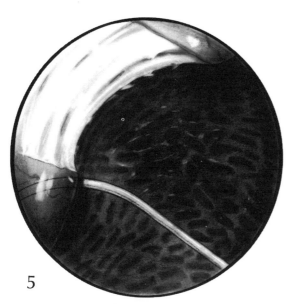

5

5

The first cut has been made, exposing the circular muscle fibres which mark the plane between the hyperplastic portion and the 'surgical capsule', i.e. true prostate. The adenoma is thinnest anteriorly, usually not more than one or two bites deep. Beginning anteriorly enables the resectionist to identify the external limits of the operation early. Using the circular fibres as a landmark, the loop follows the plane of cleavage exactly as the enucleating finger does in open prostatectomy.

6

As resection proceeds, bleeding arterial branches are spot-fulgurated. Generalized searing devitalizes large areas of prostatic tissue and is to be avoided. Resection carried deeply into the circular fibres may cause bleeding from venous sinuses which is often difficult to control. Deep resection may also lead to perforation and extravasation. The appearance of fatty tissue is a danger sign.

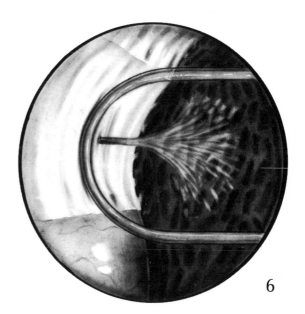

6

7

After the right side of the bladder neck has been resected, the identical procedure is carried out on the left, beginning at 1 o'clock. Midline tissue on the floor between 5 and 7 o'clock is then resected, with the aim of lowering the bladder neck to the level of the trigone. A sizeable middle lobe has to be handled with special care to avoid damaging the ureteric orifices or trigone. It is in this area that the latter may be undermined, leading to perforation and extravasation.

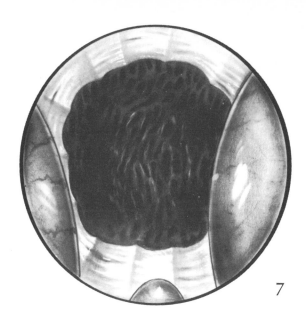

7

8

Attention is now turned to the right lateral lobe. If this is large, it is usually advantageous to establish the plane of cleavage peripherally at the outset, again using the loop in a manner similar to the enucleating finger. This speeds up subsequent resection of the lobe and also facilitates control of bleeding. With smaller lobes not more than three to four bites thick, identifying the cleavage plane initially is not always necessary. The verumontanum is an important landmark in avoiding damage to the external sphincter.

8

9

With the right lobe out of the way, removal of the left one is much easier. Systematic resection is accomplished in the same manner as on the other side.

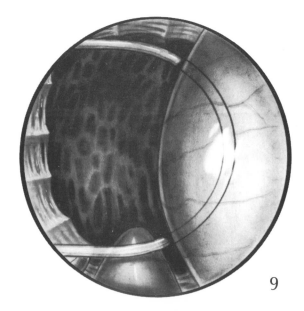

9

10

Following removal of middle and lateral lobes, the remaining tissue at the apex is carefully resected, taking care to preserve the verumontanum. Final trimming is accomplished and bleeding vessels are fulgurated. All loose fragments are evacuated from the bladder. Terminal inspection of the fossa with the resectoscope situated just distal to the verumontanum should present a well coned-out appearance without residual adenoma. A 22 or 24 Fr Foley catheter is inserted and the bag inflated with 20–30 ml, taking care that this is done in the bladder, *not* the prostatic fossa. This will permit the muscular layer of the surgical capsule to contract, thereby minimizing any ooze which may be present. Return irrigations should be clear or pink-tinged at the conclusion of the operation. Approximately 100 ml of irrigant is left indwelling when the patient is sent to the recovery room.

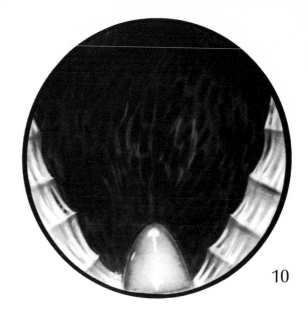

10

Postoperative care

Upon arrival in the recovery room the catheter is attached to straight drainage. Gentle irrigation with 30–60 ml of sterile saline or water at room temperature is carried out at intervals, using a bulb syringe. Frequency of irrigation will depend on the degree of bleeding, but should be kept to a minimum in order to allow blood vessels to seal off. Mannitol is useful in promoting diuresis for purposes of self-irrigation. Catheter traction is usually unnecessary, but may help if bleeding is moderate to severe.

The use of three-way catheters and continuous drip irrigation is favoured by some urologists, but this requires constant monitoring to be certain the bladder does not inadvertently become distended as the result of obstructing clots or tissue debris in the outflow channel.

Severe bleeding in the immediate postoperative period, which cannot be controlled by moderate traction on the catheter requires reinsertion of the resectoscope, evacuation of blood and clots, and a search for bleeding vessels. Sometimes simple bladder decompression will control bleeding by permitting the distended fossa to contract.

In the uncomplicated case the urethral catheter can usually be removed in 48–72 hours. Antibiotic coverage is provided while the catheter is in place and for varying periods after its removal, depending on urine cultures.

The patient is ordinarily discharged one week after surgery, and returns for his first postoperative visit in 3–4 weeks. Further check-ups are scheduled as needed.

Illustrations by Arthur E. Cottrell and Douglas P. Hammersley

Litholapaxy, lithotrity and evacuation of foreign bodies from the bladder

J. P. Mitchell CBE, TD, MS, FRCS, FRCS(Ed)
Honorary Professor of Surgery (Urology), University of Bristol, UK

Preoperative

Indications for litholapaxy and lithotrity

Phosphate calculi up to 3 cm in diameter in the bladder can be crushed and evacuated in fragments. The blind lithotrite can be used for large stones, as this is a stronger instrument and the size of the stone makes it easier to find without any visual aid. Smaller stones of 2 cm or less diameter will require a viewing lithotrite, for it can be a tedious and time-consuming operation trying to detect and grasp smaller stones with a blind lithotrite.

Contraindications

Stones larger than 3 cm diameter are best removed by suprapubic lithotomy. Some surgeons may attempt to crush stones up to 5 cm diameter, but suprapubic removal of larger stones is quicker, less traumatic and carries considerably less risk of inducing septicaemia. Stones in a diverticulum generally cannot be grasped with either the blind or the viewing lithotrite.

If the prostate is considerably enlarged, lithotrity may be difficult and postoperative retention is very likely to occur; calculi associated with prostatic hypertrophy, therefore, are better removed at open operation concom-

itant with prostatic enucleation. If a transurethral resection is preferred, a two-stage procedure should be considered when the litholapaxy or lithotrity is likely to require more than half an hour: the risk of septicaemia becomes greater with prolonged manipulation.

In the presence of infection litholapaxy should be delayed until the infection is under control and the patient has a therapeutic serum level of antibiotics.

If the urethra is too small to admit the lithotrite readily, suprapubic lithotomy should be used.

Preparation of the patient and anaesthesia

The patient should be shaved, prepared and positioned as for cystoscopy. A recent intravenous pyelogram should be available to give a clear visualization of the number of stones, their approximate size, and whether they are lying in a diverticulum. General or epidural anaesthesia is essential. Preliminary cystoscopy is performed to inspect the vesical calculi, the bladder and the prostatic urethra.

If infection is present, the patient should be given antibiotics preoperatively; even if the urine is sterile on culture, the risk of infection within the bladder calculus makes it advisable to give antibiotic cover empirically during the procedure and for 5 days after litholapaxy.

Instruments

Blind lithotrite

The locking device on the blind lithotrite varies considerably and the surgeon is advised to familiarize himself with the method of locking before introducing the instrument into the urethra.

1

Endoscopic lithotrity forceps

Small bladder stones, up to 1 cm in diameter, can be crushed with the simple lithotrity forceps. This instrument is passed through the 23 Fr cystoscopy sheath. Larger stones cannot be grasped in the jaws, which are set on a fulcrum. Any stone more than 1 cm in size will slide out of the jaws. Also, the fulcrum is not strong enough to crush hard stones for which the conventional type of lithotrite is more suitable by virtue of its stouter construction.

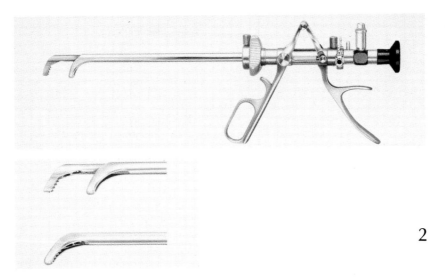

1

2

Endoscopic lithotrite

Again the surgeon should familiarize himself with the mechanism of this instrument. He should also know how to strip the instrument down should the blades jam while attempting to crush the stone. This instrument is more delicately constructed than the blind lithotrite but stronger than the endoscopic lithotrity forceps. It should never be used, therefore, for large calculi (more than 2 cm in diameter). The instrument should be tested to ensure that both blades of the lithotrite are well within the field of vision before it is introduced into the urethra. This visual test of blades must be carried out underwater. Certain lithotrites require a 30° fore-oblique telescope, while others need a 70° or even a 90° angle of view.

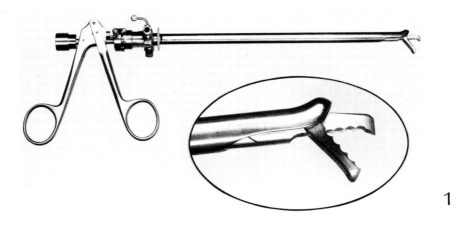

2

3

The hydraulic lithotriptor and ultrasonic lithotriptor

Larger stones (more than 2 cm in diameter) may be fragmented, either by high-frequency discharge of explosive gases or by high-intensity ultrasonic bombardment. The principles of the hydraulic lithotriptor is to generate a small bubble of hydrogen and oxygen from electrolytic hydrolysis and to explode this bubble by a spark across the electrodes. This explosive discharge can be regulated up to a frequency of 80 cycles per second. It should be noted that mucosal damage can occur with the hydraulic lithotriptor if its electrodes are allowed to come nearer than 1 cm to the mucosa.

Alternatively, by applying the transducer head directly to the bladder stone the ultrasonic stone destructor will fragment the calculus without the risk of damage to the bladder mucosa.

Both these sophisticated instruments are expensive and require the special technical expertise only likely to be available in a well-equipped department of urology. The reader is advised to refer to other literature for details of the technique of using these instruments.

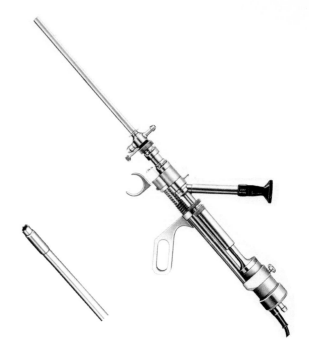

3

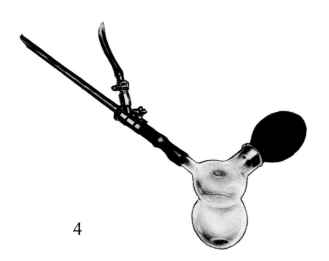

4

4

Evacuator

A glass vessel fitted with a rubber evacuating bulb, such as the Ellick evacuator, will be needed to wash out the fragments of the calculus after it has been crushed.

Metal catheters with a larger lumen (26 Fr), complete with an obturator for passage along the urethra, can be used with the evacuator, but an adaptor may be required to connect the two instruments. Preferably a resectoscope sheath of the same calibre (26 Fr) should be used with the appropriate connector for the Ellick evacuator.

The operations

BLIND LITHOTRITY FOR STONES MORE THAN 2 cm IN DIAMETER

5 & 6

After preliminary cystoscopy, the bladder is left distended with some fluid so that there are no folds in the bladder wall. Gentle dilatation of the urethra may be necessary; then, having ensured that the jaws are tightly closed, the lithotrite is introduced slowly and carefully into the bladder. The jaws are separated and the beak of the instrument is guided into the most dependent part of the bladder so that the stone can roll between the jaws, which should be pointing upwards away from the bladder mucosa. The beak of the lithotrite is moved gently from side to side and, at the same time, the jaws, still pointing towards the vault (i.e. away from the mucosa of the bladder base), are opened and closed gently. During this manoeuvre the stone will be felt as it rolls between the jaws, which are closed firmly on the stone and locked. While the stone is grasped the handle of the instrument is dipped so that the beak is raised and lies approximately in the middle of the bladder, well away from the mucosa. The lithotrite is then rotated gently through 180° in each direction. It is possible to feel whether the jaws have caught on the bladder mucosa, which will give a slight dragging sensation. Only after ensuring that the bladder mucosa is free should the jaws be screwed together to crush the stone. This process is repeated until all fragments have been crushed. Before removing the lithotrite the blades should be completely closed again, ensuring that the bladder mucosa is not caught.

After evacuating the fragments any remaining calculi are inspected by cystoscopy (hence the value of using the resectoscope sheath so that evacuation and endoscopy can be performed via the same sheath). Providing no damage has been done to the bladder mucosa, an adequate view is easily obtained. If there are still any large fragments, the blind lithotrite should be reinserted to crush them. If only small fragments remain, these can be crushed with the endoscopic lithotrity forceps or the endoscopic lithotrite. Free lubrication of the lithotrite each time it is reinserted reduces the risk of damage to the urethral mucosa.

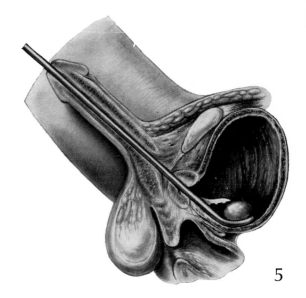

5

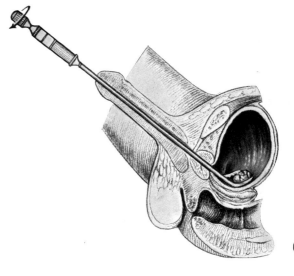

6

7

REMOVAL OF STONES BY ENDOSCOPIC LITHOTRITY FORCEPS

Small stones (less than 1 cm in diameter) can be crushed between the blades of the small lithotrity forceps. These forceps have the advantage of being constructed to fit into the standard 23 Fr cystoscopy sheath or the 24 Fr resectoscope sheath. These avoid the repeated passage of different instruments down the urethra – first to crush, then to evacuate, then to inspect and so on. Care must be taken not to use too much force on the handle if the stone will not crush easily. The fulcrum on which the crushing blade is mounted may buckle or break if too much force is used. If the stone is hard, the stronger endoscopic lithotrite should be used, even though the stone may only be small in size.

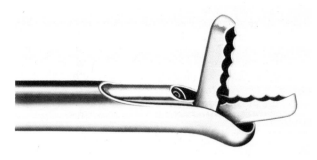

7

ENDOSCOPIC (VIEWING) LITHOTRITY

8

The viewing lithotrite is introduced without the telescope, which is replaced by an obturator. When the instrument is in the bladder, the obturator is removed and the water nozzle is attached. The telescope, carrying its own illumination, is then inserted. The stone can be viewed and grasped by the jaws of the lithotrite, pointing in any direction towards the stone. The operator can ensure by direct vision that the mucosa of the bladder is free and well clear of the jaws of the lithotrite.

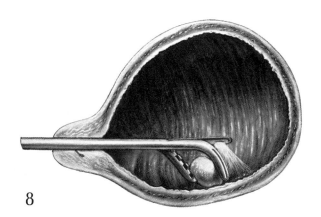

8

9

The jaws are raised clear of the mucosa and the stone is crushed. This should be repeated until all the fragments have been reduced to a size small enough to be evacuated through the metal catheter or resectoscope sheath. Some stones may become partially pulverized, which temporarily obscures the view. Evacuation will clear the view as well as removing the smaller fragments. The lithotrite can then be reinserted and the remaining fragments crushed. Crushing should never be attempted without a clear view.

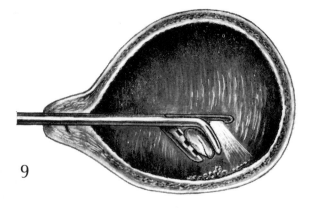

9

EVACUATION OF FRAGMENTS

A thin-walled metal catheter or preferably the resectoscope sheath of 26 Fr size is inserted into the urethra (a 28 Fr may be used only if the urethra will accommodate it easily). The Ellick evacuator filled with fluid is attached to the end of the catheter and the fragments are aspirated by compressing and releasing the rubber bulb. The flow and return can be improved if some fluid is left in the bladder. As the fragments are aspirated into the glass receiver of the evacuator they drop into the lower bulb. When all fragments appear to have been evacuated the metal catheter or sheath is removed and the bladder reinspected by cystoscopy. If further fragments remain, the process of lithotrity and evacuation is repeated.

In all cases of litholapaxy, a catheter (18 Fr) should be left indwelling for at least 48 hours. In view of the risk of bacteraemia from repeated instrumentation, 10 ml of antiseptic gel (chlorhexidine 1:200 in methyloxycellulose jelly) should be injected from the external urinary meatus and milked down the urethra before inserting the catheter. If there is any suspicion of damage to the bladder wall during the litholapaxy, then 5 days' catheter drainage is advisable.

Postoperative care and complications

Haemorrhage

Bleeding may occur from damage to the bladder mucosa by the blades of the lithotrite. For this reason a catheter should be left indwelling until the urine is clear.

Bacteraemia

This may occur from absorption of infected urine via the traumatized bladder or urethral mucosa. Hence it is advisable to provide the patient with antibiotic cover during the operation and in the immediate postoperative period, as many vesical calculi are associated with urinary tract infection.

Urethral and bladder antiseptics such as chlorhexidine gel inserted into the urethra will reduce the risk of instrumental bacteraemia. Before the catheter is removed 50 ml of chlorhexidine solution (1:5000) should be introduced into the bladder via the catheter and left in the bladder so that, at the first act of micturition following removal of the catheter, the risk of bacterial absorption from the bladder mucosa is reduced.

Stone in diverticulum

The stone may fall into a diverticulum where it cannot be grasped with the blades of a lithotrite. In this event the only treatment is open operation, removing the stone by suprapubic lithotomy. The diverticulum can be removed at the same operation.

After litholapaxy, fragments of stone may lodge in saccules, or in a small diverticulum of the bladder wall, and may require prolonged and thorough evacuation with the Ellick evacuator to wash out all the pieces from the bladder.

Adherent stones

Vesical calculi may occasionally be adherent to the bladder mucosa. The calculus must be pulled off the bladder wall with the lithotrite before crushing in order to be certain that it is not calcification over a bladder tumour, or a dumb-bell shaped stone protruding from a saccule or diverticulum. If the stone does not dislodge easily, then further radiological investigation – a cystogram – may be necessary. Having excluded the possibility of calcification over a neoplasm, suprapubic lithotomy is advisable.

After removal of an adherent calculus, it is wise to take a biopsy of the adherent area of bladder wall.

Obstruction

If the bladder neck is hypertrophied or the prostate is enlarged, postoperative urinary obstruction may occur as a result of oedema from manipulation of the lithotrite in the urethra.

Stricture

Stricture of the urethra may occur as a later complication resulting from damage to the anterior urethral mucosa.

Cause of calculus

After removal of the stone from the bladder, the aetiology of the calculus formation should be determined by appropriate metabolic and anatomical studies.

Evacuation of foreign bodies

Most foreign bodies introduced into the bladder *per urethram* lend themselves to evacuation or extraction by one or other of the methods outlined above, but floating objects (e.g. paraffin wax) and elongated or sharp implements (pencils, safety pins, etc) may have to be removed by open operation.

Long thin objects, such as electric light flex, or thermometers, which may have been introduced for sexual stimulation, can usually be manipulated so that one end of the object is grasped by the rongeur forceps, Lowsley forceps or endoscopic lithotrity forceps and extracted *per urethram*. Care must be taken not to fragment any breakable part of a foreign body such as a thermometer. It may be possible to guide one end of the foreign body into the 22 or 24 Fr sheath of a cystoscope or resectoscope so that it slides down the sheath as the telescope is withdrawn.

If these objects have been in the bladder for any length of time, considerable phosphatic encrustation may have occurred, which will prevent the extraction of the object *per urethram* and require suprapubic cystotomy. Preliminary X-ray followed by endoscopy will show whether the object is embedded in the mucosa of the bladder wall, in which case transurethral removal is not likely to be possible.

A foreign body which has been introduced via the urethra will almost certainly have carried infection into the urinary tract. Any manipulation, whether transurethral or suprapubic, should be covered by an appropriate antibiotic.

Illustrations by Gary M. James

Extraction of ureteric calculi

J. P. Mitchell   CBE, TD, MS, FRCS, FRCS(Ed)
Honorary Professor of Surgery (Urology), University of Bristol, UK

Preoperative

Indications

Only calculi in the lower third of the ureter are suitable for extraction by way of a urological endoscope. The nearer the stone is situated to the ureteric orifice the more successful is the extraction likely to be. Attempts at removing ureteric calculi at levels higher than the lower third of the ureter are nearly always unsuccessful and have not infrequently resulted in the instrument with the stone becoming impacted in the ureter.

Calculi which have become arrested in the intramural ureter or are presenting at the orifice itself may require a simple and limited meatotomy, but this will be at the risk of subsequent ureteric reflux. If the stone does not fall into the bladder easily when the orifice has been opened adequately by meatotomy, then the endoscopic lithotrite forceps can be used to lift the calculus out of the ureteric orifice.

Preoperative preparation

The patient and the instruments are prepared as for cystoscopy.

Special instruments

1

The operation is carried out via the operating cystoscope sheath, equipped with an Albarran-type lever (bridge).

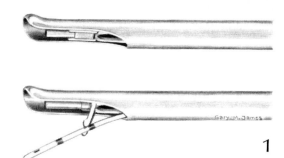

1

2

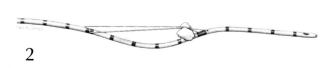

2

Various types of extractor have been designed, all of which work on the principle of passing the implement up the ureter beyond the calculus and then attempting to catch the calculus as the extractor is withdrawn. The simplest form of extractor is a ureteric catheter with a fine piece of monofilament nylon attached to the tip (Davis loop). This is threaded back down the inside of the ureteric catheter so that, when the catheter is in position, it bends as the nylon thread is pulled.

3

One of the more successful designs is the Dormia extractor which, having been passed beyond the stone, extrudes a basket or cage of wire. On withdrawal the stone is intended to fall into the basket. The extractor should be marked in centimetres to indicate the distance it has been passed up the ureter. Overhead X-ray on the cystoscopy table is invaluable to obtain visual control of the extractor and the calculus. Continuous screening with an image intensifier is often less successful than repeated still X-ray pictures, as a small ureteric calculus may be difficult to identify on the image intensifer when the extractor is in close apposition.

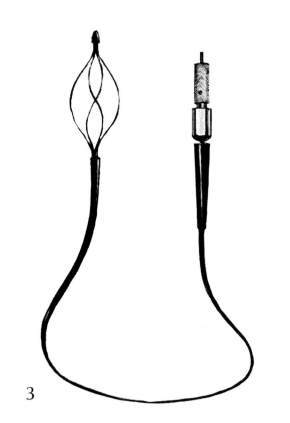

3

The operation

The extractor is passed up the ureter via the cystoscope in the same way as a ureteric catheter. The extractor should be well lubricated with liquid paraffin. The introduction of 2 ml of thin (not viscid) liquid paraffin via a ureteric catheter or Braasch bulb catheter introduced into the ureter as far as the stone before attempting to use the extractor can help to lubricate the Dormia extractor as it is manipulated past the calculus. Repeated gentle oscillations in and out longitudinally in the line of the ureter will be more successful in negotiating the instrument past the calculus than the use of force. If the operator feels that he has been successful in passing the tip of the extractor beyond the stone, he should then estimate the distance the instrument has been passed up the ureter and, if this distance is equal to the rough estimate of the distance as seen on preoperative X-ray, then the basket should be extruded and an X-ray taken on the table. The distance between the ureteric calculus and the orifice at the lower end of that ureter can be deceptive, as the ureter traverses the pelvis posteriorly as well as anteriorly, and in the two-dimensional X-ray the distance may appear shorter. It helps to remember that the length of the ureter below the brim of the pelvis is more than 15 cm. An X-ray taken on the table will clearly show whether the basket is beyond, level with or short of the stone and a very accurate estimate can be made of the correction needed.

Having adjusted the basket to the level of the stone, another X-ray can be taken to see if the stone has engaged in the basket. Once again, oscillatory movements in and out can help to engage the stone. Under no circumstances should rotary movements be attempted once the basket has been extruded, as such movements would be liable to close the wires around a portion of ureteric wall, with disastrous results when the instrument is withdrawn. The extractor should be pulled from the ureter centimetre by centimetre, being oscillated in and out gently with each centimetre of extracting movement.

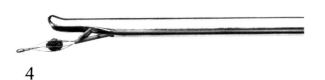

4

4

If the extraction is successful, the stone will often drop out of the basket as it enters the bladder, and can then be removed from the bladder by grasping it with Rongeur forceps or endoscopic lithotrite forceps.

Delayed passage of a ureteric calculus

Occasionally, when the Dormia extractor has failed to catch the stone, it will pass spontaneously the following day, as though the passage of the extractor, the stimulation and possible dilatation of the ureter, and the lubrication with liquid paraffin may all have helped the stone on its way down the ureter.

Ureteric meatotomy

5

Using a pointed diathermy electrode or a Colling's knife with a cutting current via the cystoscope or resectoscope, the meatus can be enlarged gradually until the stone is free and can be grasped by endoscopic forceps. The electrode can be inserted into the orifice, lifting up its margin, and the cut made with a brief touch of the diathermy pedal. Alternatively, if the stone can be seen, the electrode is pressed into the margin of the orifice, where the stone is bulging, and the cut made directly onto the stone.

Meatotomy should be restricted to the minimal amount of cutting which successfully releases the stone, as there is a serious risk of subsequent vesicoureteric reflux of urine when the normal valvular mechanism of the lower end of the ureter has been damaged.

Occasionally a Dormia extractor will bring the stone successfully to the ureteric orifice, where both stone and extractor may become impacted. A diathermy electrode, passed down the second operating channel of the endoscope, may be used to carry out a small meatotomy to liberate the stone and extractor. Care must be taken not to make contact between the electrode and one of the wires of the basket, otherwise the wire is liable to fuse and snap.

Postoperative care and complications

Impaction of the extractor

Before attempting the use of a Dormia extractor, it is always wise to warn the patient that open operation for the stone may be necessary. The surgeon is then free to go ahead with ureterolithotomy if the stone and extractor become impacted in the attempts at removal.

It may be possible to remove the extractor complete with the stone, if left in place for 24 hours. In this case the catheter sheath of the extractor and the chuck gripping the wire core of the extractor should both be removed, leaving only the basket and its length of wire *in situ*. This will release the endoscope, which can also be removed. Occasionally, the extractor may be eased out 24 hours later complete with stone. Again, this should only be done

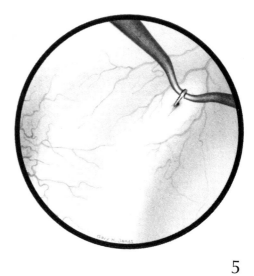

5

under careful X-ray control. If the stone shows no sign of movement at this stage, there is no alternative but open operation, removing the stone and extractor together at ureterolithotomy.

Meatotomy may be attempted if the stone and extractor become impacted at the orifice (*see* previous paragraph).

Rupture of the ureter

The tip of the extractor may perforate the ureter, but fortunately this usually amounts to mucosal damage only. If, however, the extractor penetrates the full thickness of the wall of the ureter, or if the basket closes onto a fold in the wall of the ureter which then tears on extraction of the instrument, urine may leak into the retroperitoneal tissues. This leakage will be aggravated by obstruction below the site of the perforation, due to oedema around the area where the stone is impacted. Fortunately, it is very rare for the extractor to penetrate the peritoneal cavity. Occasionally such a urinary leak may require a laparotomy and drainage of the retroperitoneal tissues.

Further reading

Blandy, J. P. Operative urology. Oxford: Blackwell Scientific, 1978: 88–90

Medical Defence Union. Surgical problems: Dormia damage. Medical Defence Union Annual Report 1982: 38

Mitchell, J. P. Endoscopic operative urology. John Wright and Sons, 1981: 200–203

Illustrations by Gary M. James

Urethral catheterization

J. P. Mitchell   CBE, TD, MS, FRCS, FRCS(Ed)
Honorary Professor of Surgery (Urology), University of Bristol, UK

Preoperative

Indications

It may be necessary to pass a catheter for the following reasons:

1. For the relief of acute or chronic retention of urine due either to obstruction of the urethra or to neurogenic paralysis of the bladder. A period of catheter drainage is required for recovery of tone in the bladder musculature following prolonged chronic retention.
2. For the relief of clot retention.
3. To empty the bladder before pelvic operations such as abdominoperineal resection of rectum and gynaecological procedures.
4. To provide postoperative drainage after prostatectomy or operations on the bladder.
5. For certain radiological or urodynamic investigations, such as micturating cystourethrography and the measurement of intravesical pressure.
6. In order to irrigate the bladder with mild antiseptic solutions when there has been prolonged accumulation of pus and debris in the bladder.
7. For the collection of a sample of urine, though usually either a midstream specimen or one collected by suprapubic puncture is preferable.
8. In order to measure urinary output hour by hour when an accurate fluid balance is essential.
9. As a form of urinary diversion following urethrotomy by the endoscopic route.

Contraindications

Catheterization of the urethra should not be attempted when a stricture of the urethra is known to be present or is suspected from resistance to gentle attempts to pass the catheter. A catheter forced against a stricture face can result in a false passage. If there is local urethral sepsis, catheterization should either be avoided or covered by a broad-spectrum antibiotic given systemically.

Preparation and positioning of the patient

The male patient should lie supine, with the legs flat and separated and at a comfortable angle. For the female the knees should be flexed, with the feet together and the thighs abducted and rotated externally as far as possible.

Catheterization should be regarded as a procedure demanding full aseptic and antiseptic precautions. If the catheter is to remain indwelling, the genitalia should be shaved. All the skin should be thoroughly cleansed with soap and water, including beneath the prepuce in the male and between the labia in the female. The soap should then be washed away carefully with a solution of chlorhexidine 1:5000. In the female a swab of chlorhexidine is left between the labia; in the male, the penis with the prepuce retracted is wrapped in a clean dry swab. Three sterile towels are placed around the genitalia, exposing only the smallest area of skin required to pass the catheter.

1

Anaesthesia and antisepsis

A solution of 5 ml of local anaesthetic, combined with chlorhexidine (Hibitane) or some other equally effective urethral antiseptic, is instilled into the urethra (2 per cent lignocaine in 0.05 per cent chlorhexidine in methyloxycellulose gel). If this local anaesthetic is prepared in 'toothpaste' tubes, only the nozzle need be sterilized; the tube itself can be wrapped in a sterile gauze swab. After the instillation, the external urinary meatus is occluded by gentle pressure and the gel is milked down the anterior urethra, so that some of the local anaesthetic flows into the posterior urethra. Anaesthesia of the posterior urethra is uncertain as the gel tends to flow straight through to the bladder, but some should remain in contact for a sufficient length of time to give partial anaesthesia.

A penile clamp is applied in the region of the corona for 2 min to prevent the local anaesthetic and antiseptic gel spilling from the external urinary meatus. The procedure in the female is similar, though reflux of the gel from the external meatus can be prevented only by gentle digital pressure to occlude the meatus.

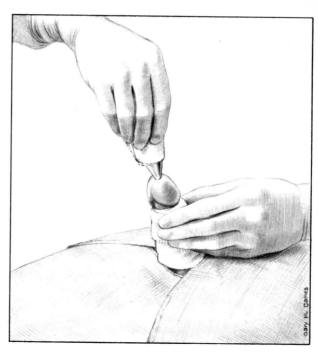

1

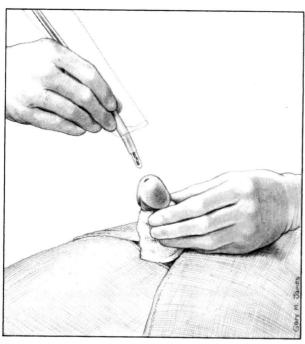

2

Choice of catheter

2

Catheters are constructed of latex, polythene or silicone. Polythene catheters have a thinner wall and provide a larger internal lumen for the comparable external calibre of the catheter. Latex produces some urethral reaction, while with polythene the reaction is minimal. The most inert is silicone, which should be used when the catheter is likely to remain indwelling for more than 5 days.

Each catheter should have a double sterile enclosure so that the inner sterile cover can be used to protect the catheter while it is being passed. This inner cover should slide easily over the catheter without sticking to the outer wall of the catheter.

Harris and Tiemann catheters

3

The non self-retaining catheter which is most commonly used today is the Harris (Nelaton) catheter. This catheter has a hollow tip for use with the introducer (*see below*) and a wide internal lumen. The Tiemann catheter is specially shaped with a Coudé tip which can help negotiate a difficult urethra or bladder neck. This catheter has a thicker wall and a correspondingly smaller lumen and is therefore more rigid so that no introducer is required. Moreover if suction is applied, the walls of the catheter will not collapse. The Jacques catheter is similar to the Harris but the tip is solid to the level of the first eye of the catheter.

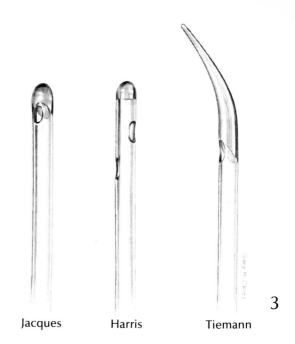

Jacques   Harris   Tiemann

3

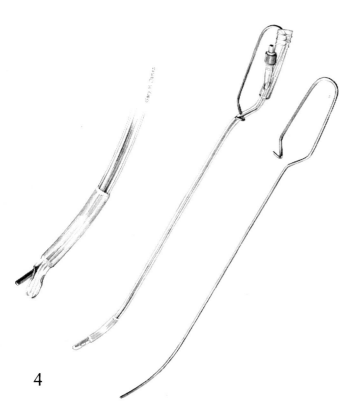

4

4

The introducer

If it is necessary to use an introducer, the catheter must have a hollow tip so that the beak of the introducer can lodge securely inside and not escape through one of the eyes of the catheter (as would occur with a Jacques or Tiemann) and thereby impale the wall of the urethra. An introducer should slide easily inside the lumen of the catheter. A little lubricant gel, injected by syringe, into the lumen of the catheter may be helpful.

Introducers should be used only with the greatest care and skill. No force should be applied. The catheter, when loaded on an introducer, should slide down the urethra and into the bladder with ease. More false passages have been made by catheters mounted on introducers than by any other urethral instrument. An introducer should be constructed in 9 Fr gauge steel wire, with the curvature at the end similar to the tip of a Clutton sound.

5

Foley catheter

The most popular catheter for temporary bladder drainage is the Foley, which has an inflatable balloon (capacity either 5 or 30 ml) to retain the catheter in the bladder. The inflating channel for the balloon reduces the calibre of the catheter lumen. If constructed in polythene, the Foley catheter has a thinner wall and a proportionately larger lumen, but the balloon is still made of latex, which tends to distort with traction and will dissolve if inadvertently lubricated with liquid paraffin. The self-retaining balloon, which has been in contact with liquid paraffin, will burst within an hour or two so that the catheter falls out. Silicone catheters are constructed with the balloon also made of silicone, whereas silicone-coated catheters have a latex balloon.

Kinder catheter

The Kinder catheter is designed with an additional irrigation channel (three-way catheter) to keep the drainage eye free of blood clot.

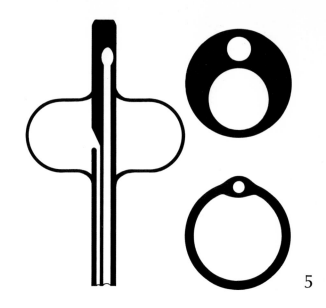

5

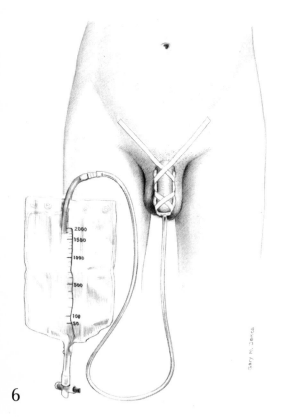

6

6

Gibbon catheter

Apart from the material with which the catheter is made, the reaction of the urethral mucosa is directly proportional to the size of the catheter. If it is to be left indwelling for anything more than 4 or 5 days, a very small catheter, such as the Gibbon type, is preferable (6, 9 or 12 Fr). The catheter which is more than 4 feet long provides an unbroken seal from bladder to drainage bottle or bag and therefore reduces the risk of contamination. The catheter is retained by straps fixed to its wall at the anticipated level of the external meatus in the male. These straps are laid along either side of the shaft of the penis and anchored with adhesive plaster.

Catheterization procedure

As small as possible a size of catheter should be used, compatible with the drainage required. If the urine is clear, a size 10, 12 or 14 Fr catheter should be large enough. If the urine is cloudy or blood clots are present, then a larger size catheter (18 or 22 Fr) may be necessary. The passage of the catheter should be smooth and free of resistance, and no force should be used. If there is any difficulty, this indicates either that the catheter is passing in the wrong direction or that it has met with an obstruction, such as a stricture of the urethra or a large middle lobe of prostate. If a polythene catheter does not feel soft and pliable, it may be immersed briefly in a bowl of warm sterile water.

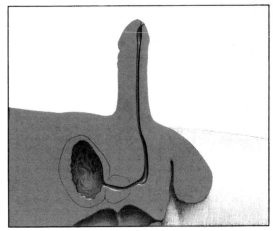

7

The penis should be drawn upwards as far as possible in order to straighten the posterior recess of the bulbous urethra and encourage the catheter to pass easily through the triangular ligament.

Sites where the tip of the urethral catheter may 'catch'

8

It should also be remembered that the urethra lies on the ventral aspect of the navicular fossa, so the tip of a fine catheter does not damage the mucosa. It sometimes helps ease the passage of a catheter through the posterior urethra if the patient is encouraged to take a few deep breaths, warning him at the same time that he will feel a little more discomfort when the tip of the catheter reaches the posterior urethra. This portion of the urethra does not hold the local anaesthetic gel in contact with the mucosa, as well as the anterior urethra.

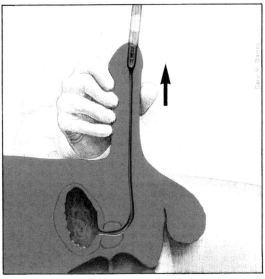

7

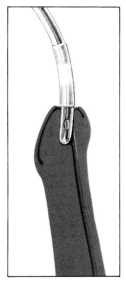

8

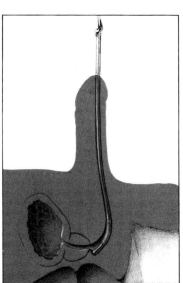

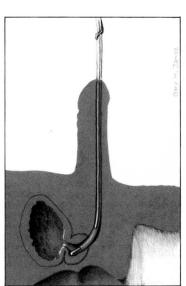

9

A finger *per rectum*, providing gentle pressure over the tip of the catheter as it advances towards the bladder neck, may help to negotiate an enlarged middle lobe or a raised bladder neck.

(For postoperative catheterization after endoscopic urethrotomy, *see* chapter on 'Dilatation and endoscopic urethrotomy for urethral stricture', pp. 724–728).

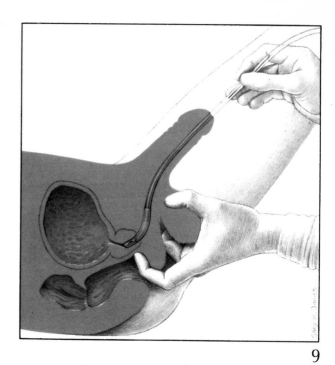

9

Securing the catheter

When continuous drainage is required, a self-retaining catheter of the Foley type offers many advantages. The balloon should be inflated with either 5 or 20 ml of sterile water, depending on the prescribed capacity. If the fluid inflating the balloon is stained with a concentrate of methylene blue, rupture of the balloon can be detected by discolouration of the drainage fluid before the catheter falls out.

A 5 ml balloon is adequate for most conditions, except in the male patient with a very large prostate, in whom a small balloon is liable to slip down into the prostatic urethra. Similarly, in a few females, the 5 ml balloon may not be large enough, if the urethra is very capacious. Otherwise a balloon of 5 ml can be an efficient retainer, provided it inflates equally on all sides into a complete sphere and does not distort.

The external urinary meatus and protruding catheter are loosely covered with gauze which can easily be removed for meatal toilet.

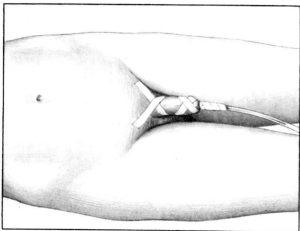

10

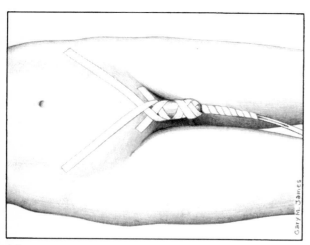

11

10 & 11

Harris, Tiemann and Gibbon catheters should be retained with adhesive strapping. Various methods can be used, but it is questionable whether complete enclosure of the external meatus is advisable, since this usually results in maceration of the skin and an increase in the urethral discharge. Any encircling ring of strapping around the penis should be avoided as this inevitably results in oedema of the tip of the penis. Therefore all strapping should be fitted in a spiral fashion.

12

Fixation of other than Foley catheters in the female is even more difficult. A cruciate series of tapes is recommended two passing anteriorly into the groin and two passing posteriorly into the natal folds.

Toilet to the external meatus in the male should be carried out every 12 hours and is more convenient when a Foley type self-retaining catheter has been used. Meatal toilet consists of cleaning away the urethral discharge, which may be sterile and only the result of foreign body reaction in the presence of the catheter. If Cetrimide is used to clean away this discharge it should be half strength to avoid a chemical balanitis as the mucosa of the glans is particularly sensitive. The Cetrimide should then be removed with a swab containing 1:5000 chlorhexidine. The penis is retracted so that the catheter is exposed for an extra 1 cm from the external meatus. One millilitre of chlorhexidine gel is applied to this exposed portion of the catheter and the external meatus is allowed to slide back over the gel.

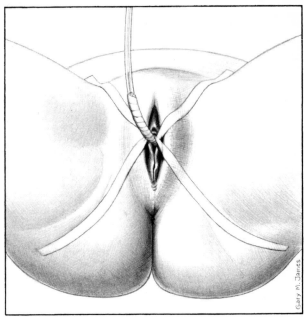

12

Connection of the closed drainage apparatus

The closed drainage of the catheter should be maintained without any break in continuity between the bladder and the drainage bottle or plastic bag. If a bottle is used, this should contain 50 ml of formaldehyde solution or hydrogen peroxide to sterilize the urine as it reaches the bottle. The inlet and air outlet tubes of the bottle should both end just below the neck of the bottle, and neither of these should pass under the fluid level; otherwise regurgitation of urine plus the antiseptic into the bladder may occur when the bottle is raised above body level for turning the patient, either for toilet or rectal examination.

If a bag is used, this should have a non-return flutter valve, to prevent reflux of urine from the bag to the catheter, and this in turn will also prevent ascending infection. The bag can be maintained as a reservoir and emptied intermittently. Provided the non-return valve is effective, the introduction of 50 ml of one of the phenolic derivatives or chlorhexidine at a concentration of 1:1000 into the bag each time it is emptied ensures that the inside of the bag is repeatedly sterilized. Hydrogen peroxide has also been shown to sterilize urinary drainage bags effectively.

Postoperative care

Before the catheter is removed, it is essential to see that the bowels are open. A febrile reaction may occur shortly after removal of the catheter, due to bacteraemic absorption from the urethral mucosa. The introduction of 50 ml of 1:5000 chlorhexidine into the bladder via the catheter just prior to its removal will reduce the risk of this bacterial absorption. If the urine is infected at the time of catheter removal, it is advisable to provide the patient with antibiotic cover.

Index